NUTRITION
ALMANAC
THIRD EDITION

Lavon J. Dunne

Nutrition Search, Inc.•John D. Kirschmann, Director

McGRAW-HILL, PUBLISHING COMPANY

New York   St. Louis   San Francisco   Auckland   Bogotá
Caracas   Lisbon   London   Madrid   Mexico   Milan
Montreal   New Delhi   Paris   San Juan   São Paulo
Singapore   Sydney   Tokyo   Toronto

Library of Congress Cataloging-in-Publication Data

Nutrition almanac/Nutrition Search, Inc., John D. Kirschmann,
    director; Lavon J. Dunne.—3rd ed.
        p. cm.
        "Third McGraw-Hill paperback edition"—T.p. verso.
        Bibliography: p.
        Includes index.
        ISBN 0-07-034912-6
        1. Nutrition. 2. Health. 3. Food—Composition—Tables.
    I. Kirschmann, John D. II. Dunne, Lavon J. III. Nutrition Search,
    Inc.
    RA784.N837 1990
    641.1—dc20   89-33019

        13   DOW/DOW   95

    ISBN 0-07-034912-6

First McGraw-Hill Paperback edition, 1975
Revised McGraw-Hill Paperback edition, 1979
Second McGraw-Hill Paperback edition, 1984
Third McGraw-Hill Paperback edition, 1990

This book was set in Times Roman. It was composed by
Techna Type, Inc.
Printed and bound by R. R. Donnelley & Sons Company.

Contents

Suggestions for Using This Book

The system presented in this book can be employed in two ways. It can help the reader work out a total plan for personal nutrition, or it can quickly answer simple questions regarding food, nutrition, and health.

Nutrients (p. 9). This section discusses over 40 vitamins and minerals in terms of description, absorption and storage, dosage and toxicity, deficiency effects and symptoms, beneficial effect on ailments, human tests, and animal tests. A list of ailments for which the nutrients may be beneficial follows the discussion of each vitamin or mineral. In order to obtain a more complete understanding of the function of nutrients in relation to total health, the reader should refer to related sections of the book. This section also presents extensive coverage of drinking water—its value to the body as well as the types and consequences of pollution.

Nutrients That Function Together (p. 108). Many vitamins and minerals prove to be more or less effective when taken simultaneously with other nutrients. This section provides an easy-to-follow guide for understanding which nutrients are compatible and which substances are their antagonists.

Vitamin and Mineral Supplements and Supplementation (p. 116). This section may be of interest to persons who wish to determine which supplements are best suited to their needs. Vitamin and mineral supplements are explained in terms of source (natural or synthetic) and dosage requirements, and an explanation of the physical forms and sources is given.

Ailments (p. 130). It is a proven fact that many common ailments and weight problems are a result of unbalanced intake of nutrients. In this section, common ailments are discussed and explained in layman's language. The discussion of each ailment is accompanied by a list of nutrients that have proven beneficial in treatment of the ailment. When quantities for a particular nutrient are given, it must be remembered that these quantities are *not prescriptive* but merely represent research findings. This section can be best utilized when cross-referenced with the ''Nutrients'' and ''Foods'' sections.

Herbs (p. 229). This section introduces the world of herbs with a brief commentary and a short summary of a number of common herbs.

Foods, Beverages, Supplementary Foods, and Eating Right to Feel Right (p. 239). The discussions of foods and supplemental foods give valuable information about specific foods or classes of foods and supplements. The list of ''Rich Sources of Nutrients'' shows at a glance what foods are good sources of the vitamins and minerals. Putting it all together—eating right—is the key to feeling right. Therefore, this section now includes a selection of recipes that allow home preparation of wholesome foods with *natural* ingredients.

Table of Food Composition (p. 265).   The "Table of Food Composition" gives the complete nutrient analysis of over 600 foods. This simple guide makes it possible for the reader to compare food values and analyze and prepare meals balanced in nutrients and calories.

Nutrient Allowance Chart (p. 309).   The "Nutrient Allowance Chart" gives a complete breakdown of the nutrient needs for each person in view of body size, metabolism, and calorie requirements.

In summary, this "Almanac" is not the type of book that one would read from front cover to back cover as one would a novel, but it can be a very useful tool if a reader takes time to understand the importance of the various sections. Like the individual B-complex vitamins, each section of this book is important in its own right; when used simultaneously, *all* sections have a much more beneficial effect.

NOTE: The information contained in this book is not intended to be prescriptive. Any attempt to diagnose and treat an illness should come under the direction of a physician who is familiar with nutritional therapy. It is possible that some individuals may suffer allergic reactions from the use of various dietary supplement preparations or the media in which they are contained; if such reactions occur, consult your physician. Nutrition Search, Inc., and the publisher assume no responsibility.

Nutrition and Health

Nutrition is the relationship of foods to the health of the human body. Proper nutrition means that all the essential nutrients—that is, carbohydrates, fats, protein, vitamins, minerals, and water—are supplied and utilized in adequate balance to maintain optimal health and well-being. Nutritional deficiencies result whenever inadequate amounts of essential nutrients are provided to tissues that must function normally over a long period of time. Good nutrition is essential for normal organ development and functioning, for normal reproduction, growth, and maintenance; for optimum activity level and working efficiency; for resistance to infection and disease; and for the ability to repair bodily damage or injury.

No single substance will maintain vibrant health. Although specific nutrients are known to be more important in the functions of certain parts of the body, even these nutrients are totally dependent upon the presence of other nutrients for their best effects. Every effort should therefore be made to attain and maintain an adequate, balanced daily intake of all the necessary nutrients throughout life.

DIGESTION, ABSORPTION, AND METABOLISM

The foods eaten by humans are chemically complex. They must be broken down by the body into simpler chemical forms so that they can be taken in through the intestinal walls and transported by the blood to the cells. There they provide energy and the correct building materials to maintain human life. These are the processes of digestion, absorption, and metabolism.

DIGESTION

Digestion is a series of physical and chemical changes by which food, taken into the body, is broken down in preparation for absorption from the intestinal tract into the bloodstream. These changes take place in the digestive tract, which includes the mouth, pharynx, esophagus, stomach, small intestine, and large intestine.

The active materials in the digestive juices which cause the chemical breakdown of food are called "enzymes," complex proteins that are capable of inducing chemical changes in other substances without themselves being changed. Each enzyme is capable of breaking down only a single specific substance. For example, an enzyme capable of breaking down fats cannot break down proteins or carbohydrates, or vice versa. Enzymatic action originates in four areas of the body: the salivary glands, the stomach, the pancreas, and the wall of the small intestine.

Digestion actually begins in the mouth, where chewing breaks large pieces of food into smaller pieces. The salivary glands in the mouth produce saliva, a

1

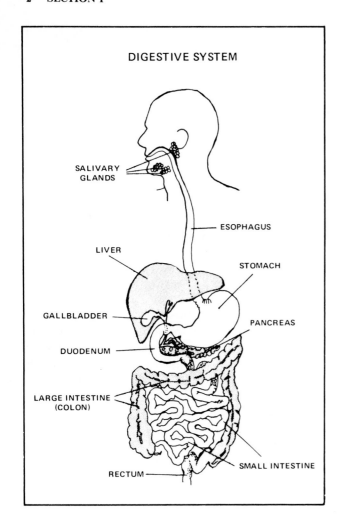

DIGESTIVE SYSTEM

SALIVARY GLANDS

ESOPHAGUS

LIVER

STOMACH

GALLBLADDER

PANCREAS

DUODENUM

LARGE INTESTINE (COLON)

SMALL INTESTINE

RECTUM

the stomach and enter the small intestine in the following order: carbohydrates, protein, and fat—which takes the longest to digest.

When chyme enters the small intestine, the pancreas secretes its digestive juices. If fats are present in the food, bile, an enzyme produced by the liver and stored in the gallbladder, is also secreted. Bile separates the fat into small droplets so that the pancreatic enzymes can break it down. The pancreas also secretes a substance that neutralizes the digestive acids in the food, and it secretes additional enzymes that continue the breakdown of proteins and carbohydrates.

The remaining undigested products enter the large intestine and eventually are excreted. No digestive enzymes are secreted in the large intestine, and little change occurs there except for the absorption of water.

ABSORPTION

Absorption is the process by which nutrients in the form of glucose (from carbohydrates), amino acids (from protein), and fatty acids and glycerol (from fats) are taken up by the intestines and passed into the bloodstream to facilitate cell metabolism.

Absorption takes place primarily in the small intestine. The lining of the small intestine is covered with small fingerlike projections called "villi." These villi contain lymph channels and tiny blood vessels called "capillaries" which are the principal channels of absorption, depending upon the type of nutrient. Fats and fat-soluble vitamins move through the blood to the cells. Other nutrients are carried away from the villi by the capillaries, which funnel them into the portal vein leading to the liver.

In the liver, many different enzymes help change the nutrient molecules into new forms for specific purposes. Unlike earlier changes, which prepared nutrients for absorption and transport, the reactions in the liver produce the products needed by individual cells. Some of the products are used by the liver itself, but the rest are held in storage by the liver, to be released into the body as needed. The remainder go into the bloodstream, where they are picked up by the cells and put to work. Water-soluble vitamins and minerals are also absorbed into the bloodstream in the small intestine.

fluid that moistens food for swallowing and which contains ptyalin, the enzyme necessary for carbohydrate breakdown. The masticated food mass passes back to the pharynx under voluntary control, but from there on and through the esophagus, the process of swallowing is carried on by peristalsis, a slow wavelike motion occurring along the entire digestive tract, which moves the food into the stomach.

Active chemical digestion begins in the middle portion of the stomach, where the food is mixed with gastric juices containing hydrochloric acid, water, and enzymes that break up protein and other substances.

After 1 to 4 hours, depending upon the combination of foods ingested by the system, peristalsis pushes the food, now in the liquid form of chyme, out of the stomach and into the small intestine. Foodstuffs leave

METABOLISM

At this point the handling of food within the body has reached its final stage. The process of metabolism involves all the chemical changes that nutrients undergo from the time they are absorbed until they become a part of the body or are excreted from the body. Metabolism is the conversion of the digested nutrients into building material for living tissue or energy to meet the body's needs.

Metabolism occurs in two general phases that occur simultaneously, *anabolism* and *catabolism*. Anabolism involves all the chemical reactions that the nutrients undergo in the construction or building up of body chemicals and tissues, such as blood, enzymes, hormones, glycogen, and others. Catabolism involves the reactions in which various compounds of the tissues are broken down to supply energy. Energy for the cells is derived from the metabolism of glucose, which combines with oxygen in a series of chemical reactions to form carbon dioxide, water, and cellular energy. The carbon dioxide and water are waste products, carried away from the cells by the bloodstream. Energy can also be derived from the metabolism of essential fatty acids and amino acids, although the primary effect of the metabolism of amino acids is to provide material for growth and the maintenance and repair of tissues. The waste products of essential fatty acid and amino acid metabolism are also carried away from the cells by the bloodstream.

The process of metabolism requires that extensive systems of enzymes be maintained to facilitate the thousands of different chemical reactions and regulate the rate at which these reactions proceed. These enzymes often require the presence of specific vitamins and minerals to perform their functions.

FACTORS INHIBITING DIGESTION

The movements of the stomach are interfered with by nervousness and anxiety. Eating while agitated, fatigued, or worried may give rise to gastrointestinal disturbances. Hurried meals under tense conditions are not conducive to normal digestion. Weather variations and physical disorders such as diabetes or other illnesses may inhibit the proper digestion of foods.

EXERCISE

A healthy body is the result of proper nutrition combined with a regular pattern of physical exercise. Exercise imparts vigor and activity to all organs and secures and maintains healthful integrity of all their functions. Exercise improves the tone and quality of muscle tissue and stimulates the processes of digestion, absorption, metabolism, and elimination. It also strengthens blood vessels, lungs, and heart, resulting in improved transfer of oxygen to the cells and increased circulation of the blood and lymph systems. Exercise develops grace, poise, and symmetry of the body, helps in correcting defective development or injuries, and stimulates the mind.

The key to any type of exercise is a strong will and a sincere desire to improve one's physical condition. It is important to have a program that fits individual needs and capacities. A beginning exercise program should be light; it should increase in difficulty gradually as endurance increases. Exercise should not be done for at least an hour after eating because physical exertion may impede digestion. Exercise should be self-motivating and fun. An ideal exercise program may include many different forms of the following physical activities.

Calisthenics

Calisthenics consists of light exercises or gymnastics including sit-ups, push-ups, jumping jacks, etc., which promote grace and health. The emphasis of calisthenics is on building skeletal muscles.

Dancing

Dancing or rhythmic exercise is often an enjoyable way to exercise the body thoroughly and refresh the mind. Besides toning muscles, joints, glands, the respiratory system, and digestive organs, it gives everyday movements grace and poise.

Isometrics

Isometric exercise involves the pressure of a muscle or group of muscles against each other or against an immovable object. It is especially good for reducing because it can be applied to specific areas. Isometrics primarily tone and build the skeletal muscles.

Jogging

Jogging is a form of exercise that consists of alternately walking and running. It is an excellent exercise for improving the heart, lungs, and circulatory system by expanding their capacity to handle stress. It can help build muscle tone, reduce hips and thighs, redistribute weight, and flatten the abdomen.

Stretching

Stretching is natural exercise that should be practiced on a regular basis. A good habit to develop is stretching upon rising in the morning and throughout the day. Stretch exercises tend to increase both energy and endurance for all parts of the body. Stretching tends to relieve many aches and pains; loosen up ligaments, joints, and muscles; and increase coordination and suppleness. Stretching stimulates circulation and alleviates the stiffness of contracted muscles.

Walking

Walking is one of the best overall exercises and helps the entire system function better. The metabolism is increased while walking; thus fat is burned up and weight loss is promoted. Blood pressure, blood cholesterol, and sugar levels tend to fall. Walking builds up the heart muscle and keeps the arteries clear and elastic. Walking helps increase the oxygen supply to the blood, thus bringing more oxygen to the heart. It also increases the capacity of the lungs, making more oxygen available to the circulatory system.

Weight Lifting

Weight lifting is a form of exercise involving the lifting of weights and is often used by athletes to strengthen muscle tone.

Yoga

Yoga is a series of stretching movements that are performed slowly and methodically. Some postures are quite advanced and complicated for the average person, at least at first; however, there are simple yoga exercises that can be practiced by people of all ages with great benefit. The prime goal of yoga is to relieve the body of tension. Yoga, if practiced consistently, gives elasticity to the spine, firms the skin, tones flabby muscles, and improves poor posture. Many people feel that yoga increases their endurance and flexibility for participation in other more strenuous activities.

Above all, do not forget the recreational exercises, such as golf, tennis, riding, skating, skiing, etc. There are endless sports that can improve the functioning of the body. The important thing is to remember to exercise *regularly* and maintain a nutritionally balanced diet of good, healthy food.

EXPENDITURE OF CALORIC ENERGY PER HOUR

Activity	Calories Expended per Hour
Ballroom dancing	330
Bed making	234
Bicycling 5½ mph	210
Bowling	264
Bricklaying	240
Carpentry	408
Desk work	132
Driving a car	168
Farm work in field	438
Gardening	220
Golf	300
Handball and squash	612
Horseback riding (trot)	480
Ironing (standing up)	252
Lawn mowing (hand mower)	462
Painting at an easel	120
Piano playing	150
Preparing a meal	198
Roller skating	350
Running 10 mph	900
Scrubbing floors	216
Sitting and eating	84
Sitting and knitting	90
Sitting in a chair reading	72
Skiing	594
Sleeping (basal metabolism)	60
Standing up	138
Sweeping	102
Swimming (leisurely)	300
Tennis	420
Volleyball	350
Walking (2.5 miles per hour)	216
Walking downstairs	312

Sources of Calories: Carbohydrates, Fats, and Protein

Carbohydrates, fats, and proteins are the primary sources of energy to the body because they supply fuel necessary for body heat and work. Their fuel potential is expressed in *calories,* a term that signifies the amount of chemical energy that may be released as heat when food is metabolized. Therefore foods that are high in energy value are high in calories, while foods that are low in energy value are low in calories. Fats yield approximately 9 calories per gram, and carbohydrates and proteins yield approximately 4 calories per gram.

CARBOHYDRATES

Carbohydrates are the chief source of energy for all body functions and muscular exertion and are necessary to assist in the digestion and assimilation of other foods. Carbohydrates provide us with immediately available calories for energy by producing heat in the body when carbon in the system unites with oxygen in the bloodstream. Carbohydrates also help regulate protein and fat metabolism; fats require carbohydrates for their breakdown within the liver.

The principal carbohydrates present in foods are sugars, starches, and cellulose. Simple sugars, such as those in honey and fruits, are very easily digested. Double sugars, such as table sugar, require some digestive action, but they are not nearly as complex as starches, such as those found in whole grain. Starches require prolonged enzymatic action in order to be broken down into simple sugars (glucose) for digestion. Cellulose, commonly found in the skins of fruits and vegetables, is largely indigestible by humans and contributes little energy value to the diet. It does, however, provide the bulk necessary for intestinal action and aids elimination.

All sugars and starches are converted by the body to a simple sugar such as "glucose or fructose." Some of the glucose, or "blood sugar," is used as fuel by tissues of the brain, nervous system, and muscles. A small portion of the glucose is converted to glycogen and stored by the liver and muscles; the excess is converted to fat and stored throughout the body as a reserve source of energy. When fat reserves are reconverted to glucose and used for body fuel, weight loss results.

Carbohydrate snacks containing sugars and starches provide the body with almost instant energy because they cause a sudden rise in the blood sugar level. However, the blood sugar level drops again rapidly, creating a craving for more sweet food and possibly fatigue, dizziness, nervousness, and headache.

Overindulgence in starchy and sweet foods may crowd out other essential foods from the diet and can therefore result in nutritional deficiency as well as in obesity and tooth decay. Diets high in refined carbohydrates are usually low in vitamins, minerals, and cellulose. Such foods as white flour, white sugar, and polished rice are lacking in the B vitamins and other nutrients. Excessive consumption of these foods will perpetuate any vitamin B deficiency an individual may have. Enriched products may include some of the B vitamins. If the B vitamins are absent, carbohydrate combustion cannot take place, and indigestion, symptoms of heartburn, and nausea can result. Research continues as to whether or not such problems as diabetes, heart disease, high blood pressure, anemia, kidney disorders, and cancer can be linked to an overabundance of refined carbohydrate foods in the diet.

Carbohydrates can be manufactured in the body from some amino acids and the glycerol component of fats; therefore the National Research Council lists no specific requirement for carbohydrates in the diet.[1]

Differences in basal metabolism, amount of activity, size, and weight will influence the amount of carbohydrates the body needs to get from an outside source. However, a total lack of carbohydrates may produce ketosis, loss of energy, depression, and breakdown of essential body protein.

FATS

Fats, or lipids, are the most concentrated source of energy in the diet. When oxidized, fats furnish more than twice the number of calories per gram furnished by carbohydrates or proteins. One gram of fat yields approximately 9 calories to the body.

In addition to providing energy, fats act as carriers for the fat-soluble vitamins, A, D, E, and K. By aiding in the absorption of vitamin D, fats help make calcium available to body tissues, particularly to the bones and teeth. Fats are also important for the conversion of carotene to vitamin A. Fat deposits surround, protect, and hold in place organs, such as the kidneys, heart, and liver. A layer of fat insulates the body from environmental temperature changes and preserves body heat. This layer also rounds out the contours of the body. Fats prolong the process of digestion by slowing down the stomach's secretions of hydrochloric acid. Thus fats create a longer-lasting sensation of fullness after a meal.

The substances that give fats their different flavors, textures, and melting points are known as the "fatty acids." There are two types of fatty acids, saturated and unsaturated. Saturated fatty acids are those that are usually hard at room temperature and which, except for coconut oils, come primarily from animal sources. Unsaturated fatty acids, including polyunsaturates, are usually liquid at room temperature and are derived from vegetable, nut, or seed sources, such as corn, safflowers, sunflowers, and olives. Vegetable shortenings and margarines have undergone a process called "hydrogenation" in which unsaturated oils are converted to a more solid form of fat. Other sources of fat are milk products, eggs, and cheese.

There are three "essential" fatty acids: linoleic, arachidonic, and linolenic, collectively known as unsaturated fatty acids. Arachidonic and linolenic acids can be synthesized from linoleic acid if it is sufficiently supplied to the body through diet. They are unsaturated fatty acids necessary for normal growth and healthy blood, arteries, and nerves. Also, they keep the skin and other tissues youthful and healthy by preventing dryness and scaliness. Essential fatty acids may be necessary for the transport and breakdown of cholesterol.

Cholesterol is a lipid or fat-related substance necessary for good health. It is a normal component of most body tissues, especially those of the brain and nervous system, liver, and blood. It is needed to form sex and adrenal hormones, vitamin D, and bile, which is needed for the digestion of fats. Cholesterol also seems to play a part in lubricating the skin.

[1]National Academy of Sciences, *Recommended Dietary Allowances,* 9th ed. (Washington, D.C.: National Academy of Sciences, 1980), p. 33.

Although a cholesterol deficiency is unlikely to occur, abnormal amounts of cholesterol may be stored throughout the body if fats are eaten excessively. Research continues, as to the relationship of increased cholesterol storage to the development of arteriosclerosis. Lecithin has been found to decrease cholesterol levels in some individuals.

Fat and fat-containing foods should be stored in covered containers, away from direct light, and in a cool place to prevent rancidity caused by oxidation. Some protection from rancidity will be provided by vitamin E, a fat-soluble vitamin that is a natural antioxidant and is present in most fat-containing foods.

Although a fat deficiency rarely occurs in man, such a deficiency would lead to a deficiency in the fat-soluble vitamins. A deficiency of fatty acids may produce eczema or other skin disorders. An extreme deficiency could lead to severely retarded growth.

Excessive amounts of fat in the diet may lead to abnormal weight gain and obesity if more calories are consumed than are needed by the body. In addition to obesity, excessive fat intake will cause abnormally slow digestion and absorption, resulting in indigestion. If a lack of carbohydrates is accompanied by a lack of water in the diet, or if there is a kidney malfunction, fats cannot be completely metabolized and may become toxic to the body.

The National Research Council sets no Recommended Dietary Allowance for fats because of the widely varying fat content of the diet among individuals. Linoleic acid, however, should provide about 2 percent of the calories in the diet. Vegetable fats, such as corn, safflower, and soybean oils, are high in linoleic acid. Nutritionists suggest that an intake of fat providing 25 to 30 percent of the calories is compatible with good health.

PROTEIN

Next to water, protein is the most plentiful substance in the body. Protein is one of the most important elements for the maintenance of good health and vitality and is of primary importance in the growth and development of all body tissues. It is the major source of building material for muscles, blood, skin, hair, nails, and internal organs, including the heart and the brain.

Protein is needed for the formation of hormones, which control a variety of body functions such as growth, sexual development, and rate of metabolism. Protein also helps prevent the blood and tissues from becoming either too acid or too alkaline and helps regulate the body's water balance. Enzymes, substances necessary for basic life functions, and antibodies, which help fight foreign substances in the body, are also formed from protein. In addition, protein is important in the formation of milk during lactation and in the process of blood clotting.

As well as being the major source of building material for the body, protein may be used as a source of heat and energy, providing 4 calories per gram of protein. However, this energy function is spared when sufficient fats and carbohydrates are present in the diet. Excess protein that is not used for building tissue or energy can be converted by the liver and stored as fat in the body tissues.

During digestion the large molecules of proteins are decomposed into simpler units called "amino acids." Amino acids are necessary for the synthesis of body proteins and many other tissue constituents. They are the units from which proteins are constructed and are the end products of protein digestion.

The body requires approximately twenty-two amino acids in a specific pattern to make human protein. All but eight of these amino acids can be produced in the adult body. The eight that cannot be produced are called "essential amino acids" because they must be supplied in the diet. In order for the body to properly synthesize protein, all the essential amino acids must be present simultaneously and in the proper proportions. If just one essential amino acid is low or missing, even temporarily, protein synthesis will fall to a very low level or stop altogether. The result is that *all* amino acids are reduced in the same proportion as the amino acid that is low or missing.

Foods containing protein may or may not contain all the essential amino acids. When a food contains all the essential amino acids, it is termed "complete protein." Foods that lack or are extremely low in any one of the essential amino acids are called "incomplete protein." Most meats and dairy products are complete-protein foods, while most vegetables and fruits are incomplete-protein foods. To obtain a complete-protein meal from incomplete proteins, one must combine foods carefully so that those weak in an essential amino acid will be balanced by those adequate in the same amino acid.

The minimum daily protein requirement, the smallest amino acid intake that can maintain optimum growth and good health in man, is difficult to determine. Protein requirements differ according to the nutritional status, body size, and activity of the individual. Dietary calculations are usually based on the National Research Council's Recommended Dietary Allowances. The protein recommendations are considered to cover individual variations among most persons living in the United States under usual environmental stress. The National Research Council recommends that 0.42 gram of protein per day be consumed for each pound of body weight. To figure out individual protein requirements, simply divide body weight by 2, and the result will indicate the approximate number of grams of protein required each day. For example, a person weighing 120 pounds requires approximately 60 grams of protein daily. However, total daily protein needs in grams per pound will be reduced if the daily limited amino acid requirements are met. (See "Table of Food Composition," p. 239.)

Protein deficiency may lead to abnormalities of growth and tissue development. The hair, nails, and skin especially will be affected, and muscle tone will be poor. A child whose diet is deficient in protein may not attain his potential physical stature. Extreme protein deficiency in children results in kwashiorkor, a disease characterized by stunted mental and physical growth, loss of hair pigment, and swelling of the joints. It is often fatal. In adults, protein deficiency may result in lack of vigor and stamina, mental depression, weakness, poor resistance to infection, impaired healing of wounds, and slow recovery from disease.

Loss of body protein occurs as a result of particular bodily stresses, such as surgery, hemorrhage, wounds, or prolonged illness. At times of stress, it is necessary to consume extra protein in order to rebuild or replace used or worn-out tissues. However, excessive intake of protein may cause fluid imbalance.

Nutrients

Knowledge of the nutrients and their functions in the body is necessary for understanding the importance of good nutrition. The six nutrients—carbohydrates, fats, protein, vitamins, minerals, and water—are present in the foods we eat and contain chemical substances that function in one or more of three ways: they furnish the body with heat and energy, they provide material for growth and repair of body tissues, and they assist in the regulation of body processes.

Each nutrient has its own specific functions and relationship to the body, but no nutrient acts independently of other nutrients. All of the nutrients must be present in the diet in varying quantities in order for the body to maintain basic life processes. Although all persons need the same nutrients, each person is different in his or her genetic and physiological makeup. Therefore their quantitative nutritional needs will differ.

"Actually there is little justification in nutritional thinking for the concept that a representative prototype of *Homo sapiens* is one who has average requirements with respect to all essential nutrients and thus exhibits no unusually high or low needs. In the light of contemporary genetic and physiologic knowledge and the statistical interpretations thereof, the typical individual is more likely to be one who has average needs with respect to many essential nutrients *but who also exhibits some nutritional requirements for a few essential nutrients which are far from average.*"[1]

The reasons for this are as yet not completely understood. However, it is known that some people, as indicated above, may have unusual nutritional needs because of genetics. Genetic dependency is described as a condition that exists when normal levels of nutrients are not sufficient for proper body functioning, and therefore very large doses of the needed nutrients are required. Another reason seems to be that there are barriers within the bodies of some individuals that prevent the proper assimilation of the foods that are eaten, resulting, again, in more-than-normal requirements of certain nutrients.

The amounts of the nutrients required by an individual are also influenced by age, sex, body size, environment, level of activity, and nutritional status. Processing, storage, and preparation of food may influence the nutritional value of food. Proper understanding of the nutrients and the means of balancing a diet of the foods that contain them will result in optimum health for the body and mind.

---

[1]B. T. Burton, ed., *The Heinz Handbook of Nutrition* (New York: McGraw-Hill, 1959).

VITAMINS

All natural vitamins are organic food substances found only in living things, that is, plants and animals. Less than twenty substances have been discovered so far that are believed to be active as vitamins in human nutrition. Each of these vitamins is present in varying quantities in specific foods, and each is absolutely necessary for proper growth and maintenance of health. With a few exceptions, the body cannot synthesize vitamins; they must be supplied in the diet or in dietary supplements.

Vitamins function with chemicals called enzymes, which have numerous essential functions within the body. Enzymes are made up of two parts: one is a protein molecule and the other is a coenzyme. This coenzyme is often a vitamin, or it may contain a vitamin, or it may be a molecule that has been manufactured from a vitamin. Enzymes are responsible for the oxidation process within the body. Oxidation first begins when oxygen enters the bloodstream and is transported to the cells, where oxidation actually occurs. Then the wastes are removed—carbon dioxide via the lungs and other waste products via the urine. Enzymes are also a major factor in biochemical processes such as growth, metabolism, cellular reproduction, and digestion. Most enzymes remain within the cell, acting as a catalyst; in other words, they initiate chemical reactions that enable other materials to continue their work. Because vitamins work on the cellular level, a lack of one or several can cause many varied symptoms.

"A cell which is poorly nourished may actually have many enzymes without the proper (vitamin) coenzyme part. Enough functional enzymes will remain for the cell itself to function, perhaps for a long time. However, the cell will go through its paces more and more slowly until either proper nourishment is received or it dies. This explains why no vitamin lack strikes overnight or in a day or two, in contrast to the quick manner of infectious diseases or foreign poisons. Many weeks, or even many months, are usually required for signs of a vitamin deficiency to appear. The cells continue to function, but at reduced efficiency due to lower enzyme levels. Then as they decline further or die, different tissues and organs will slowly be affected."[2]

Much work has been done to determine requirements of vitamins for various age groups and in circumstances of additional needs, such as pregnancy and lactation. The Recommended Dietary Allowances (RDA) of the nutrients mentioned in this book are based on the standards established by the Food and Nutrition Board of the National Research Council. Desirable levels for those vitamins whose requirements are known to be essential to healthy humans are based upon available scientific knowledge and are considered adequate to meet the known nutritional needs of practically all healthy persons. These levels are intended to apply to persons whose physical activity is considered "light" and who live in temperate climates, and they provide a safety margin for each vitamin above the minimum level that will maintain health.

Where there is doubt that the requirements for certain nutrients are being met through the diet alone, supplements may be ingested to offset any deficiency. Vitamin therapy does not produce results overnight. Regeneration or the alteration in body chemistry necessary for repair takes weeks and sometimes months before the full benefits are felt. A change in food habits may also be necessary.

Vitamins taken in excess of the finite amount utilized in the metabolic processes are valueless and will be either excreted in the urine or stored in the body. Excessive ingestion of some nutrients may result in toxicity, and risks associated with ingestion of excessive quantities of nutrients are mentioned at appropriate points in the text.

Vitamins are usually distinguished as being water-soluble or fat-soluble. The water-soluble vitamins, B-complex vitamins, vitamin C, and the compounds termed "bioflavonoids," are usually measured in milligrams. The fat-soluble vitamins, A, D, E, and K, are measured in units of activity known as "International Units" (IU) or "United States Pharmacopoeia Units" (USP). (Vitamins A, D, E, and K are expressed in International Units (IU) throughout this

[2]Dr. Harold Rosenberg, *The Doctor's Book of Vitamin Therapy* (New York: G. P. Putnam's Sons, 1974), p. 279.

book.) An exception is beta-carotene, a water-soluble form of vitamin A, which is expressed in IU also.

MINERALS

Minerals are nutrients that exist in the body and in food in organic and inorganic combinations. Approximately seventeen minerals are essential in human nutrition. Although only 4 or 5 percent of the human body weight is mineral matter, minerals are vital to overall mental and physical well-being. All tissues and internal fluids of living things contain varying quantities of minerals. Minerals are constituents of the bones, teeth, soft tissue, muscle, blood, and nerve cells. They are important factors in maintaining physiological processes, strengthening skeletal structures, and preserving the vigor of the heart and brain as well as all muscle and nerve systems.

Minerals, just like vitamins, act as catalysts for many biological reactions within the human body, including muscle response, the transmission of messages through the nervous system, digestion, and metabolism or utilization of nutrients in foods. They are important in the production of hormones.

Minerals coexist with vitamins and their work is interrelated. For example, some B-complex vitamins are absorbed only when combined with phosphorus. Vitamin C greatly increases the absorption of iron, and calcium absorption would not occur without vitamin D. Zinc helps vitamin A to be released from the liver. Some minerals are even part of vitamins: vitamin B_1 contains sulfur and B_{12} contains cobalt.

Minerals help to maintain the delicate water balance essential to the proper functioning of mental and physical processes. They keep blood and tissue fluids from becoming either too acid or too alkaline and permit other nutrients to pass into the bloodstream. They also help draw chemical substances in and out of the cells and aid in the creation of antibodies. All of the minerals known to be needed by the human body must be supplied in the diet.

Calcium, chlorine, phosphorus, potassium, magnesium, sodium, and sulfur are known as the "macrominerals" because they are present in relatively high amounts in body tissues. They are measured in milligrams. Other minerals, termed "trace minerals," are present in the body only in the most minute quantities but are essential for proper body functioning. Trace minerals are measured in micrograms.

Although the minerals are discussed separately, it is important to note that their actions within the body are interrelated; no one mineral can function without affecting others. Physical and emotional stress causes a strain on the body's supply of minerals. A mineral deficiency often results in illness, which may be checked by the addition of the missing mineral to the diet.

HOW VITAMINS AND MINERALS ARE EXPLAINED IN THIS BOOK

Vitamins and minerals are explained in this book in terms of description, absorption and storage, dosage and toxicity, deficiency effects and symptoms, and beneficial effect on ailments. Human and animal tests are described at the end of some listed nutrients. A table listing the ailments that are associated with a specific nutrient follows the discussion of each nutrient.

Description

The description of the vitamin or mineral defines the nutrient—whether or not it is water- or fat-soluble (if it is a vitamin) and its function in the body—and lists the major foods in which it is contained.

Absorption and Storage

The section on absorption and storage explains the places where the nutrient is absorbed and stored in the body, the synthesis of body processes, and if possible, the time factor involved. Any variables that may stimulate or interfere with absorption and storage of the nutrient are also mentioned together with the way the nutrient is excreted.

Dosage and Toxicity

Dosage is given in accordance with the Recommended Dietary Allowances as suggested by the National Research Council's Food and Nutrition Board. Symptoms and effects are given for those nutrients that may be toxic.

Deficiency Effects and Symptoms

If nutrient intake is insufficient to meet requirements for a prolonged period of time, the ability to respond to stress is lessened and depletion and deterioration eventually occur, despite the effectiveness of the various mechanisms that prolong survival. The effects and symptoms of a deficiency are stated for each nutrient.

Beneficial Effect on Ailments

Those ailments that have been successfully treated with a specific nutrient are mentioned here. Additional information, including dosages, is provided in the section "Ailments and Other Stressful Conditions." Dosages listed in the "Ailments" section should not be taken as prescriptive but merely as representations of research findings. In many instances, nutrients should not be taken alone: they are more beneficial when accompanied by other nutrients.

Human Tests

Examples of tests on humans, in clinical situations, are those involving nutritional therapy. Dosages used in these tests should not be taken as prescriptive but merely as examples of how specific nutrients affect some people. Nutritional therapy applied to one individual may not work as well on others. Sources of further information are provided.

Animal Tests

Before results are applied to humans, animal tests are often done because there are some biological similarities between humans and animals in nutritional therapy.

Chart of Beneficial Effects on Ailments

A chart listing the ailments that are associated with a specific vitamin or mineral follows the discussion of each nutrient. These include ailments for which, according to nutritional studies, this particular nutrient may be beneficial.

VITAMINS

VITAMIN A

Description

Vitamin A is a fat-soluble nutrient that occurs in nature in two forms: preformed vitamin A and provitamin A, or carotene. Preformed vitamin A is concentrated only in certain tissues of animal products in which the animal has metabolized the carotene contained in its food into vitamin A. One of the richest natural sources of preformed vitamin A is fish-liver oil, which is classified as a food supplement. Some animal products, such as cream and butter, may contain both preformed vitamin A and carotene.

Carotene is a substance that must be converted into vitamin A before it can be utilized by the body. Carotene is abundant in carrots, from which its name is derived, but it is present in even higher concentrations in certain green leafy vegetables, such as beet greens, spinach, and broccoli. If, owing to any disorder, the body is unable to use carotene, a vitamin A deficiency may arise.

Vitamin A aids in the growth and repair of body tissues and helps maintain smooth, soft, disease-free skin. Internally it helps protect the mucous membranes of the mouth, nose, throat, and lungs, thereby reducing susceptibility to infection. This protection also aids the mucous membranes in combating the effects of various air pollutants. The soft tissue and all linings of the digestive tract, kidneys, and bladder are also protected. In addition, vitamin A prompts the secretion of gastric juices necessary for proper digestion of proteins. Other important functions of vitamin A include the building of strong bones and teeth, the formation of rich blood, and the maintenance of good eyesight. Heavy use of the eyes for watching television and working under glaring lights require more vitamin A. It is essential in the formation of visual purple, a substance in the eye which is necessary for proper night vision.

RNA production is greatly enhanced by vitamin A. RNA (ribonucleic acid) is a nucleic acid that transmits to each cell of the body instructions on how to perform so that life, health, and proper function can be maintained. The body must be able to synthesize new RNA or cell degeneration begins. Studies have revealed that new RNA can be produced in vitamin A deficient bodies; however, the rate of production of new RNA is much less than if sufficient A is available. One of the best sources of RNA is yeast.

Absorption and Storage

The upper intestinal tract is the primary area of absorption of vitamin A; it is here that the fat-splitting enzymes and bile salts convert carotene into a usable nutrient. This conversion is stimulated by thyroxine, a hormone obtained from the thyroid gland. Once converted into vitamin A, carotene is absorbed in the same way as is the preformed vitamin. Vitamin A is carried through the bloodstream, readily accessible to tissues throughout the body. Preformed vitamin A as found in fish-liver oil or other animal products is absorbed by the body 3 to 5 hours after ingestion, whereas the conversion and absorption of carotene takes 6 to 7 hours.

The conversion of carotene into vitamin A is not 100 percent complete; approximately one-third of the carotene in food is converted into vitamin A. Less than one-fourth of the carotene in carrots and root vegetables undergoes conversion, and about one-half of the carotene in leafy green vegetables undergoes conversion. Some unchanged carotene is absorbed into the circulatory system and stored in the fat tissues rather than in the liver. Unabsorbed carotene is excreted in the feces.

The ability of the body to utilize carotene varies with the food and the form in which the food is ingested. Cooking, pureeing, or mashing of vegetables ruptures the cell membranes and therefore makes the carotene more available for absorption.

Factors interfering with absorption of vitamin A and carotene include strenuous physical activity performed with 4 hours of consumption, intake of mineral oil, excessive consumption of alcohol, excessive consumption of iron, and the use of cortisone and other drugs. The intake of polyunsaturated fatty acids with carotene results in rapid destruction of carotene unless antioxidants also are present. Even cold weather can hinder the transport and metabolism of both vitamin A and carotene. Diabetics may not be able to convert carotene into vitamin A.

Approximately 90 percent of the body's vitamin A is stored in the liver, with small amounts deposited in the fat tissues, lungs, kidneys, and retinas of the eyes. Under stressful conditions the body will use this reserve supply if it is not receiving enough vitamin A from the diet. An adequate supply of zinc is needed so the liver can mobilize vitamin A out of its storage depots. Gastrointestinal and liver disorders, infections of any kind, or any condition in which the bile duct is obstructed may limit the body's capacity to retain and use vitamin A. Factors affecting absorption of vitamin A include the quantity given, influence of other substances present in the intestines, and amount of the vitamin stored in the body. A diet low in fat, resulting in little bile reaching the intestine, can cause carotene and vitamin A to be lost in the feces. For these reasons, the recommended dietary amounts vary for each individual.

Dosage and Toxicity

Recommended Dietary Allowances of vitamin A, as established by the National Research Council, are 1500–4000 International Units (IU) for children and 4000–5000 IU for adults. These amounts increase during disease, trauma, pregnancy, and lactation. Requirements vary for people who smoke, those who live in highly polluted areas, people who easily absorb vitamin A, and those who have had their stored supply of vitamin A depleted by pneumonia or nephritis.

Recommended amounts of vitamin A may be supplied through food sources; e.g., ½ pound of calf's liver contains approximately 74,000 IU preformed vitamin A, whereas a carrot contains 11,000 IU of carotene.

Toxicity symptoms include nausea, vomiting, diarrhea, dry skin, hair loss, headaches, appetite loss, sore lips, and flaky, itchy skin. Bone fragility, thickening of long bones, deep bone pain, enlargement of the liver and spleen, blurred vision, and skin rashes are symptoms of prolonged excessive intake. Excessive daily use of vitamin A also may lead to reduced thyroid activity and abnormalities in the skin, eyes, and mucous membranes. Excessive serum calcium can be an indication of vitamin A overdose.

If toxicity is detected, the symptoms will disappear in a few days if the vitamin is withdrawn. Vitamin C can help prevent the harmful effects of vitamin A toxicity.

Deficiency Effects and Symptoms

The eyes are well-known indicators of vitamin A deficiency. One of the first symptoms is night blindness, an inability of the eyes to adjust to darkness. Another eye-related deficiency symptom is xerosis, a disease in which the eyeball loses luster, it becomes dry and inflamed, and visual acuity is reduced.

Other signs of deficiency include rough, dry, or prematurely aged skin; loss of sense of smell; loss of appetite; frequent fatigue; skin blemishes; sties in the eye; and diarrhea. Vitamin A may be lacking when the hair loses its sheen and luster, when dandruff accumulates and fingernails become brittle. A drastic drop of serum A has been found in severely injured patients. More severe symptoms are corneal ulcers and softening of bones and teeth. Deficiency of vitamin A leads to the rapid loss of vitamin C.

Vitamin A deficiency may occur when an inadequate dietary supply exists; when the body is unable to absorb or store the vitamin (as in ulcerative colitis, cirrhosis of the liver, and obstruction of the bile ducts); when an ailment interferes with the conversion of carotene to vitamin A (as in diabetes mellitus and hypothyroidism); and when any rapid bodily loss of the vitamin occurs (as in pneumonia, hyperthyroidism, chronic nephritis, scarlet fever, and some respiratory infections).

Beneficial Effect on Ailments

Many people are unaware of the importance of vitamin A in fighting infections. By giving strength to cell walls, it helps protect the mucous membranes against invading bacteria. People who live in environments with high air-pollution counts are more susceptible to infections and colds than are people who live in environments with cleaner air. If infection has already occurred, therapeutic doses of vitamin A will help keep it from spreading.

Vitamin A can be used successfully in treating several eye disorders, such as Bitot's spots (white, elevated, sharply outlined patches on the white of the eye), blurred vision, night blindness, cataracts, crossed eyes, and nearsightedness. Therapeutic dosages of vitamin A are necessary for treatment of glaucoma and conjunctivitis, an inflammation of the mucous membrane that lines the eyelids.

Administration of vitamin A has helped shorten the duration of communicable diseases—measles, scarlet fever, the common cold, and infections of the eye, middle ear, intestines, ovaries, uterus, and vagina. It also has been effective in reducing high cholesterol levels and atheroma, fatty degeneration or thickening of the wall of the larger arteries.

Vitamin A has proved successful in treating cases of brochial asthma, chronic rhinitis, and dermatitis. Vitamin A has also been helpful in treating patients suffering from tuberculosis, cirrhosis of the liver, emphysema, gastritis, and hyperthyroidism. Patients with nephritis (inflammation of the kidney), migraine headaches, and tinnitus (ringing in the ear) have benefited from vitamin A therapy.

Vitamin A protects the epithelial tissues like the skin, the stomach, and the lungs from becoming cancerous. Little research has been done to discover just what happens to the cells of the body from the time of exposure to a cancer-causing agent to the actual development of a malignancy. This period of time can be as much as 20 years or more. It is known that many cells repair themselves during this period. Vitamin A has been found to be extremely important in this repair process. Studies of animals have shown that carcinogens remain much more active when there is a vitamin A deficiency. Researchers also believe that the vitamin counters the cancerous process by activating the body's immune system and preventing the thymus gland from shrinking. When animals injected with a tumor-virus are given large doses of vitamin A, their tumors diminish and the thymus returns to normal size.

There is increasing evidence that vitamin A is related to sexual development and reproduction. Studies conducted on men having varying levels of sperm deficiency showed that when vitamin A along with Vitamin E was given to them, their sperm levels returned to normal. Dr. Thomas Moore in Cambridge, England, reports that experiments done on animals deficient in vitamin A resulted in undersized, shrunken, and flabby testicles. He also states that a deficiency of vitamin A in females causes an inability to conceive and a higher susceptibility to miscarriage. In animal studies, females that were vitamin A deficient yet able to conceive still had problems such as difficult births, death of the fetus, cleft palate, or other congenital defects.

Vitamin A is essential in the chemical process whereby cholesterol is converted into female estrogens and male androgens. Insufficient supply of these sex hormones results in degeneration of the sex organs. Vitamin A given to animals in this condition resumed normal hormone activity. Diabetic men have a higher incidence of impotence than nondiabetics. As diabetics are unable to convert carotene to vitamin A, their impotence could possibly be related to a vitamin A deficiency.

Externally, vitamin A is used in treating acne; when applied locally, it can clear up impetigo, boils, carbuncles, and open ulcers. Vitamin A applied directly to open wounds hastens the healing process in cases where healing has been retarded because cortisone has been used. It also stimulates the production of mucus, which in turn prevents scarring. A treatment using injections of vitamin A has proved effective in the removal of plantar warts.

Human Tests

1. Vitamin A and Stress Ulcers. Dr. Merril S. Chernov and his associates, Dr. Harry W. Hale, Jr., and Dr. MacDonald Wood, did a two-part study of severely injured patients to determine whether administration of vitamin A would prevent formation of stress ulcers. According to Chernov, serum vitamin A levels dropped "sharply and profoundly" in severely injured patients. (*Medical World News,* January 7, 1972.)

The first part of the study involved 35 patients suffering from burns covering more than 25 percent of their bodies or major injuries to two or more organs. Vitamin A levels in the serum fell dramatically in 29 of the patients within 24 to 72 hours after hospitalization.

In the second part of the study, 14 of 36 similarly stressed patients received 10,000 to 400,000 IU of water-soluble vitamin A daily. Their care was the same as that of the other 22 patients.

Results. Evidence of stress ulcers was seen in 15 of the 22 untreated patients in the second group (69 percent). Massive intestinal bleeding developed in 7 of these patients, and serious intestinal bleeding developed in another 7. Of the 14 patients treated with massive doses of vitamin A, upper gastrointestinal bleeding occurred in only 2.

Dr. Chernov stated, "The sudden and marked depletion of vitamin A is directly related to the corresponding depression of the serum protein, and particularly that fragment of the serum protein involved in transport of vitamin A. This results initially in the development of superficial mucosal erosions followed later by frank ulceration and hemorrhage." The results of Dr. Chernov's study suggest that treatment with high doses of vitamin A reduced the risk of gastroduodenal ulceration in these severely stressed patients. (J. I. Rodale, ed., *Prevention,* April 1972.)

2. Vitamin A and Acne. One hundred acne patients were given oral doses of 100,000 IU of vitamin A at bedtime.

Results. Thirty-six patients were completely relieved of acne, and 43 were relieved except for an occasional pustule. In most cases, responses occurred in less than 9 months. (Jon V. Straumfjord, M.D., Astoria, Oregon, reported in Rodale, ed., *Prevention,* November 1968.)

3. Vitamin A and Acne Lesions. Seventy-five patients who failed to respond to other forms of treatment were given 100,000 IU of vitamin A per day.

Results. Disappearance of the lesions occurred for 30 patients in 2½ months, for another 30 in 3 months, and for 10 more in 5½ months. All could be regarded as cured at the end of 3 months. Drawbacks stated: (1) treatment could take up to a year; (2) dosage given was very high and could have toxic effects. (Dr. K. D. Larharl, *Journal of the Indian Medical Association,* March 1954; reported in Rodale, ed., *Prevention,* November 1968.)

4. Vitamin A and Asthma. Five thousand cases suffering from bronchial dermatitis, bronchial asthma, and chronic rhinitis were treated with vitamins A and D and bone meal.

Results. There was success in relieving the symptoms of 75 percent of the patients, including 1000 patients suffering from bronchial asthma. (Dr. Carl J. Reich, 1972; reported in Rodale, ed., *Prevention,* September 1970.)

5. Vitamin A and Premenstrual Symptoms. Twenty-four patients were given large doses of vitamin A.

Results. There were improvements in premenstrual symptoms. Seventeen patients were partially relieved of symptoms, and all breast tenderness was eliminated. Three more noticed considerable improvement but had some distress. Four patients did not respond to the therapy. (Dr. Alexander Pou, *American Journal of Obstetrics and Gynecology,* June 1951.)

Animal Tests

1. Vitamin A and Tumors. Hamsters given high doses of vitamin A before being subjected to benzpyrene (a carcinogen in smoke) were protected against the appearance of squamous tumors on the lung. Hamsters given a similar high dosage after the development of lung cancer showed a complete block of the cancer process.

Results. Of the 60 treated animals, 5 developed tumors and 4 of these were noncancerous. Of the 53 untreated animals, 16 developed lung cancer. (Dr. Umberto Saffioto of the National Cancer Institute, Bethesda, Maryland, as reported in Rodale, ed., *Prevention,* December 1969.)

2. Vitamin A and Reproductive Processes. Bulls deficient in vitamin A suffered degeneration of their seminiferous tubules. They reportedly regained full potency after receiving strong doses of vitamin A. (J. L. Madsen, *Journal of Animal Science,* reported in Rodale, ed., *Prevention,* January 1971.)

VITAMIN A MAY BE BENEFICIAL FOR THE FOLLOWING AILMENTS:*

Body Member	Ailment or Other Stressful Condition*
Bladder	Cystitis
Blood/Circulatory system	Angina pectoris
	Arteriosclerosis
	Atherosclerosis
	Diabetes
	Hemophilia
	Jaundice
	Mononucleosis
	Stroke (cerebrovascular accident)
Bones	Fracture
	Osteomalacia
	Rickets
Bowel	Celiac disease
	Colitis
	Diarrhea
Brain/Nervous system	Alcoholism
	Epilepsy
	Meningitis
Ear	Ear infection
Eye	Amblyopia
	Bitot spots
	Cataracts
	Conjunctivitis
	Eyestrain
	Glaucoma
	Night blindness
Gallbladder	Gallstones
Glands	Cystic fibrosis
	Diabetes
	Goiter
	Hyperthyroidism
	Prostatitis
	Swollen glands

* The word "ailment" used in subsequent tables of beneficial effects of nutrients is intended to include other stressful conditions.

Body Member	Ailment or Other Stressful Condition*
Hair/Scalp	Hair problems
Head	Fever
	Headache
	Sinusitis
Heart	Angina pectoris
	Arteriosclerosis
	Atherosclerosis
	Congestive heart failure
	Myocardial infarction
Intestine	Celiac disease
	Constipation
	Hemorrhoids
	Worms
Joints	Arthritis
	Gout
Kidney	Kidney stones (renal calculi)
	Nephritis
Leg	Varicose veins
Liver	Cirrhosis of liver
	Hepatitis
	Jaundice
Lungs/Respiratory system	Allergies
	Asthma
	Bronchitis
	Common cold
	Croup
	Emphysema
	Hay fever (allergic rhinitis)
	Influenza
	Sinusitis
	Tuberculosis
Mouth	Canker sore
	Halitosis
Muscles	Muscular dystrophy
Nails	Nail problems
Reproductive system	Impotence
	Prostatitis
	Reproduction
	Vaginitis

Body Member	Ailment or Other Stressful Condition*
Skin	Abscess
	Acne
	Athlete's foot
	Bedsores
	Boil (furuncle)
	Burns
	Carbuncle
	Dandruff
	Dermatitis
	Dry skin
	Eczema
	Impetigo
	Psoriasis
	Shingles (herpes zoster)
	Ulcers
	Warts
Stomach	Gastritis
	Gastroenteritis
	Stomach ulcer (peptic)
Teeth/Gums	Pyorrhea
	Tooth and gum disorders
General	Alcoholism
	Chicken pox
	Fatigue
	Fever
	Infection
	Kwashiorkor
	Measles
	Pregnancy
	Rheumatic fever
	Rhinitis
	Scurvy
	Stress

* The word "ailment" used in subsequent tables of beneficial effects of nutrients is intended to include other stressful conditions.

VITAMIN B COMPLEX

Description

All B vitamins are water-soluble substances that can be cultivated from bacteria, yeasts, fungi, or molds. The known B-complex vitamins are B_1 (thiamine), B_2 (riboflavin), B_3 (niacin), B_5 (pantothenic acid), B_6 (pyridoxine), B_{12} (cyanocobalamin), B_{15} (pangamic acid), biotin, choline, folic acid, inositol, and PABA (para-aminobenzoic acid).   The grouping of these water-soluble compounds under the term "B complex" is based upon their common source distribution, their close relationship in vegetable and animal tissues, and their functional relationships.

The B-complex vitamins are active in providing the body with energy, basically by converting carbohydrates into glucose, which the body "burns" to produce energy.   They are vital in the metabolism of fats and protein.   In addition, the B vitamins are necessary for normal functioning of the nervous system and may be the single most important factor for health of the nerves.   They are essential for maintenance of muscle tone in the gastrointestinal tract and for the health of skin, hair, eyes, mouth, and liver.

All the B vitamins are natural constituents of brewer's yeast, liver, and whole-grain cereals.   Brewer's yeast is the richest natural source of some of the B-complex group.   Another important source of some of the B vitamins is production by the intestinal bacteria.   These bacteria grow best on milk sugar and small amounts of fat in the diet.   Maintaining milk-free diets or taking sulfonamides and other antibiotics may destroy these valuable bacteria.

Absorption and Storage

Because of the water-solubility of the B-complex vitamins, any excess is excreted and not stored.   Therefore they must be continually replaced.   All B vitamins mixed with salve absorb readily.

Sulfa drugs, sleeping pills, insecticides, and estrogen create a condition in the digestive tract which can destroy the B vitamins.   Certain B vitamins are lost through perspiration.

Dosage and Toxicity

The most important thing to remember is that all the B vitamins should be taken together.   They are so interrelated in function that large doses of any one of them may be therapeutically valueless or may cause a deficiency of others.   For example, if extra B_6 is taken in 50-milligram potencies, it is important that a complete B complex accompany it, not all in 50-milligram potencies, but each B vitamin increased proportionately according to the amounts established by the National Academy of Sciences for normal maintenance.   For instance, the adult RDA for vitamin B_6 is 2 milligrams.   Fifty milligrams is 25 times the RDA.   The B vitamins accompanying B_6 should then all be increased 25 times.   Using folic acid as an example, the adult RDA for this B vitamin being 400 micrograms, multiplying by 25 would give an amount of 10,000 micrograms, or 10 milligrams.   In nature, we find the B-complex vitamins in yeast, green vegetables, etc., but nowhere do we find a single B vitamin isolated from the rest.   Most preparations of single B vitamins are synthetic or at least no longer in their natural form.   These synthetic B vitamins are used primarily to overcome severe deficiencies or serious physical conditions in which rapid results are needed.   When taking supplements, it is very important to remember that the B vitamins exert many different effects upon each other; therefore excesses and insufficiencies may be harmful.

Deficiency Effects and Symptoms

The thirteen or more B vitamins are so meagerly supplied in the American diet that almost every American lacks some of them.   If a person is tired, irritable, nervous, depressed, or even suicidal, suspect a vitamin B deficiency.   Gray hair, falling hair, baldness, acne, or other skin troubles indicate a lack of B vitamins.   A poor appetite, insomnia, neuritis, anemia, constipation, or high cholesterol level may be an indicator of a vitamin B deficiency.   Having an enlarged tongue (including the buds on each side) that is shiny, bright red, and full of grooves means B vitamins are needed.

One reason there is so much B-vitamin deficiency in the American population is that Americans eat so many processed foods from which the B vitamins have often been removed.   Some times some, but not all, of the B vitamins are replaced by the manufacturer.

Another reason for widespread deficiency is the high amount of sugar consumed.   Sugar produces an abnormal intestinal flora from which some of the B vitamins are manufactured.   Sugar also is pure carbohydrate with no vitamins or minerals or enzymes to aid in its digestion.   Therefore it takes nutrient supplies, including the B vitamins, from other parts of the body, depleting those storage areas.

Alcoholics and individuals who consume excessive

amounts of carbohydrates require a higher intake of B vitamins for proper metabolism. Alcohol has a tendency to destroy some of the B vitamins such as thiamine and folic acid. Like sugar, alcohol contains large amounts of carbohydrates but no vitamins or minerals, making it very difficult for the body to utilize the carbohydrates found in alcohol.

The caffeine in coffee is known to destroy the B vitamin thiamine, which is, among other things, essential for the health of the nervous system.

The need for the B-complex vitamins increases during infection or stress. Children and pregnant women need extra B vitamins for normal growth.

Beneficial Effect on Ailments

The B vitamins have been used in the treatment of barbiturate overdosage, alcoholic psychoses, and drug-induced delirium. An adequate dose has been found to control migraine headaches and attacks of Ménière's syndrome. Some heart abnormalities have responded to use of B complex because the nerves affecting the heart need the B-complex vitamins for smooth, quiet functioning. Massive dosages of the B-complex vitamins have been helpful in polio, to improve the condition of hypersensitive children who fail to respond favorably to drugs such as Ritalin, and to improve cases of shingles. Nervous individuals and persons working under tension can greatly benefit from taking larger than normal doses of B vitamins.

Postoperative nausea and vomiting, resulting from anesthesia, can be successfully treated with B vitamins. The amount of B vitamins needed seems to be related to the amount of female sex hormones available. Menstrual difficulty is often relieved with small doses. The B vitamins may also help these ailments: beriberi, pellagra, constipation, burning feet, tender gums, burning and drying eyes, fatigue, lack of appetite, skin disorders, cracks at the corner of the mouth, and anemia.

Human Tests

1. B Vitamins and Ménière's Syndrome. A person testified that the therapy of Dr. Mills Atkinson, which consisted of heavy intakes of the B-complex vitamins four times daily, reversed his case of Ménière's syndrome (see "Ailments," p. 115), which had lasted almost 4 months.

Results. Within 2 months the B-vitamin treatment relieved the dizziness, double vision, nausea, and inability to concentrate associated with this ailment. ("Migraine, Ménière's and Mealtime," Rodale, ed., *Prevention,* August 1971.)

2. B Vitamins and Senile Dementia (Deteriorative Mental State of the Aged). Patients in mental hospitals and convalescent homes who were suffering from senile dementia exhibited a dramatic improvement in their mental condition 24 to 48 hours after large doses of B vitamins were administered. (Bicknell and Prescott, *Vitamins in Medicine,* as reported in Linda Clark, *Know Your Nutrition,* 1973, p. 67.)

VITAMIN B COMPLEX MAY BE BENEFICIAL FOR THE FOLLOWING AILMENTS:

Body Member	Ailment
Bladder	Cystitis
Blood/Circulatory system	Anemia
	Angina pectoris
	Arteriosclerosis
	Atherosclerosis
	Cholesterol level, high
	Diabetes
	Hypertension
	Hypoglycemia
	Leukemia
	Stroke (cerebrovascular accident)
Bowel	Diarrhea
Brain/Nervous system	Alcoholism
	Bell's palsy
	Epilepsy
	Insomnia
	Meningitis
	Mental illness
	Multiple sclerosis
	Neuritis
	Parkinson's disease
	Stroke (cerebrovascular accident)
	Vertigo
Ear	Ménière's syndrome
Eye	Amblyopia
	Cataracts
	Conjunctivitis

Body Member	Ailment	Body Member	Ailment
	Eyestrain	Nails	Nail growth
	Glaucoma	Reproductive	Prostatitis
	Night blindness	system	Vaginitis
Gallbladder	Gallstones	Skin	Abscess
Glands	Adrenal exhaustion		Acne
	Cystic fibrosis		Bedsores
	Hyperthyroidism		Bruises
	Prostatitis		Burns
	Swollen glands		Dandruff
Hair/Scalp	Baldness		Dermatitis
	Dandruff		Eczema
	Hair problems		Psoriasis
Head	Fever		Shingles (herpes zoster)
	Headache		Ulcers
Heart	Angina pectoris	Stomach	Gastritis
	Arteriosclerosis		Gastroenteritis
	Atherosclerosis		Indigestion (dyspepsia)
	Congestive heart failure		Stomach ulcer (peptic)
	Hypertension	Teeth/Gums	Pyorrhea
	Myocardial infarction	General	Aging
Intestine	Celiac disease		Alcoholism
	Constipation		Arthritis
	Diverticulitis		Backache
	Hemorrhoids		Beriberi
	Indigestion (dyspepsia)		Cancer
	Worms		Edema
Joints	Arthritis		Fatigue
	Bursitis		Fever
	Gout		Hypoxia
Kidney	Nephritis		Infection
Leg	Leg cramp		Overweight and obesity
	Phlebitis		Pellagra
	Sciatica		Pregnancy
	Varicose veins		Stress
Liver	Cirrhosis of liver		Stroke (cerebrovascular accident)
	Hepatitis		
Lungs/Respiratory system	Common cold		
	Emphysema		
	Hay fever (allergic rhinitis)		
	Influenza		
	Pneumonia		
Mouth	Canker sore		
	Halitosis		
Muscles	Parkinson's disease		

VITAMIN B$_1$ (THIAMINE)

Description

Thiamine, or vitamin B$_1$, is a water-soluble vitamin that acts as a coenzyme participating in the complex process of glucose conversion into energy. Thiamine is vulnerable to heat, air, and water in cooking.

Thiamine is a component of the germ and bran of wheat, the husk of rice, and that portion of all grains which is commercially milled away to give the grain a lighter color and finer texture.

Known as the "morale vitamin" because of its relation to a healthy nervous system and its beneficial effect on mental attitude (see Human Test 1), thiamine is also linked with improving individual learning capacity. It is necessary for consistent growth in children and for the improvement of muscle tone in the stomach, the intestines, and the heart. Thiamine is essential for stabilizing the appetite by improving food assimilation and digestion, particularly that of starches, sugars, and alcohol.

A diet rich in brewer's yeast, wheat germ, blackstrap molasses, and bran will provide the body with adequate thiamine and will help prevent undue accumulation of fatty deposits in the artery walls.

Absorption and Storage

Thiamine is rapidly absorbed in the upper and lower small intestine. It is then carried by the circulatory system to the liver, kidneys, and heart, where it may combine further with manganese and specific proteins to become active enzymes. These are the enzymes that break down carbohydrates into simple sugars.

Thiamine is not stored in the body in any great quantity and therefore must be supplied daily. It is excreted in the urine in amounts that reflect the intake and the quantity stored. Because the amount of thiamine stored in the body is not very great, body tissues deplete rapidly when a deficiency occurs.

Eating sugar will cause a thiamine depletion, as will smoking and drinking alcohol. Thiamine can be destroyed by an enzyme present in raw clams, oysters and raw fish.

Dosage and Toxicity

Individual thiamine needs are determined by body weight, the quantity of the vitamin synthesized in the intestinal tract, and daily calorie intake. As the calorie intake, especially of carbohydrates, increases, the proportion of thiamine ingested increases. The National Research Council recommends 0.5 milligram of thiamine per 1000 calories daily for all ages.

There is evidence suggesting that older people use thiamine less efficiently; hence a higher intake, along with the other B vitamins, may be advantageous. A thiamine intake of 1.4 milligrams daily is recommended during pregnancy and lactation. The need for additional B_1 increases during severe diarrhea, fever, stress, and surgery. There are no known toxic effects with thiamine, although large doses may cause B-complex imbalances.

Deficiency Effects and Symptoms

A deficiency of thiamine not only makes it difficult for a person to digest carbohydrates but also leaves too much pyruvic acid in the blood. This causes loss of mental alertness, labored breathing, and cardiac damage. A mild deficiency of thiamine is difficult to diagnose and easily attributed to other problems. First signs include easy fatigue, loss of appetite, irritability, and emotional instability. If the deficiency is not arrested, confusion and loss of memory appear, followed closely by gastric distress, abdominal pains, and constipation. Heart irregularities crop up, and finally, prickling sensations in the lower extremities, impaired fibratory sense, and tenderness of calf muscles will occur. A thiamine deficiency can also lead to inflammation of the optic nerve. Without thiamine, the function of the central nervous system, which depends upon glucose for energy, is impaired.

A thiamine deficiency can result in decreased coordination, body-reaction time, eye-hand coordination, motor speed and manual steadiness. A thiamine deficiency affects the cardiovascular system as well. The heart muscles are weakened, and cardiac failure may occur. The gastrointestinal tract is also affected, and symptoms such as indigestion, severe constipation, anorexia (a loss of appetite), and gastric atony (loss of muscle tone in the stomach) may occur. "Some researchers believe that the lack of thiamine may be the first link in a chain leading by way of the liver and female hormones to cancer of the uterus."[3]

Beneficial Effect on Ailments

Thiamine is used in the treatment of beriberi, a deficiency disease associated with malnutrition. Thiamine

[3]Ernest Ayre and W. A. G. Gauld, *Science,* April 12, 1946; also J. I. Rodale, *The Encyclopedia for Healthful Living* (Emmaus, Pa.: Rodale Books, 1970), p. 117.

intake has improved the excretion of fluid stored in the body, decreased rapid heart rate, shrunken enlarged hearts, and normalized electrocardiograms.

Nutrients such as thiamine and niacin have been used together to treat multiple sclerosis patients. Dr. George Schumacher tells of his use of thiamine hydrochloride given intraspinally to two multiple sclerosis patients with noted improvement. Dr. Frederick Kleuner used large doses (100 milligrams) of B_1, B_3, and B_6 with reported success.[4]

Thiamine and a multivitamin program have been used in the treatment of myasthenia gravis.

Alcoholism has been successfully treated with thiamine: "Cade (1972) reported that alcoholics admitted to his hospital are routinely given intravenous multivitamins containing at least 200 mg. thiamine. They may require this twice a day. In spite of a great increase in the number of alcoholic admissions to the hospital, there has been steady improvement until the death rate has fallen to zero. In 1945–50, before thiamine treatment was used, eighty-six patients died of alcoholism complications. In 1956–60, eight people died, but no deaths have occurred from 1966 to now. Cade concluded 'that because the mode of death was identical with that in beriberi, because thiamine deficiency has been demonstrated in a significant proportion of sick alcoholics, because deaths no longer occur when they are given thiamine, and because there have been no other discernible significant changes in treatment which are likely to have been responsible, thiamine is the therapeutic agent which is literally lifesaving in a significant proportion of patients.' Thus thiamine—Vitamin B_1—has been clearly shown to have saved lives among alcoholics."[5]

Many other ailments have been aided by the administration of thiamine. Thiamine is essential in the manufacture of hydrochloric acid, which aids in digestion. It helps in eliminating nausea, especially that caused by air or sea sickness. It has improved people's dispositions by alleviating fatigue. Thiamine helps improve muscle tone in the stomach and intestines, which in turn relieves constipation. Herpes zoster (shingles), a painful clustering of blisters behind the ear or elsewhere, has been successfully treated with thiamine.[6]

[4]Prevention Magazine Staff, *Encyclopedia of Common Diseases* (Emmaus, Pa.: Rodale Books, 1969), pp. 786–77.

[5]Abram Hoffer, M.D., *Orthomolecular Nutrition*, p. 121.

[6]Betty Lee Morales, ed., *Cancer Control Journal*, vol. 2, no. 3, p. 13, June 1974.

Dentists have found B_1 useful. Dental postoperative pain is promptly and completely relieved in many patients by the administration of thiamine. Pain can often be prevented before the operation by administration of B_1 to the patient. Thiamine therapy has reduced the healing time of dry tooth sockets. Evidence shows that replacement of thiamine to injured and diseased nerves not only restores proper functioning but also relieves pain.[7]

Human Tests

1. Vitamin B_1 and Morale. Over several years, Horwitt and coworkers studied the psychological effects of thiamine deficiency on psychiatric patients in an institution. The subjects received varying amounts of thiamine in an adequate diet. They were tested for various deficiency effects.

Results. When approximately 0.4 milligram of thiamine was administered, specific conditions, including loss of inhibitory emotional control, paranoid trends, manic-depressive features, and confusion, were helped. (M. K. Horwitt et al., "Investigations of Human Requirements of B-Complex Vitamins," *National Research Council Bull.* 116, 1948.)

2. Vitamin B_1 and Herpes Zoster. Twenty-five patients were given intramuscular injections of 200 milligrams of thiamine hydrochloride daily.

Results. Herpes zoster, a stubborn, painful clustering of small blisters, was successfully treated. (A. L. Oriz, *Medical World,* November 1958.)

3. Vitamin B_1 and Mental Ability. An experiment was conducted by Dr. Ruth Flinn Harrell which involved 104 children from nine to nineteen years of age. Half of the children were given a vitamin B_1 pill each day, and the other half received a placebo. The test lasted 6 weeks.

Results. It was found by a series of tests that the group that was given the vitamin gained one-fourth

[7]J. L. O. Bock, *U.S. Armed Forces Medical Journal,* March 1953.

more in learning ability than did the other group. (Dr. Ruth Flinn Harrell, "Effect of Added Thiamine on Learning," as reported in Rodale and Staff, *The Health Seeker,* pp. 18, 19.)

VITAMIN B₁ MAY BE BENEFICIAL FOR THE FOLLOWING AILMENTS:

Body Member	Ailment
Blood/Circulatory system	Anemia
	Diabetes
Bowel	Constipation
	Diarrhea
Brain/Nervous system	Alcoholism
	Bell's palsy
	Mental illness
	Multiple sclerosis
	Neuritis
Ear	Ménière's syndrome
Eye	Amblyopia
	Night blindness
Head	Fever
	Headache
Heart	Congestive heart failure
Intestine	Worms
Leg	Leg cramp
	Sciatica
Lungs/Respiratory system	Influenza
Skin	Shingles (herpes zoster)
Stomach	Indigestion (dyspepsia)
General	Alcoholism
	Beriberi
	Myasthenia gravis
	Pellagra
	Stress

VITAMIN B₂ (RIBOFLAVIN)

Description

Vitamin B₂, also known as riboflavin, is a water-soluble vitamin occurring naturally in those foods in which the other B vitamins exist. Riboflavin is stable to heat, oxidation, and acid although it disintegrates in the presence of alkali or light, especially ultraviolet light.

Riboflavin functions as part of a group of enzymes that are involved in the breakdown and utilization of carbohydrates, fats, and proteins. Riboflavin is necessary for cell respiration because it works with enzymes in the utilization of cell oxygen. It also is necessary for the maintenance of good vision, skin, nails, and hair.

The amount of B₂ found in most foods is so little that it normally is quite difficult to obtain a sufficient supply without supplementing the diet. Good sources of riboflavin are liver, tongue, and other organ meats, milk, eggs, and brewer's yeast.

Absorption and Storage

Riboflavin is easily absorbed through the walls of the small intestine. It is then carried by the blood to the tissues of the body and excreted in the urine. The amount excreted depends upon the intake and relative need of the tissues and may be accompanied by a loss of protein from the body. Small amounts of riboflavin are found in the liver and kidneys, but it is not stored to any great degree in the body and therefore must be supplied regularly in the diet.

Dosage and Toxicity

According to the National Research Council, the daily riboflavin requirements are related to body size, metabolic rate, and rate of growth. These factors are directly related to the protein and calorie intake of the individual. The Recommended Dietary Allowance is 1.6 milligrams for the adult male and 1.2 milligrams for the female. Pregnancy and lactation requirements are 1.5 and 1.7 milligrams, respectively.

There is no known toxicity of riboflavin. However, prolonged ingestion of large doses of any one of the B-complex vitamins, including riboflavin, may result in high urinary losses of other B vitamins. Therefore it is important to take a complete B complex with any single B vitamin.

Deficiency Effects and Symptoms

Riboflavin deficiency may result from one or several of these factors: (1) long-established faulty dietary habits; (2) food idiosyncrasies ("I won't eat liver!"); (3) alcoholism; (4) arbitrarily selected diets for relief of symptoms of digestive trouble; and (5) prolonged following of a restricted diet in the treatment of a disease such as peptic ulcer or diabetes.

The most common symptoms of a lack of B_2 are cracks and sores in the corners of the mouth; a red, sore tongue; a feeling of grit and sand on the insides of the eyelids; burning of the eyes; eye fatigue; dilation of the pupil; changes in the cornea; sensitivity to light; lesions of the lips; scaling around the nose, mouth, forehead, and ears; trembling; sluggishness; dizziness; dropsy; inability to urinate; vaginal itching; oily skin; and baldness. A vitamin B_2 deficiency can cause some types of cataracts.[8] Experimental studies have shown that some forms of cancer may be related to B_2 deficiency.[9]

A lack of stamina and vigor, retarded growth, digestive disturbances and impaired lactation are results of a riboflavin deficiency. Hair and weight losses also frequently result. Underweight persons feeling tense and depressed may need more riboflavin.

Beneficial Effect on Ailments

Riboflavin plays an important role in the prevention of some visual disturbances, especially cataracts. Undernourished women during the end of pregnancy often suffer from conditions such as visual disturbances, burning sensations in the eyes, excessive watering of eyes, and failing vision. These conditions can be helped by supplementing the diet with large doses of B_2.

Riboflavin has brought relief to children suffering from eczema. Increased dosages of riboflavin are needed for hyperthyroidism, fevers, stress of injury or surgery, and malabsorption.

Human Test

1. B_2 (Riboflavin) and Visual Disturbances. Forty-seven patients suffered from a variety of visual disturbances. They were sensitive to light; they suffered from eyestrain, burning sensations in their eyes, and

visual fatigue; and their eyes watered easily. Six of them had cataracts.

Results. Within 24 hours after the administration of riboflavin, symptoms began to improve. After 2 days, the burning sensations and other symptoms began to disappear. All disorders were gradually cured. When riboflavin was removed, the symptoms gradually appeared again and once again were cured with administration of riboflavin. (Dr. Syndensticker, as reported in Rodale, ed., *Prevention,* November 1970.)

VITAMIN B_2 MAY BE BENEFICIAL FOR THE FOLLOWING AILMENTS:

Body Member	Ailment
Blood/Circulatory system	Diabetes
Bowel	Diarrhea
Brain/Nervous system	Multiple sclerosis
	Neuritis
	Parkinson's disease
	Vertigo
Ear	Ménière's syndrome
Eye	Cataracts
	Conjunctivitis
	Glaucoma
	Night blindness
Glands	Adrenal exhaustion
Hair/Scalp	Baldness
Intestine	Worms
Joints	Arthritis
Kidney	Nephritis
Leg	Leg cramp
Lungs/Respiratory system	Influenza
Reproductive system	Vaginitis
Skin	Acne
	Bedsores
	Dermatitis
	Ulcers
Stomach	Indigestion (dyspepsia)
	Stomach ulcer (peptic)
General	Alcoholism
	Cancer
	Pellagra
	Retarded growth
	Stress

[8]Linda Clark, *Know Your Nutrition* (New Canaan, Conn.: Keats Publ., 1973), p. 78.
[9]Boris Sokoloff, *Cancer: New Approaches, New Hope* (New York: Devin-Adair).

NIACIN (B$_3$, NICOTINIC ACID, NIACINAMIDE, NICOTINAMIDE)

Description

Niacin, a member of the vitamin B complex, is water-soluble. It is more stable than thiamine or riboflavin and is remarkably resistant to heat, light, air, acids, and alkalies. There are also three synthetic forms of niacin: niacinamide, nicotinic acid, and nicotinamide. As a coenzyme, niacin assists enzymes in the breakdown and utilization of proteins, fats, and carbohydrates. Niacin is effective in improving circulation and reducing the cholesterol level in the blood. It is vital to the proper activity of the nervous system and for formation and maintenance of healthy skin, tongue, and digestive-system tissues. Niacin is necessary for the synthesis of sex hormones.

Relatively small amounts of pure niacin are present in most foods. The niacin "equivalent" listed in dietary tables means either pure niacin or adequate supply of tryptophan, an amino acid that can be converted into niacin by the body. Lean meats, poultry, fish, and peanuts are rich daily sources of both niacin and tryptophan, as are such dietary supplements as brewer's yeast, wheat germ, and desiccated liver. Niacin is difficult to obtain except from these foods.

Absorption and Storage

Niacin is absorbed in the intestine and is stored primarily in the liver. Any excess is eliminated through the urine. Excessive consumption of sugar and starches will deplete the body's supply of niacin, as will certain antibiotics.

Dosage and Toxicity

The National Research Council suggests that daily allowances of niacin be based on caloric intake; 6.6 milligrams of niacin per 1000 calories is recommended. Tryptophan may provide part or all of the daily niacin requirements; 60 milligrams of tryptophan yield 1 milligram of niacin. The Recommended Dietary Allowance is 16 milligrams for men, 13 milligrams for women, and 9 to 16 milligrams for children. During pregnancy, lactation, illness, tissue trauma, and growth periods and after physical exercise, daily requirements are increased.

No real toxic effects are known, but large doses, usually 100 or more milligrams, may cause passing side effects such as tingling and itching sensations, intense flushing of the skin, and throbbing in the head due to a dilation of the blood vessels. The flush is not considered dangerous. It lasts for approximately 15 minutes and then disappears. By taking a synthetic form of niacin, niacinamide, a person gets all the benefits of niacin but avoids the above side effects.

Niacinamide may, however, cause depression in some people. It has also been known to cause liver damage in doses starting at 2 grams per day. Because niacin is involved in the release of stomach acid, patients using large doses should take the vitamin on a full stomach. Niacin can also precipitate a gout attack by competing with the excretion of uric acid.

Deficiency Effects and Symptoms

The symptoms of niacin deficiency are many. In the early stages, muscular weakness, general fatigue, loss of appetite, indigestion, and various skin eruptions occur. A niacin deficiency may also cause bad breath, small ulcers, canker sores, insomnia, irritability, nausea, vomiting, recurring headaches, tender gums, strain, tension, and deep depression. Severe niacin deficiency results in pellagra, which is characterized by dermatitis; dementia; diarrhea; rough, inflamed skin; tremors; and nervous disorders. Many digestive abnormalities causing irritation and inflammation of mucous membranes in the mouth and gastrointestinal tract develop from a niacin deficiency.

Beneficial Effect on Ailments

The amazing thing about niacin is the speed with which it can reverse disorders. Diarrhea has been cleared up in 2 days. Atherosclerosis, attacks of Ménière's syndrome (vertigo), and some cases of progressive deafness have improved or even disappeared. Niacin is often used to reduce high blood pressure and increase circulation in cramped, painful legs of the elderly. It also helps to stimulate the production of hydrochloric acid to aid impaired digestion. Acne has been successfully treated with niacin.

Lewis J. Silvers, M.D., writes: "Many a migraine

headache can be prevented from developing into the excruciating painful stage by taking niacin at the first sign of attack.''[10]

Niacin is very important for brain metabolism. In studies, niacin along with other vitamins relieved such schizophrenic symptoms as paranoia and hallucinations. Large doses of niacin have helped elderly patients who are mentally confused.

Drs. Richard M. Halpern and Robert A. Smith have reported research indicating that the flushless nicotinamide may be a factor in preventing cancer, due to enzyme regulation that protects normal cells and prevents them from becoming malignant. Investigators have found niacin able to cure pellagra, a disease that affects the skin, intestinal tract, and nervous system. When given in high doses, niacin may bring complete relief from delirium within 24 to 48 hours.

Niacin can be helpful for weight reduction because of its ability to elevate and stabilize blood sugar levels. For this reason it is also beneficial for hypoglycemics. Smokers can benefit from niacin because it widens blood vessels and removes lipids from arterial walls, opposite actions of nicotine. Fluid loss from severe burns can be lessened with niacin. Many insomniacs respond well to the sleep-inducing effects of niacin.

Niacin has been very effective in the treatment of alcoholism. Arthritics have experienced increased joint mobility, decreased joint stiffness and pain, as well as greater muscle strength and lessened fatigue with the administration of niacin. In most cases, long-term treatment is needed for optimum benefits.

Niacin can decrease the effects of hallucinogens like LSD and mescaline. Because of its calming properties, niacin can reduce the amount of tranquilizers needed or may even be able to replace them.

Human Tests

1. Niacin and Acne. Twenty cases of acne were treated with 100 milligrams three times daily. This treatment continued for 2 or 3 weeks or until the patients experienced regular flushing.

Results. The niacin treatment provided definite relief in all 20 cases. (Lewis J. Silvers, M.D., as reported in Clark, *Know Your Nutrition,* pp. 83–84.)

[10]Clark, *Know Your Nutrition,* pp. 83–84.

2. Niacin and Cancer. Drs. Richard M. Halpern and Robert A. Smith reported that malignancy is, in some way, associated with a deficiency of niacin. To prove that niacin could help prevent cancer, they exposed isolated malignant cells in their laboratory to nicotinamide and watched the vitamin suppress the malignancy. The doctors did not state dosages since individual needs vary so greatly. (Drs. Richard M. Halpern and Robert A. Smith, Molecular Biology Institute, as reported in Clark, *Know Your Nutrition,* p. 84.)

NIACIN MAY BE BENEFICIAL FOR THE FOLLOWING AILMENTS:

Body Member	Ailment
Blood/Circulatory system	Arteriosclerosis
	Atherosclerosis
	Cholesterol level, high
	Diabetes
	Hemophilia
	Hypertension
	Hypoglycemia
	Phlebitis
Bowel	Diarrhea
Brain/Nervous system	Dizziness
	Epilepsy
	Headache
	Insomnia
	Mental illness
	Multiple sclerosis
	Neuritis
	Parkinson's disease
Ear	Ménière's syndrome
Eye	Conjunctivitis
	Night blindness
Hair/Scalp	Baldness
Heart	Arteriosclerosis
	Atherosclerosis
	Hypertension
Intestine	Constipation
Joints	Arthritis
Leg	Phlebitis
Lungs/Respiratory system	Tuberculosis
Mouth	Canker sore
	Halitosis

Body Member	Ailment
Skin	Acne
	Bedsores
	Dermatitis
Stomach	Indigestion (dyspepsia)
Teeth/Gums	Pyorrhea
General	Alcoholism
	Cancer
	Stress

PANTOTHENIC ACID (B₅)

Description

Pantothenic acid, a part of the vitamin B complex, is water-soluble. It occurs in all living cells, being widely distributed in yeasts, molds, bacteria, and individual cells of all animals and plants. Organ meats, brewer's yeast, egg yolks, and whole-grain cereals are the richest sources. Pantothenic acid is synthesized in the body by the bacterial flora of the intestines.

There is a close correlation between pantothenic acid tissue levels and functioning of the adrenal cortex. Pantothenic acid stimulates the adrenal glands and increases production of cortisone and other adrenal hormones important for healthy skin and nerves.

Pantothenic acid plays a vital role in cellular metabolism. As a coenzyme it participates in the release of energy from carbohydrates, fats, and proteins and in the utilization of other vitamins, especially riboflavin. Pantothenic acid is an essential constituent of coenzyme A, which forms active acetate and, as such, acts as an activating agent in metabolism. Pantothenic acid is essential for the synthesis of cholesterol, steroids (fat-soluble organic compounds), and fatty acids. It is important in maintaining a healthy digestive tract.

Pantothenic acid can improve the body's ability to withstand stressful conditions. Adequate intake of pantothenic acid reduces the toxicity effects of many antibiotics. It aids in the prevention of premature aging and wrinkles. It also protects against cellular damage caused by excessive radiation.

Absorption and Storage

Pantothenic acid is found in the blood, particularly in the plasma, which is the liquid part of the lymph. Pantothenic acid is excreted daily in the urine.

Approximately 33 percent of the pantothenic acid content of meat is lost during cooking and about 50 percent is lost by the milling of flour. It is easily destroyed by acid, such as vinegar, or alkali, such as baking soda.

Dosage and Toxicity

Individual needs for pantothenic acid vary according to periods of stress, daily food intake, and urinary excretion levels. Several sources, including the National Research Council, suggest 5 to 10 milligrams daily for adults and children, respectively. *The Heinz Handbook of Nutrition* suggests daily requirements to be 10 to 15 milligrams.

Therapeutic dosages usually range from 50 to 200 milligrams per day. In some studies, 1000 and more milligrams were given daily for 6 months without side effects.[11] It is presumed that folic acid aids in the assimilation of pantothenic acid. There are no known toxic effects with pantothenic acid.

A more-than-normal amount of pantothenic acid may be needed after injury, severe illness, or antibiotic therapy.

Deficiency Effects and Symptoms

Pantothenic acid is so widely distributed in foods that deficiency is rare. The means of detecting deficiencies are limited, although low intakes may slow down many metabolic processes.

Symptoms of a deficiency may include vomiting, restlessness, abdominal pains, burning feet, muscle cramps, sensitivity to insulin, decreased antibody formation, and upper respiratory infections.

Pantothenic acid is essential for proper functioning of the gastrointestinal tract. In some individuals, including postoperative patients, intestinal gas and abdominal distension can be relieved by more-than-average amounts of pantothenic acid.

A deficiency may lead to skin disorders, adrenal exhaustion, and low blood sugar (hypoglycemia). The list of deficiency symptoms reflects impaired health of cells in many tissues. A lack of pantothenic acid

[11]Paavo Airola, *How to Get Well* (Phoenix, Ariz.: Health Plus Pub., 1974), p. 265.

may result in duodenal ulcers. Deficiencies may occur when the body lacks the intestinal flora needed to synthesize pantothenic acid. The function of the adrenal gland is diminished, which may lead to physical and mental depression, insufficient secretions of hydrochloric acid in the stomach, and disturbances of the motor nerves. Because the brain contains one of the highest concentrations of pantothenic acid, mental symptoms such as insomnia, fatigue, and depression can be the result of a deficiency.

Beneficial Effect on Ailments

Pantothenic acid has been used successfully to treat paralysis of the gastrointestinal tract after surgery.[12] It appears to stimulate gastrointestinal movement and aids in the prevention of nerve degeneration due to a deficiency. Nerve degeneration includes peripheral neuritis, nerve disorders, and epilepsy.

Blood pantothenic acid levels decrease during rheumatoid arthritis; the more severe the symptoms, the lower the acid level. Daily injections of pantothenic acid may lead to a rise in blood pantothenic acid levels. Pantothenic acid is important in the prevention of arthritis.[13] It is probably the greatest defense against stress and fatigue, and it also helps build antibodies for fighting infection.

Animal Tests

1. Pantothenic Acid and Duodenal Ulcers. Rats were kept on a diet deficient in pantothenic acid.

Results. Increased hormonal activity was shown to cause ulcers in 11 to 14 weeks. The same hormonal activity in rats that had been fed pantothenic acid did not produce any ulcers. (*Drug Trade News,* March 11, 1957, as reported in J. I. Rodale, ed., *Best Health Articles from Prevention Magazine,* pp. 231, 232.)

2. Pantothenic Acid and Infection. Rats were divided into two groups: one with a diet containing pantothenic acid and one without any. They were then exposed to an infection source.

[12]Helen A. Guthrie, *Introductory Nutrition,* 2d ed. (St. Louis: C. V. Mosby Co., 1971), p. 262.
[13]Roger J. Williams, *Nutrition against Disease* (New York: Pitman Publ., 1971), p. 126.

Results. Spontaneous infections were widespread in the rats whose diet did not contain pantothenic acid. No infections were seen in the rats whose diet was complete. In the rats (deficient in pantothenic acid) that were inoculated with the infection source, 100 percent infection was noted. The rats whose diet included this vitamin showed an infection incidence of only 1 in 45 when given the same inoculation. (*Nutrition Review,* February 1957, as reported in Rodale, *Encyclopedia for Healthful Living,* p. 951.)

3. Pantothenic Acid and Life-Span. Mice were divided into two groups. They were treated alike except that each animal in the control group received 0.3 milligram of extra pantothenate per day in its drinking water. This amount was several times the amount that mice supposedly require.

Results. The 41 mice on the regular diet lived an average of 550 days. The 33 mice who received extra pantothenate lived an average of 653 days (550 days is equivalent to 75 years for humans, and 653 days is equivalent to 89 years). (Williams, *Nutrition against Disease,* pp. 141, 142.)

PANTOTHENIC ACID MAY BE BENEFICIAL FOR THE FOLLOWING AILMENTS:

Body Member	Ailment
Blood/Circulatory system	Anemia
	Hypoglycemia
Bladder	Cystitis
Bones	Fracture
Bowel	Diarrhea
Brain/Nervous system	Epilepsy
	Fainting spells
	Insomnia
	Mental illness
	Multiple sclerosis
	Neuritis
Eye	Cataracts
Foot	Burning and tingling sensations
Glands	Adrenal exhaustion
Hair/Scalp	Baldness
Head	Headache
Intestine	Worms
	Flatulence

Body Member	Ailment
Joints	Arthritis
	Gout
Leg	Leg cramp
	Phlebitis
Lungs/Respiratory system	Allergies
	Asthma
	Tuberculosis
Muscles	Muscular dystrophy
Skin	Acne
	Psoriasis
Stomach	Gastritis
	Indigestion (dyspepsia)
	Nausea
General	Alcoholism
	Cancer
	Depression
	Fatigue
	Infection
	Retarded growth
	Stress

VITAMIN B₆ (PYRIDOXINE)

Description

Vitamin B_6 is a water-soluble vitamin consisting of three related compounds: pyridoxine, pyridoxal, and pyridoxamine. It is required for the proper absorption of vitamin B_{12} and for the production of hydrochloric acid and magnesium. It also helps linoleic acid function better in the body. Pyridoxine plays an important role as a coenzyme in the breakdown and utilization of carbohydrates, fats, and proteins. It must be present for the production of antibodies and red blood cells. The release of glycogen for energy from the liver and muscles is facilitated by vitamin B_6. It also aids in the conversion of tryptophan, an essential amino acid, to niacin and is necessary for the synthesis and proper action of DNA and RNA.

Vitamin B_6 helps maintain the balance of sodium and potassium, which regulates body fluids and promotes the normal functioning of the nervous and musculoskeletal systems. The best sources of vitamin B_6 are meats and whole grains. Desiccated liver and brewer's yeast are the recommended supplemental sources.

Absorption and Storage

A daily supply of vitamin B_6, together with the other B-complex vitamins, is necessary because it is excreted in the urine within 8 hours after ingestion and is not stored in the liver. Fasting and reducing diets can deplete the body's supply of vitamin B_6 if proper supplements are not taken.

Dosage and Toxicity

Vitamin B_6 seems to be another B vitamin that, if administered alone, can cause an imbalance or deficiency of other B vitamins. The Recommended Dietary Allowance of vitamin B_6 is 2 milligrams per day. The need for vitamin B_6 increases during pregnancy, lactation, exposure to radiation, cardiac failure, aging, and use of oral contraceptives. Intravenous doses of 200 miligrams have proved nontoxic, and daily oral doses of 100 to 300 milligrams have been administered to alleviate drug-induced neuritis without side effects.[14] However, too-high amounts taken for a prolonged time have resulted in nerve damage in some people.

Because B_6 is involved in the production of hydrochloric acid, people with stomach ulcers should seek a doctor's advice before taking the vitamin in large doses.

Deficiency Effects and Symptoms

In cases of B_6 deficiency there is low blood sugar and low glucose tolerance, resulting in a sensitivity to insulin. Deficiency may also cause loss of hair, water retention during pregnancy, cracks around the mouth and eyes, numbness and cramps in arms and legs, slow learning, visual disturbances, neuritis, arthritis, heart disorders involving nerves, temporary paralysis of a limb, and an increase in urination.

If a vitamin B_6 deficiency is allowed to continue through late pregnancy, stillbirths or postdelivery infant mortality may result. Infants born to B_6 deficient mothers may have convulsions. Studies have shown that pregnant women retain more B_6 than nonpregnant

[14]National Academy of Sciences, *Toxicants Occurring Naturally in Foods* (Washington, D.C.: National Research Council, 1973), p. 246.

women; therefore supplemental doses may be needed to make sure the fetus is adequately supplied.

A certain type of anemia characterized by red blood cells that are too small, apparently the result of a defective heredity factor, responds very well to vitamin B_6. Some people may have an unbalanced metabolism caused by a genetic dependency on B_6. Too much B_6 without zinc can lead to numbness and tingling of the fingers and toes. Reducing the dosage and adding brewer's yeast and zinc or a multiple vitamin (without copper) can eliminate the symptoms.

Kryptopyrrole, also known as the mauve factor, found in large quantities in the urine of many schizophrenics and less often in normal people, has been shown to bind pyridoxine, resulting in a deficiency of the vitamin. Some patients with this mauve factor may need as much as 250–3000 milligrams per day. The treatment should include zinc; and manganese and niacin may also be helpful. B_6 and zinc have also helped people with kryptopyrrole to remember their dreams (a part of treatment).

Symptoms of a B_6 deficiency are similar to those seen in niacin and riboflavin deficiencies and may include muscular weakness, nervousness, irritability, depression, and dermatitis. Tingling hands, shoulder-hand syndrome, wrist-hand syndromes, and arthritis associated with menopause also may be present.

Beneficial Effect on Ailments

There is evidence that suggests a relationship between vitamin B_6 and cholesterol metabolism; therefore B_6 may be involved in the control of atherosclerosis. Vitamin B_6 has been used in the treatment of nervous disorders and in the control of nausea and vomiting during pregnancy.

Vitamin B_6 has been successfully used to help treat male sexual disorders, eczema, thinning and loss of hair, elevated cholesterol level, diarrhea, hemorrhoids, pancreatitis, ulcers, muscular weakness, some types of heart disturbances, burning feet, some types of kidney stones, acne, tooth decay, and diabetes. It is needed to prevent and treat shoulder-hand syndrome. Administration of B_6 to mentally retarded children has helped relieve convulsize seizures. It also appears to be beneficial in treating stress, along with zinc.

As a natural diuretic, vitamin B_6 aids in the prevention of water buildup in the tissues. It has helped

women who suffer from temporary premenstrual changes such as edema and may be effective in helping problems of overweight caused by water retention. Reduction of the pain and size of the reddened knots on the sides of finger joints occurring in women during menopause has responded to daily ingestion of B_6. Individuals who are especially photosensitive to sunlight and quickly sunburn have been treated successfully with B_6.

Human Tests

1. Vitamin B_6 and Parkinson's Disease. It was found that Parkinson's disease, a nervous disorder that causes trembling hands, responded to B_6 treatments. A case of the disease which had existed for 25 years responded to B_6 injections within 2 months. This is one of the unexpected results of B_6—whereas it may take a long time to derive benefits from some vitamins, B_6 seems to bring results quickly and dramatically. (Dr. Douw G. Stern, University of South Africa, as reported in Clark, *Know Your Nutrition,* p. 91.)

2. Vitamin B_6 and Painful Finger Joints. Vitamin B_6 was given to women and men near the age of menopause who had developed painful spurs or knots on the sides of their finger joints.

Results. There was a dramatic change after the administration of B_6. Finger joints ceased to be painful, and finger sensitivity and hand flexion improved within 6 weeks. (John M. Ellis, "The Doctor Who Looked at Hands," as reported in Clark, *Know Your Nutrition,* p. 91.)

Animal Tests

1. Vitamin B_6 and Cleft Palates. Cleft palates developed in 85 percent of the offspring of mice injected with cortisone four times daily during pregnancy.

Results. When pyridoxine was injected along with the cortisone, such abnormalities were reduced to 45 percent, and the addition of folic acid reduced the occurrence of cleft palate to 20 percent. On the basis of these experiments, folic acid and pyridoxine were given to human mothers who had previously borne cleft palate children, and all children subsequently born to these mothers were normal. (Dr. Lyndon A. Peer, 22d Annual Meeting of International College of Surgeons, as reported in Rodale, *The Health Seeker,* p. 194.)

VITAMIN B₆ MAY BE BENEFICIAL FOR THE FOLLOWING AILMENTS:

Body Member	Ailment
Blood/Circulatory system	Anemia
	Cholesterol level, high
	Diabetes
	Hypoglycemia
	Jaundice
	Pernicious anemia
Bladder	Cystitis
Bowel	Colitis
	Diarrhea
Brain/Nervous system	Bell's palsy
	Carpal tunnel syndrome
	Epilepsy
	Insomnia
	Infantile autism
	Mental illness
	Multiple sclerosis
	Neuritis
	Parkinson's disease
Ear	Dizziness
Eye	Conjunctivitis
Glands	Prostatitis
Hair/Scalp	Baldness
	Dandruff
Head	Headache
Intestine	Celiac disease
	Hemorrhoids
	Worms
Joints	Arthritis
Kidney	Kidney stones (renal calculi)
Lungs/Respiratory system	Asthma
	Common cold
	Influenza
	Tuberculosis
Mouth	Halitosis
Muscles	Muscular dystrophy
	Rheumatism

Body Member	Ailment
Reproductive system	Prostatitis
	Vaginitis
Skin	Acne
	Dandruff
	Dermatitis
	Eczema
	Psoriasis
	Shingles (herpes zoster)
Stomach	Gastritis
	Indigestion (dyspepsia)
	Nausea of pregnancy
Teeth/Gums	Pyorrhea
General	Alcoholism
	Edema
	Overweight and obesity
	Stress

VITAMIN B₁₂

Description

Vitamin B₁₂, a water-soluble vitamin, is unique in being the first cobalt-containing substance found to be essential for longevity, and it is the only vitamin that contains essential mineral elements. It cannot be made synthetically but must be grown, like penicillin, in bacteria or molds. Animal protein is almost the only source in which B₁₂ occurs naturally in foods in substantial amounts. Liver is the best source; kidney, muscle meats, fish, and dairy products are other good sources.

Vitamin B₁₂ is necessary for normal metabolism of nerve tissue and is involved in protein, fat, and carbohydrate metabolism. B₁₂ is closely related to the actions of four amino acids, pantothenic acid, and vitamin C. It also helps iron function better in the body and aids folic acid in the synthesis of choline. B₁₂ helps the placement of vitamin A into body tissues by aiding carotene absorption or vitamin A conversion. It also aids in the production of DNA and RNA, the body's genetic material.

Absorption and Storage

Vitamin B₁₂ is prepared for absorption by two gastric secretions. It is poorly absorbed from the gastrointestinal tract unless the "intrinsic factor," a mucoprotein enzyme, is present. Autoimmune reactions in the body can bind the intrinsic factor, preventing B_{12} absorption. The intrinsic factor itself may not even be made because autoimmune reactions prevent the cells' ability to produce it. A defect in the molecule that transports B_{12} from the blood to the tissues can cause a deficiency even when a normal serum B_{12} level is read.

B_{12} needs to be combined with calcium during absorption to benefit the body properly. The presence of hydrochloric acid aids in the absorption of B_{12} given orally, and a properly functioning thyroid gland also helps B_{12} to be better absorbed.

After absorption, B_{12} is bound to serum protein (globulins) and is transported in the bloodstream to various tissues. The highest concentrations of B_{12} are found in the liver, kidneys, heart, pancreas, testes, brain, blood, and bone marrow. These body members are all related to red blood cell formation.

People deficient in B_{12} usually lack one or more gastric secretions necessary for its absorption. Many people lack the ability to absorb it at all.

The actual amount of B_{12} absorbed is regulated by the intrinsic factor. When intake is low, 60 to 80 percent of the vitamin is absorbed. When high amounts are taken, the absorption decreases to 5 to 10 percent. Absorption of B_{12} is better when it is taken with several meals instead of one. Absorption of B_{12} appears to decrease with age and with iron, calcium, and B_6 deficiencies; absorption increases during pregnancy. The use of laxatives depletes the storage of B_{12}.

Because of its close relationship with folic acid, both vitamins taken together could be of benefit in many cases.

Dosage and Toxicity

Human requirements are minute but essential. The Recommended Dietary Allowance of vitamin B_{12} is 3 micrograms for adults and 4 micrograms for pregnant and lactating women. Infants require a daily intake of 3 micrograms, and growing children need 1 to 2 micrograms. A vegetarian diet frequently is low in vitamin B_{12} and high in folic acid, which may mask a vitamin B_{12} deficiency. No cases of vitamin B_{12} toxicity have been reported, even with large doses.

Deficiency Effects and Symptoms

Symptoms of a vitamin B_{12} deficiency may take 5 or 6 years to appear, after the body's supply from natural sources has been restricted.[15] A deficiency of vitamin B_{12} is usually due to an absorption problem caused by a lack of the intrinsic factor. It can also be the result of fish tapeworm infestation or excessive bacteria in the stomach and intestines. Symptoms of a deficiency begin with changes in the nervous system such as soreness and weakness in the legs and arms, diminished reflex response and sensory perception, difficulty in walking and speaking (stammering), and jerking of limbs.

Lack of B_{12} has been found to cause a type of brain damage resembling schizophrenia. This brain damage may be detected by the following symptoms: sore mouth, numbness or stiffness, a feeling of deadness, shooting pains, needles-and-pins, or hot-and-cold sensations. The *British Medical Journal* (March 26, 1966) stated editorially, "It is true that vitamin B_{12} deficiency may cause severe psychotic symptoms which may vary in severity from mild disorders of mood, mental slowness, and memory defect to severe psychotic symptoms . . . occasionally, these mental disturbances may be the first manifestations of B_{12} deficiency. . . ."

Vitamin B_{12} deficiency also manifests itself in nervousness, neuritis, unpleasant body odor, menstrual disturbances, and difficulty in walking.

If a deficiency is not detected in early stages, it *may* result in permanent mental deterioration and paralysis. When symptoms become serious, do not try to treat them yourself. Consult a doctor.

Beneficial Effect on Ailments

Injections of B_{12} can be used to treat patients suffering from pernicious anemia, an ailment characterized by insufficient red blood cells in the bone marrow. Injections rather than oral doses of B_{12} are used to bypass the absorption defect in pernicious anemic patients. B_{12} helps the red blood cells to mature up to a certain point, and after that, protein, iron, vitamin

[15]Marie V. Krause and Martha A. Hunscher, *Food, Nutrition and Diet Therapy*, 5th ed. (Philadelphia: W. B. Saunders Co., 1972), p. 141.

C, and folic acid help to finish the development of the cells so that they can mature. Like folic acid, vitamin B_{12} has been effective in the treatment of the intestinal syndrome sprue.

The *Medical Press* reported remarkable results in the treatment of osteoarthritis, a degenerative joint disease, and osteroporosis, a softening of the bone, with vitamin B_{12} (see Human Tests). The condition known as "tobacco amblyopia," a dimness of vision or a loss of vision due to poisoning by tobacco, has been improved with injections of vitamin B_{12} whether or not the patient stopped smoking. Symptoms are blackouts, headaches, and farsightedness.

B_{12} has provided relief of the following symptoms: fatigue, increased nervous irritability, mild impairment in memory, inability to concentrate, mental depression, insomnia, and lack of balance. B_{12} also has been used successfully in the treatment of hepatitis, bursitis, and asthma.

Studies have confirmed that B_{12} improves the growth rate of children. In animal experiments, pregnant females' resistance to infection was considerably enhanced when given more-than-normal amounts of the vitamin. Vitamin B_{12} is important in reproduction and lactation. It helps to reduce the effects of bruising and black eyes. It has been successfully used for hangovers, leg paralysis, and atrophy of the brain's cerebellum. Under certain circumstances, B_{12} can protect the liver from injury caused by toxic substances.

Human Tests

1. Vitamin B_{12} and Cancer. Cancerous children were treated with B_{12} so that it could be shown that B_{12} could reduce the growth rate of cancer of the nervous system in children.

Results. Among 82 children who were treated with B_{12}, 32 (39 percent) survived up to 12 years. With conventional treatment, 8 out of 25 (32 percent) survived. (*Archives of Disease in Childhood,* December 1963, as reported in *Cancer,* March 28, 1964.)

2. Vitamin B_{12} and Osteoarthritis and Osteoporosis. Thirty-three cases of osteoarthritis and 2 cases of osteoporosis were treated with vitamin B_{12}. The injected dosages varied between 30 and 900 micrograms, but the optimum dose was 100 micrograms per week.

Results. Twenty patients benefited from the treatment within the first week; 7 obtained complete relief. At the end of the second week, 4 more showed partial relief. By the end of the third week, all but 3 of the patients showed some benefit. Three cases of rheumatoid arthritis did not react at all to the vitamin. (*Medical Press,* March 12, 1952, as reported in Rodale, *The Encyclopedia for Healthful Living,* p. 942.)

3. Vitamin B_{12} and Mental Confusion. A seventy-six-year-old patient was suffering from ailments relating to a poor system of blood vessels and heart. He was unable to walk without pain in his legs, and he showed signs of extreme depression and mental confusion. Finally he came down with a siege of pneumonia and sciatica, severe leg pain. Dr. Grabner prescribed 400 micrograms daily of injected vitamin B_{12}.

Results. After the fourth injection the patient exhibited a more pleasant attitude, and his state of confusion had improved. After 2 weeks, the dosage was reduced to 200 micrograms daily; then that was cut to every other day; and finally the patient was receiving 200 micrograms twice weekly. The doctor described his condition as healthy and completely normal mentally. (Dr. Grabner, *"Munchener Medizenische Wochenschrift,"* Munich Medical Weekly, October 31, 1958, as reported in Rodale, *The Encyclopedia for Healthful Living,* 1970, p. 946.)

4. Vitamin B_{12} and Bursitis. Injections of 1000 micrograms of vitamin B_{12} were given to subjects suffering from all types of bursitis. They were given the doses daily for 3 weeks, then once or twice a week for 2 or 3 weeks depending upon clinical observations.

Results. Rapid relief was achieved in all cases. Calcium deposits, if present, were absorbed, and there were no side effects or toxicity. Dr. Klemes reported that over a 5-year period, only 3 patients failed to respond to vitamin B_{12} therapy for treatment of bursitis. (Dr. I. S. Klemes, *Industrial Medicine and Surgery,* June 1957, as reported in Rodale, *The Encyclopedia for Healthful Living,* pp. 108–110.)

VITAMIN B$_{12}$ MAY BE BENEFICIAL FOR THE FOLLOWING AILMENTS:

Body Member	Ailment
Blood/Circulatory system	Anemia
	Angina pectoris
	Arteriosclerosis
	Atherosclerosis
	Diabetes
	Hypoglycemia
	Pernicious anemia
Bones	Osteoporosis
Brain/Nervous system	Epilepsy
	Insomnia
	Multiple sclerosis
	Neuritis
	Vertigo
Glands	Adrenal exhaustion
Heart	Angina pectoris
	Arteriosclerosis
	Atherosclerosis
Intestine	Celiac disease
	Worms
Joints	Arthritis
	Bursitis
Liver	Cirrhosis of liver
Lungs/Respiratory system	Allergies
	Asthma
	Tuberculosis
Muscles	Muscular dystrophy
Skin	Pellagra
	Psoriasis
	Shingles (herpes zoster)
	Ulcers
Stomach	Gastritis
	Stomach ulcer (peptic)
General	Alcoholism
	Overweight and obesity

PANGAMIC ACID (B$_{15}$)

Description

Pangamic acid is a water-soluble nutrient that was originally isolated in extracted apricot kernels and later was obtained in crystalline form from rice bran, rice polish, whole-grain cereals, brewer's yeast, steer blood, and horse liver. Pangamic acid promotes oxidation processes and cell respiration and stimulates glucose oxidation. The chief merit of pangamic acid is its ability to eliminate the phenomenon of hypoxia, an insufficient supply of oxygen in living tissue. This is especially true in the cardiac and other muscles.

Pangamic acid is essential in promoting protein metabolism, particularly in the muscles of the heart. It regulates fat and sugar metabolism, which partly accounts for its effects on atherosclerosis and diabetes. In some treatments, the action of pangamic acid is improved by the addition of vitamins A and E.

Pangamic acid is helpful in stimulating the glandular and nervous system and is helpful in treating high blood cholesterol levels, impaired circulation, and premature aging. It can help protect against the damaging effect of carbon monoxide poisoning.

Little is actually known about pangamic acid, and only small quantities are used in the United States although it is used widely in Russia and other European countries. Pharmaceutical pangamic acid is derived from ground apricot pits. Good natural sources of pangamic acid are brewer's yeast, whole brown rice, whole grains, pumpkin seeds, and sesame seeds.

Absorption and Storage

Little is known about the absorption and storage of pangamic acid, but excessive amounts are excreted through the kidneys and bowels and in perspiration.

Dosage and Toxicity

The Recommended Dietary Allowance has not been established. According to Dr. Ernest T. Krebs, Jr., pangamic acid has no undesirable effects and its toxic level for man is 100,000 times the therapeutic dose.[16] Clinical tests in which intramuscular injections of pangamic acid were given in doses of 2.5 to 10 milligrams daily proved completely nontoxic. After injections, some patients experienced a flushing of the skin. Similar effects were noted with niacin, but no labora-

[16]Ya. Yu. Shpirt, *Vitamin B$_{15}$ (Pangamic Acid) Indications for Use and Efficacy in Internal Disease* (Moscow: V/O Medexport, 1968), p. 7.

tory changes were reported.[17] The valuable quality of the substance is its nontoxicity.

Deficiency Effects and Symptoms

A deficiency of pangamic acid may cause diminished oxygenation of cells, heart disease, and glandular and nervous disorders.

Beneficial Effect on Ailments

Many claims have been made concerning the therapeutic value of pangamic acid. In widespread Soviet clinical tests, over one-half of hospitalized sclerosis patients responded to pangamic acid therapy. Even patients who have had serious heart attacks have been restored to good health with treatments of pangamic acid.[18] Most tests on pangamic acid have been conducted in the USSR.

People complaining of headaches, chest pains, shortness of breath, tension, insomnia, and other common symptoms of advancing atherosclerosis have benefited from additional pangamic acid. Pangamic acid has been found to alleviate hypoxia and has been used in cases of coronary artery insufficiency. It has been shown to relieve symptoms of angina, cyanosis (a discoloration of skin due to poor oxidation), and asthma.[19]

Good results have been obtained in the treatment of rheumatism, rheumatic heart disease, and acute and chronic cases of alcoholism.[20] Some alcoholics have lost their craving for alcohol when treated with pangamic acid. Pangamic acid has been helpful in treating chronic hepatitis and early stages of liver cirrhosis.

Betty Lee Morales, a pangamic acid researcher, has had success using pangamic acid in treating conditions such as circulatory problems, emphysema, and premature aging.[21] Dr. Ya. Yu. Shpirt, a Russian, developed a combination of vitamins A and E (AEVIT) which has proved to be therapeutically successful in treating severe cases of atherosclerosis of the lower limbs.[22]

There are indications that pangamic acid may be a preventive substance in the treatment of cancer.

[17]"The Life-Saving Banned Vitamin," *Prevention*, May 1968.
[18]*Northern Neighbors*, November 1969, p. 6.
[19]"The Life-Saving Banned Vitamin," *Prevention*, May 1968.
[20]Ibid.
[21]Clark, *Know Your Nutrition*, p. 127.
[22]"The Life-Saving Banned Vitamin," *Prevention*, May 1968.

Dr. Felix Warburg states: "The primary cause of cancer is the replacement of the respiration of oxygen in normal body cells by a fermentation of sugar. All normal body cells meet their energy needs by respiration of oxygen, whereas cancer cells meet their energy needs in great part by fermentation, an oxidative decomposition of complex substances through the action of enzymes. All normal cells require oxygen and cancer cells can thrive without oxygen."[23] According to Warburg's theory, because of the lack of oxygen the cell is faced with death. The cells without oxygen are able to change their metabolism and to derive their energy from glucose fermentation. These cells may become malignant. Thus a preventive treatment against deoxidation of cells is inclusion of sufficient pangamic acid in the diet.

Russian investigators have used pangamic acid on retarded children with considerable success. After treatment of 20 milligrams three times daily, the patients showed improvement in speech development, increased vocabulary, and improved mental states, intellectual activity, concentration, and interest in extracurricular activities.

Human Tests

1. Pangamic Acid and Circulatory Disturbance. Forty-two patients suffering from circulatory problems were given pangamic acid in the form of calcium pangamate. They were given 30 milligrams three times daily orally, for a total of 90 milligrams daily. The treatment lasted 20 days.

Results. All patients showed improvement in their clinical conditions. The pains in the heart subsided or disappeared. (Clark, *Know Your Nutrition*, pp. 127, 128.)

2. Pangamic Acid and Cholesterol Level. A study was conducted on the general cholesterol levels of the same 42 cases mentioned in Test 1. They were measured before treatment, after 10 days of treatment, and at the end of 20 days of treatment.

Results. In most cases a drop of the cholesterol was noticed as early as 10 days after the treatment began

[23]Ibid.

and continued over the following period. Ten days after the end of treatment with pangamic acid, the general level of cholesterol was greatly reduced. (Clark, *Know Your Nutrition,* p. 128.)

3. Pangamic Acid and Coronary Sclerosis. A group of 118 patients, all over fifty years of age, having coronary sclerosis, were observed after being treated with calcium pangamate. Both subjective symptoms and objective characteristics (EGG, biochemical analysis of the blood, and oscillation findings) were taken as criteria of the effectiveness of the treatment.

Results. Of all 118 cases, good results were obtained in 49 and satisfactory results in 55; in 11 cases the treatment had no effect; deterioration was noted in 3 cases. [Shpirt, *Vitamin B_{15} (Pangamic Acid) Indications,* p. 10.]

4. Pangamic Acid and Muscles of Injured Legs. Groups of athletes were given various amounts of substances to stimulate energy in muscular activity. Then they were given 300 milligrams of pangamic acid on successive days.

Results. The pangamic acid was effective in early healing of muscles of injured legs. (Clark, *Know Your Nutrition,* p. 129.)

5. Pangamic Acid and Cardiopulmonary Insufficiency. Sixteen patients suffering from cardiopulmonary insufficiency due to pneumosclerosis and bronchial asthma were treated with calcium pangamate. It was administered for 20 to 30 days orally in a dosage of 120 to 160 milligrams per day and as an aerosol in a dosage of 80 milligrams per day.

Results. Four patients obtained good results, 10 obtained satisfactory results, and 2 showed no effects of the treatment. [Shpirt, *Vitamin B_{15} (Pangamic Acid) Indications,* pp. 24, 25.]

6. Pangamic Acid and Atherosclerosis. Twenty-seven patients were receiving calcium pangamate for treatment of atherosclerosis. They were given 120 to 150 milligrams daily for 15 to 30 days.

Results. Fifteen patients showed good results, 8 showed satisfactory results, 2 showed no effects of

treatment, and 2 showed relapse. [Shpirt, *Vitamin B_{15} (Pangamic Acid) Indications,* p. 25.]

PANGAMIC ACID MAY BE BENEFICIAL FOR THE FOLLOWING AILMENTS:

Body Member	Ailment
Blood/Circulatory system	Angina pectoris
	Atherosclerosis
	Cholesterol level, high
	Hypertension
Brain/Nervous system	Hypertension
	Multiple sclerosis
Head	Headache
Heart	Angina pectoris
	Atherosclerosis
	Hypertension
Liver	Cirrhosis of liver
Lungs/Respiratory system	Asthma
	Emphysema
General	Alcoholism
	Autism
	Cancer
	Hepatitis
	Hypoxia
	Rheumatic fever
	Rheumatism

BIOTIN

Description

Biotin is a water-soluble B-complex vitamin. As a coenzyme, it assists in the making of fatty acids and in the oxidation of fatty acids and carbohydrates. Without biotin the body's fat production is impaired. Biotin also aids in the utilization of protein, folic acid, pantothenic acid, and vitamin B_{12}.

Biotin is an essential nutrient that appears in trace amounts in all animal and plant tissue. Some rich sources of biotin are egg yolk, beef liver, unpolished rice, brewer's yeast, cauliflower and mushrooms.

Absorption and Storage

Biotin is synthesized by the intestinal bacteria. Some of the vitamin is absorbed in the intestines, but much is excreted in the urine. Biotin is stored mainly in the liver, kidney, brain, and adrenal glands.

Raw egg white contains the protein avidin, which binds with biotin in the intestine and prevents its absorption by the body. However, since eggs are usually eaten in a cooked form and avidin is inactivated by heat, there is no real danger of a deficiency resulting from the ingestion of a cooked egg.

Dosage and Toxicity

The National Research Council indicates that 150 to 300 micrograms of biotin (the RDA) will meet the body's daily needs. Additional amounts are required during pregnancy and lactation. There are no known toxic effects of this nutrient.

Deficiency Effects and Symptoms

Deficiency states have been reported in man only when the diet contained large amounts of raw egg white and when too many antibiotics were taken. Antibiotics interfere with the production of the intestinal bacteria from which biotin is produced.

A deficiency of biotin in man causes muscular pain, poor appetite, dry skin, lack of energy, sleeplessness, and a disturbed nervous system. Dermatitis, grayish skin color, and depression are other symptoms of a biotin deficiency. In severe deficiency there may be impairment of the body's fat metabolism. Lowered hemoglobin level, a raised cholesterol level, and a decrease in biotin excretion are signs of a biotin deficiency.

Beneficial Effect on Ailments

Dermatitis has shown improvement when treated with biotin. The use of biotin has been beneficial in treating baldness.

Human Tests

1. Biotin and Seborrheic Dermatitis and Leiner's Disease. Nine cases of seborrheic dermatitis and 2 cases of Leiner's disease in infants were given 5 milligrams of biotin injected intramuscularly daily for 7 to 14 days. Milder cases were given 2 to 4 milligrams orally for 2 to 3 weeks.

Results. Both ailments showed marked improvement when treated with biotin. (*Journal of Pediatrics,* November 1957.)

2. Biotin and Biotin Deficiency Symptoms. Persons who were suffering from dermatitis, a grayish pallor of the skin and mucous membranes, diminuation of hemoglobin, a striking rise in serum cholesterol, depression, and muscle pain were given 150 or more milligrams of biotin, injected intravenously daily. The excretion of biotin in the urine was much below that of a person on a normal diet.

Results. After the injections the symptoms became less evident. The ashy pallor disappeared in 4 days, serum cholesterol was reduced, and urinary excretion of biotin increased. (Margaret S. Chaney and Margaret L. Ross, *Nutrition,* Houghton Mifflin Co., Boston, 1971, p. 307.)

BIOTIN MAY BE BENEFICIAL FOR THE FOLLOWING AILMENTS:

Body Member	Ailment
Hair/Scalp	Baldness
Muscles	Muscle pains
Skin	Dermatitis
	Eczema
	Infant dermatitis
General	Depression

CHOLINE

Description

Choline is considered one of the B-complex vitamins. It functions with inositol as a basic constituent of lecithin. It is present in the body of all living cells and is widely distributed in animal and plant tissues. The richest source of choline is lecithin, but other rich dietary sources include egg yolk, liver, brewer's yeast, and wheat germ.

Choline appears to be associated primarily with the utilization of fats and cholesterol in the body. It prevents fats from accumulating in the liver and facilitates the movement of fats into the cells. Choline combines with fatty acids and phosphoric acid within the liver to form lecithin. It is essential for the health of the liver and kidneys.

Choline is also essential for the health of the myelin sheaths of the nerves; the myelin sheaths are the principal component of the nerve fibers. It plays an important role in the transmission of the nerve impulses. It also helps to regulate and improve liver and gallbladder functioning and aids in the prevention of gallstones.

Absorption and Storage

Choline is synthesized by the interaction of B_{12} and folic acid with the amino acid methionine.

Dosage and Toxicity

Daily requirements for choline are not known. The average diet has been estimated to contain 500 to 900 milligrams of choline per day, according to the 1968 revision of the Recommended Dietary Allowances. Dr. Paavo Airola has estimated the daily dietary intake to be 1000 or more milligrams. Usual therapeutic daily doses range from 500 to 6000 milligrams; prolonged ingestion of massive doses of isolated choline may induce a deficiency of vitamin B_6.[24] It is important to remember that the B-complex vitamins function better when all are taken together.

Deficiency Effects and Symptoms

A choline deficiency is associated with fatty deposits in the liver, resulting in bleeding stomach ulcers, heart trouble, and blocking of the tubes of the kidneys. Insufficient supplies of choline may cause hemorrhaging of the kidneys. A deficiency can also result when too little protein is in the diet. Prolonged deficiencies may cause high blood pressure, cirrhosis and fatty degeneration of the liver, atherosclerosis, and hardening of the arteries.[25]

Beneficial Effect on Ailments

Choline has been successful in reducing high blood pressure because it strengthens weak capillary walls. Symptoms such as heart palpitation, dizziness, head-

[24]Airola, *How to Get Well*, p. 266.
[25]Ibid.

aches, ear noises, and constipation have been relieved or removed entirely within 5 to 10 days after administration of choline treatments. Insomnia, visual disturbances, and blood flow to the eyes have also benefited from choline therapy.

Because choline is a fat and cholesterol dissolver, it is used to treat atherosclerosis and hardening of the arteries. It can be used to treat fatty livers, liver damage, cirrhosis of the liver, and hepatitis. Choline is also used in kidney damage, hemorrhaging of the kidneys, and nephritis, as well as for eye conditions such as glaucoma.

Human Tests

1. Choline and Atherosclerosis. Of 230 patients hospitalized for atherosclerosis, half were given conventional medication but no choline after discharge from the hospital; the other half received choline daily for 1 to 3 years.

Results. Among the untreated patients, the 3-year death rate was nearly 30 percent. Only 12 percent of the choline-treated patients died. (Dr. L. M. Morrison and W. F. Gonzalez, *Proceedings of the Society of Biology and Medicine,* vol. 73, pp. 37–38, 1950, as reported in Rodale, *The Encyclopedia for Healthful Living,* pp. 457, 458.)

CHOLINE MAY BE BENEFICIAL FOR THE FOLLOWING AILMENTS:

Body Member	Ailment
Blood/Circulatory system	Angina pectoris
	Cholesterol level, high
	Hepatitis
	Hypoglycemia
	Stroke (cerebrovascular accident)
Brain/Nervous system	Dizziness
	Multiple sclerosis
Eye	Glaucoma
Glands	Hyperthyroidism
Hair/Scalp	Hair problems
Heart	Arteriosclerosis
	Atherosclerosis
	Hypertension
Intestine	Constipation
Liver	Cirrhosis of liver

Body Member	Ailment
Lungs/Respiratory system	Asthma
Muscles	Muscular dystrophy
Skin	Eczema
General	Alcoholism

FOLIC ACID (FOLACIN)

Description

Folic acid is part of the water-soluble vitamin B complex and functions as a coenzyme, together with vitamins B_{12} and C, in the breakdown and utilization of proteins. Folic acid performs its basic role as a carbon carrier in the formation of heme, the iron-containing protein found in hemoglobin, necessary for the formation of red blood cells. It also is needed for the formation of nucleic acid, which is essential for the processes of growth and reproduction of all body cells.

Folic acid is necessary for proper brain function, being concentrated in the spinal and extracellular fluids. It is essential for mental and emotional health. It also increases the appetite and stimulates the production of hydrochloric acid, which helps prevent intestinal parasites and food poisoning. In addition, it aids in performance of the liver. Folic acid is easily destroyed by high temperature, exposure to light, and being left at room temperature for long periods of time.

In surveys conducted, folic acid was shown to be one of the nutrients most often deficient in our diets. The best sources of folic acid are green leafy vegetables, liver, and brewer's yeast.

Absorption and Storage

Folic acid is absorbed in the gastrointestinal tract by active transport and diffusion and is stored primarily in the liver. Sulfa drugs may interfere with the bacteria in the intestine which manufacture folic acid. Aminoperin and streptomycin destroy folic acid.

Any disease such as sprue, celiac disease, or any illness accompanied by vomiting or diarrhea that interferes with the absorption of food can result in a deficiency. Oral contraceptives interfere with the absorption of folic acid.

Dosage and Toxicity

The Recommended Dietary Allowance of folic acid is 400 micrograms for adults, 800 micrograms during pregnancy, and 600 micrograms during lactation.

Requirements can vary with individual metabolic rate. Hemolytic anemia and hyperthyroidism need higher quantities. Stress and disease increase the body's need for folic acid, as does the consumption of alcohol. There is no known toxicity of this vitamin, although an excessive intake of folic acid can mask a vitamin B_{12} deficiency.

Deficiency Effects and Symptoms

Deficiency of folic acid results in poor growth, graying hair, glossitis (tongue inflammation), and gastrointestinal-tract disturbances arising from inadequate dietary intake, impaired absorption, excessive demands by tissues of the body, and metabolic disturbances. Because of the role folic acid plays in the formation of red blood cells, a deficiency could lead to anemia that cannot be corrected by supplementary iron.

A folate deficiency can lead to irritability, forgetfulness, and mental sluggishness. It can be the cause of lesions at the corners of the mouth called cheiloses. A deficiency has been found in mentally retarded children, the aged, and in people with ailments such as Hodgkin's disease and leukemia where the requirement for folic acid is above normal.

Alcohol, phenobarbital and anticonvulsants can produce a folic acid deficiency. Low serum and cerebrospinal fluid folate levels have been observed in epileptics administered anticonvulsant medication.

In the past few years there have been a number of studies implicating folic acid deficiency as a contributing factor in mental illness. Studies have shown that prolonged folic acid deficiency can cause neurological changes and mental deterioration. Because of their close interrelationship, vitamin B_{12}, in almost every case, should accompany any folic acid therapy.

A need for the vitamin is especially increased during pregnancy. The fetus, meeting its need for rapid growth, easily depletes the mother's reserves. The World Health Organization reports that one-third to one-half of pregnant women are folic acid deficient in the last three months of pregnancy. Almost any interference with the metabolism of folic acid in the fetus encourages deformities such as cleft palate, brain damage, or slow development and poor learning ability in the child.[26] In addition, deficiency of folic acid may lead to toxemia, premature birth, afterbirth hemorrhaging, and megaloblastic anemia in both mother and child.

Beneficial Effect on Ailments

Folic acid is not limited to treatment of anemia. It is beneficial in treating diarrhea, sprue, dropsy, stomach ulcers, menstrual problems, leg ulcers, and glossitis. Circulation may be improved in patients suffering from atherosclerosis. Folic acid may prevent the graying of hair when used with PABA and pantothenic acid.[27] During pregnancy, folacin-rich foods should be stressed in the diet so that the fetal and maternal needs are met and megaloblastic anemia is prevented.

Human Tests

1. Folic Acid and Toxicity. Twenty healthy young adults were given 15 milligrams of folic acid daily for 1 month and were matched with a control group given placebos.

Results. No ill effects were detected. Physicians have given 150 milligrams of folic acid to children and 450 milligrams to adults, both daily, with no report of toxicity. (Davis, *Let's Get Well.*)

2. Folic Acid and Megaloblastic Anemia. A sixty-nine-year-old woman was suffering from megaloblastic anemia. She was brought to the hospital with a history of pallor, fatigue, forgetfulness, and lack of energy. According to tests, she lacked vitamin B_{12}, and some was administered before she came to the hospital. She was then given folic acid.

Results. Her condition improved immediately and she was soon discharged from the hospital. Tests 6 months later showed her in good health; all symptoms of megaloblastic anemia had disappeared. (*Journal of the American Medical Association,* July 31, 1972.)

---

[26]Rodale Press Editors, *Be a Healthy Mother, Have a Healthy Baby* (Emmaus, Pa.: Rodale Press, 1973), p. 29.
[27]Adelle Davis, *Let's Get Well* (New York: Harcourt, Brace & World, 1965), p. 166.

3. Folic Acid and Atherosclerosis. Seventeen elderly patients were treated with 5 to 7.5 milligrams of folic acid daily.

Results. Fifteen patients responded with increased capillary blood flow, resulting in improved vision due to better blood supply to the retina. In many cases there was increased skin temperature. (Roger J. Williams, *Nutrition Against Disease,* Pitman Publ., New York, 1971, pp. 75–76.)

Animal Tests

1. Folic Acid and Cleft Palate. Pregnant mice were first injected with cortisone, which can cause interference with vital life chemistry, four times daily. Cleft palates developed in 85 percent of their offspring. Pyridoxine and folic acid were separately injected with the cortisone.

Results. When pyridoxine was injected, the abnormalities were reduced to 45 percent; the folic acid in the combination reduced the cleft palate cases to 20 percent. (Dr. Lyndon A. Peer, *Chicago Daily Tribune,* September 11, 1957.)

FOLIC ACID MAY BE BENEFICIAL FOR THE FOLLOWING AILMENTS:

Body Member	Ailment
Blood/Circulatory system	Anemia
	Leukemia
	Pernicious anemia
Bowel	Diarrhea
Brain/Nervous system	Alcoholism
	Mental illness
Glands	Adrenal exhaustion
Hair/Scalp	Baldness
Heart	Arteriosclerosis
	Atherosclerosis
Intestine	Celiac disease
	Diverticulitis
Joints	Arthritis
Lungs/Respiratory system	Emphysema
Nails	Nail problems
Skin	Psoriasis
	Ulcers

Body Member	Ailment
Stomach	Gastritis
	Indigestion (dyspepsia)
General	Alcoholism
	Anemia
	Bruises
	Fatigue
	Kwashiorkor
	Pellagra
	Pregnancy
	Scurvy
	Stress
	Tonsilitis

INOSITOL

Description

Inositol is recognized as part of the vitamin B complex and is closely associated with choline and biotin. Like choline, inositol is found in high concentrations in lecithin. Animal studies have shown that the vitamins B_6, folic acid, pantothenic acid, and PABA also have a close working association with inositol.

Both animal and plant tissues contain inositol. In animal tissues it occurs as a component of phospholipids, substances containing phosphorus, fatty acids, and nitrogenous bases. In plant cells it is found as phytic acid, an organic acid that binds calcium and iron in an insoluble complex and interferes with their absorption. Inositol is found in unprocessed whole grains, citrus fruits, brewer's yeast, crude unrefined molasses, and liver.

Inositol is effective in promoting the body's production of lecithin. Fats are moved from the liver to the cells with the aid of lecithin; therefore inositol aids in the metabolism of fats and helps reduce blood cholesterol. In combination with choline, it prevents the fatty hardening of arteries and protects the liver, kidneys, and heart.

Inositol is also found to be helpful in brain cell nutrition. Large quantities of inositol are found in the spinal cord nerves and in the brain and cerebral spinal fluid. It is needed for the growth and survival of cells in bone marrow, eye membranes, and the intes-

tines. It is vital for hair growth and can prevent thinning hair and baldness.

Absorption and Storage

About 7 percent of ingested inositol is converted to glucose; inositol is only one-third as effective as glucose in alleviating ketosis, the incomplete metabolism of fatty acids.

There is some disagreement as to whether inositol is synthesized by the intestinal flora. One reliable source indicates it is,[28] while another claims that synthesis occurs within the individual cell rather than by intestinal organisms.[29] The amount the body excretes daily in the urine is small, averaging 37 milligrams. The diabetic excretes more inositol than does the nondiabetic. Large amounts of coffee may deplete the body's storage of inositol.

Dosage and Toxicity

The Recommended Dietary Allowance has not yet been established, but most authorities recommend consuming the same amount of inositol as choline. The daily consumption of inositol in food is about 1 gram. The human body contains more inositol than any other vitamin except niacin. One tablespoon of yeast provides approximately 40 milligrams each of choline and inositol. Therapeutic doses range from 500 to 1000 milligrams daily. Fifty grams have been given by mouth and 1 gram intravenously with no side effects. There is no known toxicity of inositol.

Deficiency Effects and Symptoms

Tests on yeast cells have shown that when they are deprived of inositol, metabolic processes are prevented from functioning and consequently most of the cells die. In other studies, inositol deficiency in yeast cells led to abnormal cell walls and an inability of daughter cells to separate from the parent cells. Also found was the inhibition of fermentation and oxidation actions as well as a lower level of nucleotide coenzymes.

Caffeine may create an inositol shortage in the body.

[28]J. I. Rodale, *The Health Seeker* (Emmaus, Pa.: Rodale Books, 1962), p. 869.
[29]John Hoover, ed., *Remington's Pharmaceutical Sciences* (Easton, Pa.: Mack Publishing, 1970), p. 1029.

The use of sulfonamides increases the need for inositol. Diuresis, as in diabetes insipidus and an excess intake of water, can cause a loss of inositol.

An inositol deficiency may cause constipation, eczema, and abnormalities of the eyes. The deficiency contributes to hair loss and a high blood cholesterol level, which may result in artery and heart disease.

Beneficial Effect on Ailments

Inositol is beneficial in the treatment of constipation because it has a stimulating effect on the muscular action of the alimentary canal. It also is recommended for men who are becoming bald and is vital in helping to lower cholesterol levels in the blood. Inositol aids in eliminating liver fats from patients about to be operated on for stomach cancer.

Dr. Carl Pfeiffer, at his Brain Bio Center, has been studying the effect of inositol on brain waves. Results have shown that the vitamin has an antianxiety effect similar to Librium. Dr. Pfeiffer believes that people who take Valium or Librium can discontinue the use if sufficient inositol is taken.[30]

Because inositol has a sedative-like effect, it can be beneficial for insomnia. Inositol relieves mild hypertension by gradually lowering the blood pressure; 1 gram in the morning and at night is recommended. Inositol is helpful for schizophrenia, hypoglycemia, and for people with high serum copper and low serum zinc levels. The phosphate ester of inositol impedes zinc absorption, so pure inositol is recommended.

Animal Tests

1. Inositol and Cholesterol. Two groups of rabbits were fed a capsule of cholesterol daily. One group of rabbits received just cholesterol and a regulation diet. The other group of rabbits received a capsule of inositol in addition to the cholesterol.

Results. At the end of the feeding period, the first group of rabbits showed an increase of 337 percent in the cholesterol content in their blood. Those that had received inositol showed a cholesterol increase of only 181 percent. (*Newsweek,* September 11, 1950, Dr. Louis B. Potte, Dr. William C. Felch, and Stephanie J. Ilka of St. Luke's Hospital, New York; reported in Rodale, *The Encyclopedia for Healthful Living.*)

INOSITOL MAY BE BENEFICIAL FOR THE FOLLOWING AILMENTS:

Body Member	Ailment
Blood/Circulatory system	Arteriosclerosis
	Atherosclerosis
	Cholesterol level, high
	Hypertension
	Hypoglycemia
	Stroke (cerebrovascular accident)
Bowel	Constipation
Brain/Nervous system	Dizziness
	Schizophrenia
Eye	Glaucoma
Hair/Scalp	Baldness
Intestine	Constipation
Liver	Cirrhosis of the liver
Lungs/Respiratory system	Asthma
Stomach	Gastritis
General	Insomnia
	Overweight and obesity

PARA-AMINOBENZOIC ACID (PABA)

Description

Para-aminobenzoic acid, an integral part of the vitamin B complex, is water-soluble and is considered unique in that it is a "vitamin within a vitamin," occurring in combination with folic acid.[31] PABA is found in liver, yeast, wheat germ, and molasses.

PABA stimulates the intestinal bacteria, enabling them to produce folic acid, which in turn aids in the production of pantothenic acid. As a coenzyme, PABA functions in the breakdown and utilization of proteins and in the formation of blood cells, especially red blood cells. PABA plays an important role in determining skin health, hair pigmentation, and health

[30]Carl D. Pfeiffer, Ph.D., M.D., *Mental and Elemental Nutrients,* p. 145.

[31]Krause and Hunscher, *Food, Nutrition and Diet Therapy,* p. 140.

of the intestines.[32] PABA acts as a sunscreen and is incorporated into some sunscreen ointments.[33]

Absorption and Storage

PABA is stored in the tissues but is manufactured by friendly bacteria in the intestines if conditions in the intestines are favorable.

Dosage and Toxicity

The need for PABA in human nutrition has not yet been established. PABA is available in supplements in potencies higher than 30 milligrams, but these higher doses are used for therapeutic purposes. Continued ingestion of high doses of PABA is not recommended and can be toxic to the liver, heart, and kidneys. Symptoms of toxicity are nausea and vomiting.

Deficiency Effects and Symptoms

A deficiency of PABA may result from the use of sulfa drugs. Because sulfas resemble PABA in structure, they kill the intestinal bacteria by substituting for the PABA they need. Deficiency symptoms include fatigue, irritability, depression, nervousness, headache, constipation, and other digestive disorders.

Beneficial Effect on Ailments

PABA is used in treating vitiligo, a condition characterized by depigmentation of some areas of the skin. PABA is used in treating some parasitic diseases, including Rocky Mountain spotted fever. In certain laboratory animals, PABA, when combined with pantothenic acid, has helped restore color to hair that was turning gray and has prevented further graying. Research continues as to whether PABA has this effect on human hair. According to Adelle Davis, the administration of PABA and folic acid has restored graying or white hair to its natural color. A daily intake of folic acid and PABA should be continued so that the restored hair is prevented from returning to its previous color.

PABA often soothes the pain of burns even more

effectively than vitamin E.[34] PABA ointment has been effective in preventing and treating sunburn. Persons normally susceptible to sunburn have been able to remain many hours in the sun after applying PABA ointment. PABA alleviates the pain of sunburn and other burns immediately.[35] Adelle Davis has stated that PABA ointment may delay old-age skin changes such as wrinkles, dry skin, and dark spots.

Dr. Carl Pfeiffer reports that large doses of PABA, 2 grams per day, have been used with good results in schizophrenia. He speculates that PABA may prevent certain amines from forming hallucinogens.[36]

Human Tests

1. PABA and Lupus Erythematosus (a severe skin disorder). Thirty-three patients with lupus erythematosus were given 1 to 4 grams of para-aminobenzoic acid at 2- to 3-hour intervals.

Results. Two of 10 with chronic discord lupus showed no improvement, 1 patient had a poor response, and 7 showed good to excellent responses. Improvement occurred in all of 7 patients with scleroderma, a skin disorder; the sclerodermatous areas gradually softened and became thinner and more pliable. (*Zarafonetis: Ann. Intern. Med.,* vol. 30, p. 1188, 1949.)

PABA MAY BE BENEFICIAL FOR THE FOLLOWING AILMENTS:

Body Member	Ailment
Blood/Circulatory system	Anemia
Bowel	Constipation
Brain/Nervous system	Schizophrenia
Hair/Scalp	Baldness
Head	Headache
Skin	Burns
	Sunburn
	Vitiligo

[32]*The Vitamins Explained Simply,* 5th ed. (Melbourne: Science of Life Books, 1972), p. 28.

[33]Hoover, ed., *Remington's Pharmaceutical Sciences,* p. 1041.

[34]Davis, *Let's Get Well,* p. 37.

[35]Ibid., p. 154.

[36]Pfeiffer, *Mental and Elemental Nutrients,* p. 183.

VITAMIN C (ASCORBIC ACID)

Description

Vitamin C, also known as ascorbic acid, is a water-soluble nutrient. Although fairly stable in acid solution, it is normally the least stable of vitamins and is very sensitive to oxygen. Its potency can be lost through exposure to light, heat, and air, which stimulate the activity of oxidative enzymes.

A primary function of vitamin C is maintaining collagen, a protein necessary for the formation of connective tissue in skin, ligaments, and bones. Vitamin C plays a role in healing wounds and burns because it facilitates the formation of connective tissue in the scar. Vitamin C also aids in forming red blood cells and preventing hemorrhaging. In addition, vitamin C fights bacterial infections and reduces the effects on the body of some allergy-producing substances. For these reasons, vitamin C is frequently used in preventing and treating the common cold.

Vitamin C has significant relationships with other nutrients. It aids in the metabolism of the amino acids phenylalanine and tyrosine. Vitamin C converts the inactive form of folic acid to the active form, folinic acid, and may have a role in calcium metabolism. In addition, vitamin C protects thiamine, riboflavin, folic acid, pantothenic acid, and vitamins A and E against oxidation. It protects the brain and spinal cord from destruction by free radicals.

Large concentrations of vitamin C are found in the adrenal glands, and the vitamin is essential in the formation of adrenalin. During stress, the level of adrenal ascorbic acid is rapidly used up.

The intestinal absorption of iron is greatly increased by adequate vitamin C. Vitamin C is present in most fresh fruits and vegetables.

Absorption and Storage

The level of ascorbic acid in the blood reaches a maximum in 2 or 3 hours after ingestion of a moderate quantity, then decreases as it is eliminated in the urine and through perspiration.[37] Most vitamin C is out of the body in 3 or 4 hours. Increased urinary output of vitamin C resulting from larger intake of the vitamin does *not* mean body tissues are saturated. The blood level of vitamin C will return to its average level in 12 to 13 hours regardless of the amount ingested. To maintain adequate serum level, the vitamin should be taken throughout the day. Excess vitamin C carried to the bladder may prevent bladder cancer.

Because vitamin C is a "stress vitamin," it is used up even more rapidly under stressful conditions. Man, apes, and guinea pigs are among the very few animals that need vitamin C in their foodstuffs, because they are unable to meet body needs by synthesis and must rely upon a dietary source.

Taken orally, most of the vitamin is absorbed through the mucous membranes of the mouth, stomach, and upper part of the small intestine. The larger the dose, the less is absorbed. For example, 80 percent of less than 250 milligrams ingested is absorbed; a dose of up to 2 grams results in about 50 percent absorption. Therefore it is best to take vitamin C in small doses several times a day. In therapeutic treatment, injection of several grams of sodium ascorbate into the bloodstream is more effective than the same amount taken by mouth.

The normal human body when fully saturated contains about 5000 milligrams of vitamin C, of which 30 milligrams are found in the adrenal glands, 200 milligrams in the extracellular fluids, and the rest distributed in varying concentrations throughout the cells of the body. The body's ability to absorb vitamin C is reduced by smoking, stress, high fever, prolonged administration of antibiotics or cortisone, inhalation of DDT or fumes of petroleum, and ingestion of aspirin or other pain killers. Sulfa drugs increase urinary excretion of vitamin C by two or three times the normal amount. Baking soda creates an alkaline medium that destroys vitamin C. In addition, drinking excessive amounts of water will deplete the body's vitamin C. Cooking in copper utensils will destroy the vitamin C content of foods.

Dosage and Toxicity

The National Research Council recommends 60 milligrams of vitamin C for adults. The requirement may vary due to differences in weight, amount of activity,

---

[37]Linus C. Pauling, *Vitamin C and the Common Cold* (New York: Bantam Books, 1971), pp. 63, 64.

rate of metabolism, ailments, and age. Periods of stress, such as anxiety, infection, injury, surgery, burns, or fatigue, increase the body's need for this vitamin.

Individuals who are hypoglycemic or are on a high-protein diet need more vitamin C, as these conditions interfere with the vitamin's metabolism. Persons with high copper or iron blood levels need a larger intake of vitamin C. Any condition that elevates the serum copper increases the need for sufficient C, including schizophrenia, smoking, use of the contraceptive pill, menstruation, and the last months of pregnancy.

It is better to take frequent small doses of the vitamin instead of a single large dose, because the body can absorb only a certain amount during a given period of time. Ingestion of above 100 milligrams of vitamin C at one time results in decreased efficiency of absorption and an increased rate of excretion of unmetabolized ascorbic acid.

When vitamin C is given for therapeutic reasons, dosage is very important. Too little will have little or no effect. Dr. Frederick Klenner recommends 30 grams a day as necessary for proper response. When megavitamin doses of vitamin C are given it is important that calcium intake be increased.

Large doses may have side effects in some persons. Symptoms can be a slight burning sensation during urination, loose bowels, intestinal gas, and/or skin rashes. When any symptom occurs, dosage should be reduced. It may help to take the vitamin after a meal, which is also better for proper assimilation. If symptoms persist, various kinds of C may be tried.

Large doses of C should not be taken by people with a tendency to formation of oxalate stones, or cystinuria, unless it is in the form of sodium ascorbate. Sodium ascorbate does not affect the acidity of the urine and aids in oxalate excretion.

Some people have a rare genetic disease that forms kidney stones when large amounts of C are taken. These people need to reduce their intake of the vitamin.

Vitamin C can give blood sugar tests, except the hexokinase test, or glucose oxidase test, a false reading. Lowering the dose level of vitamin C after ingestion of high doses can result in symptoms of scurvy. Therefore, reduction of the vitamin should be done slowly over a period of time until the body has adjusted.

Deficiency Effects and Symptoms

Signs of deficiency are shortness of breath, impaired digestion, poor lactation, bleeding gums, weakened enamel or dentine, tendency to bruising, swollen or painful joints, nosebleeds, anemia, lowered resistance to infections, and slow healing of wounds and fractures. Severe deficiency results in scurvy. Breaks in the capillary walls are signs of vitamin C deficiency, and clots usually form at the point of the break. Therefore a lack of vitamin C is a probable cause of heart attacks and strokes initiated by clots. The blood level of ascorbic acid is known to be lowered by smoking. Nicotine added to a sample of human blood of known ascorbic acid content decreased the ascorbic acid content of the blood by 24 to 31 percent.[38]

Alcoholics have a very low C serum level because so much of the vitamin is used to destroy the toxic effects.

Beneficial Effect on Ailments

Vitamin C plays an important role in preventing and relieving scurvy. Vitamin C promotes fine bone and tooth formation while protecting the dentine and pulp. It reduces the effects on the body of some allergy-producing substances. Vitamin C is frequently used in the prevention and treatment of the common cold.

The lubricating fluid of joints (synovial fluid) becomes thinner (allowing freer movement) when the serum levels of ascorbic acid are high. Therefore arthritic patients given vitamin C may find some relief of pain. It is an important nutrient in treating wounds because it speeds up the healing process. Ascorbic acid may lower blood cholesterol content of patients with arteriosclerosis. The serum cholesterol level in individuals has been reduced 35 to 40 percent by vitamin C.

The need for vitamin C increases with age due to a greater need to regenerate collagen. With age, the sex glands develop a greater need for vitamin C and will draw it from other tissues, leaving these tissues

[38]Rodale, *The Encyclopedia for Healthful Living*, p. 953.

vulnerable to disease. Therefore proper supplementation will help reduce depletion. Vitamin C is important in all stressful conditions. The tissue requirements for ascorbic acid are increased under conditions of increased metabolism.

Vitamin C stimulates the production of interferon and acts as an inactivator against viruses including herpes, vaccinia, hepatitis, polio, encephalitis, measles, and pneumonia. This is accomplished because vitamin C, catalyzed by copper ions, reduces oxygen molecules to molecules that, in turn, attack the nucleic acid of the virus. This same mechanism, plus the fact that vitamin C increases the power of the body's defense systems, works against bacteria, including the bacterias responsible for tuberculosis, diphtheria, tetanus, staphylococcus, and typhoid fever.

If enough vitamin C has been given to saturate the tissues, it will enter cells where dormant viruses are and destroy them. For more than 25 years, Dr. Frederick Klenner of Reidsville, North Carolina, has been using vitamin C to treat viral diseases. His treatment involves administration, either intravenously or by mouth, of 20 to 40 grams vitamin C daily.

Massive doses of vitamin C have been used to cure drug addicts, including users of heroin, methadone, and barbiturates. Chiropractor Alfred F. Libby of Santa Ana, California, has successfully administered 25 to 85 grams of sodium ascorbate, a version of vitamin C, for 4 days, then reduced the dose to 5 grams of sodium ascorbate and 5 grams of ascorbic acid. The treatment eases heroin withdrawal, helps to restore proper appetite and restfulness, and helps to eliminate abnormal thought patterns.

Vitamin C has been found to be of value in minimizing the effects of environmental pollution, including carbon monoxide, cadmium, mercury, lead, iron, copper, arsenic, benzene, and some pesticides.

Physicians in Scotland report that vitamin C counteracts bleeding in the gastrointestinal tract caused by aspirin or alcohol. The bleeding may also continue or restart if sufficient C is not available for wound healing.

Vitamin C prevents the formation of carcinogenic nitrosamines from nitrites and nitrates found in some foods. Vitamin C has been successfully used to treat snake and spider bites, insect stings and rabies. Vitamin C is important for recovery from heart attacks by preventing free radical damage. However, the heart

will take so much of the vitamin from other body tissues that sufficient supplementation is essential.

Dr. Carl Pfeiffer reports that vitamin C has an anti-anxiety effect on the nervous system. He uses the vitamin in treating schizophrenia. Studies have shown that psychiatric patients have an unusually high need for vitamin C. Vitamin C treatment results in improvement of depression and paranoia.

Vitamin C is essential for stimulating the immune system, enabling the body to resist diseases including cancer. Some individuals taking 10 grams of C a day have reportedly been cured of their cancer. Other terminal cancer patients lived four times longer than those in a control group.

Dr. James Greenwood at Baylor University has reported from his observations that a more-than-average intake of vitamin C helps preserve the integrity of intervertebral disks and helps prevent back problems. Vitamin C has been used in tests determining its effect on intelligence. A study using control groups of children resulted in a 3.6 IQ rise when a 50 percent increase of vitamin C intake was administered.

Low outdoor temperatures increase the body's need for vitamin C. The vitamin, in part, improves the metabolism of tyrosine and phenylalanine, precursors of such heat-raising hormones as the thyroid.

Laboratory tests on monkeys have shown that vitamin C can protect against frostbite. Russian studies have shown vitamin C to slow the aging process. Russian athletes use the vitamin to build muscle tissue. Vitamin C can reduce the amount needed of some drugs, including L-Dopa and painkillers given to cancer patients. The vitamin prevents certain enzymes from breaking down the natural painkilling compounds of the brain.

Vitamin C helps victims of shock from injury, electric shock, and lightning. It prevents prickly heat and heat stroke. Leukemia, pancreatitis, and rheumatic heart disease respond well to vitamin C therapy. Powdered vitamin C mixed with water to form a paste and then applied on the skin will clear up poison ivy or oak in 24 hours if adequate oral doses of the vitamin are taken at the same time.

Human Tests

1. Vitamin C and Whooping Cough. Ninety children with whooping cough were given vitamin C orally or were injected with 5000 milligrams daily for 7 days, with the dosage being gradually reduced until a daily level of 100 milligrams was reached. A control group was given whooping-cough vaccine.

Results. The duration of the disease in the children receiving ascorbic acid was 15 to 20 days, while the average duration for the children receiving vaccine was 34 days. When ascorbic acid therapy was started during the catarrhal stage, the spasmodic stage was prevented in 75 percent of the cases. (*Journal of the American Medical Association,* November 4, 1950, as reported in Rodale, *The Encyclopedia for Healthful Living,* p. 956.)

2. Vitamin C and Prickly Heat. Thirty children were divided into two groups of 15. One group was given vitamin C in proportion to body weight; the other group was given placebos, in this case, sugar pills. Only the pharmacist knew who had which. After 2 weeks, Dr. Hindson and the pharmacist compared their notes:

Vitamin C Group	Placebo Group
1 same	9 same
4 improved	4 improved
10 free from lesions	2 worse

The 15 patients given the placebos were then given vitamin C following the first comparison. Within 2 months, no lesions were seen on any of the 30 children. (Dosage for a child of 38 pounds: 250 milligrams a day.) (Dr. C. Hindson, as reported in Rodale, ed., *Prevention,* July 1972.)

3. Vitamin C and Iron Deficiency. Thirty females ages fourteen to forty-two were suffering from iron deficiency. They were given one tablet of 200 milligrams of ascorbic acid daily.

Results. After 60 days of treatment, the iron deficiency was alleviated. A chronic deficiency of iron is often complicated by the side effect of scurvy. In order to influence absorption of iron, a vitamin C intake of at least 200 to 500 milligrams per day is needed. (Enil Margo Schleicher, Director of Hematology at St. Barnabas Hospital, Minneapolis, as reported in Rodale, ed., *Prevention,* August 1970.)

4. Vitamin C and Nicotine. Fourteen smokers and 14 nonsmokers having similar characteristics and dietary habits were placed on vitamin C–deficient diets. Blood samples of all were taken. Then the subjects were given 1.1 grams of vitamin C and high doses of water-soluble vitamins to facilitate absorption. This process continued for 5 days, until the subjects' bodies were saturated with vitamin C. For 3 days vitamin C intakes were carefully limited, and the urine was closely examined.

Results. Blood tests showed that the smokers had about 30 percent less vitamin C in their blood than the nonsmokers. (Omar Pelletier of the Nutrition Research Division of the Food and Drug Directorate in Ottawa, Canada, as reported in Rodale, ed., *Prevention,* July 1969.)

5. Vitamin C and Inflammation of the Urethra. Twelve men were suffering from painful inflammation of the urethra. The patients were examined, and each was given 3 grams of vitamin C daily for 4 days. The irritation was caused by phosphatic crystals formed in the urine due to insufficient acidity.

Results. The large doses of vitamin C proved to be a safe way of introducing enough acidity to force the crystals back into solution. What cured the patients was the "wasted" vitamin C, the part not stored in the body and spilled into the urine. The excess vitamin C in the urine proved to be 100 percent effective in relieving the symptoms. (Rodale, ed., *Prevention,* July 1973.)

Animal Tests

1. Vitamin C and Tooth Formation. In vitamin C–deficient guinea pigs, the dentine near the developing teeth ceased to form and the pulp was separated from the dentine by liquid. Either dentine ceased being manufactured, or it was of inferior quality. The pulp itself shrunk and once free from the dentine, was apparently floating in a liquid.

Results. Rapid repair followed the administration of vitamin C. (*Journal of Dentistry for Children,* Third Quarter, 1943, as reported in Rodale, *The Encyclopedia for Healthful Living,* pp. 953, 954.)

2. Vitamin C and Mercury Poisoning. Twenty guinea pigs were given 200 milligrams of vitamin C daily for 6 days (equivalent to 14 grams per day for humans). On the sixth day, each pig was given what should have been a fatal dosage of mercury. After the poisoning, they were put back on their regular diet, which included 200 milligrams of vitamin C daily.

Results. After 2 days, they lost weight but ate and behaved normally. The experiment was finally terminated. After 20 days the animals were considered saved. (Momcilo Mokranjae and Ceda Petrovic in the *C. R. Acad. Sc. Paris,* 1964, as reported in Rodale, ed., *Prevention,* July 1972, p. 82.)

3. Vitamin C and Oxygen Starvation. Forty-two rats were placed in a decompression chamber until the atmospheric pressure equaled that at an altitude of 33,000 feet. All died within 13 minutes. A second group of rats were injected with vitamin C before being placed in the decompression chamber. The dosage given was equivalent to a human dosage of 7 grams.

Results. Three rats did not die; the others stayed alive for an average of 23.7 minutes. A third group of 44 rats were injected with double the vitamin C dosage of the second group (equivalent to a human dosage of 14 grams) and then were put in the decompression chamber.

Results. Twenty-one rats did not die, and the others stayed alive for nearly an hour. The investigators admitted that they did not know why the vitamin C had this effect. (Kazuo Asahina and Katsumi Asano, Toho University School of Medicine, Tokyo, as reported in Rodale, ed., *Prevention,* July 1972.)

VITAMIN C MAY BE BENEFICIAL FOR THE FOLLOWING AILMENTS:

Body Member	Ailment
Bladder	Cystitis
Blood/Circulatory system	Alcoholism
	Anemia
	Angina pectoris
	Arteriosclerosis
	Bruising
	Cholesterol level, high
	Diabetes
	Hemophilia
	Hypertension
	Hypoglycemia
	Jaundice
	Leukemia
	Mononucleosis
	Pernicious anemia
	Phlebitis
	Stroke (cerebrovascular accident)
	Varicose veins
Bones	Fracture
	Osteomalacia
	Osteoporosis
	Rickets
Bowel	Celiac disease
	Colitis
	Cystic fibrosis
	Diarrhea
	Worms
Brain/Nervous system	Dizziness
	Epilepsy
	Fatigue
	Hypertension
	Hypoxia
	Insomnia
	Meningitis
	Mental illness
	Multiple sclerosis
	Parkinson's disease
	Schizophrenia
	Shingles (herpes zoster)
	Stroke (cerebrovascular accident)
Ear	Ear infection
Eye	Amblyopia
	Cataracts
	Conjunctivitis
	Eyestrain
	Glaucoma
	Vision and focus disorders
Gallbladder	Gallstones
Glands	Adrenal exhaustion
	Cystic fibrosis
	Goiter

Body Member	Ailment
	Prostatitis
	Swollen glands
Hair/Scalp	Baldness
	Hair problems
Head	Headache
Heart	Angina pectoris
	Arteriosclerosis
	Hypertension
Intestine	Celiac disease
	Constipation
	Hemorrhoids
Joints	Arthritis
	Bursitis
	Gout
Kidney	Kidney stones (renal calculi)
	Nephritis
Leg	Leg cramp
	Phlebitis
	Varicose veins
Liver	Cirrhosis of liver
	Hepatitis
	Jaundice
Lungs/Respiratory system	Allergies
	Bronchitis
	Common cold
	Croup
	Emphysema
	Hay fever (allergic rhinitis)
	Influenza
	Pneumonia
	Tuberculosis
Mouth	Canker sore
	Halitosis
Muscles	Muscular dystrophy
	Rheumatism
Reproductive system	Prostatitis
Skin	Abscess
	Acne
	Athlete's foot
	Bedsores
	Boil (furuncle)
	Bruises
	Burns

Body Member	Ailment
	Carbuncle
	Eczema
	Impetigo
	Psoriasis
	Scurvy
	Shingles (herpes zoster)
Stomach	Gastritis
	Gastroenteritis
	Stomach ulcer (peptic)
Teeth/Gums	Pyorrhea
	Tooth and gum disorders
General	Alcoholism
	Arthritis
	Backache
	Beriberi
	Cancer
	Chicken pox
	Fever
	Infection
	Influenza
	Kwashiorkor
	Overweight and obesity
	Polio
	Pregnancy
	Rheumatic fever
	Snake and insect bites
	Stress
	Stroke (cerebrovascular accident)

VITAMIN D

Description

Vitamin D is a fat-soluble vitamin, and it can be acquired either by ingestion or by exposure to sunlight. It is known as the "sunshine" vitamin because the action of the sun's ultraviolet rays activates a form of cholesterol, which is present in the skin, converting it to vitamin D.

The provitamins D are found in both plant and animal tissue. Vitamin D_2 is known as calciferol, a synthetic; vitamin D_3 is the natural form as it occurs in fish-liver oils. D_3 can be made synthetically by ultraviolet irradiation of 7-dehydrocholesterol, a derivative of cholesterol.

Vitamin D aids in the absorption of calcium from the intestinal tract and the breakdown and assimilation of phosphorus, which is required for bone formation. It helps synthesize those enzymes in the mucous membranes which are involved in the active transport of available calcium. Vitamin D is necessary for normal growth in children, for without it bones and teeth do not calcify properly.

Adults also benefit from vitamin D. It is valuable in maintaining a stable nervous system, normal heart action, and normal blood clotting because all these functions are related to the body's supply and utilization of calcium and phosphorus. Vitamin D is best utilized when taken with vitamin A. Fish-liver oils are the best natural source of vitamins A and D.

Absorption and Storage

Ingested vitamin D is absorbed with the fats through the intestinal walls with the aid of bile. Vitamin D from dehydrocholesterol by sun radiaion is formed in the skin and absorbed into the circulatory system. Pigmentation is a factor in the absorption of ultraviolet rays. The more pigment there is in the skin, the less vitamin D is produced in the body by irradiation.

After absorption from the intestine or formation in the skin, vitamin D is transported to the liver for storage; other deposits are found in the skin, brain, spleen, and bones. The body can store sizable reserves of vitamin D. Mineral oil can destroy the vitamin D already stored in the intestinal tract.

Dosage and Toxicity

Most of the body's needs for vitamin D can be met by sufficient exposure to sunlight and from the ingestion of small amounts of food, but the sun's action on the skin can be inhibited by such factors as air pollution, clouds, window glass, or clothing. The National Research Council sets the dietary allowance of vitamin D at 400 IU per day to meet the requirements of practically all healthy individuals who have little or no exposure to ultraviolet light. This same dosage is recommended for infants, provided the calcium consumption at the same time is adequate. During pregnancy and lactation women need to include extra

vitamin D in their diets. According to the National Research Council, there are no vitamin D recommendations for adults over twenty-two years of age since there are no data available upon which to base such a recommendation.

The adult rate of calcium and phosphorus loss from the skeletal system is thought to be less rapid than that of the growing organism.

It must be emphasized that good will result from the provision of adequate vitamin D *only* when the calcium and phosphorus requirements are met. No extra benefit is obtained from taking more than 400 IU daily except for therapeutic reasons; then dosages may range from 1500 to 2800 IU daily for several months. Increased heart activity requires increased calcium, which is not supplied unless there is enough vitamin D in the system.

It is known that "hypervitaminosis D" can occur and can cause pathological changes in the body. Excessive amounts may cause high levels of calcium and phosphorus in the blood and excessive excretion of calcium in the urine; this leads to calcification of soft tissues and of the walls of the blood vessels and kidney tubules, which is hypercalcemia.

Symptoms of acute overdosage are increased frequency of urination, loss of appetite, nausea, vomiting, diarrhea, muscular weakness, dizziness, weariness and calcification of the soft tissues of the heart, blood vessels, and lungs. These symptoms will disappear within a few days when the overdosage is terminated.

Some infants react hyperactively to the amounts of vitamin D found in fortified milk. This reaction to the vitamin could result in further medical complications. Hypercalcemia that has developed in children ingesting average supplementation of D may be an indication of hyperreactivity to the vitamin.

Large doses of vitamin D given to rheumatoid arthritic patients resulted in deposition of calcium in the arteries. This condition can cause kidney dysfunction and high blood pressure.

Deficiency Effects and Symptoms

A deficiency of vitamin D leads to inadequate absorption of calcium from the intestinal tract and retention of phosphorus in the kidney, leading to faulty mineralization of bone structures. The inability of the soft bones to withstand the stress of weight results in skeletal malformations.   Rickets, a bone disorder in children, is a direct result of vitamin D deficiency. Signs of rickets are softening of the skull; softening of the fragile bones with bowing of the legs and spinal curvature; enlargement of the wrist, knee, and ankle joints; poorly developed muscles; and nervous irritability.

A deficiency is most commonly seen in premature babies or children who have too little exposure to sunshine. "Adult rickets," called osteomalacia, may also occur.

It is believed that vitamin D and parathyroid hormones work together to regulate the transport of calcium.   A deficiency may cause tetany, a condition characterized by muscular numbness, tingling, and spasm.

Dr. Arthur A. Knapp, an ophthalmologist, reported tests indicating that a vitamin D deficiency may cause myopia, or nearsightedness.   An imbalance in calcium is the root of this disorder (see Animal and Human Tests).   A vitamin D deficiency may also lead to faulty development of tooth structure.

The severe low calcium levels found in kidney disease have been attributed to the body's inability to properly metabolize vitamin D.   Significant improvement in absorption has been observed in patients receiving 100 IU of supplemental vitamin D.

Beneficial Effect on Ailments

Vitamin D helps prevent and cure rickets, a disease resulting from insufficient calcium, phosphorus, or vitamin D.   It also aids in repairing osteomalacia in adults.

Vitamin D plays an important role in dentition. Besides being necessary for proper tooth eruption and linear growth, it continually strengthens the teeth. According to Adelle Davis, vitamin D helps in preventing tooth decay and pyorrhea, an inflammation of the sockets of the teeth.

Vitamins D and A have been beneficial in reducing the incidences of colds.   The two vitamins taken along with vitamin C act as a preventive measure.   Researchers have reported that the acidity of gastric juices is affected by the amount of vitamin D in the diet.   These juices are named as a cause of stomach ulcers.   Therefore an ulcer patient should be checked to see whether his diet has a sufficient supply of vitamin D.

Human Tests

1. Vitamin D and Myopia.   50,000 USP units of vitamin D in capsule and 1 gram of calcium, in the form of milk or dicalcium phosphate tables, were given daily to selected patients.

Results.   In one group, 18 of 52 vitamin-fed patients showed a reduction in myopia, and 8 remained unchanged.   (Rodale, ed., *Prevention,* May 1973, p. 95.)

2. Vitamin D and Conjunctivitis.   Forty-one patients suffering from allergic conjunctivitis were given 50,000 units of vitamin D daily for 7 weeks.

Results.   Twenty-nine patients experienced complete relief with vitamin D therapy, 11 showed marked improvement, and 1 remained unchanged.   (Dr. Arthur A. Knapp, Columbia College of Physicians and Surgeons, as reported in Rodale, ed., *Prevention,* September 1969, pp. 80–82.)

3. Vitamins D and A and Colds.   54 patients suffering from frequent colds, accompanied by high fever, were put into three groups.   Group 1 received only vitamin A; Group 2 received only vitamin D; Group 3 received both vitamins A and D.   Children under twelve were given half the adult dosage.

Results.   None of the patients who received either vitamin D or A alone benefited by the treatment. In the group that received both vitamins, 80 percent showed a significant reduction in both the number and severity of common colds.

Animal Tests

1. Vitamin D and Myopia.   Animals fed diets deficient in vitamin D and calcium developed axial myopia, keratoconus (a conical protrusion of the cornea), cataracts, and even arteriosclerosis comparable to the senile type observed clinically in human beings.   (Dr. Arthur A. Knapp, Columbia College of Physicians and Surgeons, as reported in Rodale, ed., *Prevention,* September 1969, pp. 80–82.)

2. Vitamin D and Bone Growth.   Experiments in which the calcium intake varied in rats showed that vitamin D was responsible for suppressing growth when dietary calcium was high and for stimulating growth when dietary calcium intake was low. (H. Steenback and D. C. Herting, *Nutrition Reviews,* vol. 14, p. 191, 1956.)

VITAMIN D MAY BE BENEFICIAL FOR THE FOLLOWING AILMENTS:

Body Member	Ailment
Bladder	Cystitis
Blood/Circulatory system	Cholesterol level, high
	Diabetes
Bones	Fracture
	Osteomalacia
	Osteoporosis
	Rickets
Brain/Nervous system	Epilepsy
	Meningitis
Eye	Bitot spots
	Cataracts
	Eyestrain
	Glaucoma
	Vision and focus disorders
Gallbladder	Gallstones
Glands	Cystic fibrosis
Head	Fever
Intestine	Celiac disease
	Constipation
	Worms
Joints	Arthritis
Leg	Leg cramp
	Sciatica
Liver	Cirrhosis of liver
	Jaundice
Lungs/Respiratory system	Allergies
	Bronchitis
	Common cold
	Emphysema
	Tuberculosis
Mouth	Canker sores
Muscles	Tetany
Reproductive system	Vaginitis
Skin	Acne
	Bedsores
	Burns
	Carbuncles

Body Member	Ailment
	Eczema
	Psoriasis
	Shingles (herpes zoster)
Teeth/Gums	Pyorrhea
General	Aging
	Alcoholism
	Backache
	Cancer
	Fatigue
	Insomnia
	Kwashiorkor
	Pregnancy
	Rheumatic fever
	Stress

VITAMIN E (TOCOPHEROL)

Description

Vitamin E, a fat-soluble vitamin, is composed of a group of compounds called tocopherols. Seven forms of tocopherol exist in nature: alpha, beta, delta, epsilon, eta, gamma, and zeta. Of these, alpha tocopherol is the most potent form of vitamin E and has the greatest nutritional and biological value. Tocopherols occur in highest concentrations in cold-pressed vegetable oils, all whole raw seeds and nuts, and soybeans. Wheatgerm oil is the source from which vitamin E was first obtained.

Vitamin E is an antioxidant, which means it opposes oxidation of substances in the body. Oxidation involves a compound called an oxidizer which attacks another compound, removing an electron from it. Vitamin E prevents saturated fatty acids and vitamin A from breaking down and combining with other substances that may become harmful to the body. Fat oxidization results in the formation of free radicals. Free radicals are highly destructive molecules that can cause extensive damage to the body, from cancer to blood clots to damage of DNA.

The vitamin B complex and ascorbic acid are also protected against oxidation when vitamin E is present in the digestive tract. Fats and oils containing vitamin E are less susceptible to rancidity than those devoid of vitamin E. Vitamin E has the ability to unite with oxygen and prevent it from being converted into toxic peroxides; this leaves the red blood cells more fully supplied with the pure oxygen that the blood carries to the heart and other organs.

Vitamin E plays an essential role in cellular respiration of all muscles, especially cardiac and skeletal. Vitamin E makes it possible for these muscles and their nerves to function with less oxygen, thereby increasing their endurance and stamina. It also causes dilation of the blood vessels, permitting a fuller flow of blood to the heart. Vitamin E is a highly effective antithrombin in the bloodstream, inhibiting coagulation of blood by preventing clots from forming. It also aids in bringing nourishment to the cells, strengthening the capillary walls, and protecting the red blood cells from destruction by poisons, such as hydrogen peroxide, in the blood.

Vitamin E prevents both the pituitary and adrenal hormones from being oxidized and promotes proper functioning of linoleic acid, an unsaturated fatty acid. Because aging in the cells is due primarily to oxidation, vitamin E is useful in retarding this process. It is also necessary for proper focusing of the eyes in middle-aged persons. A sufficient amount of vitamin E allows greater storage and reduces the requirement for vitamin A.

Vitamin E is effective in the prevention of elevated scar formation on the body surface and within the body. In ointment form it is used on burns to promote healing and lessen the formation of scars. It stimulates urine excretion, which helps heart patients whose body tissues contain an excessive amount of tissue fluid (edema). As a diuretic, vitamin E helps lower elevated blood pressure. It protects against the damaging effects of many environmental poisons in the air, water, and food. It protects the lungs and other tissues from damage by polluted air.

The vitamin prevents ozone from oxidizing lung lipids in the body. In this process, vitamin E itself is used up and needs to be replaced in order for it to continue its protection. In animal studies, vitamin E has a dramatic effect on the reproductive organs: it helps prevent miscarriages, increases male and female fertility, and helps restore male potency.

Vitamin E may possibly be involved in calcium metabolism, correcting deposition in the body of either too little or too much. Removal of abnormal calcium deposits from the walls of hardened arteries and deposition of calcium into weak bones, a disease called fragilitas osseum, has been observed.[39]

Absorption and Storage

Vitamin E, as other fat-soluble vitamins, is absorbed in the presence of bile salts and fat. From the intestines, it is absorbed into the lymph and is transported in the bloodstream as tocopherol to the liver, where high concentrations of it are stored. It is also stored in the fatty tissues, heart, muscles, testes, uterus, blood, and adrenal and pituitary glands. Vitamin E in ointment form can be absorbed through the skin and mucous membranes. Excessive amounts of vitamin E are excreted in the urine, and all effects of vitamin E disappear within three days.

There are several substances that interfere with, or even cause a depletion of, vitamin E in the body. For example, when the inorganic form of iron and vitamin E are administered together, the absorption of both substances is impaired. Dr. Wilfred Shute, in *Vitamin E for Ailing and Healthy Hearts,* suggests that vitamin E should be taken in one dose and all iron taken 8 to 12 hours later for proper absorption. The best time to take vitamin E is before mealtime or bedtime. Chlorine in drinking water, ferric chloride, rancid oil or fat, and inorganic iron compounds destroy vitamin E in the body. Mineral oil used as a laxative depletes vitamin E. Vegetable oils dissolve alpha tocopherol and readily release it in the body, whereas mineral oil dissolves it but does not readily release it.

Large amounts of polyunsaturated fats or oils in the diet increase the rate of oxidation of vitamin E; the more unsaturated fats or oils consumed, the more vitamin E is necessary. The female hormone estrogen is a vitamin E antagonist. Intake of this hormone makes it very difficult to estimate the amount of alpha tocopherol the individual is lacking.

Improper absorption may be partly responsible for muscular problems, such as muscular dystrophy and poor performance in athletes, and digestive problems, such as peptic ulcers and cancer of the colon. Poor absorption can impair the survival of red blood cells.

[39]Dr. Wilfred E. Shute, *Health Preserver* (Emmaus, Pa.: Rodale Press, 1977), p. 84.

Dosage and Toxicity

The daily intake of vitamin E recommended by the National Research Council is based upon the metabolic body size and the level of polyunsaturated fatty acids in the diet rather than upon weight or calorie intake. The requirements increase with gains in polyunsaturated fatty acids in the diet. Air pollution also increases the need for vitamin E. The RDA for infants is 4 to 5 IU daily; for children and adolescents the range is 7 to 12 IU; for adult males, 15 IU; for adult females, 12 IU; in pregnancy and lactation, needs increase to 15 IU daily. Many nutritionists consider these daily allowances exceedingly low. Adelle Davis recommends 30 IU daily for infants and children and 100 IU for adolescents and adults.[40] In cases of illness, doctors recommend 300 to 600 IU daily, although 2000 IU have been used therapeutically with excellent results.

Vitamin E has a tendency to raise blood pressure when it is given in large doses to someone whose body is not accustomed to it; therefore initial intake should be small, and as tolerance rises, the dosage should be gradually increased. It has been suggested that men start with 100 IU and gradually increase to 600 IU when used for preventive purposes. Women should begin with 100 IU and gradually increase to 400 IU.[41] The best way to determine the correct dosage is with the help of a doctor who is learned in vitamin E therapy.

Vitamin E is considered nontoxic except in two conditions: in high blood pressure patients, it elevates the pressure; starting a chronic rheumatic heart disease patient on high doses can lead to rapid deterioration or death. It is best to begin with small doses, gradually increasing the amount. When using vitamin E externally, Shute states that it is a good idea to take it orally while simultaneously applying it to the body. These methods complement each other.[42]

Deficiency Effects and Symptoms

The first clinical sign of a vitamin E deficiency is the rupture of red blood cells, which results from their increased fragility. A deficiency could result in a reduction of membrane stability and a shrinkage in collagen, connective tissue. A vitamin E deficiency may result in a tendency toward muscular wasting or abnormal fat deposits in the muscles and an increased demand for oxygen. Without sufficient amounts of vitamin E in the body, the essential fatty acids are altered so that blood cells break down and hemoglobin formation is impaired. In addition, several amino acids cannot be utilized, and pituitary and adrenal glands reduce their level of functioning. Iron absorption and hemoglobin formation also are impaired. A severe deficiency can cause damage to the kidneys and liver.

Perhaps the widest incidence of vitamin E deficiency among adults in the United States is in gastrointestinal disease, where prolonged deficiency can cause faulty absorption of fat and of fat-soluble vitamins, possibly resulting in cystic fibrosis, blockage of the bile ducts, and chronic inflammation of the pancreas.[43] Poor utilization of the vitamin or an increased vitamin E demand peculiar to the individual can cause anemia and edema in premature and malnourished infants. Serious deficiencies of vitamin E in men may lead to degeneration of tissues in the testes. No amount of vitamin E therapy can repair the permanent damage, and such men may become sterile.[44] Women who are severely deficient in vitamin E cannot carry a pregnancy term successfully and often have miscarriages. Premature births frequently result from insufficient intake of vitamin E during pregnancy, leaving the infants more susceptible to anemia.[45] Hemorrhaging can occur in newborn infants who lack vitamin E. The blood cells of vitamin E–deficient babies are prone to weakness (hemolysis).

Vitamin E deficiencies can result in nephritis. This occurs when kidney tubules plug up with dead cells so that urine is unable to pass; dropsy and progressive degeneration then occur. Vitamin E deficiency appears to make red blood cells more susceptible to damage frcm medication and from environmental stresses.

A deficiency of vitamin E can produce heart disease. Approximately 25,000 children are born with heart defects every year in the United States, where 50 per-

[40]Davis, *Let's Get Well,* p. 398.

[41]Carlson Wade, *The Rejuvenated Vitamin* (New York: Award Books, 1970), p. 21.

[42]Wilfred E. Shute and Harold J. Taub, *Vitamin E for Ailing and Healthy Hearts* (New York: Pyramid House, 1969), pp. 75–77.

[43]Martin Ebon, *The Truth about Vitamin E* (New York: Bantam Books, 1972), p. 7.

[44]Ibid., p. 30.

[45]Davis, *Let's Get Well,* p. 281.

cent of all deaths result from heart-related ailments. Evidence is accumulating to indicate that a lack of sufficient vitamin E may be a contributing factor in atherosclerosis and cancer.

According to Dr. Wilfred Shute, the lack of vitamin E in the American diet is partially due to the milling process which eliminates the highly perishable wheat germ, a significant source of vitamin E. About 90 percent of the vitamin E is lost in the milling process.

Beneficial Effect on Ailments

Vitamin E works to treat and prevent heart diseases such as coronary thrombosis, a heart attack in which the vessels are blocked by blood clots and part of the heart is deprived of its blood supply. Vitamin E causes arterial blood clots to disintegrate. Angina pectoris, a chest pain resulting from an insufficient supply of blood to the heart tissues, is successfully treated with alpha tocopherol.

According to Shute, rheumatic heart disease is responsible for 90 percent of defective hearts among children. Vitamin E aids rheumatic heart disease and early stages of cardiac complications by returning abnormal capillaries to normal and reducing fluid accumulation within and between cells. This promotes normal gas interchange across the cell membranes, which seems to arrest the disease.[46] Congenital heart disease results in structural defects of the heart. Vitamin E cannot alter the defective structure, but its oxygen-saving effects and its antithrombin activity are vital for patients who are not treated surgically. Many congenital heart disease patients have cyanosis, insufficient supply of oxygen in the blood, and with adequate dosage of vitamin E the cyanosis has disappeared.

Vitamin E is able to bring relief to intermittent claudication, a severe pain in calf muscles which results from inadequate blood supply caused by arterial spasm, "restless legs," atherosclerosis, or arteriosclerosis. Vitamin E is beneficial to persons with atherosclerosis if vitamin E therapy is used before irreparable damage has occurred. It relieves pain in the extremities, speeds up blood flow, and reduces clotting tendencies.[47]

Vitamin E can aid in the healing of burned tissue, skin ulcers, and abrasions. It prevents or dissolves scar tissues. Vitamin E helps remove old acne scars, particularly if x-ray treatments have been given. It is needed also to help dissolve scars in the arterial walls caused by toxic substances.

Free radicals cause a process called cross-linking which can result in skin wrinkles. Adequate intake of vitamin E, a free radical scavenger, could be helpful in counteracting premature aging of the skin.[48] It is useful to apply vitamin E to the skin in ointment form while taking it orally, because it affects the cell formation by replacing the cells on the outer layer of the skin. Vitamin E also helps counter the gradual decline in metabolic processes during aging. Dry, itchy skin is often part of the aging process; vitamin E ointment is able to relieve the itching.

Under normal conditions vitamin E reduces the formation of thrombin, a clotting agent; this tends to reduce the likelihood of thrombosis, the formation of a blood clot. The intake of estrogen, found in contraceptive pills, may neutralize the effect of vitamin E. Intake of estrogen causes the collection of fibrin, an insoluble protein that promotes blood clotting by forming a fibrous network, to become greater. The greater amount of fibrin increases the chances of thromboembolism, the blocking of blood vessels.

Vitamin E has been successful in regulating excessive or scanty flows during menstruation.[49] When vitamin E is added to the diet, it can correct menstrual rhythm. Vitamin E is recognized as a treatment for hot flashes and headaches during menopause. It has helped relieve itching and inflammation of the vagina when applied in ointment form and simultaneously ingested.

Vitamin E has been successfully used as treatment of noncancerous breast tissue known as fibrocystic breast disease. Vitamin E decreases the breast tenderness women experience during premenstruation.

Because the vitamin is an antioxidant, it reportedly eliminates perspiration odor. Bursitis, wry-neck, gout, and arthritis have improved with vitamin E therapy. Ingestion of large amounts has improved conditions of nearsightedness and crossed eyes. Vitamin E has also been used to prevent calcification of the kidneys caused by excessive vitamin D or other toxic sub-

[46]Shute and Taub, *Vitamin E for Ailing and Healthy Hearts,* pp. 61–64.
[47]Ibid., pp. 70–73.

[48]Durk Pearson and Sandy Shaw, *Life Extension,* p. 406.
[49]Ebon, *The Truth about Vitamin E,* p. 80.

stances. Oxygen toxicity in preemies has reportedly been prevented by vitamin E.

Vitamin E has been used to help treat varicose veins, as an alternative to surgery. It also can relieve the pain of varicose veins by decreasing the amount of oxygen needed by the tissues involved.

Vitamin E has been successful in treating thrombosis and phlebitis, which are clots in the veins. In large doses it prevents clots from spreading, dissolves existing clots, and provides indirect circulation around obstructed veins. It should be used to prevent initial attacks of clotting after operations or childbirth.[50]

Individuals suffering from muscular dystrophy have benefited from massive doses of vitamin E.[51] Vitamin E may be able to clear up or control many forms of kidney disease, including nephritis. It also aids in restoring the functions of damaged livers.[52]

Vitamin E helps promote body defenses against virus infections and in some cases may be utilized as a flu vaccine. High doses may build both the serum and the cellular levels of the body to high levels of immunity against flu.

Vitamin E therapy has been able to help diabetics. After administration of the vitamin, some patients found that their blood sugar levels became normal or near normal, and the amount of insulin required was reduced. Vitamin E has also been used to prevent and treat gangrene in diabetics.

Vitamins A and E may be beneficial in lowering blood cholesterol by preventing fat deposits. The vitamins help offset the high cholesterol accumulations deposited on the arterial walls.

Vitamin E is used for easing headaches because it preserves the oxygen in the blood for an extended period. This results in more efficiency as the blood is pumped through the blood vessels of the head. Vitamin E has also relieved migraine attacks. Vitamins C and E work together to keep blood vessels flexible, healthy, and less subject to painful disturbances.

Test animals given vitamin E have shown a reduced death rate and an increased life span. It is possible that the vitamin assists the body's immune system by preventing membrane oxidation, thereby slowing down the aging process.

Intravenous injections of vitamin E (200 to 400 milligrams) plus 200 to 300 milligrams taken orally have successfully prevented digitalis intoxication.[53] Vitamin E supplementation is essential for smokers. The carbon monoxide in the smoke from cigarettes destroys the oxygen-carrying ability of hemoglobin in the blood.

Vitamin E can help reduce side effects from some painkillers such as codeine, morphine, and aminopyrine. It is possible that vitamin E also influences enzymatic actions that detoxify many drugs.

Human Tests

1. Vitamin E and Menopause. A woman had undergone a complete hysterectomy due to cancer of an ovary. The patient suffered from hot flashes. She was given 75 IU of alpha tocopherol daily.

Results. Administration of the vitamin proved valuable in diminishing or entirely removing the hot flashes. (*Journal of the American Medical Association,* vol. 167, p. 1806, 1958, as reported in Rodale, *The Encyclopedia for Healthful Living,* p. 980.)

2. Vitamin E and Varicose Veins. Fifty-one patients with varicose veins were given 300 to 500 milligrams of vitamin E daily. They were kept on this treatment from 2 months to 3 years, depending upon the severity of the ailment.

Results. Nine of the patients showed improvement within 30 days; 7 were completely healed; and the other 35 all showed some relief of congestion, pain, and edema. No side effects were noted. (*La Riforma Medical,* Vol. 69, pp. 853–56, 1955, as reported in Rodale, *The Encyclopedia for Healthful Living,* p. 978.)

3. Vitamin E and Menstrual Pain. One hundred women between eighteen and twenty-one years of age were suffering from pain and discomfort during their menstrual periods. They were divided into two groups. Each woman in the first group was given 50 milligrams of vitamin E daily for 10 days before

[50]Ibid.

[51]Herbert Bailey, *Vitamin E, Your Key to a Healthy Heart* (New York: Arc Books, 1971), pp. 97–98.

[52]Ibid., p. 99.

[53]Carl C. Pfeiffer, *Mental and Elemental Nutrients* (New Canaan, Conn.: Keats Publishing, 1975), p. 206.

menstruation and for the next 4 days. Each woman in the second group was given a placebo. Treatment lasted 3 months.

Results. Of the women in the first group 76 percent noted improvement; only 29 percent of the women in the second group noted any improvement in 3 months. The patients experienced a recurrence of their pain 2 to 6 months after treatment ceased. (*The Lancet,* vol. I, pp. 844–47, 1955, as reported in Rodale, *The Encyclopedia for Healthful Living,* p. 988.)

4. Vitamin E and Coronary Occlusion (Blood Clot in the Coronary Artery). A forty-year-old male suffering from a coronary occlusion was treated with 60 IU of alpha tocopherol daily.

Results. The symptoms of angina (sense of suffocation) disappeared completely in 4 weeks. (Shute, *Vitamin E for Ailing and Healthy Hearts,* p. 39.)

5. Vitamin E and Athletic Performance. In a controlled study athletes were given large doses of alpha tocopherol.

Results. Their muscle performance, endurance, and speed of recovery improved. The effect was transient but persisted as long as the treatment was maintained. ("Resolving the Vitamin E Controversy," *Percival,* Summary 3.55, 1951.)

Animal Test

1. Vitamin E and Muscular Stamina in Racehorses. Dr. Evan Shute and William Gutterson devised an experiment with vitamin E and its effect on racehorses.

Results. The percentage of wins for each horse given vitamin E was 2.7, compared to 2.3 the year before, when a smaller dose of vitamin E was given. Two years before, when no vitamin E was given, the percentage of wins per horse had been 1.8. Although there was an improvement in the first year, the horses hit their peak the following year, when the dosages were doubled or tripled. (*The Summary,* December 1956, published by the Shute Foundation for Medical Re-search, London, Canada, as reported in Rodale, *The Encyclopedia for Healthful Living,* p. 777.)

VITAMIN E MAY BE BENEFICIAL FOR THE FOLLOWING AILMENTS:

Body Member	Ailment
Bladder	Cystitis
Blood/Circulatory system	Anemia
	Angina pectoris
	Arteriosclerosis
	Atherosclerosis
	Bruising
	Coronary thrombosis
	Diabetes
	Hypertension
	Pernicious anemia
	Phlebitis
	Stroke (cerebrovascular accident)
	Thrombophlebitis
	Varicose veins
Bones	Osteoporosis
Bowel	Colitis
Brain/Nervous system	Epilepsy
	Mental illness
	Multiple sclerosis
	Parkinson's disease
	Stroke (cerebrovascular accident)
Ear	Ménière's syndrome
Eye	Amblyopia
	Cataracts
	Eyestrain
Gallbladder	Gallstones
Glands	Cystic fibrosis
	Hyperthyroidism
	Prostatitis
Hair/Scalp	Baldness
	Dandruff
Head	Headache
	Sinusitis
Heart	Angina pectoris
	Arteriosclerosis
	Atherosclerosis
	Congestive heart failure
	Coronary thrombosis
	Hypertension
	Myocardial infarction

Body Member	Ailment
Intestine	Celiac disease
	Constipation
	Hemorrhoids
Joints	Arthritis
	Bursitis
	Gout
Kidney	Kidney stones (renal calculi)
	Nephritis
Leg	Leg cramp
	Phlebitis
	Sciatica
	Varicose veins
Lungs/Respiratory system	Allergies
	Bronchitis
	Common cold
	Emphysema
	Hay fever (allergic rhinitis)
Muscles	Muscular dystrophy
	Rheumatism
Reproductive system	Miscarriage
	Prostatitis
	Vaginitis
Skin	Abscess
	Acne
	Athlete's foot
	Bedsores
	Boil (furuncle)
	Bruises
	Burns
	Carbuncle
	Impetigo
	Ulcers
	Warts
Stomach	Gastritis
	Stomach ulcer (peptic)
General	Backache
	Cancer
	Measles
	Overweight and obesity
	Pregnancy
	Sunburn
	Thrombophlebitis

VITAMIN K

Description

There are three main K vitamins: K_1 and K_2 are fat-soluble and can be manufactured in the intestinal tract in the presence of certain intestinal flora (bacteria); K_3 is produced synthetically for the treatment of patients who are unable to utilize naturally occurring vitamin K because they lack bile, an enzyme necessary for the absorption of all fat-soluble vitamins.

If yogurt, kefir (a preparation of curdled milk), or acidophilus milk (fermented milk used to change intestinal bacteria) is included in the diet, the body may be able to manufacture sufficient amounts of vitamin K. In addition, unsaturated fatty acids and a low-carbohydrate diet increase the amounts of vitamin K produced by intestinal flora.

Vitamin K is necessary for the formation of prothrombin, a chemical required in blood clotting. Vitamin K is involved in a body process, phosphorylation, in which phosphate, when combined with glucose, is passed through the cell membranes and converted into glycogen, a form in which carbohydrates are stored in the body. It is also vital for normal liver functioning and is an important vitality and longevity factor.

Some natural sources of vitamin K are kelp, alfalfa, green plants, and leafy green vegetables. Cow's milk, yogurt, egg yolks, blackstrap molasses, safflower oil, fish-liver oils, and other polyunsaturated oils are other good sources. The most dependable supply is the intestinal bacteria.

Vitamin K can be safely used as a preservative to control fermentation in foods. It has no bleaching effect, no unpleasant odor, and when added to naturally colored fruits, helps maintain a stable and effective condition of the food.

Absorption and Storage

Vitamin K is absorbed in the upper intestinal tract with the aid of bile or bile salts and is transported to the liver, where it is essential for synthesis of prothrombin and several related proteins involved in the clotting of blood. Vitamin K is stored in very small amounts, and considerable quantities are excreted after administration of therapeutic doses.

Factors interfering with absorption of vitamin K include any obstruction of the bile duct limiting the secretion of fat-emulsifying bile salts; failure of the liver to secrete bile; and dicumarol, an anticoagulant that reduces the activity of prothrombin in the blood plasma.

Rancid fats, radiation, x-rays, aspirin, and industrial air pollution all destroy vitamin K. Excessive use of antibiotics can destroy the intestinal flora. Ingestion of mineral oil will cause rapid excretion of vitamin K.

Dosage and Toxicity

The National Research Council states that the abundance of vitamin K in most diets, along with synthesis by the intestinal bacteria, provides adequate intake of vitamin K. The newborn infant needs a daily intake of 1 to 5 milligrams to prevent hemorrhagic disease, which is abnormal bleeding.[54] It is estimated that the average daily intake is between 300 and 500 micrograms, which is considered an adequate supply of vitamin K.[55]

Therapeutic dosages of vitamin K are often given before and after operations to reduce blood losses. Vitamin K injections are sometimes given to women prior to labor to protect against hemorrhaging.

Abnormal blood clotting can occur in persons taking anticoagulant drugs and high doses of vitamin K. Excessive doses of synthetic vitamin K can cause toxic reactions because the supplements will build up in the blood. Toxicity brings about a form of anemia that results in an increased breakdown in the red blood cells. In infants, kernicterus, a condition in which yellow pigment infiltrates the spinal cord and brain areas, can result, usually developing during the second to eighth day of life. Heinz bodies, or granules in the red blood cells resulting from damage to the hemoglobin molecules, are seen in infants suffering from an overdose. Toxicity has occurred when large dosages of synthetic vitamin K were injected into pregnant women. Flushing, sweating, and chest constrictions are symptoms of synthetic vitamin K toxicity. Natural vitamin K is stored in the body and produces no toxicity signs.

Deficiency Effects and Symptoms

Deficiencies of vitamin K usually result from inadequate absorption or the body's inability to utilize vitamin K in the liver. Vitamin K deficiency is common in diseases such as celiac disease (intestinal malabsorption), sprue (malabsorption in adulthood), and colitis, which affect the absorbing mucosa of the small intestine and cause a rapid loss of intestinal contents. In such cases, intravenous administration of vitamin K may be needed.

In a deficiency, a condition of hypoprothrombinemia can occur, causing blood-clotting time to be greatly or even indefinitely prolonged. A deficiency can cause hemorrhages in any part of the body, including the brain, spinal cord, and intestinal tract. A vitamin K deficiency can cause miscarriages and nosebleeds and can also be a factor in cellular disease and diarrhea.

Beneficial Effect on Ailments

Vitamin K is necessary to promote blood clotting, especially when jaundice is present. It is administered to heart patients who are using anticoagulant drugs to thin the consistency of their blood. Carefully measured doses of vitamin K are given to these patients to raise the prothrombin level slightly while not allowing it to completely counteract the effect of the anticoagulant.[56]

Vitamin K has proved beneficial in reducing the blood flow during prolonged menstruation; clots either diminish or disappear. It has often lessened or relieved menstrual cramps.

Vitamin K is frequently used with vitamin C in the prevention and improvement of hemorrhages in various parts of the eye.[57] Vitamin K is also used

[54]Guthrie, *Introductory Nutrition*, p. 216.

[55]Robert S. Goodhart and Maurice E. Shils, *Modern Nutrition in Health and Disease*, 5th ed. (Philadelphia: Lea & Febiger, 1973), p. 172.

[56]Prevention Magazine Staff, *Complete Book of Vitamins*, p. 439.

[57]J. I. Rodale, *The Health Builder* (Emmaus, Pa.: Rodale Books, 1957), p. 341.

to prevent hemorrhaging following gallbladder operations and to prevent cerebral palsy.[58]

VITAMIN K MAY BE BENEFICIAL FOR THE FOLLOWING AILMENTS:

Body Member	Ailment
Blood/Circulatory system	Bruising
	Hemorrhage
Gallbladder	Gallstones
Glands	Cystic fibrosis
Intestine	Celiac disease
	Worms
Liver	Cirrhosis of liver
	Jaundice
Skin	Ulcers
General	Aging
	Alcoholism
	Cancer
	Hepatitis
	Kwashiorkor

BIOFLAVONOIDS (VITAMIN P)

Description

Bioflavonoids, known as vitamin P, are water-soluble and are composed of a group of brightly colored substances that often appear in fruits and vegetables as companions to vitamin C. The components of the bioflavonoids are citrin, hesperidin, rutin, flavones, and flavonals.

Bioflavonoids were first discovered as a substance in the white segments, not in the juices, of citrus fruits. There is ten times the concentration of bioflavonoids in the edible part of the fruit that there is in the strained juice. Sources of bioflavonoids include lemons, grapes, plums, black currants, grapefruit, apricots, buckwheat, cherries, blackberries, and rose hips.

Bioflavonoids are essential for the proper absorption and use of vitamin C. They assist vitamin C in keeping collagen, the intercellular cement, in healthy condition. Bioflavonoids act as an antioxidant, keeping vitamin C and adrenalin from being oxidized by copper-con-

taining enzymes. The bioflavonoids also chelate copper from the body. They are vital in their ability to increase the strength of the capillaries and to regulate their permeability. These actions help prevent hemorrhages and ruptures in the capillaries and connective tissues and build a protective barrier against infections.

Absorption and Storage

The absorption and storage properties of bioflavonoids are very similar to those of vitamin C. The bioflavonoids are readily absorbed from the gastrointestinal tract into the bloodstream. Excessive amounts are excreted through urination and perspiration.

Dosage and Toxicity

There is no Recommended Dietary Allowance for this vitamin. Since bioflavonoids occur with vitamin C in natural food sources, synthetic vitamin C does not contain the bioflavonoids. When ingested together, bioflavonoids and C are more helpful than vitamin C taken alone. Rutin, which comes from buckwheat leaves, is a good food source of bioflavonoids. Bioflavonoids are reportedly nontoxic.

Deficiency Effects and Symptoms

Symptoms of a bioflavonoid deficiency are closely related to those of a vitamin C deficiency. Especially noted is the increased tendency to bleed or hemorrhage and bruise easily. A deficiency of vitamins C and P may contribute to rheumatism and rheumatic fever.[59]

Beneficial Effect on Ailments

The body's utilization of vitamin C is increased when bioflavonoids are present. They are helpful in strengthening the capillaries and may help prevent colds and influenza. Bioflavonoids have proved to be beneficial in treating various degrees of capillary injury and have been found to minimize bruising that occurs in contact sports.

Rutin is especially helpful in the prevention of recurrent bleeding arising from weakened blood vessels. It is sometimes used in the treatment of hemorrhoids

---

[58]Clark, *Know Your Nutrition*, p. 61.

[59]Rodale, *The Health Seeker*, p. 76.

and helps prevent the walls of the blood vessels from becoming fragile.

Bioflavonoids have been used successfully to treat ulcer patients and those suffering from dizziness caused by labyrinthitis, a disease of the inner ear. Weakness of the capillaries was found to be a major causative factor in both of these ailments.[60] Asthma has been successfully treated by the administration of bioflavonoids. Bioflavonoids have also been used as a protective agent against the harmful effects of x-rays.[61]

Bioflavonoids and vitamin C when taken together may help prevent habitual miscarriages. They are helpful in the treatment of disorders such as bleeding gums, eczema, and susceptibility to hemorrhaging. Rheumatism and rheumatic fever seem to be helped by vitamins C and P. The blood-vessel disorder of the eye which affects diabetics seems to respond to bioflavonoid-vitamin C treatment.[62] Administered together, these vitamins have also been beneficial in the treatment of muscular dystrophy because they help lower blood pressure moderately.

Dr. Carl Pfeiffer has used rutin, at an oral dose of 50 milligrams, for depressed patients. His studies have shown that rutin has a sedative-stimulant effect on the brain. There are also indications that rutin, in oral doses of 60 milligrams, raises blood histamine and lowers serum copper in the body, helpful for schizophrenics.[63]

In France, bioflavonoids have been used successfully for a number of women's gynecological problems. Physicians have found the flavone compounds effectively replace hormone therapy in cases of irregular or painful menstrual flow not caused by anatomical damage. Some of the compounds have prevented bleeding and regulated menstrual flow after insertion of intrauterine contraceptive devices.

Human Tests

1. Bioflavonoids and Rheumatoid Arthritis. A fifty-two-year-old woman with rheumatoid arthritis in both hands, wrists, and elbows and in the right shoulder, knees, and ankles was given 3000 milligrams of bioflavonoid complex.

Results. In 7 days she "felt better." Two weeks later the pain had practically disappeared, her digestion was improved, and bowel action was normal. Her blood pressure dropped from 190 to 176, and by the end of 5 weeks she had more action in her joints and a great deal more endurance. (Dr. James R. West, Morrell Memorial Hospital, Lakeland, Florida, as reported in Rodale, *The Encyclopedia for Healthful Living,* p. 30.)

2. Bioflavonoids and Duodenal Ulcers. Thirty-six cases of bleeding duodenal ulcers were treated with bioflavonoids and a diet consisting of an orange juice-milk-gelatin mixture given in doses of 4 to 6 ounces every 2 hours with bioflavonoid capsules, until bleeding was arrested. The bioflavonoid capsules were administered orally at the rate of three to nine capsules daily.

Results. All bleeding ceased on the fourth day. Then the patients were put on a bland diet. Vitamin supplements and bioflavonoid rations were added to the diet. All 36 patients responded with a return of mucous membrane and duodenal contour to a normal state. Total treatment took from 12 to 22 days. No recurrence of bleeding in 2 years or more occurred in 23 of the 36 cases. Twelve cases remained ulcer-free for 1 year or more, and the remaining cases were successfully treated and ulcer-free for 4 months. (Drs. Samuel Weiss, Jerome Weiss, and Bernard Weiss, *American Journal of Gastroenterology,* July 1958, as reported in Rodale, *The Encyclopedia for Healthful Living,* pp. 70–71.)

3. Bioflavonoids and Labyrinthitis (Disease of the Inner Ear). Nine cases were treated with four to six capsules of bioflavonoids daily with decreased salt intake.

Results. Positive results occurred in 3 to 6 days. The symptoms of dizziness, loss of balance, and nausea were successfully treated with no recurrence. (Dr. Theodore R. Miller, *Eye, Ear, Nose and Throat Monthly,* September 1958, as reported in Rodale, *The Encyclopedia for Healthful Living,* pp. 72–73.)

[60]Rodale, *Encyclopedia for Healthful Living,* p. 70.
[61]Paavo Airola, *Are You Confused?* (Phoenix, Ariz.: Health Plus, 1974), p. 161.
[62]Rodale, *The Health Seeker,* p. 76.
[63]Pfeiffer, *Mental and Elemental Nutrients,* p. 186.

BIOFLAVONOIDS MAY BE BENEFICIAL FOR THE FOLLOWING AILMENTS:

Body Member	Ailment
Blood/Circulatory system	Arteriosclerosis
	Atherosclerosis
	Bruising
	Cholesterol level, high
	Hemophilia
	Hypertension
	Leukemia
	Stroke (cerebrovascular accident)
	Varicose veins
Heart	Arteriosclerosis
	Atherosclerosis
	Hypertension
	Hypoxia
Intestine	Hemorrhoids
Joints	Arthritis
	Rheumatic fever
	Rheumatism
Lungs/Respiratory system	Pneumonia
Skin	Ulcers
Teeth/Gums	Pyorrhea
	Scurvy
General	Common cold
	Menstruation
	Schizophrenia

UNSATURATED FATTY ACIDS (UFA)

Description

Unsaturated fatty acids, UFA, usually come in the form of liquid vegetable oils, while saturated fatty acids are usually found in solid animal fat. The saturated fatty acids are more slowly metabolized by the body than are the unsaturated fatty acids.

The body cannot manufacture the essential unsaturated fatty acid, linoleic; linolenic and arachidonic acids can be synthesized from linoleic acid if it is sufficiently supplied to the body through diet. Wheat germ; seeds; natural golden vegetable oils, such as safflower, soy, and corn; and cod-liver oil contain lecithin and are the best sources of the unsaturated fatty acids.

Unsaturated fatty acids are important for respiration of vital organs and make it easier for oxygen to be transported by the bloodstream to all cells, tissues, and organs. They also help maintain resilience and lubrication of all cells and combine with protein and cholesterol to form living membranes that hold the body cells together.

UFA help to regulate the rate of blood coagulation and perform a vital function in breaking up cholesterol deposited on arterial walls. They are essential for normal glandular activity, especially of the adrenal glands and the thyroid gland. They nourish the skin cells and are essential for healthy mucous membranes and nerves.

The unsaturated fatty acids function in the body by cooperating with vitamin D in making calcium available to the tissues, assisting in the assimilation of phosphorus, and stimulating the conversion of carotene into vitamin A. Fatty acids are related to normal functioning of the reproductive system.

Absorption and Storage

The stomach, small intestine, and pancreas normally produce liberal amounts of fat-splitting digestive enzymes necessary for conversion of fats into fatty acids and glycerols (broken-down fatty acids). These are absorbed through the walls of the intestinal tract and are then transported through the portal vein to the liver, where they are usually metabolized as a source of energy. These changes must take place before the nutrients can enter the blood without causing food allergies.[64]

The digested fat is taken from the gastrointestinal tract as fatty acids and glycerol. These then enter fat-collecting ducts that finally carry the fat to the lymphatic system, which is primarily concerned with collecting body fluids and returning them to the general circulatory system. The fatty acids are stored in the adipose (containing massive amounts of fat cells) tissues.

Absorption of fat is decreased when there is increased movement in the gastrointestinal tract and when there is an absence of bile to break down the fat. X-ray treatments and radiation destroy the essential fatty acids within the body, although destruction

[64]Davis, *Let's Get Well*, p. 171.

can be prevented if large doses of vitamin E are taken. UFA are easily destroyed when exposed to air and may become rancid.

Dosage and Toxicity

The National Research Council states that the fat intake should include essential unsaturated fatty acids to the extent of at least 1 percent of the total calories. The level of essential fatty acids needed by infants has been set at 3 percent of the total calories.[65] The need for essential fatty acids is usually met when 2 percent of the calories are produced by linoleic acid, which is found in food sources such as the vegetable oils of soy, corn, sunflower, and wheat germ.

The need for linoleic acid increases in proportion to the amount of solids eaten. If the intake of saturated fats is high, a deficiency of linoleic acids can occur even though oils are included in the diet, and increased consumption of such foods as butter, cream, and saturated fat increases the need for UFA. Eating a great deal of carbohydrates also increases the need for unsaturated fatty acids. When there is sufficient linoleic acid in the diet, the other two essential fatty acids can be synthesized from it.

In order to get the full benefit of UFA, one should take vitamin E with it at mealtimes. This ensures the best absorption. In addition, it is important that as the amount of oils and fats is increased, the dosage of vitamin E is increased.

A diet including UFA should include the antioxidants, such as vitamins A, C, and E and zinc and selenium. These antioxidants prevent the formation of harmful peroxides that result when oxygen and the UFA interact in the body. If the peroxides or free radicals are allowed to form, serious damage to various body proteins can result.

There are no known toxic effects of UFA; however, excessive amounts of saturated fats may cause metabolic disturbances and abnormal weight gain.

Deficiency Effects and Symptoms

UFA deficiency causes changes to occur in the structure and enzyme function within the nucleus of the cells, resulting in a number of disorders. A deficiency

[65]Guthrie, *Introductory Nutrition*, p. 44.

may be responsible for brittle and lusterless hair, nail problems, dandruff, and allergic conditions. In addition, diarrhea, varicose veins, underweight, and gallstones may be a result of UFA deficiency. Skin disorders such as eczema, acne, and dry skin have been linked with UFA deficiency; also ailments, such as diseases of the heart, circulatory system, and kidneys, associated with faulty fat metabolism. Without UFA, growth is retarded, teeth do not form properly, and prostaglandins, a group of fatty acids found in tissues of the prostate gland, brain, kidney, and seminal and menstrual fluid, cannot be made by the cells.

Beneficial Effects on Ailments

Unsaturated fatty acids have been used to treat external ulcers, especially leg ulcers, with good results. The unsaturated fat preparation causes rapid granulation and regeneration of the skin. It can also be used orally and externally for treating infantile eczema and the nonallergenic eczema that occurs in adolescents and adults. Psoriasis can benefit from treatment with unsaturated fatty acids. Arachidonic acid is effective in curing dermatitis.

Linoleic acid is effective in restoring growth. Hay fever has been successfully treated with UFA. It is also essential for the prevention and treatment of bronchial asthma and rheumatoid arthritis.

UFA have been used in preventing heart disease. They keep cholesterol soft and prevent it from forming any hard deposits in the lumen of the blood vessels or under the skin. This is especially important for the atherosclerosis patient. Because UFA lower blood cholesterol, they help prevent high blood pressure and hardening of the arteries.

Unsaturated fatty acids have helped prevent diarrhea and underweight. They have been useful in preventing prostate trouble and arthritis. Any person who has gallbladder problems or has had one removed needs to take extra bile in the form of a food supplement so as to ensure proper breakdown of fats.

Human Tests

1. Unsaturated Fatty Acids and Prostate Glands. Nineteen cases of prostate gland disorders were treated with unsaturated fatty acids.

Results. All 19 cases had a lessening of residual urine, that is, the urine that cannot be released from the bladder due to pressure from the enlarged prostate gland. In 12 cases there was no residual urine at the end of treatment. There was also a decrease in leg pains, fatigue, kidney disorders, and excessive urination at night. (James P. Hart and William de Grande Cooper, *Lee Report,* No. 1, as reported in Rodale, *The Health Builder,* p. 352.)

2. Fatty Acids and Asthma. Two doctors observed the effects of a diet supplement plus fatty acids in patients suffering from asthma.

Results. Forty percent of the patients were either entirely relieved of asthmatic symptoms or noticed some improvement. The other 60 percent did not respond to treatment. (*The Journal of Applied Nutrition,* Spring 1955, as reported in Rodale, *The Health Builder,* p. 357.)

3. Unsaturated Fatty Acids and Eczema. Eighty-seven chronic eczema patients were treated daily with corn oil (rich in unsaturated fatty acids) for a period of over 4½ years.

Results. Standard treatments had been used but not with the same success that corn oil had on the patients. All patients responded and showed improvement with the corn oil treatment. (Lee Foundation Report, February 1942, as reported in Rodale, *The Encyclopedia for Healthful Living,* p. 777.)

UFA MAY BE BENEFICIAL FOR THE FOLLOWING AILMENTS:

Body Member	Ailment
Blood/Circulatory system	Cholesterol level, high
	Diabetes
Bowel	Colitis
	Diarrhea
Brain/Nervous system	Mental illness
	Multiple sclerosis
Ear	Ménière's syndrome
Glands	Prostatitis
Heart	Coronary thrombosis
Intestine	Constipation
Joints	Arthritis
Legs	Leg cramp
Lungs/Respiratory system	Asthma
	Bronchitis
Skin	Acne
	Dermatitis
	Eczema
	Psoriasis
Teeth/Gums	Tooth and gum disorders
General	Allergies
	Common cold
	Overweight and obesity
	Underweight

MINERALS

ALUMINUM

Description

Aluminum is a trace mineral, but it can be dangerous, even fatal, if consumed in excessive amounts. There is no established function of aluminum in human nutrition. Aluminum weakens the living tissue of the alimentary canal, the digestive tube from the mouth to the anus. Many of aluminum's harmful effects result from its destruction of vitamins. It binds with many other substances and is never found alone in nature.

Aluminum is found in many plant and animal foods. It can be found in tap water because aluminum sulfate is used in the water purification process and not all of the aluminum is filtered out. Aluminum is added to most table salt to prevent caking. It is used in certain stomach antacids. Aluminum is also used in foil, deodorants, baking powder, as an emulsifier in some processed cheeses, and as a bleaching agent to whiten flour.

Absorption and Storage

Aluminum is easily absorbed by the body and is accumulated in the arteries. Highest concentrations are found in the lungs, liver, thyroid, and brain. Usually, most of the aluminum taken into the body is ultimately excreted. Adelle Davis reports that magnesium can displace aluminum in the body. A patient with aluminum toxicity was relieved of irritability and poor memory and concentration after taking magnesium supplements. Foods cooked in aluminum utensils may absorb minute quantities of the mineral.

Dosage and Toxicity

The total aluminum content of the adult body is from 50 to 150 milligrams. The daily amount ingested in the average diet ranges from 10 milligrams to more than 100 milligrams.

Excessive amounts of aluminum can result in symptoms of poisoning. These symptoms include constipation, colic, loss of appetite, nausea, skin ailments, twitching of leg muscles, excessive perspiration, and loss of energy. Patients with aluminum poisoning should discontinue the use of aluminum cookware. Doctors often recommend that the drinking of tap water be discontinued.

Small quantities of soluble salts of aluminum present in the blood cause a slow form of poisoning characterized by motor paralysis and areas of local numbness, with fatty degeneration of kidney and liver. There are also anatomical changes in the nerve centers and symptoms of gastrointestinal inflammation. These symptoms result from the body's effort to eliminate the poison.

It has been found that aluminum hydroxide gel, a stomach antacid, can reduce blood phosphate, leading bones to dissolve and causing aching and weak muscles. Persons particularly prone to osteoporosis should be careful of aluminum ingestion.

Trace amounts of aluminum applied to the brain surface of animals resulted in seizures and fits. Other studies demonstrated that aluminum salts injected into the fluid surrounding the brain produced changes that are similar to those occurring in senile dementia. In further animal studies, cats given aluminum became slow learners at experimental tasks. The level of aluminum in the cats' brains was equivalent to the amount found in the brains of persons who have a type of senility called Alzheimer's disease.

Deficiency Effects and Symptoms

No available information.

Beneficial Effect on Ailments

No available information.

BERYLLIUM

Description

Beryllium is a mineral that has definite adverse effects on the human body. This mineral can deplete the body's store of magnesium, allowing disease to result. When beryllium is absorbed into the bloodstream, it often lodges in vital organs and keeps them from performing their functions. It interferes with a number of the body's enzyme systems. It does not allow the enzyme system to carry on its function in the body.

Beryllium is used in neon signs, electronic devices, some alloys including steel, bicycle wheels, fishing rods, and many common household products.

Beryllium is a dangerous substance in industrial toxicology. Beryllium dust makes breathing difficult. This condition may lead to injury of the lungs, causing scarring or fibrosis. Some victims of beryllium poisoning become completely disabled by serious lung destruction.

BISMUTH

Description

Bismuth is a mineral which has no known function in the human body. It has been used in treating syphilis and been given to patients undergoing a colostomy. Bismuth is also contained in certain rectal suppositories and antidiarrhea medicines.

Bismuth overdose can resemble mental illness, resulting in a staggering gait, poor memory, body tremors, visual and hearing disturbances, difficulty in judging time and distance, and in some cases occurrence of auditory and visual hallucination. Symptoms disappear when use of the mineral is discontinued. It is possible that bismuth can interfere with the absorption of zinc.

CADMIUM

Description

Cadmium is a toxic trace mineral that has many structural similarities to zinc. There is no biological function for this element in humans. Its toxic effects are kept under control in the body by the presence of zinc.

Refining processes disturb the important cadmium-zinc balance. In whole wheat, cadmium is present in proportion to zinc in a ratio of 1 to 120.

Cadmium is found primarily in refined foods such as flour, rice, and white sugar. It is present in the air as an industrial contaminant. In addition, soft water usually contains higher levels of cadmium than does hard water. Soft water, especially if it is acid, leaches cadmium from metal water pipes.

Absorption and Storage

The liver and kidneys are storage areas for both cadmium and zinc. The total body concentration of cadmium increases with age and varies in different areas of the world.

When a deficit of zinc occurs in the diet, the body may make it up by storing cadmium instead. If the daily intake of zinc is high, zinc will be stored and cadmium will be excreted.

Dosage and Toxicity

Daily intakes of cadmium have been estimated at 0.2 to 0.5 milligram, with considerable variation according to sources and types of food. Cadmium's toxic effects may stem from its being stored for use in the body in place of zinc when the proportion between the two metals is unfavorably out of balance. Zinc is a natural antagonist to cadmium. Cadmium can also interfere with the metabolism of copper.

Dr. Henry A. Shroeder, a trace mineral researcher, has developed a theory about cadmium being a major causative factor in hypertension and related heart ailments.[66] Testing his theories on rats because of their biological similarity to humans, Dr. Schroeder found that regular high doses of cadmium caused increased tension. When he stopped administering the cadmium to the rats, they returned to normotension.

In humans, the urine of hypertensive patients contains up to 40 percent more cadmium than does the urine of normotensive persons. These findings may lend credibility to the theory that excessive cadmium can directly lead to hypertension.[67]

Cadmium poisoning is a very subtle process. It deposits in the kidneys, causing kidney damage, and settles into arteries, raising the blood pressure and resulting in atherosclerosis.

Cigarette smoke contains substantial amounts of cadmium. One pack of cigarettes deposits 2 to 4 micrograms into the lungs of a smoker while some of the smoke passes into the air to be inhaled by smokers and nonsmokers alike. The cadmium in cigarette smoke can cause emphysema.

Deficiency Effects and Symptoms

No available information.

Beneficial Effect on Ailments

No available information.

CALCIUM

Description

Calcium is the most abundant mineral in the body. About 99 percent of the calcium in the body is deposited in the bones and teeth. One percent is involved in the blood-clotting process, in nerve and muscle stimulation, parathyroid hormone function, and metabolism of vitamin D.

The ratio of calcium to phosphorus in the bones is 2.5 to 1. To function properly, calcium must be accompanied by magnesium, phosphorus, and vitamins A, C, D, and very possibly vitamin E.

The major function of calcium is to act in cooperation with phosphorus to build and maintain bones and teeth. It is essential for healthy blood, eases insomnia, and helps regulate the heartbeat. An important calcium partner in cardiovascular health is magnesium.

In addition, calcium assists in the process of blood clotting and helps prevent the accumulation of too

[66]Prevention Magazine Staff, *Complete Book of Minerals for Health*, p. 413.

[67]Ibid., p. 277.

much acid or too much alkali in the blood. It also plays a part in muscle growth, muscle contraction, and nerve transmission. Calcium aids in the body's utilization of iron, helps activate several enzymes (catalysts important for metabolism), and helps regulate the passage of nutrients in and out of the cell walls.

Calcium is present in significant amounts in a very limited number of foods. Milk and dairy products are dependable sources. Those who are unable to use bone meal may use calcium gluconate or calcium lactate, natural derivatives of calcium which are even easier to absorb than is bone meal.

Absorption and Storage

Calcium absorption is very inefficient, and usually only 20 to 30 percent of ingested calcium is absorbed. About 100 to 200 milligrams are filtered through the blood and excreted in the urine. Another 125 to 180 milligrams are excreted in the feces. Some is lost in sweat. Absorption takes place in the duodenum and ceases in the lower part of the intestinal tract when the food content becomes alkaline.

Many other factors influence the actual amount of calcium absorbed. When in need, the body absorbs calcium more effectively; therefore the greater the need and the smaller the dietary supply, the more efficient the absorption. Absorption is also increased during periods of rapid growth.

Calcium needs acid for proper assimilation. If acid in some form is not present in the body, calcium is not dissolved and therefore cannot be used as needed by the body. Instead it can build up in tissues or joints as calcium deposits, leading to a variety of disturbances.

Calcium absorption also depends upon the presence of adequate amounts of vitamin D, which works with the parathyroid hormone to regulate the amount of calcium in the blood. In hyperparathyroidism, too much calcium is taken from the bones.

Phosphorus is needed in at least the same amount as calcium. The body uses calcium and phosphorus together to give firmness to bones. If excessive amounts of either mineral is taken, as in the typical American diet of too little calcium and too much phosphorus, that excess cannot be used efficiently.

Vitamins A and C are necessary for calcium absorp-

tion. Fat content in moderate amounts, moving slowly through the digestive tract, helps facilitate absorption.

Certain substances interfere with the absorption of calcium. When excessive amounts of fat combine with calcium, an insoluble compound is formed which cannot be absorbed. Oxalic acid, found in chocolate, spinach, and rhubarb, when combined with calcium makes another insoluble compound and may form into stones in the kidney or gallbladder. Large amounts of phytic acid, present in cereals and grains, may inhibit the absorption of calcium by the body. Other interfering factors include lack of exercise, excessive stress, excitement, depression, and too rapid a flow of food through the intestinal tract.

Dosage and Toxicity

The National Research Council recommends 800 milligrams as a daily calcium intake; since only 20 to 30 percent is absorbed, 800 milligrams would maintain the necessary balance. During pregnancy and lactation, this amount increases to 1200 milligrams. With age, it seems the requirement also increases because the rate of absorption is reduced. If the calcium intake is high, the magnesium levels also need to be high. Too little magnesium results in calcium accumulation in muscles, heart, and in the kidney, causing kidney stones.

A high intake of calcium and vitamin D is a potential source of hypercalcemia. This condition may result in excessive calcification of the bones and some tissues, such as the kidney's. Too much calcium can interfere with the functioning of the nervous and muscular systems. When an excess of calcium is added to blood plasma, coagulation does not take place. Animal studies show that too much calcium can decrease the body's absorption of zinc.

Deficiency Effects and Symptoms

One of the first signs of a calcium deficiency is a nervous affliction, tetany, characterized by muscle cramps and numbness and tingling in the arms and legs. A calcium deficiency can result in bone malformation, causing rickets in children and osteomalacia in adults. Another calcium deficiency ailment is osteoporosis, in which the bones become porous and fragile because calcium is withdrawn from the bones and other body areas faster than it is deposited in them.

Moderate cases of calcium deficiency may lead to cramps, joint pains, heart palpitation, slow pulse rates, tooth decay, insomnia, impaired growth, and excessive irritability of nerves and muscles. In extreme cases of deficiency, brittle or porous bone and tooth formation, slow blood clotting, or hemorrhaging may result.

Confinement, most commonly experienced in bed rest following an illness, depletes calcium from the bones and nitrogen from muscle tissue. To prevent this condition from becoming serious, gradual exercise should be undertaken as soon as possible.

Beneficial Effect on Ailments

Calcium has been successfully used in the treatment of osteoporosis. The hormones involved are stimulated by the concentration of calcium ions in the blood. Calcium is a natural tranquilizer and tends to calm the nerves.

Calcium has been beneficial in the treatment of cardiovascular disorders. In addition, calcium is a recognized aid for cramps in the feet or legs. It also helps patients suffering from "growing pains."

Calcium has been used in the treatment and prevention of sunburn. In addition to giving protection against effects of sun damage such as redness and subsequent peeling, it also protects against sun-caused skin cancers. Calcium helps the skin to remain healthy. Vitamin A and calcium are a good combination for protection of the skin. This combination can also be used as a neutralizing agent against the poison of a black widow spider or a bee sting.

Arthritis, structural rigidity often caused by depletion of bone calcium, can be helped with regular supplements of calcium. Early consumption of calcium may help prevent arthritis. Rheumatism can also be treated successfully with calcium therapy.

Problems of menopause, such as nervousness, irritability, insomnia, and headaches, have been overcome with administration of calcium, magnesium, and vitamin D. When there is not enough calcium in the body to be absorbed, the output of estrogen decreases. Calcium can help prevent premenstrual tension and menstrual cramps.

High intakes of calcium may relieve the symptoms commonly associated with aging. Some of the disorders include bone pain, backaches, insomnia, brittle teeth with cavities, and tremors of the fingers.

The parathyroid glands located in the neck help adjust the body's storage of calcium. If these glands are not functioning properly, calcium accumulation may occur. The remedy for this situation is to renew the proper function of the parathyroid glands rather than to cut down on calcium intake.

Calcium treatments have been used successfully in treating rickets in children and osteomalacia in adults. In addition, nephritis has been cleared up with administration of calcium and other nutrients. Tooth and gum disorders are also relieved by higher intakes of calcium in the diet. A high dietary intake of calcium may protect against the harmful effects of radioactive strontium 90.

CALCIUM MAY BE BENEFICIAL FOR THE FOLLOWING AILMENTS:

Body Member	Ailment
Blood/Circulatory system	Anemia
	Diabetes
	Hemophilia
	Pernicious anemia
Bones	Fracture
	Osteomalacia
	Osteoporosis
	Rickets
Bowel	Colitis
	Diarrhea
Brain/Nervous system	Dizziness
	Epilepsy
	Insomnia
	Mental illness
	Parkinson's disease
Ear	Ménière's syndrome
Eye	Cataracts
Head	Fever
Heart	Arteriosclerosis
	Atherosclerosis
	Hypertension
Intestine	Celiac disease
	Constipation
	Hemorrhoids
	Worms
Joints	Arthritis

Body Member	Ailment
Kidney	Nephritis
Leg	Leg cramp
Lungs/Respiratory system	Allergies
	Common cold
	Tuberculosis
Muscles	General muscle cramps
	Tetany
Nails	Nail problems
Skin	Acne
Stomach	Stomach ulcer (peptic)
Teeth/Gums	Pyorrhea
	Tooth and gum disorders
General	Aging
	Fever
	Overweight and obesity
	Sunburn

CHLORINE (CHLORIDE)

Description

Chlorine is an essential mineral, occurring in the body mainly in compound form with sodium or potassium. It is widely distributed throughout the body in the form of chloride in amounts less than 15 percent of the total body weight. Chlorine compounds such as sodium chloride, or salt, are found primarily within the cells.

Chlorine helps regulate the correct balance of acid and alkali in the blood and maintains pressure that causes fluids to pass in and out of cell membranes until the concentration of dissolved particles is equalized on both sides. It stimulates production of hydrochloric acid, an enzymatic juice needed in the stomach for digestion of protein and rough, fibrous foods.

Chlorine stimulates the liver to function as a filter for wastes and helps clean toxic waste products out of the system. It aids in keeping joints and tendons in youthful shape, and it helps to distribute hormones.

Chlorine in the diet is provided by sodium chloride, or table salt. Some form of chlorine is also found in kelp, dulse, rye flour, ripe olives, sea greens, and most foods. Chlorine is sometimes added to water for purification purposes because it destroys waterborne diseases such as typhoid and hepatitis.

Absorption and Storage

Chlorine is absorbed in the intestine and excreted through urination and perspiration. The highest body concentrations are stored in the cerebrospinal fluid and in the secretions of the gastrointestinal tract. Muscle and nerve tissues are relatively low in chloride. Excess chlorine is excreted; additional loss may be caused by conditions such as vomiting, diarrhea, or sweating.

There has been much controversy over the relative merits of adding chlorine to drinking water supplies because it is a highly reactive chemical and may join with inorganic minerals and other chemicals to form possibly harmful substances. It is known that chlorine in the drinking water destroys vitamin E. It also destroys many of the intestinal flora that help in the digestion of food.

Dosage and Toxicity

There is no Recommended Dietary Allowance for chlorine because the average person's salt intake is high and usually provides between 3 and 9 grams daily. Diets sufficient in sodium and potassium provide adequate chlorine. Daily intake of 14 to 28 grams of salt is considered excessive.[68]

Deficiency Effects and Symptoms

A deficiency of chlorine can cause hair and tooth loss, poor muscular contraction, and impaired digestion.

Beneficial Effect on Aliments

Chlorine is beneficial in treating diarrhea and vomiting.

CHLORINE MAY BE BENEFICIAL FOR THE FOLLOWING AILMENTS:

Body Member	Ailment
Bowel	Diarrhea
Stomach	Vomiting

[68]National Academy of Sciences, *Toxicants Occurring Naturally in Foods*, p. 30.

CHROMIUM

Description

Chromium is an essential mineral found in concentrations of 20 parts of chromium per 1 billion parts of blood. It has functions in both animal and human nutrition. Organic chromium is an active ingredient of a substance called GTF (glucose tolerance factor); niacin and amino acids complete the formula.

Chromium stimulates the activity of enzymes involved in the metabolism of glucose for energy and the synthesis of fatty acids and cholesterol. Chromium appears to increase the effectiveness of insulin and its ability to handle glucose, preventing hypoglycemia (too much insulin) or diabetes (too little insulin). In the blood it competes with iron in the transport of protein. Chromium may also be involved in the synthesis of protein through its binding action with RNA molecules.

Measuring chromium content of food can be misleading because of the different forms in which it occurs and their varying absorption rate by the body. Inorganic chromium is only 1 percent or less absorbable. The chromium in eggs is in a form that can not be completely utilized. The chromium-containing foods most biologically available to the body are brewer's yeast (the best), liver, beef, whole-wheat bread, beets and beet sugar molasses, and mushrooms.

Absorption and Storage

Chromium is difficult to absorb. Only about 3 percent of dietary chromium is retained in the body. The mineral is stored primarily in the spleen, kidneys, and testes; small amounts are also stored in the heart, pancreas, lungs, and brain. Chromium has been found in some enzymes and in RNA. Excretion occurs mainly through urination, with minor amounts lost in the feces. The amount of chromium stored in the body decreases with age.

Dosage and Toxicity

There is no Recommended Dietary Allowance for chromium. The daily chromium intake of humans is estimated to range from 80 to 100 micrograms.

Deficiency Effects and Symptoms

Even a very slight chromium deficiency will have serious effects on the body. Tests indicate systematic deficiency of chromium to be common in the United States, although it rarely occurs in other countries. Americans tend to be deficient because their soil does not contain an adequate supply and thus chromium cannot be absorbed by the crops or reach the water supply. The refining of foods is another probable cause of chromium loss.

A chromium deficiency may be a factor that will upset the function of insulin and result in depressed growth rates and severe glucose intolerance in diabetics. It is also believed that the interaction of chromium and insulin is not limited to glucose metabolism but also applies to amino acid metabolism. Chromium may inhibit the formation of aortic plaques, and a deficiency may contribute to atherosclerosis.

Pregnant women are particularily susceptible to chromium deficiency because the fetus uses so much. Postoperative patients receiving glucose intravenously for nourishment need extra chromium. Studies have shown that blood chromium drops greatly when 60 grams of glucose are administered. If the patient also has a virus infection, the blood chromium drops even more.[69]

Beneficial Effect on Ailments

Chromium helps to regulate sugar levels in the blood. Infants suffering from kwashiorkor have benefited from oral administration of chromium. Schizophrenics need extra niacin and have impaired glucose tolerance; therefore it is possible they may greatly benefit from chromium supplementation, creating the formation of more GTF.

CHROMIMUM MAY BE BENEFICIAL FOR THE FOLLOWING AILMENTS:

Body Member	Ailment
Blood/Circulatory system	Diabetes
General	Heart disease
	Hypoglycemia
	Kwashiorkor

[69]Pfeiffer, *Mental and Elemental Nutrients*, p. 292.

COBALT

Description

Cobalt is considered an essential mineral and is an integral part of vitamin B_{12}, or cobalamin. Vitamin B_{12} and cobalt are so closely connected that the two terms can be used interchangeably.

Cobalt activates a number of enzymes in the body. It is necessary for normal functioning and maintenance of red blood cells as well as all other body cells.

The body does not have the ability to synthesize cobalt and must depend on animal sources for an adequate supply of this nutrient. For this reason, strict vegetarians are more susceptible to cobalt deficiency than are meat eaters. The best sources are meats, especially liver and kidney, oysters, clams, and milk. Cobalt is present in ocean and sea vegetation but is lacking in almost all land green foods, although cobalt-enriched soil can yield minute amounts.

Absorption and Storage

Cobalt is not easily assimilated, and most of it passes through the intestinal tract unabsorbed. Most of what is absorbed is excreted in the urine after being used by the body. Cobalt is stored in the red blood cells and plasma; some storage occurs also in the liver, kidneys, pancreas, and spleen.

Dosage and Toxicity

There is no Recommended Dietary Allowance for cobalt because the dietary need for it is low and can be supplied in protein foods. The average daily intake of cobalt is 5 to 8 micrograms.

There is evidence that high intakes of cobalt may result in an enlarged thyroid gland. Reduction in the cobalt intake should allow an enlarged thyroid to return to normal size.

In animal tests, excessive cobalt results in too many blood cells, a condition called polycythemia. Less severe symptoms include paleness, fatigue, diarrhea, heart palpitations, and numbness in fingers and toes. It has been found that high-quality protein in the diet helps to protect against the toxic effects of cobalt.

Deficiency Effects and Symptoms

A deficiency of cobalt may be resonsible for the symptoms of pernicious anemia and a slow rate of growth. If cobalt deficiency is not treated, permanent nervous disorders may result.

Beneficial Effect on Ailments

Therapeutic doses of cobalt have been beneficial in the treatment of pernicious anemia. This action is attributed to cobalt's importance as a builder of the red blood cells.

COBALT MAY BE BENEFICIAL FOR THE FOLLOWING AILMENTS:

Body Member	Ailment
Blood/Circulatory system	Pernicious anemia

COPPER

Description

Copper is a trace mineral found in all body tissues. Copper assists in the formation of hemoglobin and red blood cells by facilitating iron absorption.

Copper is present in many enzymes that break down or build up body tissue. It aids in the conversion of the amino acid tyrosine into a dark pigment that colors the hair and skin. It is also involved in protein metabolism and in healing processes. Copper is required for the synthesis of phospholipids, substances essential in the formation of the protective myelin sheaths surrounding nerve fibers. Copper helps the body to oxidize vitamin C and works with this vitamin in the formation of elastin, a chief component of the elastic muscle fibers throughout the body. Copper is necessary for proper bone formation and maintenance. It is also necessary for the production of RNA.

Among the best food sources of copper are liver, whole-grain products, almonds, green leafy vegetables, and dried legumes. The amounts vary in plant sources, according to the mineral content in the soil in which they were grown. Most seafoods are also good sources of copper.

Absorption and Storage

Approximately 30 percent of ingested copper is used by the body; absorption takes place in the stomach and upper intestine. The copper moves from the intestine into the bloodstream 15 minutes after ingestion. Most of the dietary copper is excreted in the feces and bile, with very little lost in the urine.

Copper is stored in the tissues; highest concentrations of copper are in the liver, kidneys, heart, and brain. Bones and muscles have lower concentrations of copper, but because of their mass they contain over 50 percent of the total copper in the body.

Dosage and Toxicity

The National Research Council recommends a daily dietary intake of 2 milligrams of copper for adults. The average person ingests 2.5 to 5.0 milligrams per day. Drinking water may be a major source of copper, which leaches from copper piping.

The possibility of copper toxicity occurs with Wilson's disease, a rare genetic disorder that results from abnormal copper metabolism, bringing about excess copper retention in the liver, brain, kidney, and corneas of the eyes.[70] Too much copper in the body can result in serious physical and mental illness. Serum copper levels increase with the use of birth control pills. High levels are found in patients who have heart attacks, high blood pressure, and in those who smoke.

Copper may also be a factor in paranoid and hallucinatory schizophrenia, hypertension, stuttering, autism, childhood hyperactivity, toxemia of pregnancy, premenstrual tension, depression, insomnia, senility, and functional hypoglycemia.[71]

Studies of pregnant women indicate that high copper levels cause a decrease in body iron and a deficiency of molybdenum. Certain anemia not helped by iron may be an indication of elevated copper levels.

Serum copper, elevated by estrogens, rises progressively during pregnancy. After delivery, it takes 2 to 3 months before the copper level lowers to an acceptable amount. This high level may cause the depression and psychosis that women often experience after giving birth.

In studies using rats, high levels of copper increased

[70]Guthrie, *Introductory Nutrition,* p. 165.
[71]Pfeiffer, *Mental and Elemental Nutrients,* p. 337.

liver and brain copper and caused some deaths. The function of a zinc-containing enzyme was impaired. The adrenal glands increased in weight, an indication of stress.

Supplemental zinc and manganese in a ratio of 20 to 1 have proved to increase copper excretion via the urine. In studies on sheep, molybdenum prevents copper absorption.

Deficiency Effects and Symptoms

Although copper deficiencies are relatively unknown, low blood levels of copper have been noted in children with iron-deficiency anemia, edema, and kwashiorkor. Symptoms of deficiency include general weakness, impaired respiration, and skin sores. Premature infants and patients receiving intravenous feeding have also shown a deficiency.

Beneficial Effect on Ailments

Copper works with iron to form hemoglobin, thereby helping in the treatment of anemia. Copper is beneficial in the prevention and treatment of edema and kwashiorkor in children.

COPPER MAY BE BENEFICIAL FOR THE FOLLOWING AILMENTS:

Body Member	Ailment
Blood/Circulatory system	Anemia
	Leukemia
Bones	Osteoporosis
Hair	Baldness
Skin	Bedsores
General	Edema

FLUORINE (FLUORIDES)

Description

Fluorine is an essential trace mineral that is present in minute amounts in nearly every human tissue but is found primarily in the skeleton and teeth. Fluorine occurs in the body in compounds called fluorides. There are two types of fluorides: sodium fluoride is added to drinking water and is not the same as calcium fluoride, which is found in nature.

Recent research indicates that fluorine increases the deposition of calcium, thereby strengthening the bones. Fluorine also helps to reduce the formation of acid in the mouth caused by carbohydrates, thereby reducing the likelihood of decayed tooth enamel. Although traces of fluorine are beneficial to the body, excessive amounts are definitely harmful. Fluorine can destroy the enzyme phosphatase, which is vital to many body processes including the metabolism of vitamins. Fluorine inhibits the activities of other important enzymes and appears to be especially antagonistic toward brain tissues.

Fluoridated water supplies are by far the most common source of this mineral, although this form (sodium fluoride) may be toxic. Toxic levels occur when the content of fluorine in drinking water exceeds 2 parts per million. Calcium is an antidote for fluoride poisoning. Other rich sources of fluorine include seafoods, cheese, meat, and tea. The fluorine content in plant foods varies according to environmental conditions such as type of soil, intensity of prevailing winds, and use of fertilizers and sprays that contain fluorine.

Absorption and Storage

Fluorine is absorbed primarily in the intestine, although some may be taken up by the stomach. About 90 percent of ingested fluorine appears in the bloodstream. Half of this is excreted in the urine, and the other half is readily absorbed by the teeth and bones.

Substances interfering with absorption include aluminum salts of fluorine and insoluble calcium.

Dosage and Toxicity

An average diet will provide 0.25 to 0.35 milligram of fluorine daily. In addition, the average adult may ingest 1.0 to 1.5 milligrams from drinking and cooking water containing 1 part per million (ppm) of fluorine. Dental fluorosis may occur at fluoride concentrations of 2 to 8 ppm; osteosclerosis, at 8 to 20 ppm. Higher levels can depress growth, cause calcification of the ligaments and tendons, and bring about degenerative changes in the kidneys, liver, adrenal glands, heart, central nervous system, and finally the reproductive organs. Fatal poisoning can occur at 50 ppm, or 2500

times the recommended level.[72] There are some areas in the United States where fluorine levels in the water are high and tooth mottling (enamel discoloration) is epidemic, and there are other areas where fluorine is not added to the water and dental decay is high.

Dr. Ionel Rapaport, a University of Wisconsin researcher, suggests that there is a direct relationship between the incidence of mongolism and fluoridated drinking water.[73] Higher than average incidences of mongolism have been noted in areas where mottled teeth indicate an excess concentration of fluorides in the water.[74]

Deficiency Effects and Symptoms

A diet deficient in fluorine may lead to poor tooth development and subsequent dental caries. Fluorine deficiencies are unusual in the American diet.

Beneficial Effect on Ailments

Fluorides have been used in the treatment and prevention of osteoporosis and dental caries. They have also been used to stop the loss of hearing that occurs in otosclerosis.

FLUORINE MAY BE BENEFICIAL FOR THE FOLLOWING AILMENTS:

Body Member	Ailment
Bones	Osteoporosis
Teeth/Gums	Tooth decay
	Tooth and gum disorders

IODINE (IODIDE)

Description

Iodine is a trace mineral most of which is converted into iodide in the body. Iodine aids in the development and functioning of the thyroid gland and is an integral part of thyroxine, a principal hormone produced by the thyroid gland. It is estimated that the body contains 25 milligrams of iodine, about 0.0004 percent of the total weight.

[72]Guthrie, *Introductory Nutrition*, p. 171.
[73]Prevention Magazine Staff, *Complete Book of Minerals for Health*, pp. 367–370.
[74]Ibid.

Iodine plays an important role in regulating the body's production of energy, promotes growth and development, and stimulates the rate of metabolism, helping the body burn excess fat. Mentality; speech; and the condition of hair, nails, skin, and teeth are dependent upon a well-functioning thyroid gland. The conversion of carotene to vitamin A, the synthesis of protein by ribosomes, the absorption of carbohydrates from the intestine all work more efficiently when thyroxine production is normal. The synthesis of cholesterol is stimulated by thyroxine levels.

Both types of sea life, plant and animal, absorb iodine from seawater and are excellent sources of this mineral. Mushrooms and Irish moss are good sources, too, but only if they are grown in soil rich in iodine.

Absorption and Storage

Iodine is readily absorbed from the gastrointestinal tract and is transported via the bloodstream to the thyroid gland, where it is oxidized and converted to thyroxine. About 30 percent of the iodide in the blood is absorbed by the thyroid gland; the rest is absorbed by the kidneys and excreted in the urine.

Dosage and Toxicity

The National Research Council has suggested that an intake of 1 microgram of iodine per kilogram of body weight is adequate for most adults. They recommend a daily intake of 150 micrograms for men and 150 micrograms for women, 175 micrograms during pregnancy, and 200 micrograms during lactation.

There have been no reported cases of toxicity resulting from too much iodine as it naturally occurs in food or water. However, iodine prepared as a drug or medicine must be carefully prescribed, because an overdose can be serious.[75] Sudden large doses of iodine administered to humans with a normal thyroid may impair the synthesis of thyroid homones. For individuals on low-salt therapeutic diets, iodine supplements may be desirable.

Deficiency Effects and Symptoms

An iodine deficiency results in simple goiter, characterized by thyroid enlargement and hypothyroidism (an

[75]Ibid., p. 215.

abnormally low rate of secretion of thyroid hormones, including thyroxine).

Iodine deficiency may lead to hardening of the arteries, obesity, sluggish metabolism, slowed mental reactions, dry hair, rapid pulse, heart palpitation, tremor, nervousness, restlessness, and irritability. An iodine deficiency may also result in cretinism, which is a congenital disease characterized by physical and mental retardation in children born to mothers who have had a limited iodine intake during adolescence and pregnancy. Polio has also been associated with iodine deficiency. The higher rate of occurrence of polio cases in the summer may be caused in part by higher losses of iodine through perspiration.

An iodine deficiency may be caused by certain compounds present in some raw foods, such as cabbage and nuts, which may interfere with the utilization of iodine in thyroid-hormone production. This will not occur unless excessive amounts of these raw foods are eaten and the intake of iodine is low to begin with.

Beneficial Effect on Ailments

Iodine therapy has been used successfully in the treatment and prevention of simple goiter.

Hardening of the arteries occurs when a disturbance in normal fat metabolism allows cholesterol to collect in the arteries instead of being used or expelled. Iodine is needed to prevent this metabolic malfunction. Sufficient dietary iodine will also reduce the danger of radioactive iodine collecting in the thyroid gland.

Iodine is beneficial to children suffering from cretinism, if treatment is started soon after birth. Many of the symptoms are reversible, but if conditions persist beyond childbirth or possibly early infancy, the mental and physical retardation will be permanent.

IODINE MAY BE BENEFICIAL FOR THE FOLLOWING AILMENTS:

Body Member	Ailment
Blood/Circulatory system	Angina pectoris
Hair	Hair problems
Heart	Arteriosclerosis
	Atherosclerosis
Joints	Arthritis
Thyroid	Goiter
	Hyperthyroidism
	Hypothyroidism

Body Member	Ailment
General	Cretinism
	Loss of physical and mental vigor

IRON

Description

Iron is a mineral concentrate in the blood which is present in every living cell. All iron exists in the body combined with protein.

The major function of iron is to combine with protein and copper in making hemoglobin, the coloring matter of red blood cells. Hemoglobin transports oxygen in the blood from the lungs to the tissues, which need oxygen to maintain the basic life functions. Thus iron builds up the quality of the blood and increases resistance to stress and disease. Iron is also necessary for the formation of myoglobin, which is found only in muscle tissue. Myoglobin is also a transporter of oxygen; it supplies oxygen to the muscle cells for use in the chemical reaction that results in muscle contraction.

Iron is present in enzymes that promote protein metabolism, and it works with other nutrients to improve respiratory action. Calcium and copper must be present for iron to function properly.

The best source of dietary iron is liver, with oysters, heart, lean meat, and tongue as second choices. Leafy green vegetables, whole grains, dried fruits, legumes, and molasses are rich in iron.

Absorption and Storage

The body can utilize either ferric or ferrous iron, but evidence indicates that naturally occurring ferrous iron is used more efficiently and that most iron is reduced to ferrous iron before being absorbed. It is absorbed from food in regulated amounts into the blood and bone marrow. Ninety percent of the iron ingested never reaches the blood and remains unabsorbed.

Absorption occurs in the upper part of the small intestines. Iron is usually absorbed within 4 hours after ingestion; from 2 to 4 percent of the iron found in the food is used by the body. It is primarily stored in the liver, spleen, bone marrow, and blood.

The iron in the body is normally used efficiently. It is neither used up nor destroyed, but it is conserved to be used repeatedly. Only very small amounts are normally excreted from the body. Iron is excreted in small amounts in the urine, feces, during menstruation, and through perspiration and exfoliation of the skin.

There are many factors that influence the absorption of iron. Ascorbic acid enhances absorption by helping reduce ferric to ferrous iron. The iron found in animal protein is more readily absorbed than the iron in vegetables. The degree of gastric acidity regulates the solubility and availability of the iron in food.

The balance of calcium, phosphorus, and iron is very important. Excess phosphorus hinders iron absorption, although if calcium is present in sufficient amounts, it will combine with the phosphates and free the iron for use. In addition, the lack of hydrochloric acid; the administration of alkalis; a high intake of cellulose, coffee, and tea; the presence of insoluble iron complexes (phytates, oxalates, and phosphates); and increased intestinal mobility all interfere with iron absorption.

Dosage and Toxicity

The National Research Council suggests a daily iron intake of 18 milligrams for women and 10 milligrams for men. The need for iron increases during menstruation, hemorrhage, periods of rapid growth, or whenever there is a loss of blood. Additional iron is required during pregnancy, when the developing fetus builds up its own reserve supply of iron in the liver.

A toxic level of iron may occur in an individual due to a genetic error of metabolism, due to blood transfusion, due to a prolonged oral intake of iron, in persons who consume large amounts of red wine containing iron, and in those addicted to certain iron tonics.

Excessive deposits of iron may result from such conditions as cirrhosis of the liver, diabetes, pancreas insufficiency, the presence of other diseases, hemolytic or aplastic anemia, early hepatitis, and a vegetarian diet.

Too much iron, accumulating over the years, occurs often in older men. Iron overload can result in siderosis, damage to the heart, liver, and pancreas. Studies have shown that arthritic patients insufficiently metabolize iron, possibly resulting in deposition of the mineral in the joints.

These diseases caused by iron toxicity are due to the inability of the digestive tract to eliminate excess iron. Iron deposited in body tissues eventually turns the skin a grayish color. Symptoms of iron overload include headache, shortness of breath, fatigue, dizziness, and loss of weight.

Deficiency Effects and Symptoms

The most common deficiency of iron is iron-deficiency anemia (hypochromic anemia), in which the amount of hemoglobin in the red blood cells is reduced and the cells consequently become smaller. As in other forms of anemia, iron-deficiency anemia reduces the oxygen-carrying capacity of the blood, resulting in pale skin and abnormal fatigue. Symptoms of anemia may include constipation, lusterless, brittle nails, and difficult breathing.

A deficiency of B_6 and zinc can cause blood disorders that mimic an iron deficiency. Measuring serum iron, not the hemoglobin, is the most efficient way to diagnose an iron deficiency.

Hemorrhagic anemia, marked by internal hemorrhaging, may not be detected for some time, especially when associated with the bleeding that may occur in peptic ulcers. Excessive donation of blood may cause this type of anemia.

Infections and peptic ulcers may also lead to anemia.

Beneficial Effect on Ailments

When iron-deficiency anemia, with its symptoms of pallor, easy fatigue, and decreased resistance to disease, is diagnosed, a diet high in iron-rich foods with a concurrent intake of vitamin C will speed up the restoration of hemoglobin levels to normal.

Iron is the most important mineral for the prevention of anemia during menstruation. Iron may also be beneficial in the treatment of leukemia and colitis.

IRON MAY BE BENEFICIAL FOR THE FOLLOWING AILMENTS:

Body Member	Ailment
Blood/Circulatory system	Anemia
	Diabetes
	Leukemia
	Menstruation
	Pernicious anemia
Bowel	Colitis
	Diarrhea
Brain/Nervous system	Alcoholism
Intestine	Celiac disease
	Colitis
	Worms
Joint	Gout
Kidney	Nephritis
Lungs/Respiratory system	Tuberculosis
Nails	Nail problems
Reproductive system	Menstruation
	Pregnancy
Skin	Scurvy
	Ulcers
Stomach	Gastritis
	Stomach ulcer (peptic)
Teeth/Gums	Tooth and gum disorders
General	Aging
	Alcoholism
	Bruises
	Cancer
	Pregnancy

LEAD

Description

Lead is a highly toxic trace mineral. In recent years human exposure to lead poisoning has changed in origin and probably has increased in magnitude.[76]

The human body can tolerate only 1 to 2 milligrams (about 0.00003 of an ounce) of lead without suffering toxic effects.[77] Two pounds of food contaminated by only 1 part per million of lead contain almost a milligram of lead, so there is not a very wide margin of safety.

[76]National Academy of Sciences, *Toxicants Occurring Naturally in Foods*, p. 61.
[77]Prevention Magazine Staff, *Complete Book of Minerals for Health*, p. 446.

Absorption and Storage

Lead contained in food is poorly absorbed and is excreted mainly in the feces. Lead may enter the body via the skin and the gastrointestinal tract. The lead that is absorbed enters the blood and is stored in the bones and the soft tissues, including the liver. Up to certain levels of consumption, lead excretion keeps pace with ingestion so that retention is negligible.

Dosage and Toxicity

Critical levels of intake, above which significant lead retention occurs, cannot be quoted with any accuracy.[78] Toxic intake can come from consumption of moonshine whiskey and foods stored in lead-glazed earthenware pottery that has been fired at too low a temperature, preventing sufficient fixation of the lead and allowing it to leach out.

Sources of poisoning include drinking water that is soft and acidic and erodes lead from lead piping, food from lead-lined containers, lead-based paint, cosmetics, cigarettes (because of the lead-containing insecticide applied to tobacco), the burning of coal, peeling lead-based paint or plaster and lead-based paint coating pencils often chewed on by children, and motor vehicle exhausts. The accumulation of lead in the body from motor vehicle exhausts is caused directly by inhalation and indirectly through deposition in the soil and plants along highways and in urban areas.

Acute lead toxicity is manifested in abdominal colic, encephalopathy (dysfunction of the brain), myelopathy (any pathological condition of the spinal cord), and anemia. Lead is able to cause abnormal brain function by competing with and replacing other vital minerals, such as zinc, iron, and copper, which regulate mental processes. Acute lead poisoning attacks the central nervous system and is a possible cause of hyperactivity in children.[79] Lead poisoning in children may cause learning disorders, autism, and epilepsy.

A definite relationship has been established between lead ingested from soft drinking water and mental retardation in children. The lead from drinking water ingested by pregnant women can cross the placenta and settle into the brain of the fetus.

[78]National Academy of Sciences, *Toxicants Occurring Naturally in Foods,* pp. 61–62.
[79]"Problem Children, Lead and What to Do about It," *Prevention,* October 1973, p. 87.

Lead intoxication can result from a condition in children called pica, the eating of lead-containing dirt, paper, and paint. Depression is a symptom of chronic lead poisoning, as are headaches, restlessness, irritability, inability to concentrate, impairment of memory, insomnia, hallucination, muscular aches, nausea, and indigestion. Consumption of alcohol allows higher levels of lead to settle in soft tissues, including the brain.

The usual treatment for lead poisoning during acute stages consists of a diet high in calcium plus injections of a calcium chloride solution and administration of vitamin D. Sufficient calcium prevents the accumulation of lead in the body by reducing its absorption from the intestinal tract. Too little calcium in the body results in higher levels of lead in the blood, bone, and soft tissues.

Vitamin C at doses up to 6 grams per day can help lead excretion. The amino acids cysteine and methionine and supplementation of all essential minerals also help.

An effective way that may prevent lead poisoning is to include a small amount of algin in the daily diet. Algin is a nonnutritive substance found in Pacific kelp, which is sometimes used as a thickening agent in the preparation of various foods. It attaches itself to any lead that is present and carries it harmlessly out of the system.[80]

Deficiency Effects and Symptoms

No available information.

Beneficial Effect on Ailments

No available information.

MAGNESIUM

Description

Magnesium is an essential mineral that accounts for about 0.05 percent of the body's total weight. Nearly 70 percent of the body's supply is located in the bones together with calcium and phosphorus, while 30 percent is found in the soft tissues and body fluids.

[80]Ibid.

Magnesium is involved in many essential metabolic processes. Most magnesium is found inside the cell, where it activates enzymes necessary for the metabolism of carbohydrates and amino acids. By countering the stimulative effect of calcium, magnesium plays an important role in neuromuscular contractions. It also helps regulate the acid-alkaline balance in the body.

Magnesium helps promote absorption and metabolism of other minerals, such as calcium, phosphorus, sodium, and potassium. It also helps utilize the B complex and vitamins C and E in the body. It aids during bone growth and is necessary for proper functioning of the nerves and muscles, including those of the heart. Evidence suggests that magnesium is associated with the regulation of body temperature. Sufficient amounts of magnesium are needed in the conversion of blood sugar into energy.

Magnesium appears to be widely distributed in foods, being found chiefly in fresh green vegetables, where it is an essential element of chlorophyll. Other excellent sources include raw, unmilled wheat germ, soybeans, milk, whole grains, seafoods, figs, corn, apples, and oil-rich seeds and nuts, especially almonds.

Absorption and Storage

Nearly 50 percent of the average daily intake of magnesium is absorbed in the small intestine. The rate of absorption is influenced by the parathyroid hormones, the rate of water absorption, and the amounts of calcium, phosphate, and lactose (milk sugar) in the body. Vitamin D is necessary for the proper utilization of magnesium. When the intake of magnesium is low, the rate of absorption may be as high as 75 percent; when the intake is high, the rate of absorption may be as low as 25 percent.

The adrenal gland secretes a hormone called aldosterone, which helps to regulate the rate of magnesium excretion through the kidneys. Losses tend to increase with the use of diuretics and with the consumption of alcohol.

Dosage and Toxicity

The National Research Council recommends a daily magnesium intake of 350 milligrams for the adult male and 300 milligrams for the adult female. The amount increases to 450 milligrams during pregnancy and lactation.[81] It is estimated that the typical American diet provides 120 milligrams per 1000 kilocalories, a level that will barely provide the recommended daily intake.

Evidence suggests that the balance between calcium and magnesium is especially important. If calcium consumption is high, magnesium intake needs to be high also. The amounts of protein, phosphorus, and vitamin D in the diet also influence the magnesium requirement. The need for magnesium is increased when blood cholesterol levels are high and when consumption of protein is high.

Magnesium toxicity (hypermagnesia) is rare but can occur when urinary excretion is unusually decreased, when there is a considerable increase in absorption of the mineral, and sometimes after intramuscular injection. Certain bone tumors and cancers can raise the magnesium level in the body. Toxic symtoms can result in depression of the central nervous system and in extreme cases, death.[82]

Deficiency Effects and Symptoms

Magnesium deficiency can easily occur. The mineral is refined out of many foods during processing. The cooking of food removes magnesium. Oxalic acid, found in foods like spinach, and phytic acid, found in cereals, form salts binding magnesium in the body.

Magnesium deficiency can occur in patients with diabetes, pancreatitis, chronic alcoholism, kwashiorkor, cirrhosis of the liver, arteriosclerosis, kidney malfunction, a high-carbohydrate diet, or severe malabsorption as caused by chronic diarrhea or vomiting. Some hormones when used as drugs can upset metabolism and cause local deficiencies.

Magnesium deficiency is thought to be closely related to coronary heart disease.[83] An inadequate supply of this mineral may result in the formation of clots in the heart and brain and may contribute to calcium deposits in the kidneys, blood vessels, and heart.

Symptoms of magnesium deficiency may include apprehensiveness, muscle twitch, tremors, confusion, irregular heart rhythm, depression, irritability, and disorientation.

[81]Krause and Hunscher, *Food, Nutrition and Diet Therapy*, p. 109.
[82]Pfeiffer, *Mental and Elemental Nutrients*, p. 278.
[83]Williams, *Nutrition against Disease*, p. 80.

Studies have shown that painful uterine contractions experienced by women toward the end of pregnancy could result from a deficiency of magnesium.[84]

Beneficial Effect on Ailments

Magnesium is vital in helping prevent heart attacks and severe coronary thrombosis. Magnesium seems to be important in controlling the manner in which electrical charges are utilized by the body to induce the passage of nutrients in and out of cells. It has been successfully used to treat prostate troubles, polio, and depression. It has also proved beneficial in the treatment of neuromuscular disorders, nervousness, tantrums, sensitivity to noise, and hand tremor.

In alcoholics, the magnesium levels in the blood and muscles are low. Magnesium treatment helps the body retain magnesium and often helps control delirium tremens.

Magnesium helps to protect the accumulation of calcium deposits in the urinary tract. It makes the calcium and phosphorus soluble in the urine and prevents them from turning into hard stones. Adequate amounts of magnesium can help reduce blood cholesterol and help keep the arteries healthy.

Magnesium, not calcium, helps form the kind of hard tooth enamel that resists decay. No matter how much calcium is ingested, only a soft enamel will be formed unless magnesium is present.

Magnesium therapy has been effective in treating diarrhea, vomiting, nervousness, and kwashiorkor. Since magnesium works to preserve the health of the nervous system, it has been successfully used in controlling convulsions in pregnant women and epileptic patients. Because magnesium is very alkaline, it acts as an antacid and can be used in place of over-the-counter antacid compounds.

Human Tests

1. Magnesium and Kidney Stones. A thirty-three-year-old pregnant woman had passed at least eight to twelve stones during previous pregnancies. She was

[84]Carl Pfeiffer, *Mental and Elemental Nutrients,* p. 279.

given 500 to 1500 milligrams of magnesium daily over a period of 6 weeks.

Results. The pregnancy during which she was given the oral dose of magnesium was the first one during which she did not pass a single kidney stone. (F. Peter Kohler and Charles A. W. Uhle, *Journal of Urology,* November 1966, as reported in Rodale, *Complete Book of Minerals for Health,* p. 78.)

MAGNESIUM MAY BE BENEFICIAL FOR THE FOLLOWING AILMENTS:

Body Member	Ailment
Blood/Circulatory system	Arteriosclerosis
	Atherosclerosis
	Cholesterol level, high
	Diabetes
	Hypertension
Bones	Fracture
	Osteoporosis
	Rickets
Bowel	Colitis
	Diarrhea
Brain/Nervous system	Alcoholism
	Epilepsy
	Mental illness
	Multiple sclerosis
	Nervousness
	Neuritis
	Parkinson's disease
Heart	Arteriosclerosis
	Atherosclerosis
	Hypertension
Intestine	Celiac disease
Joint	Arthritis
Kidney	Kidney stones (renal calculi)
	Nephritis
Leg	Leg cramp
Muscles	Muscular excitability
Skin	Psoriasis
Stomach	Vomiting
General	Alcoholism
	Backache
	Kwashiorkor
	Overweight and obesity

MANGANESE

Description

Manganese is a trace mineral and plays a role in activating numerous enzymes. Manganese aids in the utilization of choline and is an activator of enzymes that are necessary for utilization of biotin, thiamine, and ascorbic acid. Manganese is a catalyst in the synthesis of fatty acids and cholesterol. It also plays a part in protein, carbohydrate, and fat production; is necessary for normal skeletal development; and may be important for the formation of blood. Manganese is important for the production of milk and the formation of urea, a part of the urine. It helps maintain sex-hormone production. Manganese also helps nourish the nerves and brain. It is essential for the formation of thyroxin, a constituent of the thyroid gland.

Whole-grain cereals, egg yolks, nuts, seeds, and green vegetables are among the better sources of manganese, but the content will vary depending upon the amount present in the soil. A good portion of manganese is lost in the processing and milling of foods.

Absorption and Storage

Manganese is absorbed while in the small intestinal tract. Normally people excrete about 4 milligrams of manganese each day. This amount needs to be replaced.

Large intakes of calcium and phosphorus in the diet will depress the rate of absorption. Excretion of manganese occurs via the feces, much of it in the form of choline complex in the bile.

The adult body contains only 10 to 20 milligrams of manganese. The highest concentrations of it are in the kidney, bones, liver, pancreas, and pituitary gland.

Dosage and Toxicity

The National Research Council sets the adequate dietary intake at 2.5 to 5 milligrams for adults. The average daily diet contains approximately 4 milligrams.[85]

A high calcium and phosphorus intake will increase the need for manganese. Very high dosages of manganese result in reduced storage and utilization of iron.

Industrial workers frequently exposed to manganese dust may absorb enough of the metal in the respiratory tract to develop toxic symptoms.[86] Weakness, psychological and motor difficulties, irritability, and impotency can result from high tissue levels of manganese.

Manganese given to older schizophrenic patients to lower copper levels sometimes results in a rise in blood pressure. Giving zinc alone will normalize the blood pressure. L-Dopa has been used in treating manganese toxicity.

Deficiency Effects and Symptoms

A deficiency of manganese can affect glucose tolerance, resulting in the inability to remove excess sugar from the blood by oxidation and/or storage, causing diabetes. Low manganese levels may cause atherosclerosis and be a factor in triggering seizures in some epileptics. Tardive dyskinesia, a neuromuscular disease, requires additional manganese along with B vitamins. Ataxia, the failure of muscular coordination, has been linked with the inadequate intake of manganese. Deficiencies may also lead to paralysis, convulsion, blindness, and deafness in infants. Dizziness, ear noises, and loss of hearing may occur in adults.

Beneficial Effect on Ailments

Manganese has been beneficial in the treatment of diabetes. When combined with the B vitamins, manganese has helped children and adults who are suffering from devastating weakness by stimulating the transmission of impulses between nerve and muscle. Manganese also helps treat myasthenia gravis (failure of muscular coordination and loss of muscle strength). Research suggests that manganese may play a role in the treatment of multiple sclerosis.[87]

Many schizophrenics have high copper levels.

[85]Krause and Hunscher, *Food Nutrition and Diet Therapy,* p. 116.

[86]Prevention Magazine Staff, *Complete Book of Minerals for Health,* p. 223.

[87]Clark, *Know Your Nutrition,* pp. 166–67.

Manganese, like zinc, is effective in increasing copper excretion from the body.

MANGANESE MAY BE BENEFICIAL FOR THE FOLLOWING AILMENTS:

Body Member	Ailment
Blood/Circulatory system	Diabetes
Brain/Nervous system	Epilepsy
	Multiple sclerosis
	Schizophrenia
Lungs/Respiratory system	Allergies
	Asthma
General	Fatigue

MERCURY

Description

Mercury occurs widely in the biosphere and is a toxic element presenting occupational hazards associated with both ingestion and inhalation. Mercury has no essential function in the human body.

Pesticides and large fish are the most potent sources of mercury. The amount of mercury found in fish is directly proportional to the size of the fish. Mercury enters lakes, rivers, and oceans from industrial discharges. It settles into bacteria which are then eaten by algae; fish eat the algae and man eats the fish. The mercury is concentrated thousands of times as it moves up the chain.

Industrial workers are exposed to mercury-containing products they manufacture. Mercury is used in certain tooth fillings, contaminating the air (from high-speed drilling) and skin of dental workers.

Mercurous chloride preparations can be purchased over-the-counter, including some laxative preparations containing calomel (mercurous chloride). Continued use of these products can result in mercury accumulation in body tissues, including the brain.

Mercury compounds are also added to some cosmetics to kill bacteria. These preparations can be absorbed through the skin and into the body. Contaminated grain seeds consumed by wild game can affect persons eating the animals.

About 10 percent of the mercury ingested accumulates in the brain. Two forms of mercury, methyl and phenyl mercury, deplete the brain tissues of zinc. Methyl mercury (the kind found in fish) can produce nerve, birth, and genetic defects. Studies have found chromosome damage to persons eating mercury-poisoned fish. Symptoms of methyl mercury poisoning include loss of coordination, intellectual ability, vision, and hearing. Organic mercury can produce redness, irritation, and blistering of the skin. Chest pain, fever, coughing, and chills result from inhalation of mercury vapor.

Symptoms of subacute mercury poisoning may be excessive salivation, stomatitis, and diarrhea; or they may be neurological, such as Parkinsonian tremors, vertigo, irritability, moodiness, and depression.[88] Psychosis, loss of teeth, insomnia, fatigue, headache; numbness of lips, hands, and feet; and loss of memory can occur.

The average intake of mercury from food is estimated to be only 0.5 milligram daily. Oral ingestion of as little as 100 milligrams of mercury chloride produces toxic symptoms, and 500 milligrams is usually always fatal unless immediate treatment is given. Mercury poisoning in man has been treated by penicillamine, a chelating agent.

MOLYBDENUM

Description

Molybdenum is a trace mineral found in practically all plant and animal tissues. It is an essential part of two enzymes: xanthine oxidase, which aids in the mobilization of iron from the liver reserves, and aldehyde oxidase, which is necessary for the oxidation of fats. Molybdenum is a factor in copper metabolism.

Food sources of molybdenum include meats, legumes, cereal grains, and some of the dark-green leafy vegetables. The food's mineral content is completely dependent upon the soil content.

[88]National Academy of Sciences, *Toxicants Occurring Naturally in Foods,* p. 67.

Absorption and Storage

Molybdenum is found in minute amounts in the body, being readily absorbed from the gastrointestinal tract and excreted in the urine. Molybdenum is stored in the liver, kidneys, and bones.

Dosage and Toxicity

The National Research Council recommends 150 to 500 micrograms of molybdenum daily. Toxicity symptoms include diarrhea, anemia, and depressed growth rate. High intake may also result in a copper deficiency.[89]

Deficiency Effects and Symptoms

Because of food refining and processing, molybdenum deficiency can possibly occur. A deficiency may result in male impotence.

Beneficial Effect on Ailments

Molybdenum may play a part in the prevention of anemia. Tooth enamel contains molybdenum, and the mineral has been found to be important in the prevention of dental caries. Studies have also linked adequate molybdenum intake to decreased rates of cancer of the esophagus.

**MOLYBDENUM MAY BE BENEFICIAL
FOR THE FOLLOWING AILMENTS:**

Body Member	Ailment
Digestive system	Cancer of the esophagus
Liver	Anemia
Reproductive system	Impotence
Teeth/Gums	Tooth decay

NICKEL

Description

Nickel is an essential trace mineral found in the body. Human and animal tests show that nickel may be a

factor in hormone, lipid, and membrane metabolism. It is an activator of some enzymes and may also be involved in glucose metabolism. Significant amounts are found in DNA and RNA, and nickel may possibly act as a stabilizer of these nucleic acids.

Nickel is a by-product of many industries; it is found in heating fuel, cigarette smoke, and car exhaust. Seafood, cereals, grains, seeds, beans, and vegetables are food sources of nickel.

Absorption and Storage

The amount of nickel actually absorbed by the intestine is small. Most of it passes into the urine or feces. The kidneys appear to regulate the amount of nickel retained or excreted from the body.

Dosage and Toxicity

Daily dietary intake from food varies with the soil content of nickel; estimates range from several micrograms to several hundred milligrams.

Nickel can be toxic to humans if levels are high. Excessive levels can occur in people who experience myocardial infarction, stroke, uterine cancer, burns, and toxemia of pregnancy.

Nickel is particularly toxic when combined with carbon monoxide, producing nickel carbonyl. This element is a result of many industrial processes. It is also a component of cigarette smoke. Studies on rats revealed that the amount of nickel capable of causing lung cancer can be obtained from 15 cigarettes smoked per day over a period of 1 year.

In animals, nickel toxicity results in pigmentation changes, leg swelling, dermatitis, and fat and oxygen depletion of the liver. Nickel accumulates in the liver, bone, and aorta. It may cause lung cancer in humans. Symptoms of nickel poisoning are headache, vertigo, nausea, vomiting, chest pain, and coughing.

Deficiency Effects and Symptoms

A deficiency can result from cirrhosis of the liver, chronic kidney failure, excessive sweating, intestinal malabsorption, and stress. Iron-deficiency anemia may also be aggravated.

[89]Margaret S. Chaney and Margaret L. Ross, *Nutrition,* 8th ed. (Boston, Houghton Mifflin Co., 1971), p. 183.

Beneficial Effect on Ailments

No available information.

PHOSPHORUS

Description

Phosphorus is the second most abundant mineral in the body and is found in every cell. It often functions along with calcium, and the healthy body maintains a specific calcium-phosphorus balance in the bones of 2.5 parts calcium to 1 part phosphorus, although phosphorus is in higher ratio in the soft tissues. This balance of calcium and phosphorus is needed for these minerals to be effectively used by the body.

Phosphorus plays a part in almost every chemical reaction within the body because it is present in every cell. It is important in the utilization of carbohydrates, fats, and protein for the growth, maintenance, and repair of cells and for the production of energy. It stimulates muscle contractions, including the regular contractions of the heart muscle. Niacin and riboflavin cannot be digested unless phosphorus is present. Phosphorus is an essential part of nucleoproteins, which are responsible for cell division and reproduction and the transference of hereditary traits from parents to offspring. It is also necessary for proper skeletal growth, tooth development, kidney functioning, and transference of nerve impulses.

Phospholipids, such as lecithin, help break up and transport fats and fatty acids. They help prevent the accumulation of too much acid or too much alkali in the blood, assist in the passage of substances through the cell walls, and promote the secretion of glandular hormones. They are also needed for healthy nerves and efficient mental activity.

Foods rich in protein are also rich in phosphorus. Meat, fish, poultry, eggs, whole grains, seeds, and nuts are primary sources of phosphorus.

Absorption and Storage

Unlike calcium, which is poorly absorbed, most dietary phosphorus is absorbed from the intestine into the bloodstream. About 70 percent of the phosphorus ingested in foods is absorbed. About 88 percent of the absorbed phosphorus is stored in the bones and teeth, along with calcium, although antacids can deplete the storage. There is relatively little control over the rate of absorption, so the body content is regulated by urinary excretion.

Phosphorus absorption depends on the presence of vitamin D and calcium. Absorption can be interfered with by excessive amounts of iron, aluminum, and magnesium, which tend to form insoluble phosphates. The calcium-phosphorus balance is disturbed in the presence of white sugar. High fat diets or digestive conditions that prevent the absorption of fat increase the absorption of phosphorus in the intestine, but such conditions are not healthful because they also decrease the amount of calcium absorbed and upset the calcium-phosphorus balance.

Dosage and Toxicity

The National Research Council recommends a daily dietary intake of 800 milligrams of phosphorus for men and women. During pregnancy and lactation the amount increases to 1200 milligrams. This is equal to the daily requirement for calcium. If the phosphorus content of the body is high, additional calcium should be taken to maintain a proper balance. There is no known toxicity of phosphorus.

Deficiency Effects and Symptoms

An insufficient supply of phosphorus, calcium, or vitamin D may result in stunted growth, poor quality of bones and teeth, or other bone disorders. A deficiency in the calcium-phosphorus balance may result in diseases such as arthritis, pyorrhea, rickets, and tooth decay.

A phosphorus deficiency can cause lack of appetite and weight loss or, conversely, overweight. Irregular breathing, mental and physical fatigue, and nervous disorders may occur.

Beneficial Effect on Ailments

Dietary phosphate has speeded up the healing process in bone fractures and has reduced the expected loss of calcium in such patients. It has been used successfully in the treatment of osteomalacia and osteoporosis. It also helps to prevent or cure rickets and to prevent stunted growth in children.

Mental stress can cause an upset in the body chemistry and bring on strong arthritic symptoms such as aching joints. The calcium-phosphorus balance can help treat the stressful condition and can also help alleviate the arthritis.

Recent research has shown that phosphorus may be important in cancer prevention. Investigators have discovered that phosphorus is more easily lost from cancerous cells than from normal cells.[90] Phosphorus is essential in treating disorders of the teeth and gums.

PHOSPHORUS MAY BE BENEFICIAL FOR THE FOLLOWING AILMENTS:

Body Member	Ailment
Bones	Fracture
	Osteomalacia
	Osteoporosis
	Rickets
	Stunted growth
Bowel	Colitis
Brain/Nervous system	Mental illness
Heart	Arteriosclerosis
	Atherosclerosis
Joints	Arthritis
Leg	Leg cramp
Teeth/Gums	Tooth and gum disorders
General	Backache
	Cancer
	Pregnancy
	Stress

POTASSIUM

Description

Potassium is an essential mineral found mainly in the intracellular fluid; a small amount occurs in the extracellular fluid. Potassium constitutes 5 percent of the total mineral content of the body. Potassium and sodium help regulate water balance within the body; that is, they help regulate the distribution of fluids on either side of the cell walls.

Potassium is necessary for normal growth, to stimulate nerve impulses for muscle contraction, and to preserve proper alkalinity of the body fluids. It aids in keeping the skin healthy. Potassium assists in the conversion of glucose to glycogen, the form in which glucose can be stored in the liver. It functions in cell metabolism, enzyme reactions, and the synthesis of muscle protein from amino acids in the blood. It stimulates the kidneys to eliminate poisonous body wastes.

Potassium works with sodium to help normalize the heartbeat and nourish the muscular system. It unites with phosphorus to send oxygen to the brain and also functions with calcium in the regulation of neuromuscular activity.

Food sources of potassium include all vegetables, especially green leafy vegetables, oranges, whole grains, sunflower seeds, and mint leaves. Large amounts of potassium are found in potatoes, especially in the peelings, and in bananas.

Absorption and Storage

Potassium is rapidly absorbed from the small intestine. It is excreted mainly through urination and perspiration, and very little is lost in the feces. The kidneys are able to maintain normal serum levels through their ability to filter, secrete, and excrete potassium. Aldosterone, an adrenal hormone, stimulates potassium excretion.

Excessive potassium buildup may result from kidney failure or from severe lack of fluid.

Because sodium and potassium must be in balance, the excessive use of salt depletes the body's conservation of its often scarce potassium supplies. In addition, potassium can be depleted by prolonged diarrhea, excessive sweating, vomiting, and the use of diuretics.

Alcohol and coffee increase the urinary excretion of potassium. Alcohol is a double antagonist since it also depletes the magnesium reserve. Excessive intake of sugar is also antagonistic towards potassium.

A low blood sugar level is a stressful condition that strains the adrenal glands, causing additional potassium to be lost in the urine while water and salt are held in the tissues. An adequate supply of magnesium

[90]Rodale, *Health Builder*, p. 664.

is needed to retain the storage of potassium in the cells.

Dosage and Toxicity

A Recommended Dietary Allowance for potassium has not been established, but many authorities suggest that between 2000 and 2500 milligrams be included in the diet daily. The amount of potassium in the average American's daily diet has been estimated at 2000 to 6000 milligrams per day, since it is distributed in many different foods.

Deficiency Effects and Symptoms

Excessive urinary losses induced by high salt intake have caused potassium deficiencies to be commonplace. A potassium deficiency can result from an excessive intake of sodium chloride or from an inadequate intake of fruits and vegetables. Refined sugar can cause the urine to become alkaline so that minerals cannot be held in solution. Deficiency can be caused by prolonged intravenous administration of saline, which induces potassium excretion.[91] Vomiting, severe malnutrition, and stress, both mental and physical, may also lead to potassium deficiency.

A potassium deficiency may cause nervous disorders, insomnia, constipation, slow and irregular heartbeat, and muscle damage. When a deficiency of potassium impairs glucose metabolism, energy is no longer available to the muscles and they become more or less paralyzed.

When the body is lacking potassium, the sodium content of the heart and muscles increases. Infants suffering from diarrhea may have a potassium deficiency because the passage of the intestinal contents is so rapid that there is decreased absorption of potassium.[92] Diabetic patients are often deficient in potassium. Persons suffering from diseases of the digestive tract are frequently found to be potassium-deficient. A person loses potassium when taking water pills or hormone products such as cortisone and aldosterone. Sodium is retained and potassium is excreted when these drugs are administered.

Early symptoms of potassium deficiency include general weakness and impairment of neuromuscular function, poor reflexes, and soft, sagging muscles. In adolescents, acne can result; in older persons, dry skin may occur.

Beneficial Effect on Ailments

Potassium has been used to treat cases of high blood pressure which were directly caused by excessive salt intake. Colic in infants has disappeared after injections of potassium chloride.* Potassium chloride has also proven effective in treating allergies.

Giving potassium to patients with mild diabetes can reduce blood pressure and blood sugar levels.[93] Since potassium is essential for the transmission of nerve impulses to the brain, it has been effective in the treatment of headache-causing allergies.[94]

Potassium has also been used in the treatment of diarrhea in infants* and adults. Therapeutic doses of potassium are sometimes used to slow the heartbeat in cases of severe injury, such as burns.

POTASSIUM MAY BE BENEFICIAL FOR THE FOLLOWING AILMENTS:

Body Member	Ailment
Blood/Circulatory system	Angina pectoris
	Diabetes
	Hypertension
	Mononucleosis
	Stroke (cerebrovascular accident)
Bones	Fracture
Bowel	Colitis
	Diarrhea
Brain/Nervous system	Alcoholism
	Hypertension
	Insomnia
	Polio
Glands	Mononucleosis
Head	Fever
	Headache

*Potassium should be given to infants under the direction of a physician.

[93]Rodale, *The Health Builder*, p. 695.

[94]J. I. Rodale, *The Best Health Articles from* Prevention *Magazine* (Emmaus, Pa.: Rodale Books, 1968), p. 578.

[91]Williams, *Nutrition against Disease*, pp. 156–57.

[92]Guthrie, *Introductory Nutrition*, p. 128.

Body Member	Ailment
Heart	Angina pectoris
	Congestive heart failure
	Hypertension
	Myocardial infarction
Intestine	Constipation
	Worms
Joints	Arthritis
	Gout
Lungs/Respiratory system	Allergies
Muscles	Impaired muscle activity
	Muscular dystrophy
	Rheumatism
Skin	Acne
	Burns
	Dermatitis
Stomach	Gastroenteritis
Teeth/Gums	Tooth and gum disorders
General	Alcoholism
	Cancer
	Fever
	Stress

SELENIUM

Description

Selenium is an essential mineral found in minute amounts in the body. It works closely with vitamin E in some of its metabolic actions and in the promotion of normal body growth and fertility. Selenium is a natural antioxidant and appears to preserve elasticity of tissue by delaying oxidation of polyunsaturated fatty acids.

It is necessary for the production of prostaglandin, substances that affect blood pressure. A prostaglandin deficiency also results in a deficiency of other compounds necessary for keeping the arteries free from platelet aggregation.

Selenium improves certain energy-producing cells, including those of the heart, by ensuring adequate oxygen supply.

The selenium content of food is dependent upon the extent of its presence in the soil, whether directly, as in plant foods, or indirectly, as in animal products whose selenium levels are derived from feed. Even if selenium levels are adequate in the soil, the sulfur contained in widely used fertilizers and sulfuric compounds found in acid rain inhibit plant absorption of the mineral.

Selenium compounds in foods are easily reduced by heat, processing, and cooking. Refining of grains reduces selenium content by 50 to 75 percent, boiling by 45 percent.

Good food sources of selenium are brewer's yeast, organ and muscle meats, fish and shellfish, grains, cereals, and dairy products.

Absorption and Storage

The liver and kidneys contain four to five times as much selenium as do the muscles and other tissues. Selenium is normally excreted in the urine; its presence in the feces is an indication of improper absorption.[95] Because it binds with toxic metals, the selenium that is ingested may not be assimilated.

Dosage and Toxicity

The National Research Council recommends 50 to 200 micrograms of selenium daily. Doctors studing selenium suggest 250 to 350 micrograms may be needed. The average "good" diet may contain only 35 to 60 micrograms per day. Doses should not exceed 700 to 1110 micrograms daily for long periods of time unless under the supervision of a physician.

Male sperm cells contain high amounts of selenium. Substantial amounts are lost during sexual intercourse. For this reason, selenium requirements may be higher for men than for women.

The different selenium compounds have varying degrees of toxicity. For example, dimethyl selenium is nontoxic; sodium selenite is more toxic than organic selenium; and selenium yeast is one-third as toxic as sodium selenite.[96]

High levels of selenium in soil have caused toxicity and some deaths in animals who grazed on the grains. Selenium also contaminates water supplies located near

[95]Guthrie, *Introductory Nutrition,* p. 162.

[96]Passwater, *Selenium as Food and Medicine,* p. 198.

irrigated land. Selenium intoxication has been reported as a result of industrial inhalation.

Toxic symptoms are loss of hair, teeth, and nails; dermatitis; lethargy; and paralysis. Severe overdose produces fever, an increased respiratory and capillary rate, gastrointestinal distress, myelitis, and sometimes death.

Selenium overdoses can interfere with fluoride assimilation, which helps to prevent tooth decay.

Deficiency Effects and Symptoms

A deficiency of selenium may lead to premature aging. This is because selenium preserves tissue elasticity.

A defective selenium absorption mechanism can result in neuronal ceroid lipofuscinosis, a disease that accumulates pigment in nerve cells and is characterized by mental retardation, diminished vision, nerve disorders, and eventually death.

Selenium is essential for reproduction. Animal tests reveal that selenium-deficient rats produced immobile sperm and most of the sperm were broken near the tail. Other studies show that a selenium deficiency results in infertility.

Studies in Australia show that a selenium deficiency may relate to crib death.

Beneficial Effect on Ailments

Selenium when combined with protein is beneficial in treating kwashiorkor, a protein-deficiency disease.

Dr. Julian E. Spallholz of the Veterans Administration Hospital in Long Beach, California, has demonstrated through experiments with mice that selenium may increase resistance to disease by increasing the number of antibodies that neutralize toxins. Selenium supplements enabled mice to produce significantly more antibodies than those that were not given the trace element.

Archives of Environmental Health, September/October 1976, reports that in a study of the relationship between cancer incidence and soil distribution of selenium in the United States, areas with high selenium levels showed significantly lower overall male cancer death rates. Also in these areas, in both men and women, fewer cancers were noted in those organ systems involved with the assimilation, metabolism, and excretion of selenium.

Selenium may improve energy levels, prevent and relieve arthritis, slow down the aging process by attacking free radicals, and prevent cataracts.

It is an important element that protects against high blood pressure, stroke, heart attack, and hypertensive kidney damage. Selenium with vitamin E has been used successfully in reducing or eliminating recurrent angina attacks and increasing strength and vigor and improving electrocardiograms in heart patients.

It has been used successfully in improving the condition of persons with cystic fibrosis. Muscular dystrophy patients respond positively to selenium and vitamin E. Research in the early 1970s has proved that selenium protects against radiation. It also binds to metals such as mercury, cadmium, silver, and thallium, preventing their absorption in the body and aiding their excretion.

SELENIUM MAY BE BENEFICIAL FOR THE FOLLOWING AILMENTS:

Body Member	Ailment
Blood/Circulatory system	Hypertension
	Stroke
Glands	Cystic fibrosis
Heart	Angina pectoris
Joints	Arthritis
Muscles	Muscular dystrophy
Reproductive system	Infertility
General	Cancer
	Crib death
	Kwashiorkor

SILICON

Description

Silicon is present in the connective tissues of the body such as tendons, cartilage, and blood vessels, and it is possible that the mineral is essential for their integrity. Silicon may work with calcium to make strong bones, therefore being an important factor in osteoporosis. Studies have shown that the amount of silicon in the arteries begins to decline as atherosclerosis starts to develop. The best known sources of silicon are hard drinking water and plant fiber.

SODIUM

Description

Sodium is an essential mineral found predominantly in the extracellular fluids; the vascular fluids within the blood vessels, arteries, veins, and capillaries; and the intestinal fluids surrounding the cells. About 50 percent of the body's sodium is found in these fluids and the remaining amount is found within the bones.

Sodium functions with potassium to equalize the acid-alkali factor in the blood. Along with potassium, it helps regulate water balance within the body; that is, it helps regulate the distribution of fluids on either side of the cell walls. Sodium and potassium are also involved in muscle contraction and expansion and in nerve stimulation.

Another important function of sodium is keeping the other blood minerals soluble, so that they will not build up as deposits in the bloodstream. It acts with chlorine to improve blood and lymph health, helps purge carbon dioxide from the body, and aids digestion. Sodium is also necessary for hydrochloric acid production in the stomach.

Sodium is found in virtually all foods, especially sodium chloride, or salt. High concentrations are contained in seafoods, poultry, and meat. Kelp is an excellent supplemental source of sodium.

Absorption and Storage

Sodium is readily absorbed in the small intestine and the stomach and is carried by the blood to the kidneys, where it is filtered out and returned to the blood in amounts needed to maintain blood levels required by the body. The absorption of sodium requires energy. Any excess, which usually amounts to 90 to 95 percent of ingested sodium, is excreted in the urine.

The adrenal hormone aldosterone is an important regulator of sodium metabolism. Excessive salt in food interferes with absorption and utilization, especially in the case of protein foods. Vomiting, diarrhea, or excessive perspiration may result in a depletion of sodium. Sodium supplements to prevent sodium deficiency may be needed in such cases. The levels of sodium in the urine reflect the dietary intake; therefore when there is a high intake of sodium the rate of excretion is high, and if the intake is low the excretion rate is low.

Dosage and Toxicity

There is no established dietary requirement for sodium, but it is generally observed that the usual intake far exceeds the need. The average American ingests 3 to 7 grams of sodium and 6 to 18 grams of sodium chloride each day. The National Research Council recommends a daily sodium chloride intake of 1 gram per kilogram of water consumed.

An excess of sodium in the diet may cause potassium to be lost in the urine. Abnormal fluid retention accompanied by dizziness and swelling of such areas as legs and face can also occur. An intake of 14 to 28 grams of salt (sodium chloride) daily is considered excessive.[97]

Diets containing excessive amounts of sodium contribute to the increasing incidences of high blood pressure. The simplest way to reduce sodium intake is to eliminate the use of table salt.

Deficiency Effects and Symptoms

Deficiencies are very uncommon because nearly all foods contain some sodium, with meats containing especially high amounts. A sodium deficiency can cause intestinal gas, weight loss, vomiting, and muscle skrinkage. The conversion of carbohydrates into fat for digestion is impaired when sodium is absent. Arthritis, rheumatism, and neuralgia, a sharp pain along a nerve, may be caused by acids that accumulate in the absence of sodium.

Beneficial Effect on Ailments

An individual suffering from high blood pressure is advised to maintain a low-sodium diet, since sodium may aggravate this ailment. Resistance to heat cramps and heat strokes may be increased by moderate sodium intake. Sodium helps keep calcium in a solution that is necessary for nerve strength. Clinical studies indicate that low-sodium diets are effective in preventing or relieving the symptoms of toxemia (bacterial poisoning), edema (swelling), proteinuria (albumin in the urine), and blurred vision.

[97]National Academy of Sciences, *Toxicants Occurring Naturally in Foods,* p. 270.

STRONTIUM

Description

Strontium is apparently an essential trace mineral and is similar to calcium in chemical makeup. It may be necessary for proper bone growth and prevention of tooth decay. In studies reported by Dr. Stanley Skoryna, director of medical research at St. Mary's Hospital in Montreal, Canada, strontium may be protective of certain energy-producing structures within the cell. (Strontium should not be confused with radioactive strontium 90.) Strontium is stable and one of the least toxic of trace minerals. Dr. Skoryna believes that man's diet probably contains insufficient quantities of strontium and may need to be supplemented.

SULFUR

Description

Sulfur is a nonmetallic element that occurs widely in nature, being present in every cell of animals and plants. Sulfur makes up 0.25 percent of the human body weight. It is called nature's "beauty mineral" because it keeps the hair glossy and smooth and keeps the complexion clear and youthful.

Sulfur has an important relationship with protein. It is contained in the amino acids methionine, cystine, and cysteine, and it appears to be necessary for collagen synthesis. Sulfur is prevalent in keratin, a tough protein substance necessary for health and maintenance of the skin, nails, and hair. It is found in insulin, the hormone that regulates carbohydrate metabolism. It also occurs in carbohydrates such as heparin, an anticoagulant found in the liver and other tissues.

Sulfur works with thiamine, pantothenic acid, biotin, and lipoic acid, which are needed for metabolism and strong nerve health. In addition, sulfur plays a part in tissue respiration, the process whereby oxygen and other substances are used to build cells and release energy. It works with the liver to secrete bile. Sulfur also helps to maintain overall body balance.

The soil in many areas is deficient in sulfur; therefore plant foods vary in content. The best source of sulfur is eggs. Others are meat, fish, cheese, and milk.

Absorption and Storage

Sulfur is stored in every cell of the body. The highest concentrations are found in the joints, hair, skin, and nails. Excess sulfur is excreted in the urine and the feces.

Dosage and Toxicity

There is no Recommended Dietary Allowance for sulfur because it is assumed that a person's sulfur requirement is met when the protein intake is adequate.[98] Sulfur can be used in various forms such as ointments, creams, lotions, and dusting powders. Excessive intake of sulfur may result in toxicity.

Deficiency Effects and Symptoms

Vegetarians may become deficient in sulfur if they don't eat eggs.

Beneficial Effect on Ailments

Sulfur is important in the treatment of arthritis. The level of cystine, a sulfur-containing amino acid, in arthritic patients is usually much lower than normal.

When used topically in the form of an ointment, sulfur is helpful in treating skin disorders, such as psoriasis, eczema, and dermatitis. It also may be beneficial in treating ringworm.

[98]Chaney and Ross, *Nutrition,* p. 187.

SULFUR MAY BE BENEFICIAL FOR THE
FOLLOWING AILMENTS:

Body Member	Ailment
Intestine	Worms
Joints	Arthritis
Skin	Dermatitis
	Eczema
	Psoriasis

TIN

Description

In 1960 tin was discovered to be an essential trace element. Its specific functions are not known. Animal experiments have shown that a deficiency results in poor growth and diminished hemoglobin synthesis. Tin toxicity can cause anemia unless enough iron is present.

Tin is used widely in industry. A tin salt, stannous fluoride, is used as a preservative and is found in some toothpastes. Because appreciable amounts are part of air pollution, lung tissues have the highest concentration of tin. Estimated daily intake is from 2 to 17 milligrams. Estimated requirements are around 3 to 4 milligrams.

VANADIUM

Description

Vanadium is present in most body tissues. Because of this fact, and the fact that other elements such as zinc have similar properties, it is believed that vanadium is essential to human health. Bones, cartilage, and teeth require vanadium for proper development. Animal studies show vanadium to be important for iron metabolism and red cell growth.

Vanadium is another trace element that becomes a victim of food processing. High quantities are found in fats and vegetable oils. Whole grains, seafood, and meats such as liver are good sources of the mineral.

Absorption and Storage

Vanadium is rapidly used by the body, and most of it is excreted in the urine. Bone and liver are the main storage areas.

Dosage and Toxicity

The estimated requirement is 100 to 300 micrograms per day. Excessive intake may be toxic.

Deficiency Effects and Symptoms

Studies on animals show that vanadium deficiency results in decreased reproduction rates and increased mortality of the young.

Beneficial Effect on Ailments

Adequate amounts of vanadium can lower serum cholesterol. Animal tests have shown the mineral to be vital for proper growth.

VANADIUM MAY BE BENEFICIAL FOR THE FOLLOWING AILMENTS:

Body Member	Ailment
Blood/Circulatory system	Atherosclerosis
	Cholesterol level, high

ZINC

Description

Zinc is an essential trace mineral occurring in the body in larger amounts than any other trace element except iron. The human body contains approximately 1.8 grams of zinc compared to nearly 5 grams of iron.

Zinc has a variety of functions. It is related to the normal absorption and action of vitamins, especially the B complex. It is a constituent of at least 25 enzymes involved in digestion and metabolism, including carbonic anhydrase, which is necessary for tissue respiration. Zinc is a component of insulin, and it is part of the enzyme that is needed to break down alcohol. It also plays a part in carbohydrate digestion and phosphorus metabolism. In addition, it is essential in the synthesis of nucleic acid, which controls the formation of different proteins in the cell. Zinc is essential for general growth and proper development of the reproductive organs and for normal functioning of the prostate gland.

Recent medical findings indicate that zinc is important in healing wounds and burns. It may also be required in the synthesis of DNA, which is the master substance of life, carrying all inherited traits and directing the activity of each cell.

Soil exhaustion and the processing of food adversely affect the zinc value of the food we eat. The best sources of all trace elements in proper balance are natural unprocessed foods. Diets high in protein, whole-grain products, brewer's yeast, wheat bran, wheat germ, and pumpkin seeds are usually high in zinc.

Absorption and Storage

Zinc is readily absorbed in the upper small intestine. Uptake is only as much as the body needs at the time; the rest is unabsorbed.

The major route of excretion is through the gastrointestinal tract; little is lost in the urine. The largest storage of zinc occurs in the liver, pancreas, kidney, bones, and voluntary muscles. Zinc is also stored in parts of the eyes, prostate gland and spermatozoa, skin, hair, fingernails, and toenails as well as being present in the white blood cells.[99]

A high intake of calcium and phytic acid, found in certain grains, may prevent absorption of zinc. If the intake of calcium and phytic acid is higher, zinc consumption should be increased.

Dosage and Toxicity

The National Research Council recommends a daily dietary intake of 15 milligrams of zinc for adults. An additional 15 milligrams is recommended during pregnancy, and an additional 25 milligrams is recommended during lactation. The average "good" diet may yield only 8 to 11 milligrams of zinc per day.

Older patients have been given 660 milligrams of zinc sulfate per day with minimal side effects. Some experienced diarrhea. Nausea and vomiting are also symptoms of zinc overdose, requiring a reduction in the amount taken.

High intakes of zinc interfere with copper utilization, causing incomplete iron metabolism. Excessive intake of zinc may result in a loss of iron and copper

[99]Krause and Hunscher, *Food, Nutrition and Diet Therapy*, p. 117.

from the liver. When zinc is added to the diet, vitamin A is also needed in larger amounts.

Deficiency Effects and Symptoms

The most common cause of zinc deficiency is an unbalanced diet, although other factors may also be responsible. For example, the consumption of alcohol may precipitate a deficiency by flushing stored zinc out of the liver and into the urine. Zinc deficiency is also a factor in stress, fatigue, susceptibility to infection, injury, and decreased alertness.

Zinc deficiency can cause retarded growth, delayed sexual maturity, and prolonged healing of wounds. A deficiency of zinc, copper, and vanadium may result in atherosclerosis. Stretch marks in the skin and white spots in the fingernails may be signs of a zinc deficiency. Brittle nails and hair and hair lacking pigment, irregular menstrual cycles in teen women, impotence in young males, and painful knee and hip joints in teenagers are also indications of a deficiency.

Chronic zinc depletion can predispose body cells to cancer.

Cadmium, a toxic mineral, also plays an important role in zinc deficiencies. High intakes of cadmium will accentuate the signs of a zinc deficiency, and the cadmium will be stored in the body in the absence of zinc. This creates a detrimental situation that can be reversed by increasing the consumption of zinc.

Chelating compounds used to remove excess copper from the body also leach out zinc, which then must be replaced.

Recent studies demonstrate conclusively that zinc deficiency causes sterility and dwarfism in humans. The deficiency leads to unhealthy changes in the size and structure of the prostate gland, which contains more zinc than any other part of the human anatomy. In prostate problems, particularly prostate cancer, the levels of zinc in the prostate gland decline.

James A. Halstead and J. Cecil Smith, Jr., of the Trace Element Research Laboratory, Washington, D.C., have made interesting studies on zinc. They found low zinc levels in the blood plasma of people suffering from alcoholic cirrhosis, other types of liver disease, ulcers, heart attacks, mongolism, and cystic fibrosis. Pregnant woman and women taking oral contraceptives also had low levels of zinc in their blood plasma.

Nausea associated with pregnancy may be a result

of too-low levels of zinc and vitamin B_6. Zinc-deficient pregnant rats had many stillborn or birth-defective babies; also many offspring were mentally retarded or slow learners.

Excessive zinc excretion occurs in leukemia and Hodgkin's disease, but the causes of this are unknown. A zinc deficiency is characterized by abnormal fatigue and may cause a loss of normal taste senitivity, poor appetite, and suboptimal growth. The zinc-deficient patient has poor circulation and a tendency to faint; therefore care must be taken in anesthetic and operative situations. These people can be prone to shock, excessive bleeding, and delayed wound healing.

Beneficial Effect on Ailments

Zinc helps eliminate cholesterol deposits and has been successfully used in the treatment of atherosclerosis. Zinc may contribute to the rapid healing of internal wounds or any injury to the arteries. Zinc supplements given in therapeutic doses will speed up the rate at which the body heals certain external wounds and injuries.

Zinc is beneficial in the prevention and treatment of infertility. It also helps in the proper growth and maturity of the sex organs, in resistance to infection, improved night vision, and reduced body odor.

The administration of zinc may benefit patients suffering from Hodgkin's disease and leukemia. It also is used in treatment of cirrhosis of the liver and alcoholism.

Zinc is beneficial to the diabetic because of its regulatory effect on insulin in the blood. It has been found that the addition of zinc to insulin prolongs its effect on blood sugar.[100] A diabetic pancreas contains only about half as much zinc as does a healthy one.

ZINC MAY BE BENEFICIAL FOR THE FOLLOWING AILMENTS:

Body Member	Ailment
Blood/Circulatory system	Arteriosclerosis
	Atherosclerosis
	Cholesterol level, high
	Diabetes
	Hodgkin's disease

[100]Prevention Magazine Staff, *Encyclopedia of Common Diseases,* p. 273.

Body Member	Ailment
Brain/Nervous system	Alcoholism
	Schizophrenia
Eye	Night blindness
Glands	Prostatitis
Heart	Arteriosclerosis
	Atherosclerosis
Joints	Rheumatoid arthritis
Reproductive system	Impotency
	Menstruation
	Prostatitis
	Retarded sexual activity
Skin	Acne
	Burns
	Dermatitis
	Eczema
	Wounds
General	Alcoholism
	Pregnancy
	Retarded growth
	Ulcers

A STUDY OF DRINKING WATER

HYDROLOGICAL CYCLE, CHEMISTRY, AND BEHAVIOR

Salty ocean water comprises 97 percent of the earth's water supply. The remaining 3 percent, 33 trillion cubic feet (1 cubic foot equals 7.48 gallons), is fresh water. Of this, 75 percent is contained in glaciers, 24 percent is underground, 0.3 percent is in lakes, 0.03 percent is in rivers, 0.06 percent is in soil, and 0.035 percent is in the atmosphere. The total amount of water now in existence on this planet is believed to be the same as it was 3 billion years ago.

In its various states, drawing energy from the sun, about 95,000 cubic miles of water are circulated throughout the biosphere each year. It evaporates from the oceans and rivers into the air, condenses in the clouds to liquid drops, and descends back to earth in the form of rain, snow, or sleet. Then approximately 70 percent of this precipitation evaporates back into the atmosphere or penetrates into the soil, supplying plant life with moisture. The remainder runs off the earth's crust into nearby surface waters, ultimately reaching the oceans, or seeps to the water table, where it fills underground aquifers, which are openings in beds of rock and sand. It then travels slowly along the subterranean floors, eventually feeding into lakes, rivers, and swamps or the sea. Because of this gradual progression, most rivers continue to flow in times of little or no rainfall; also, because of the slow progression, any pollution can take decades, centuries, or millennia to be flushed.

Water comes close to being the universal solvent. The waters of the earth have been found to contain about one-half of all the known elements. It is an inert solvent, meaning that the water itself is not chemically changed by the compounds it dissolves, toxic or otherwise, thereby enabling it to be used over and over again. Emphasizing the importance of this property of solubility is the fact that the roots of plants can only absorb nutrients in solution and our human food must be dissolved in solution before it can enter the bloodstream.

A unique characteristic of water is its capillary action. This defiance of gravity enables nutrients to flow upward from the soil, nourishing plants and trees, and allows the blood, which is 83 percent water, to complete its circuit in the human body.

WATER AND THE HUMAN BODY

Emerging from the warm and watery solution of the womb, the body of a newborn baby is 77 percent water; children are 59 percent and adults are between 45 and 65 percent water. The blood is 83 percent water, kidneys 82 percent, muscles 75 percent, brain 74 percent, liver 69 percent, and bones 22 percent. Water is the principal constituent of the fluids that surround and are within all living cells.

Respiration, digestion, assimilation, metabolism, elimination, waste removal, and temperature regulation are bodily functions that can only be accomplished in the presence of water. Water is essential in dissolving and transporting nutrients such as oxygen and mineral salts via the blood, lymph, and other bodily fluids.

Water also keeps the pressure, acidity, and composition of all chemical reactions in equilibrium.

Only oxygen is more essential than water in sustaining the life of all organisms. Human beings can live around 5 weeks without protein, carbohydrates, and fats, but just 5 days without water in a moderate climate. Its circulation between the blood and bodily organs is perpetual and always maintained in proper balance; however, a certain amount is eliminated daily through evaporation or excretion and must be replaced.

Most of this water is removed by the kidneys, through which the entire blood supply passes and is filtered fifteen times each hour. Whenever the body becomes overheated, 2 million sweat glands excrete perspiration, which is 99 percent water. The heat of the blood evaporates the sweat, cooling the body and keeping the internal organs at a constant temperature. A minimal but consistent loss of water occurs during the processes of breathing and tearing. Moisture is breathed out from the water-lined nasal passages and the lungs. Dry air draws off more water than humid air. Tiny tear ducts carry a liquid solution to the upper eyelids, which lubricate the eyes 25 times every minute. The tears then pass down to the nose, where they evaporate.

To replace lost water, approximately 3 quarts is needed by the body each day under normal conditions. More strenuous activity, a high climate temperature, or a diet too high in salt may increase this requirement. The sense of thirst (as well as sleep, appetite, satiety, and sexual responses) is controlled by a part of the forebrain called the hypothalamus. Metabolic water is produced as a by-product of the food combustion process, yielding as much as a pint per day. Foods can provide up to 1½ quarts. For example, fruits and vegetables are more than 90 percent distilled water. Even dry foods like bread and crackers are 35 and 5 percent water, respectively. Drinking water is the other source of replenishment.

POLLUTION AND DRINKING WATER

Water is ingested daily by everyone, and most people get their water from the household tap, which may originate from streams, rivers, or lakes or from a well that is supplied with water from the underground aquifer system. Most water goes through various cleaning treatments at the city water plant. However, because of a lack of funds to provide the appropriate technology, many potentially harmful elements such as synthetic compounds, metals, and radionuclides are not removed. Even bacteria and viruses can escape contemporary treatment practices. Any pollutant contained in drinking water will eventually circulate throughout every cell and tissue in the body.

There are two ways toxic substances enter water supplies. The first is a relatively constant distribution by Mother Nature. These toxins do not accumulate because of the natural biological processes of dilution, oxidation, and degradation. The second is by the actions and habits of human beings. The elements reenter the environment and disrupt the natural action of organisms in such a way that the balance between accumulation and degradation can no longer be maintained.

Both surface and ground waters are habitually contaminated by such sources as fossil fuel combustion and stack emissions that descend during rainfall; industrial effluents; human wastes, including sewage and those associated with consumption of products; urban runoff (a 1974 Council on Environmental Quality reported that typical moderate-sized cities annually discharge 100,000 to 250,000 lb of lead, 6000 to 30,000 lb of mercury, 15,000 to 30,000 lb of chromium, 85,000 to 90,000 lb of copper, 140,000 to 300,000 lb of zinc, and over 10,000 lb of nickel); agricultural runoff, including pesticides and fertilizers from farmlands and animal wastes from large feedlot operations; leachate from sanitary dumps or landfills; seepage from mine tailings or abandoned mines; and accidental spills. According to the Environmental Protection Agency (EPA), municipal sewers discharge 40 billion gallons, industry 125 billion gallons, and agriculture 50 billion gallons of wastes daily into our water resources.

POLLUTION AND THE HUMAN BODY

The human system has evolved metabolic processes that can effectively assimilate toxins that are ingested periodically. However, when chronic or continual exposure occurs or when new substances are encountered that the system cannot detoxify, adverse reactions can

manifest. Chronic effects are muted, often invisible, and not immediately experienced. They can result in cancer that may be latent for 10 to 30 years and metabolic and genetic changes affecting growth, health, behavior, and resistance to disease, teratogenicity, which is the translocation of an agent across the placental membrane to the fetus, or premature death from a delayed response of a cumulative toxin. Cumulative toxins are substances taken in in sublethal doses that eventually are stored at lethal levels. The factors that determine these effects will be the inherent toxicity of the chemical, the level and length of exposure, and other stresses on the affected organism such as existing disease, exposure to other environmental pollutants, drugs, food additives, etc.

Scientists from the World Health Organization and the National Cancer Institute (NCI) estimate that between 60 and 80 percent of all cancer is caused by chemicals in the air we breathe, the food we eat, and the water we drink. Cancer will afflict one out of every four people and cost more than $15 billion annually. The NCI over 20 years ago expressed concern that the increase in carcinogens in water and our inability to remove them at the treatment plants could result in serious exposure of the general population. Epidemiological studies in Louisiana, Ohio, New Jersey, and Europe have suggested the possible association between carcinogens in drinking water and cancer mortality. Dr. Wilhelm C. Heuper of the NCI staff cautioned in 1964 that "the most common and often prolonged and therefore most dangerous contact with carcinogenic pollutants of water occurs when water thus contaminated is used for drinking purposes and in the preparation of food. It is here important that most of the agents [for example, arsenicals, chromium, radioactive substances, chlorinated hydrocarbon pesticides] are retained in the body and may accumulate in certain organs, such as the liver, skin, bones or fat tissue, from which they later on may gradually be released, thereby causing a continuous or prolonged exposure of the tissues with these carcinogens. The cancers, not infrequently, become manifest months, years, or decades after such contacts have ceased, and often the causative agents may have totally disappeared from the tissues" [David Zwick and Marcy Benstock, *Water Wasteland* (N. Grossman, 1971), p. 8].

In 1970, an ad hoc committee report to the surgeon general recommended that no level of exposure to a cancer-causing substance be recognized as toxicologically insignificant to human beings. Whether the agent in question is the ultraviolet rays of the sun or x-rays or a chemical, any health effects produced will be linear and proportional to the dose received. There is also evidence that the molecular structure of 90 percent of chemical carcinogens interacts with DNA, the genetic material in all living cells; and further, there is as yet incomplete information that a gradual accumulation of irreparable damage to DNA will ultimately result in aberrant or malignant growth. The exact role of cocarcinogens is still uncertain. Consider the interrelationship of benzpyrene and detergents, both found in waste waters. Simultaneous ingestion produces cancer; ingestion of benzpyrene alone does not.

PROBLEMS IN QUALITY CONTROL

Under the Safe Drinking Water Act, the EPA is mandated to ensure the relative safety of the nation's drinking water. The task is formidable. Standards must be established, but there is a lack of definitive information. There is also disagreement within the scientific community on such questions as the significance of human exposure to minute quantities of a hazardous substance, interpretation of animal tests in relation to people, and the identification and characterization of carcinogens. Carcinogens are chemical, physical, or biological agents which increase the probability of tumor induction. Carcinogens may act at the site of initial contact, at the site of selective organ location or accumulation, at the site of excretion, or at the site of metabolism. Some carcinogens act at single sites only; others act at multiple sites. Instruments to identify all contaminants at low-level concentrations are unavailable, and there is little biological knowledge to interpret their potential health effects.

At the present time, evaluation of the toxicity of a particular substance is developed by epidemiologists, who study the occurrence of disease in selected human populations, or by testing in animals. Several obstacles can be encountered in epidemiological studies. The precise dose to which a victim has been exposed is extremely hard to define; historical data that may reveal subtle or latent forms of disease or physiological damage are not usually available; death certificates that are used in studying chronic diseases are not always indicative of the underlying cause of death; weak toxic agents are unlikely to be detected unless there are distinct differences in exposure of the general population such as in cigarette smoking; and, at times, it is nearly impossible to maintain continuous history files that would show changes associated with jobs, diet, or water supplies.

The causes and biological processes of cancer malignancy are sometimes the same among animals and humans. But overall, humans may be more vulnerable to a toxicant than animals because of the greater number and variety of cells that are potential targets.

WATER TREATMENT

Water purification treatments such as the boiling of water, the use of wick siphons, and filtration with sand and gravel have been traced back to the prehistoric era. A history of water treatment is found in Sanskrit medical lore and Egyptian inscriptions discovered on walls dating back to the fifteenth century B.C. Hippocrates, who lived from 460 to 354 B.C., advocated the benefits of water to health but stressed the importance of boiling and straining it before ingestion.

Although water supply systems serving individuals within a community have been used for centuries, the first proof that they were a source of infection to humans was not documented until 1854 by Dr. John Snow in London, England. He tested an area where socioeconomic conditions, climate, soil, and other factors were homogeneous. This area was served by two different water companies. One company obtained its water from a supply contaminated by sewage, the other from a water supply located upstream above the sources of pollution. The results showed the incidence of cholera, a disease caused by intestinal bacteria excreted in large amounts in the feces, was higher among the homes receiving water from the more polluted source. This study is considered a classic in the field of epidemiology, and it is also noteworthy that at this time, the germ theory of disease had not yet been established.

During the seventeenth and nineteenth centuries, improvements were made in water supply systems, especially in filtration to remove turbidity and bacteria that are responsible for the communicable diseases such as cholera and typhoid fever. Chlorination was introduced in the United States in 1908 and first demonstrated in the water supply of the Chicago stockyards and subsequently in the urban water supply of Jersey City, New Jersey. Rather than undergo the expense of building a filtration plant or attempt to prevent the pollution at its source, Jersey City decided to install a chlorination system. The results produced a dramatic drop in the total bacterial count. Because chlorine is an extremely inexpensive chemical and readily adapted to the large-scale use necessary for drinking water, the process began to be utilized extensively throughout the United States.

Soon epidemiological studies began to confirm the effectiveness of chlorine. For example, in Wheeling, West Virginia, during the years 1917–1918, the incidence of typhoid fever was 155 to 200 per 100,000. After the introduction of chlorine in the latter part of 1918, only seven cases of typhoid were reported in the first 3 months of 1919. For 3 weeks in April, chlorination was discontinued, and the incidence of typhoid increased 300 percent. After the process was resumed, there were only 11 cases reported for the following 6 months. Since 1918, refinements at the engineering level have been made, but the basic concepts of water purification techniques have remained unchanged.

Prior to the enactment of the Safe Drinking Water Act in 1974, standards for water quality were limited to interstate carriers like trains and buses, and primarily focused on microbiological contaminants associated with waterborne diseases such as typhoid fever and cholera. The regulations now apply to all community water supply systems that have 15 or more connections or serve 25 or more individuals. Maximum levels of contamination are set for such substances as bacteria, arsenic, barium, cadmium, chromium, fluoride, lead, mercury, nitrate, selenium, silver, selected insecticides and herbicides, and radionuclides. There is also a limit on turbidity. Turbidity becomes a problem because substances can become imbedded in particles of turbidity and escape the chlorine action. The drinking water standard is 1 turbidity unit. However, in a 1962 study by H. E. Hudson in the *Journal of the American Waterworks Association*, a significant relation to certain diseases was shown at a turbidity concentration of a little over 0.1 unit.

The conventional treatments used in preparing water for drinking are sedimentation, filtration, and disinfection. A few systems employ lime softening and carbon filtration. None of these methods is effective in completely eliminating all toxic substances. Some may be eliminated, some reduced, but others are not removed to any significant degree.

Sedimentation, aimed at reducing turbidity and color, begins by the addition to the water of a coagulant, such as alum or iron salt (ferric sulfate), that forms the lighter particles into a mass for easier removal. The water is then passed to a settling basin. Alum coagulant is effective in reducing arsenic V, cadmium, and chromium III and ferric sulfate coagulant in reducing inorganic mercury, arsenic V, selenium IV, cadmium, and chromium III. Sand, garnet, and anthracite are usually used for filtration, removing more turbidity and floating debris; then chlorine is dispensed for disinfection against bacteria. Frequently, lime or soda to remove gross hardness, principally calcium and manganese; oxidants to remove iron and manganese; ion exchange for softening and salt removal; or carbon for removal of taste- and odor-causing organics are employed. Lime softening has shown good removal of inorganic mercury, barium, arsenic V, cadmium, and chromium III. Radium 226 is effectively removed by lime softening and ion exchange softening. Granular activated carbon sufficiently reduces a number of organic substances, including some pesticides and the trihalomethanes. The more commonly used powdered carbon, generally sprinkled into the water before coagulation, is not as effective.

Inadequate treatment is the main cause of contaminated drinking water, but there are other causes as well. Distribution systems can be at fault by inadvertent cross-connections where there is a physical connection between the distribution system and polluted water, gases, or chemicals. Backsiphonage can result from low water pressure, and contamination of the pipeline can occur during construction or repair. Water can also leach metals from the distribution pipes. Some systems store their water in inadequately protected tanks. For example, water utility officials believe that 16,000 paratyphoid cases in Riverside, California, were caused by bacteria from bird droppings that fell into the drinking water reservoir.

Fifty percent of the population in the United States uses water that in part is made up of recently discharged wastewater. The Public Advisory Committee in their report on the proposed 1974 Federal Drinking Water Standards stated that it viewed with alarm the increase in the number of wastewater discharges, the decreasing dilution of these effluents with natural waters, and the decreasing distances between these discharges and water supply intakes.

Treating wastewaters, the effluent from a city's sewers or industrial discharges, began around the 1920s. At first, the water was placed in lagoons to settle before discharge. Soon after, the trickling filter system gained popularity. The Federal Water Pollution Control Act requires a permit for any pipeline discharging wastes into a water resource. Certain standards for oxygen-demanding wastes, suspended solids, and fecal coliform must be met, usually by the implementation of various treatment processes.

Wastewater techniques usually consist of primary treatment, which is a separation of the water from solid matter in a settling tank, and secondary treatment, which filters the waste through a bed of sand or gravel upon which bacteria grow, consuming most of the organic matter. Another method using bacteria combines the sewage with air and bacteria-laden sludge in an aeration tank where the organic waste is broken down by the bacteria. However, dissolved solids such as nitrates, iron, phosphates, some acids, and industrial wastes resist such bacterial action and are not removed. Chlorination often completes the treatment. Utilized by very few plants are advanced methods such as lime precipitation, rapid sand filtration, and carbon absorption. Like the treatments for drinking water, wastewater treatments do not remove many of the toxic substances.

WATERBORNE DISEASES

Bacteria, viruses, synthetic compounds, metals, and radionuclides are the contaminants that become incorporated into our drinking waters and have the potential to cause health effects ranging from low-grade subclinical illnesses such as colds and flu to death from cancer.

Bacteria are microscopic organisms ubiquitous in nearly all natural environments, often present in large numbers (billions in a gram of soil, millions in one drop of saliva), and vital to the biochemical transformations that change complex natural substances into simple compounds that can then be easily utilized by plants, animals, and people for survival. Although most species are benign, some are pathogenic or disease-causing. Among the microbial flora most frequently found in drinking water supplies of poor quality are *Pseudomonas*, *Flavobacterium*, *Achromobacter*, *Proteus-Klebsiella*, *Bacillus*, *Serratia*, *Corynebacterium*, *Spirillum*, *Clostridium*, *Arthrobacter*, *Gallionella*, and *Leptothrix*. Many of these can precipitate illness.

Flavobacterium can become a primary pathogen in persons who have undergone surgery. Besides being prevalent in drinking water, strains have been found in water taps and drinking fountain bubbler heads. Concentrations of 10,000 to 26,000 organisms per milliliter were discovered in 23 percent of the samples taken in a study of stored emergency supplies. *Pseudomonas* organisms can become secondary pathogens in postoperation infections, burn cases, and intestinal–urinary tract infections. They can persist and grow in water containing minimal nutrients and become established in sections of the distribution lines irregularly shedding into the water supply.

Klebsiella pneumoniae produces infection of the nose, throat, and respiratory and genitourinary systems and has been reported as the cause of meningitis and septicema. The organisms collect in the slime accumulations of distribution pipes, water taps, air chambers, and aerators. Coliform organisms are generally found in the intestinal tract of humans and other warm-blooded animals and are hence a good indicator of a water supply contaminated by fecal matter. Some species are harmful. For example, *Escherichia coli* (E. coli) can cause severe inflammation of abdominal organs and membranes; *Salmonella* induces typhoid and intestinal fevers; and *Shigella* produces various forms of dysentery and enteritis. The total coliform density limit is a constituent of the Safe Drinking Water Act most frequently exceeded in drinking water surveys.

Viruses are a group of infectious agents characterized by their small size, simple composition, and the need to grow in a human, animal, plant, or bacterial cell. They have various shapes and sizes: rodlike, spherical, filamentous, spermlike, or a solid with several plane surfaces, and range from 10 to 300 millimicrons in size. (A micron is 1/25,000 of an inch.) The viruses of major concern in relation to drinking water are those of intestinal origin, excreted by infected animals or humans, which reach water resources by way of soil runoff and sewage. They include poliovirus, which is also increased by oral vaccine usage, coxsackievirus, echovirus, adenovirus, reovirus, and hepatitis virus. Human contact with any of these viruses becomes ever more likely as the reuse of wastewater for domestic purposes is increasingly practiced.

Several lab and field studies indicate that current sewage and water purification treatments do not eliminate all viruses. A survey of surface waters throughout the world revealed virus concentrations in an average of 36 percent of the samples examined. In five communities in France whose water sources are the Meurthe and Moselle Rivers, viruses were isolated after each stage of drinking water treatments of coagulation, filtration, and disinfection. The first reported viral contamination of a treated water supply in the United States occurred in 1970, when viruses were isolated from drinking water samples in two Massachusetts communities. Groundwaters can be polluted as well, as shown by the recovery of a poliovirus from a deep well in Michigan. At the present time, methods for isolating viruses occurring at low concentration levels are ineffective, and so the true extent of viral contamination in our drinking waters is difficult to determine.

Viruses invade a cell in the body and prod the cell to manufacture more new viruses. The original cell dies, releasing the new viruses to inhabit other cells. Traditional medicines such as antibiotics are ineffective because the virus hides within the cell. Most viral infections are mild and subclinical (the common cold is considered to be caused by a virus) and are generally not recognized or reported. So-called slow viruses that enter a cell and lie dormant for many years only to reappear in an often lethal form are suspected by some scientists to cause multiple sclerosis and another rare nerve disease, subacute sclerosing panencephalitis. They have also been recognized as one cause of two fatal brain diseases. Intestinal viruses have also become associated with diseases such as diabetes mellitus, spontaneous abortion, congenital heart anomalies, various malignancies, and cancer. Acute effects have been known for years, including meningitis, hepatitis, paralysis, rashes, fevers, gastroenteritis, and poliomyelitis. Although

water treatment may reduce the concentration of viruses, as little as one virus unit is all that is necessary to infect the human body.

There are two types of organics: natural and synthetic, or man-made. The natural organic content of water is derived from earthy materials such as humus substances, lignins, organic acids, and a variety of decomposition products. Tastes and odors can be created from these compounds as they decay and also as they react with chlorine. They can become potentially toxic when combined with synthetic agents or when subjected to chlorine or ozone treatment, producing either halogenated organic compounds or oxidized compounds such as peroxides or epoxides.

Then there are what Russell E. Train, former EPA administrator, in an article in the *Los Angeles Herald Examiner* in 1976, calls "strange new creatures of our own making, all around us, in our air, our water, our food, and in the things we touch. When they hit us, we don't feel a thing. Their ill effects may not show up until decades later, in the form of cancer, or generations later in the form of mutated genes." Some of these compounds break down very rapidly in the environment, others are persistent because there are no natural agents to break them down. They translocate from the environment into organisms and concentrate in food chains. Over 2 million synthetic organics are known to exist, 25,000 are added each year, and more than 30,000 are in actual commercial production. Only a fraction have been tested for their toxic properties. Unknown, too, are the synergistic effects, resulting if the combination of chemical compounds produces a greater toxic effect than each chemical by itself.

In November of 1975, the EPA listed 253 specific organic chemicals in drinking water in the United States and strongly suggested the presence of others not yet identified. These chemicals become integrated into our drinking water supplies as the result of industrial and municipal discharges, urban and rural runoff, and the water chlorination process. To get a comprehensive view of the organic content of water supplies, the EPA selected ten representative water utility companies with varying sources of their drinking water to scrutinize. The drinking water supplies investigated were in Miami and Tucson (groundwater source), Seattle and New York (uncontaminated upland source), Ottumwa, Iowa and Grand Forks, North Dakota (agricultural runoff), Philadelphia and Terrebonne Parish, Louisiana (wastewater), and Cincinnati and Lawrence, Massachusetts (industrial discharges). The following eighteen compounds occurred most frequently.

Compound	Occurrence
Bromodichloromethane	9/10
Chloral (trichloroacetaldehyde)	6/10
Chlorobenzene	9/10
Cyanogen chloride	8/10
Dibromochloromethane	9/10
Di-n-butyl phthalate	6/10
Dichloroiodomethane	7/10
Dichloromethane (methylene chloride)	9/10
Diethylphthalate	6/10
Ethylbenzene	6/10
Methanol	6/10
2-Methylpropanol (isobutyraldehyde)	7/10
Propanol (propionaldehyde)	7/10
2-Propanone (acetone)	10/10
Tetrachloromethane (carbon tetrachloride)	8/10
Tetrachloroethene (tetrachloroethylene)	8/10
Toluene	6/10
Trichloromethane (chloroform)	10/10

Inorganic compounds consist of metals and trace elements. These materials occur naturally and enter water through geochemical processes of erosion and solution. Organisms including human beings have evolved a tolerance to these natural levels. Small amounts of some are essential to health, including manganese, molybdenum, chromium, cobalt, copper, iron, vanadium, selenium, zinc, calcium, magnesium, sodium, potassium, and fluoride. However, release of additional amounts of inorganics by human activities can create degradation and health problems. Many are cumulative poisons and are concentrated above normal levels by various organisms. The different chemical forms of each element have varying toxic properties. Under certain environmental conditions, several low-toxic inorganics can be converted to a more toxic form. Also, there are synergistic effects. For example, the toxicity of some heavy metals is greater at lower levels of concentration if selenium is present.

All of the metals and trace elements can be found in industrial waste discharges. Industrial solid wastes containing metals can leach into surface waters and seep to groundwater tables. Municipal sewage, corrosion of household water distribution pipes, and water treatment processes like the use of copper for algae control and other treatments using chemicals that contain trace metals and fossil fuel combustion all contribute to the inorganic content of drinking water. A seminal study in 1971 estimated that the release and mobilization of trace elements by combustion of coal, oil, lignite, and natural gas into the atmosphere with subsequent descent into surface waters coincided with the rate of natural biological processes.

Radiation is omnipresent throughout the planet and its atmosphere and is the result of radio, ultraviolet and cosmic x-rays, naturally occurring radioisotopes such as uranium and thorium, and the radioactivity that is produced by human beings. The latter activity adds significant concentrations to the environment. As the medical field, industry, agriculture, and scientific research utilize radionuclides, their effluents and emissions, in solid, liquid, or vapor form, contaminate water supplies. Wastes are emitted from essentially all operations associated with nuclear power generation, beginning with the mining of uranium where radioactive tailings remain after the useful materials have been extracted, dissolve during precipitation, and run off into nearby streams. In a report by the EPA, radioactive gas emissions from uranium tailings buried in Colorado were escaping at a rate three times faster than when they were first dumped. Measurements taken in a residential area one-half mile from the site showed a radon gas concentration ten times greater than that occurring naturally in the area.

The United States has been accumulating thousands of tons of nuclear wastes for more than 40 years, yet does not have a permanent and safe storage for them. High levels of wastes have been dumped at sea or stored in steel tanks that have been known to corrode. Some wastes are stored underground where there is known seepage into groundwaters. Intermediate- and low-level wastes from sources such as leaking equipment, floor drains, and cleansing operations have been discharged directly into water resources or into the ground. Nuclear weapons testing above ground is prohibited in the United States, but when underground detonations are performed, occasional releases of radiation occur because of venting caused by open channels left for cables and by natural cracks and fractures created by the explosion.

Acknowledging the fact that all of life has been exposed to nominal natural background radiation levels for eons with no apparent ill-effects, artificially produced radiation infiltrates air, food, and water and eventually accumulates in the cells and tissues of the human body. Genetics Professor Sadao Ichikawa of Kyoto University has demonstrated, by using a tiny flowering plant, that supposedly harmless radiation around normally operating atomic power plants can cause mutations. He says his experiments cast doubt on reassurances from utilities that the amount of daily release of radioactivity is so small that the effect can be ignored.

Radionuclides have a biological half-life ranging from a few seconds for some to billions of years for others. The EPA bases its estimates of health reactions to radiation exposure on the assumption that there is no dose level that is harmless and that the effects will be proportional to the dose. Other factors determining damage will be the type of radiation, its penetrating ability, the body organs exposed to it, and the duration of exposure. High levels of radiation result in burn and cellular damage leading to death. Low-level exposure is usually associated with cataract formation, increase in mutations, possible teratogenic effects, damage to blood vessels, bone marrow depletion, tissue degeneration, and the development of tumor and blood cancers. The latency period for cancer can be 4 to 5 years for leukemia and up to 20 years for other forms.

There are 1 billion cells in 1 gram of cells, and approximately one cell afflicted by the proper type of radiation is sufficient to cause damage, inhibiting cell functions and/or initiating cancer. The nucleus of a cell is considered to be the crucial site of injury, especially the chromosomes, which influence cell division, growth, production of chemicals, and other metabolic activities. Radiation can induce visible alterations in the genes, which are the information units within the chromosomes. Their functions can be disrupted, providing false information to the cell. When the cell divides, the altered gene may be reproduced. Irradiation of the gene-containing cells in the reproductive organs can produce mental and physical deformities and a number of other aberrations in future generations.

It is likely that most drinking water supplies carry some kind of potential health hazard. In laboratory tests, the purification processes of distillation and reverse osmosis were the most efficient in removing and reducing the widest range of contaminants. Other methods, including charcoal types, remove only some forms of contaminants but not the full range.

REFERENCES

Akin, Elmer W., et al. *Enteric Viruses in Ground and Surface Waters: A Review of their Occurrence and Survival.* Urbana: University of Illinois, 1971.

California Department of Consumer Affairs. *Drinking Water Quality Problems Facing California Consumers*, July 1976.

Clarke, Norman A. Virus study of drinking water supplies. *J. Amer. Waterworks Asso.*, Vol. 67, April 1975, pp. 192–197.

Davis, Kenneth S. and John A. Day. *Water—The Mirror of Science.* Garden City, N.Y.: Doubleday, Inc., 1975.

Environmental Defense Fund. *The Implications of Cancer-Causing Substances in Mississippi River Water.* Washington, D.C., 1974.

Gofman, John W. and Arthur R. Tamplin. *Poisoned Power.* Emmaus, Pa.: Rodale Press, 1971.

Harris, Robert. *Carcinogenic Hazards of Organic Chemicals in Drinking Water.* Washington, D.C.: Environmental Defense Fund, 1975.

National Academy of Sciences. *Drinking Water and Health.* Washington, D.C., 1977.

North Carolina Research Triangle Universities, Environmental Protection Agency. *The State of America's Drinking Water.* Raleigh, N.C., 1974.

U.S. Environmental Protection Agency. *The Impact of Intensive Application of Pesticides and Fertilizers on Underground Water Recharge Areas Which May Contribute to Drinking Water Supplies.* Washington, D.C.: Office of Toxic Substances, 1976.

U.S. Environmental Protection Agency. *Identification of Organic Compounds in Effluents from Indus-*

trial Sources. Washington, D.C.: Office of Toxic Substances, 1975.

U.S. Environmental Protection Agency. *Preliminary Assessment of Suspected Carcinogens in Drinking Water*. Washington, D.C., 1975.

U.S. Environmental Protection Agency. *Transcript of an EPA Press Conference*, Russell Train, administrator. April 18, 1975.

Zwick, David and Marcy Benstock. *Water Wasteland*. New York: N. Grossman, 1971.

SUMMARY CHART OF NUTRIENTS

Nutrients	Importance	Deficiency Symptoms	RDA*	Toxicity Level
Carbohydrate	Provides energy for body functions and muscular exertions. Assists in digestion and assimilation of foods.	Loss of energy. Fatigue. Excessive protein breakdown. Disturbed balance of water, sodium, potassium, and chloride.	See Nutrient Allowance Chart, p. 309.	Intake should not exceed what is needed to maintain desirable weight.
Fat	Provides energy. Acts as a carrier for fat-soluble vitamins A, D, E, and K. Supplies essential fatty acids needed for growth, health, and smooth skin.	Eczema or skin disorders. Retarded growth	See Nutrient Allowance Chart, p. 309	Intake should not exceed what is needed to maintain desirable weight.
Protein	Is necessary for growth and development Acts in formation of hormones, enzymes, and antibodies. Maintains acid-alkali balance. Is source of heat and energy.	Fatigue. Loss of appetite. Diarrhea and vomiting. Stunted growth. Edema.	See Nutrient Allowance Chart, p. 309	Intake should not exceed what is needed to maintain desirable weight.
VITAMINS				
Vitamin A	Is necessary for growth and repair of body tissues. Is important to health of the eyes. Fights bacteria and infection. Maintains healthy epithelial tis-	Night blindness. Rough, dry, scaly skin. Increased susceptibility to infections. Frequent fatigue, insomnia, depression. Loss of smell and ap-	Infants: 1400–2000 IU Children: 2000–4000 IU Adults: 4000–5000 IU	

*Recommended Dietary Allowance

Nutrients	Importance	Deficiency Symptoms	RDA*	Toxicity Level
	sue. Aids in bone and teeth formation.	petite. Lusterless hair. Brittle nails. Inflamed eyelids.		
Vitamin B complex	Is necessary for carbohydrate, fat, and protein metabolism. Helps functioning of the nervous system. Helps maintain muscle tone in the gastrointestinal tract. Maintains health of skin, hair, eyes, mouth, and liver.	Dry, rough, cracked skin. Acne. Dull, dry, or gray hair. Fatigue. Poor appetite. Gastrointestinal tract disorders.	See individual B vitamins	See individual B vitamins; relatively nontoxic.
Vitamin B_1 (Thiamine)	Is necessary for carbohydrate metabolism. Helps maintain healthy nervous system. Stabilizes the appetite. Stimulates growth and good muscle tone.	Gastrointestinal problems. Fatigue. Loss of appetite. Nerve disorders. Heart disorders.	Infants: 0.3–0.5 mg Children: 0.7–1.2 mg Men: 1.4 mg Women: 1.0 mg	No known oral toxicity.
Vitamin B_2 (Riboflavin)	Is necessary for carbohydrate, fat, and protein metabolism. Aids in formation of antibodies and red blood cells. Maintains cell respiration.	Eye problems. Cracks and sores in mouth. Dermatitis. Retarded growth. Digestive disturbances.	Infants: 0.4–0.6 mg Children: 0.8–1.4 mg Men: 1.6 mg Women: 1.2 mg	No known oral toxicity.
Niacin (B_3 Nicotinic acid, Niacinamide)	Is necessary for carbohydrate, fat, and protein metabolism. Helps maintain health of skin, tongue, and digestive system.	Dermatitis. Nervous disorders. Headaches. Insomnia. Bad breath. Digestive disturbances. Sore mouth and gums.	Infants: 6–8 mg Children: 9–16 mg Men: 16 mg Women: 13 mg	
Pantothenic acid (B_5)	Aids in formation of some fats. Participates in the release of energy from carbohydrates, fats, and proteins.	Vomiting. Restlessness. Increased susceptibility to infection. Gastrointestinal disturbances.	Infants: 2–3 mg Children: 3–7 mg Adults: 5–10 mg	

*Recommended Dietary Allowance

Nutrients	Importance	Deficiency Symptoms	RDA*	Toxicity Level
	Aids in the utilization of some vitamins. Improves body's resistance to stress.	Depression. Fatigue.		
Vitamin B₆ (Pyridoxine)	Is necessary for carbohydrate, fat, and protein metabolism. Aids in formation of antibodies. Helps maintain balance of sodium and phosphorus.	Anemia. Mouth disorders. Nervousness. Muscular weakness. Dermatitis. Dandruff. Water retention.	Infants: 0.3–0.6 mg Children: 0.9–1.8 mg Men: 2.2 mg Women: 2 mg	
Vitamin B₁₂	Is essential for normal formation of blood cells. Is necessary for carbohydrate, fat, and protein metabolism. Maintains healthy nervous system	Pernicious anemia. Brain damage. Nervousness. Neuritis.	Infants: 0.5–1.5 mcg Children: 2–3 mcg Adults: 3 mcg	No known oral toxicity even with intake as high as 600–1,200 mcg.
Biotin	Necessary for carbohydrate, fat, and protein metabolism. Aids in utilization of other B vitamins.	Dermatitis. Grayish skin color. Depression. Muscle pain. Impairment of fat metabolism. Poor appetite.	Infants: 35–50 mcg Children: 65–200 mcg Adults:150–300 mcg	No known oral toxicity.
Choline	Is important in normal nerve transmission. Aids metabolism and transport of fats. Helps regulate liver and gallbladder.	Fatty liver. Hemorrhaging kidneys. High blood pressure.	No RDA, but the average diet yields 500–900 mg per day.	No known oral toxicity, even with intake as high as 50,000 mg. daily for 1 week.
Folic acid (Folacin)	Is important in red blood cell formation. Aids metabolism of proteins. Is necessary for growth and division of body cells.	Poor growth. Gastrointestinal disorders. Anemia. Poor memory.	Infants: 0.03–0.045 mg Children: 0.1–0.4 mg Adults: 0.4 mg	No toxic effects
Inositol	Is necessary for formation of lecithin. May be directly connected with metabolism of fats, including cholesterol. Is vital for hair growth.	Constipation. Eczema. Hair loss. High blood cholesterol.	No RDA, but the average diet yields 1000 mg per day.	No known toxicity.
PABA	Aids bacteria in producing folic acid. Acts as a coenzyme	Fatigue. Irritability. Depression. Nervousness.	No RDA.	Continued high ingestion may be toxic.

*Recommended Dietary Allowance

Nutrients	Importance	Deficiency Symptoms	RDA*	Toxicity Level
	in the breakdown and utilization of proteins. Aids in formation of red blood cells. Acts as a sunscreen.	Constipation. Headache. Digestive disorders. Graying hair		
Pangamic acid (B₁₅)	Helps eliminate hypoxia. Helps promote protein metabolism. Stimulates nervous and glandular system.	Diminished oxygenation of cells. Nervous disorders.	No RDA.	500 mg tolerated daily with no toxic effect.
Vitamin C	Maintains collagen. Helps heal wounds, scar tissue, and fractures. Gives strength to blood vessels. May provide resistance to infections. Aids in absorption of iron.	Bleeding gums. Swollen or painful joints. Slow-healing wounds and fractures. Bruising. Nosebleeds. Impaired digestion.	Infants: 35 mg Children: 45–50 mg Adults: 60 mg	Essentially nontoxic.
Vitamin D	Improves absorption and utilization of calcium and phosphorus required for bone formation. Maintains stable nervous system and normal heart action.	Poor bone and tooth formation. Softening of bones and teeth. Inadequate absorption of calcium. Retention of phosphorus in kidney.	Infants, children, and adults, 400 IU	
Vitamin E	Protects fat-soluble vitamins. Protects red blood cells. Is essential in cellular respiration. Inhibits coagulation of blood by preventing blood clots.	Rupture of red blood cells. Muscular wasting. Abnormal fat deposits in muscles.	Infants: 4–6 IU Children: 7–12 IU Men: 15 IU Women: 12 IU	Essentially nontoxic.
Vitamin K	Is necessary for formation of prothrombin; is needed for blood coagulation.	Lack of prothrombin, increasing the tendency to hemorrhage.	Infants: 12–20 mcg Children: 15–100 mcg Adults: 300–500 mcg	Menadione (synthetic vitamin K) may have side effects.
Bioflavonoids (Vitamin P)	Help increase strength of capillaries.	Tendency to bleed and bruise easily.	No RDA.	No known toxicity.
Unsaturated fatty acids	Is important for respiration of vital organs. Helps maintain resilience and lubrication	Brittle, lusterless hair. Brittle nails. Dandruff.	No RDA, 10% of total calories.	Intake should not exceed what is needed to maintain desirable weight.

*Recommended Dietary Allowance

Nutrients	Importance	Deficiency Symptoms	RDA*	Toxicity Level
	of cells. Helps regulate blood coagulation. Is essential for normal glandular activity.	Diarrhea. Varicose veins.		
MINERALS				
Calcium	Sustains development and maintenance of strong bones and teeth. Assists normal blood clotting, muscle action, nerve function, and heart function.	Tetany. Softening bones. Back and leg pains. Brittle bones. Insomnia. Irritability. Depression.	Infants: 360–540 mg Children: 800–1200 mg Adults: 800 mg	Excessive intakes of calcium may have side effects in certain persons. No known oral toxicity.
Chlorine	Regulates acid-base balance. Maintains osmotic pressure. Stimulates production of hydrochloric acid. Helps maintain joints and tendons.	Loss of hair and teeth. Poor muscular contractibility. Impaired digestion.	No RDA.	Daily intake of 14–28 gm of salt (sodium chloride) is considered excessive. Excess intake of chlorine may have adverse effects.
Chromium	Stimulates enzymes in metabolism of energy and synthesis of fatty acids, cholesterol, and protein. Increases effectiveness of insulin.	Depressed growth rate. Glucose intolerance in diabetics. Atherosclerosis.	Infants: 0.01–0.06 mg Children: 0.02–0.2 mg Adults: 0.05–0.2 mg	No known toxicity.
Cobalt	Functions as part of vitamin B_{12}. Maintains red blood cells. Activates a number of enzymes in the body.	Pernicious anemia. Slow rate of growth.	No RDA; average daily intake is 5–8 mcg	Excessive intakes of cobalt may have side effects in certain persons.
Copper	Aids in formation of red blood cells. Is part of many enzymes. Works with vitamin C to form elastin.	General weakness. Impaired respiration. Skin sores.	Infants: 0.5–1 mg Children: 1–3 mg Adults: 2–3 mg	Excessive intakes may have side effects.
Fluorine (Fluorides)	May reduce tooth decay by discouraging the growth of acid-forming bacteria.	Tooth decay.	Infants: 0.1–1 mg Children: 0.5–2.5 mg Adults: 1.5–4 mg	Excessive intake of fluroine may have side effects in some persons.
Iodine (Iodide)	Is essential part of	Englarged thyroid	Infants: 40–50 mcg	Up to 1000 mcg daily

*Recommended Dietary Allowance

Nutrients	Importance	Deficiency Symptoms	RDA*	Toxicity Level
	the hormone thyroxine. Is necessary for the prevention of goiter. Regulates production of energy and rate of metabolism. Promotes growth.	gland. Dry skin and hair. Loss of physical and mental vigor. Cretinism in children born to iodine-deficient mothers.	Children: 70–150 mcg Adults: 150 mcg	produced no toxic effects in persons with a normal thyroid**
Iron	Is necessary for hemoglobin and myoglobin formation. Helps in protein metabolism. Promotes growth.	Weakness. Paleness of skin. Constipation. Anemia.	Infants: 10–15 mg Children: 15–18 mg Men: 10 mg Women: 18 mg	Excessive intake may be toxic.
Magnesium	Acts as a catalyst in the utilization of carbohydrates, fats, protein, calcium, phosphorus, and possibly potassium.	Nervousness. Muscular excitability. Tremors. Depression.	Infants: 50–70 mg Children: 150–300 mg Men: 350 mg Women: 300 mg	30,000 mg daily may be toxic in certain individuals with kidney malfunctions.
Manganese	Is enzyme activator. Plays a part in carbohydrate and fat production. Is necessary for normal skeletal development. Maintains sex-hormone production.	Paralysis. Convulsions. Dizziness. Ataxia. Blindness and deafness in infants. Diabetes. Loss of hearing.	Infants: 0.5–1 mg Children: 1–5 mg Adults: 2.5–5 mg	Excessive intake may have side effects in certain persons.
Molybdenum	Acts in oxidation of fats and aldehydes. Aids in mobilization of iron from liver reserves.	Premature aging. Impotence.	Infants: 0.03–0.08 mg Children: 0.05–0.5 mg Adults: 0.15–0.5 mg	Excessive intake may be toxic.
Nickel	Is a factor in hormone, lipid, membrane, and glucose metabolism.	Aggravates iron-deficiency anemia.	No RDA.	Excessive intake may be toxic.
Phosphorus	Works with calcium to build bones and teeth. Utilizes carbohydrates, fats, and proteins. Stimulates muscular contraction.	Loss of weight and appetite. Irregular breathing. Pyorrhea. Fatigue. Nervous disorders.	Infants: 240–360 mg Children: 800–1200 mg Adults: 800 mg	No known toxicity.

*Recommended Dietary Allowance

**Goodhart and Shils, *Modern Nutrition in Health and Disease*, p. 365.

Nutrients	Importance	Deficiency Symptoms	RDA*	Toxicity Level
Potassium	Works to control activity of heart muscles, nervous system, and kidneys.	Poor reflexes. Respiratory failure. Cardiac arrest. Nervous disorders. Constipation. Irregular pulse. Insomnia.	Infants: 350–1275 mg Children: 550–4575 mg Adults: 1875–5625 mg	No known toxicity.
Selenium	Works with vitamin E. Preserves tissue elasticity.	Premature aging. Crib death.	Infants: 0.01–0.06 mg Children: 0.02–0.2 mg Adults: 0.05–0.2 mg	Excessive intake may be toxic.
Sodium	Maintains normal fluid levels in cells. Maintains health of the nervous, muscular, blood, and lymph systems.	Muscle weakness. Muscle shrinkage. Nausea. Loss of appetite. Intestinal gas.	Infants: 115–750 mg Children: 325–2700 mg Adults: 1100–3300 mg	Excessive sodium intake may have adverse effects. Intake of 14–28 gm of sodium chloride (salt) is considered excessive.
Sulfur	Is part of amino acids. Is essential for formation of body tissues. Is part of the B vitamins. Plays a part in tissue respiration. Is necessary for collagen synthesis.	Possibly sluggishness and fatigue.	The RDA of protein supplies sufficient amounts of sulfur.	Excessive intake of sulfur may be toxic.
Vanadium	Inhibits cholesterol formation. Important for bone, cartilage, and tooth development.	———	No RDA.	Excessive intake of vanadium may be toxic.
Zinc	Is component of insulin and male reproductive fluid. Aids in digestion and metabolism of phosphorus. Aids in healing process.	Retarded growth. Delayed sexual maturity. Prolonged healing of wounds. Stretch marks. Irregular menses. Diabetes. Loss of taste and appetite.	Infants: 3–5 mg Children: 10–15 mg Adults: 15 mg	Relatively nontoxic. Excessive intake may have side effects.

*Recommended Dietary Allowance

NUTRIENTS THAT FUNCTION TOGETHER

When nutrients are taken in supplemental form, they function best when taken together in particular combinations. Some nutrients are so closely interrelated that their effectiveness in the body is markedly improved when they are taken together with other nutrients. Minerals are especially important in aiding the effectiveness of specific vitamins.

For example, if one is suffering from athlete's foot, vitamin A is recommended for treatment. Vitamin A can be utilized more effectively within the body when taken with the B-complex vitamins, choline, and vitamins C, D, E, and UFA. Calcium, phosphorus, and zinc are also recommended to increase the effectiveness of vitamin A.

The following chart provides a basic guide to nutrients that function best when taken together.

A. VITAMINS

1. VITAMIN A IS MORE EFFECTIVE WHEN TAKEN WITH

Vitamin B complex	Helps preserve stored vitamin A.
Choline	
Vitamin C	Helps protect against toxic effects of vitamin A. Helps prevent oxidation.
Vitamin D	1 part vitamin D to 10 parts vitamin A.
Vitamin E	Acts as an antioxidant.
Unsaturated fatty acids	
Calcium	
Phosphorus	
Zinc	Helps in the absorption of vitamin A.

VITAMIN A ANTAGONISTS

Air pollution

Alcohol

Arsenicals

Aspirin

Corticosteroid drugs (such as prednisone and cortisone)

Dicumarol

Mineral oil

Nitrates

Phenobarbital

Thyroid

2. VITAMIN B COMPLEX IS MORE EFFECTIVE WHEN TAKEN WITH

Vitamin C

Vitamin E

Calcium

Phosphorus

VITAMIN B COMPLEX ANTAGONISTS

Alcohol

Antibiotics

Aspirin

Corticosteroid drugs

Diuretics

3. VITAMIN B$_1$ (THIAMINE) IS MORE EFFECTIVE WHEN TAKEN WITH
Vitamin B complex
Vitamin B$_2$ (riboflavin)
Folic acid
Niacin
Vitamin C   Helps protect against oxidation.
Vitamin E
Manganese
Sulfur
VITAMIN B$_1$ ANTAGONISTS
Alcohol
Antibiotics
Excess sugar

4. VITAMIN B$_2$ (RIBOVLAVIN) IS MORE EFFECTIVE WHEN TAKEN WITH
Vitamin B complex
Vitamin B$_6$ Vitamin B$_2$ and vitamin B$_6$ doses should usually be about the same.
Niacin
Vitamin C   Helps protect against oxidation.
VITAMIN B$_2$ ANTAGONISTS
Alcohol
Antibiotics
Oral contraceptives

5. NIACIN (B$_3$) IS MORE EFFECTIVE WHEN TAKEN WITH
Vitamin B complex
Vitamin B$_1$ (thiamine)
Vitamin B$_2$ (riboflavin)
Vitamin C   Helps protect against oxidation.
NIACIN ANTAGONISTS
Alcohol
Antibiotics
Excess sugar

6. PANTOTHENIC ACID (B$_5$) IS MORE EFFECTIVE WHEN TAKEN WITH
Vitamin B complex
Vitamin B$_6$ (pyridoxine)
Vitamin B$_{12}$
Biotin   Aids in the absorption of pantothenic acid.
Folic acid   Aids in the absorption of pantothenic acid.
Vitamin C   Helps protect against oxidation.
Calcium
Sulfur
PANTOTHENIC ACID ANTAGONISTS
Aspirin
Methylbromide (an insecticide
fumigant for some foods)

7. VITAMIN B_6 (PYRIDOXINE) IS MORE EFFECTIVE WHEN TAKEN WITH

Vitamin B complex

Vitamin B_1 (thiamine)   Vitamin B_1 and vitamin B_6 doses should usually be about the same.

Vitamin B_2 (riboflavin)   Vitamin B_2 and vitamin B_6 doses should usually be about the same.

Pantothenic acid

Vitamin C

Magnesium

Potassium

Linoleic acid

Sodium

VITAMIN B_6 ANTAGONISTS

Cortisone

Estrogen

Oral contraceptives

8. VITAMIN B_{12} IS MORE EFFECTIVE WHEN TAKEN WITH

Vitamin B complex

Vitamin B_6 (pyridoxine)   Helps increase absorption of vitamin B_{12}.

Choline

Folic acid

Inositol

Vitamin C   Helps increase absorption of vitamin B_{12}.

Calcium

Iron   Helps increase absorption of vitamin B_{12}.

Potassium

Sodium

VITAMIN B_{12} ANTAGONISTS

Dilantin

Oral contraceptives

9. PANGAMIC ACID (B_{15}) IS MORE EFFECTIVE WHEN TAKEN WITH

Vitamin B complex

Vitamin C

Vitamin E

10. BIOTIN IS MORE EFFECTIVE WHEN TAKEN WITH

Vitamin B complex

Vitamin B_{12}

Folic acid

Pantothenic acid

Vitamin C

Sulfur

BIOTIN ANTAGONISTS

Antibiotics

Avidin (from raw egg whites)

Sulfa drugs

11. CHOLINE IS MORE EFFECTIVE WHEN TAKEN WITH
    Vitamin A
    Vitamin B complex
    Vitamin B_{12} Helps synthesize choline.
    Folic acid   Helps synthesize choline.
    Inositol
    Linoleic acid
    CHOLINE ANTAGONISTS
    Alcohol
    Excess sugar

12. FOLIC ACID IS MORE EFFECTIVE WHEN TAKEN WITH
    Vitamin B complex
    Vitamin B_{12}
    Biotin
    Pantothenic acid
    Vitamin C   Helps protect against oxidation.
    FOLIC ACID ANTAGONISTS
    Alcohol
    Anticonvulsants
    Oral contraceptives
    Phenobarbital

13. INOSITOL IS MORE EFFECTIVE WHEN TAKEN WITH
    Vitamin B complex
    Vitamin B_{12}
    Choline
    Vitamin C
    Vitamin E
    Linoleic acid
    INOSITOL ANTAGONISTS
    Antibiotics

14. PARA-AMINOBENZOIC ACID (PABA) IS MORE EFFECTIVE WHEN TAKEN WITH
    Vitamin B complex
    Folic acid
    Vitamin C
    PABA ANTAGONISTS
    Sulfa drugs

15. VITAMIN C IS MORE EFFECTIVE WHEN TAKEN WITH
    All vitamins and minerals
    Bioflavonoids
    Calcium   Helps body utilize vitamin C.
    Magnesium   Helps body utilize vitamin C.
    VITAMIN C ANTAGONISTS
    Alcohol
    Antibiotics

Antihistamines

Aspirin

Baking soda

Barbiturates

Cortisone

DDT

Estrogen

Oral contraceptives

Petroleum

Smoking

Sulfonamides

16. VITAMIN D IS MORE EFFECTIVE WHEN TAKEN WITH

Vitamin A   10 parts vitamin A to 1 part vitamin D.

Choline   Helps to prevent toxicity.

Vitamin C   Helps to prevent toxicity.

UFA or Unsaturated fatty acids

Calcium

Phosphorus

VITAMIN D ANTAGONISTS

Alcohol

Corticosteroid drugs

Oral contraceptives

Dilantin

17. VITAMIN E IS MORE EFFECTIVE WHEN TAKEN WITH

Vitamin A

Vitamin B complex

Vitamin B_1 (thiamine)

Inositol   Helps body utilize vitamin E.

Vitamin C   Helps protect against oxidation.

Unsaturated fatty acids

Manganese   Helps body utilize vitamin E.

Selenium

VITAMIN E ANTAGONISTS

Air pollution

Antibiotics

Chlorine

Hypolipidemic drugs

Inorganic iron

Mineral oil

Oral contraceptives

Rancid fats and oils

UNSATURATED FATTY ACIDS

Vitamin A

Vitamin C

Vitamin D
Vitamin E   Helps prevent oxidation and depletion.
Phosphorus

18. VITAMIN K IS MORE EFFECTIVE WHEN TAKEN WITH
No information is available at this time.

VITAMIN K ANTAGONISTS
Air pollution
Antibiotics
Anticoagulants
Mineral oil
Radiation
Rancid oils and fats

19. BIOFLAVONOIDS (VITAMIN P) ARE MORE EFFECTIVE WHEN TAKEN WITH
Vitamin C

B. MINERALS

1. CALCIUM IS MORE EFFECTIVE WHEN TAKEN WITH
Vitamin A   Aids in absorption.
Vitamin C   Aids in absorption.
Vitamin D   Helps in the reabsorption of calcium in kidney tubules and in the retention and
                                   utilization of calcium.
Unsaturated fatty acids   Helps make calcium available to tissues.
Iron   Aids in absorption.
Magnesium   2 parts calcium to 1 part magnesium
Manganese
Phosphorus
Hydrochloric acid

CALCIUM ANTAGONISTS
Aspirin
Corticosteroid drugs
Thyroid

2. CHLORINE IS MORE EFFECTIVE WHEN TAKEN WITH
No information is available at this time.

3. CHROMIUM IS MORE EFFECTIVE WHEN TAKEN WITH
No information is available at this time.

4. COBALT IS MORE EFFECTIVE WHEN TAKEN WITH
Copper
Iron
Zinc

5. COPPER IS MORE EFFECTIVE WHEN TAKEN WITH
Cobalt
Iron
Zinc

6. FLUORINE IS MORE EFFECTIVE WHEN TAKEN WITH
No information is available at this time.

7. IODINE IS MORE EFFECTIVEW WHEN TAKEN WITH
No information is available at this time.

8. IRON IS MORE EFFECTIVE WHEN TAKEN WITH

Vitamin B_{12} Helps iron function in the body.

Folic acid

Vitamin C   Aids in absorption

Calcium

Cobalt

Copper

Phosphorus

Hydrochloric acid   Needed for assimilation of iron.

IRON ANTAGONISTS

Antacids

Aspirin

EDTA (a food preservative)

Vitamin E

9. MAGNESIUM IS MORE EFFECTIVE WHEN TAKEN WITH

Vitamin B_6

Vitamin C

Vitamin D

Calcium   1 part magnesium to 2 parts calcium.

Phosphorus

Protein

MAGNESIUM ANTAGONISTS

Alcohol

Corticosteroid drugs

Diuretics

10. MANGANESE IS MORE EFFECTIVE WHEN TAKEN WITH

Vitamin B_1 (thiamine)

Vitamin E

Calcium

Phosphorus

MANGANESE ANTAGONISTS

Antibiotics

11. MOLYBDENUM IS MORE EFFECTIVE WHEN TAKEN WITH

No information is available at this time.

12. NICKEL IS MORE EFFECTIVE WHEN TAKEN WITH
No information is available at this time.

13. PHOSPHORUS IS MORE EFFECTIVE WHEN TAKEN WITH
Vitamin A
Vitamin D

Unsaturated fatty acids

Calcium   1 part phosphorus to 2.5 parts calcium.

Iron

Manganese

Protein

PHOSPHORUS ANTAGONISTS

Alcohol

Antacids

Aspirin

Corticosteroid drugs

Diuretics

Thyroid

14. POTASSIUM IS MORE EFFECTIVE WHEN TAKEN WITH

Vitamin B_6

Sodium

POTASSIUM ANTAGONISTS

Aspirin

Corticosteroid drugs

Diuretics

Sodium

15. SELENIUM IS MORE EFFECTIVE WHEN TAKEN WITH

Vitamin E

16. SILICON IS MORE EFFECTIVE WHEN TAKEN WITH

No information is available at this time.

17. SODIUM IS MORE EFFECTIVE WHEN TAKEN WITH

Vitamin D

18. STRONTIUM IS MORE EFFECTIVE WHEN TAKEN WITH

No information is available at this time.

19. SULFUR IS MORE EFFECTIVE WHEN TAKEN WITH

Vitamin B complex

Vitamin B_1 (thiamine)

Biotin

Pantothenic acid

20. TIN IS MORE EFFECTIVE WHEN TAKEN WITH

No information is available at this time.

21. VANADIUM IS MORE EFFECTIVE WHEN TAKEN WITH

No information is available at this time.

22. ZINC IS MORE EFFECTIVE WHEN TAKEN WITH

Vitamin A

Vitamin B_6

Vitamin E

Calcium

Copper

Phosphorus

ZINC ANTAGONISTS

Alcohol

Chelating compounds (used to
remove excess copper)

Corticosteroid drugs

Diuretics

Oral contraceptives

VITAMIN AND MINERAL SUPPLEMENTS AND SUPPLEMENTATION

Taking vitamins and minerals to supplement the diet may be desirable for most individuals. The belief of the National Research Council, which established the Recommended Dietary Allowances, that the recommended amounts can be obtained by eating a well-balanced diet ignores the fact that, in reality, few people eat adequately balanced meals on a consistent basis, a practice that is essential if the body is to be maintained at a proper nutritional level. Other factors affecting adequate nutrition are insufficient soil nutrient levels resulting in nutrient-deficient food. Food processing and storage deplete foodstuffs of valuable vitamins and minerals. Many nutrients in foods are lost or diminish in strength when cooked.

As we age, the bodily processes of digestion, absorption, and assimilation become less efficient, preventing acquisition of and optimal benefit from the nutrients in food. In addition, studies show that the body's composition changes throughout life, with the amount of fat increasing and the metabolism of active tissues decreasing. This results in low basal energy metabolism. Less food is needed to meet energy needs and, consequently, the amounts of essential nutrients consumed are likely to be below desirable levels. When adequate amounts of all of the nutrients are not obtained, the body becomes unbalanced and its functions go awry, resulting in numerous ailments and dysfunctions.

NATURAL AND SYNTHETIC

Vitamin supplements come in two forms, natural and synthetic. On a molecular level in the body, natural and synthetic vitamins are equally effective. The exception is vitamin E. Synthetic forms of vitamin E do not bind tightly enough within the cellular structure.[101] Natural vitamins are organic, but not all organic vitamins are natural. Synthetic vitamins can be called organic because to be called organic, a molecule needs to have at least one carbon atom. Organic vitamins are taken from animal and plant tissues and also from raw materials such as coal tar and wood pulp. Coal tar, for example, can also be called natural because it has been formed for eons from naturally growing plant material.

Chemists isolate certain molecules from raw materials such as coal tar, then recombine them to produce pure synthetic vitamins. Natural vitamins are directly extracted from plant and animal tissues, usually with little disturbance to their basic molecular structure. Natural vitamins are usually of low potency.

Many so-called natural vitamins are not completely natural but rather are a combination of both natural and synthetic nutrients called "co-natural" vitamins. Synthetic nutrients are added to increase the potency or stability and to standardize the amount of nutrients per capsule or per batch. Synthetic vitamins and minerals often contain a salt form that is used to increase stability of the nutrient. These salt forms are palmitate, sulfate, nitrate, hydrochloride, chloride, succinate, bitartrate, acetate, and gluconate.

REQUIREMENTS FOR GOOD HEALTH

The dosage amount of each vitamin and mineral found in a supplement should correspond with the actual need of the individual taking it. The human body is a balanced system. If it does not receive enough or if it receives too much of a nutrient, its balance can be disturbed. Often, too much of a nutrient has the same effect on a particular bodily function or process as too

---

[101]*American Journal of Clinical Nutrition,* Volume 40, August 1984, pp. 240–245.

little. For instance, an intake of either too much or too little calcium will interfere with the functioning of the nervous and muscular systems. The B vitamins are essential for the health of the nerves, and deficiency causes numerous nerve problems; yet too much B_6, for example, has been known to cause nerve damage. Iodine is necessary to keep the thyroid functioning properly, but too much iodine will impair the synthesis of thyroid hormones.

Further indications of a balance is the symbiosis-like relationship between some of the nutrients. For example, too much iron hinders phosphorus absorption, and too much phosphorus hinders iron absorption. When too much molybdenum is ingested, there is a significant urinary loss of copper; too-high copper intake can cause a deficiency of molybdenum. Plasma silicon levels are affected by molybdenum intakes; plasma molybdenum levels are affected by silicon intakes.

When a nutrient is ingested in amounts above that which the body needs, especially over a prolonged period of time, it can cause stress in the body; it can cause the urinary loss of another nutrient; or it can impair, suppress, or interfere with normal physiological processes. Studies show that once a certain amount of a nutrient has produced a balance, any excess can accumulate in the body and remain unmetabolized. For instance, while 1.24 milligrams of copper ingested a day produces a balance, at 3.9 milligrams and above it begins to accumulate. An excessive amount of zinc interferes with copper utilization, causes incomplete metabolism of iron, and results in liver loss of iron and copper. Too much calcium depresses manganese and zinc absorption. Too high an intake of manganese interferes with the utilization of iron. Too much vitamin A reduces the activity of the thyroid and causes abnormalities of the mucous membranes. Too much vitamin D results in too-high levels of calcium and phosphorus in the blood, leading to calcification of soft tissues and blood vessel walls. Iron in excess interferes with vitamin A and phosphorus absorption and can accumulate in the body after prolonged ingestion.

Taking too much of any one of the B-complex vitamins will result in a deficiency of the other B vitamins. The enrichment and fortification of so many refined food products could cause a health problem because only a selected few of the B vitamins are put back by the manufacturers. Amino acids work the

same way. If there is an excess consumption of any one of the amino acids, large amounts of other amino acids are lost in the urine. Ingesting one or a select few of any of the amino acids without the accompaniment of the other amino acids could cause a serious imbalance in the body. The only valid reason for taking a single amino acid would be in response to a diagnosed deficiency.

A daily supplement that contains amounts in the range of dosage recommended by the National Academy of Sciences[102] would be in keeping with the body's natural internal equilibrium. It must be remembered that nutrients are also being obtained daily from our food. The nutrient that may be an exception is vitamin C. Above the amount needed for normal biological functioning, vitamin C is an antioxidant and may be effective in mitigating the effects of environmental pollutants that our bodies are exposed to daily in our food, water, and air. Studies show that healthy adult males have a body ascorbate (vitamin C) pool of 1500 milligrams. A body pool of only 300 milligrams results in scurvy, at 600 milligrams psychological changes are evident. In studies of ascorbic acid metabolism and elimination rates, ingestion of 77.5 milligrams a day maintains a body ascorbate pool of 1490 to 1560 milligrams. Intake of 60 milligrams of vitamin C daily results in the saturation of leukocytes or white blood cells. Ingestion of doses above 80 milligrams, for example, 100 to 250 milligrams a day, may be desirable as added protection against exposure to harmful elements in the environment. It should be noted that ingestion of vitamin C over 100 milligrams at one time results in decreased absorption of the vitamin and increased excretion.

Daily stress does not necessarily warrant ingestion of large amounts of nutrients, because the body loss of appreciable amounts of nutrients usually occurs only when the stress is severe and prolonged.[103] Managing stress involves a change in attitude or lifestyle and eating a nutritious, whole-foods diet. There are elements found in whole, unrefined foods that are essential to body health that cannot be found in a supplement. Any physical activity leads to increased energy expenditure, and therefore, the need for nutrients involving carbohydrate metabolism should be

[102]These amounts are also the levels found naturally in foods with a few exceptions, such as liver with its high vitamin A content.
[103]Davis, *Let's Get Well,* p. 23.

met through adequate consumption of complex carbo-hydrates such as whole-grain pasta and other whole-grain foods. Excessive exercising and prolonged sweating should be avoided. According to nutritional research, higher dosages of one or more nutrients become necessary when an individual has a diagnosed ailment or illness, dysfunction of a bodily process, or genetic disorder, or has an infection or is recuperating from an illness. In these situations, a physician specializing in nutrient therapy should be consulted.

ESTABLISHING THE RECOMMENDED DIETARY ALLOWANCES

The Recommended Dietary Allowances (RDAs) were established by the National Research Council of the National Academy of Sciences, an independent research organization based in Washington, D.C. The Food and Drug Administration (FDA) adapted these requirements and called them the USRDA, which are the values found on food and supplement labels. The RDAs have ten age categories plus categories for pregnant and lactating women. The USRDA are consolidated into four age categories. (See charts on pages 311–313.)

Four general procedures were followed by the Academy in establishing the requirements necessary for the maintenance of good health for the body.

1. Estimating the average requirement of a population for a given nutrient and the variability of requirement within that population.

2. Increasing the average requirement by an amount sufficient to meet the needs of nearly all members of the population.

3. Increasing the allowance to account for inefficient utilization by the body of the nutrients as consumed, such as poor absorption and poor conversion of nutrients to an active, usable form.

4. Using judgment in interpreting and extrapolating allowances when information on requirements is limited.

To arrive at what the average requirement of a nutrient

for the general population would be, a number of different methods were studied and evaluated.

1. Collection of data on nutrient intake from the food supply of apparently normal, healthy people.

2. Review of epidemiological observations when clinical consequences of nutrient deficiencies are found to be correctable by a dietary improvement.

3. Biochemical measurements that assess degree of tissue saturation or adequacy of molecular function in relation to nutrient intake.

4. Nutrient balance studies that measure nutritional status in relation to intake.

5. Studies of subjects maintained on diets containing marginally low or deficient levels of a nutrient, followed by correction of the deficit with measured amounts of that nutrient.

Although precise estimation of requirements for a nutrient may be questionable when acquired by just one of these techniques, several approaches that corroborate a figure are more convincing. The requirement established for thiamine (vitamin B_1) is an example. First, the amount needed to prevent clinical signs and symptoms was determined. Second, diets were analyzed to determine their thiamine content. Third, the amount of thiamine in the urine was measured to see how much the body kept to use and how much was disposed of as waste. And fourth, thiamine intake and its relationship to the activity of a certain enzyme found in red blood cells was measured to assess nutritional status. All of these studies when taken together indicate with some precision the body's requirement for the vitamin.

Once the basic requirement is established, it is increased to account for the difference in requirements from one individual to another. In addition, for some nutrients, requirements are increased further to compensate for inefficiency in the body, such as poor absorption. For example, only 20 to 30 percent of the calcium in food is absorbed by the body. The actual adult bodily need for calcium is between 200 and 300 milligrams, but because of the poor absorption rate of only 20 to 30 percent, the RDA requirement is increased to 800 milligrams, to make sure 200 to 300 milligrams is ultimately absorbed. This principle applies to most of the minerals. Actual adult bodily need for iron is 1 to 2 milligrams (10 to 18 milligrams RDA), magnesium, 150 to 300 milligrams (300 to 350 milligrams RDA), zinc, 6 milligrams (15 milligrams RDA), copper, 500 to 1000 micrograms (2 to 3 milligrams RDA), chromium, 6 to 9 micrograms (200 to 300 micrograms estimated requirement), and selenium, 25 to 100 micrograms (50 to 200 micrograms estimated requirement). As for other trace minerals, there is a paucity of information on their requirements and their absorption rates by the body. Generally, they have a low percentage of absorption, so the actual bodily need may be relatively small.

Other nutrients may have difficulty in converting from the food form to the form the body can use. Carotene is a good example. The vitamin A found in fruits and green and yellow vegetables such as carrots is in a form called carotene. Carotene has to be converted to pro-vitamin A in order for the body to use it. The body does not carry out this conversion process very well. It is estimated that only about 30 percent is actually converted to A; therefore, the RDA requirement for vitamin A was increased as compensation.

DAILY SUPPLEMENT GUIDELINES

There are several guidelines that can be followed in selecting a daily supplement to the regular diet. First, obtaining all of the vitamins and minerals known from sufficient evidence to be essential for the health of the body would be most desirable. All vitamins and minerals are interrelated, either directly or indirectly. All are equally valuable, for there is no one nutrient more important than another. However, there are some nutrients, for example, some trace elements, for which there is difficulty in determining what amounts are appropriate for supplement, due to a lack of adequate information.

Second, to remain in keeping with the body's natural equilibrium, the nutrients in a daily supplement for general use should be balanced in dosage, not some at excessively high and others at subnormal levels. Balance also does not mean, for example, that all B vitamins or all amino acids be of the same dosages; the body has different requirements for each one.

Third, an adjustment at the formulating level will establish the actual need by the body of a nutrient. As mentioned in the previous section, RDA values are for the expected absorption by the body of nutrients when they are found in food only. For example, the actual adult bodily need for iron is 1 milligram and 1.8 milligrams for menstruating women per day; but because the body absorbs only 10 percent of iron when it is eaten in food, the RDA had to be set at 10 and 18 milligrams in order for 1 and 1.8 milligrams ultimately to be absorbed. In other words, the RDA for iron is 10 and 18 milligrams not because the body requires those amounts but because the body will absorb only 10 percent of those amounts from the diet.

This principle applies to almost all of the minerals including calcium, 200 to 300 milligrams actual adult need, and zinc, 6 milligrams actual adult need. It is important to note that whenever absorption rates are discussed in nutrition, they are always mean averages. Because of the different internal conditions between one individual and another, precise predictions would be impossible.

Fourth, the absorption rate by the body of the various nutrient forms found in supplements is important. It is most beneficial to be able to absorb as much as possible of each nutrient. Although most vitamins generally are absorbed quite well, minerals are not. The rate depends on the form of the mineral that a vitamin company chooses. One of the most effectively absorbed forms of minerals is that which has been chelated with amino acids. Studies show that when a mineral becomes attached to an amino acid during digestion, the amino acid effortlessly carries the mineral across the intestinal wall and into the bloodstream. However, minerals that do not become attached to amino acids are, once the stomach has broken down the ingested food into a watery mass called chyme, alone and quite unstable. Any number of things can happen to them. For example, a mineral can become bound up by phytic acids, which are components found in cereal grains, which renders the mineral unavailable for transport across the intestinal wall. They can become incorporated into a mass of undigestable fibers. In studies, the loss of minerals in the feces correlates directly with the increase in dietary fiber. Some minerals require a low pH for solubility. In an alkaline or only slightly acidic environment, they will remain insoluble and therefore unabsorbable. Normally, the intestine tends to be alkaline.

Amino acids are also found along the intestinal wall acting as receptors for the minerals. Mutual attraction draws the two elements together; but even if a mineral is in the right position, it still may not have the opportunity to become attached. Chemically similar minerals compete for the same amino acid carriers. If there are not enough carriers available, the weaker minerals will lose out. Also, there are only certain sites along the way where the mineral will find its carrier. If it is moving along within a mass of food, it may pass right on by.

Chelating minerals with amino acids for use in supplements is done by several methods. (Some of the minerals because of their molecular configuration cannot be chelated but are called *complexed*.) The most effective method of chelation is accomplished in only a few specialized laboratories in the country. This method places the amino acids and the mineral together in a solution consisting of either an acid or proteolytic enzymes. The use of enzymes is preferable because it simulates the body's natural process of chelation. Acids add a harshness to the mixture and can denature the protein molecule. In addition, at the end of the process, an alkali needs to be added to neutralize the acid.

During the chelation process, minerals become bonded to amino acids when a hydrogen molecule within the amino acid structure is replaced by the mineral. The mineral then becomes part of the body of the amino acid. Chelating with a group or with the full range of amino acids is preferable to chelation with a single element such as a lysinate, citrate, or aspartate, for these latter can become vulnerable to hydrochloric acid in the stomach and separate from the mineral. Chelating with numerous peptides or polypeptides (amino acids) will surround and form a wall or protective envelope around the mineral, allowing the entire component to remain intact in the stomach.

Minerals protected by peptides and polypeptides (amino acid chelates) will not fall victim even to fiber, for the absorption sites in the intestine will reach them first. Another commonly used method of chelation places the minerals and amino acids together in a mixture of wet and dry mix or just a dry mix, neither of which is nearly as effective, the bonding being of little permanence. A mineral may also be called an amino acid chelate on a label, but only a portion is actually chelated, the rest remaining in its original salt form.

The advantages of having chelated minerals in a vitamin and mineral supplement are twofold. First, the mineral is going to have a better chance of being absorbed. It is already in a form ready to pass through the intestinal wall and into the bloodstream. Second, the presence of the amino acids themselves is helpful because they are interrelated with vitamins and minerals in many of the functions of the body. For example, the manufacture of neurotransmitters such as serotonin and acetylcholine is dependent upon amino acids and choline, a B vitamin.

Finally, supplements should contain the ingredients and the dosage amounts that are listed on their labels. Quality control in this area is probably not adequate. Dr. Michael Colgan, a New Zealand scientist and in 1982 a visiting scholar at Rockefeller University in New York City, conducted an analysis of various vitamin supplements before giving them to his patients. To his consternation, very few proved to contain exactly what their labels said they did. In the April 1982 issue of *Omni* magazine, he states his disillusionment with vitamin and mineral supplements made by drug companies and many of those found in health food stores. Because our health is at stake, vitamin companies should regularly allow independent, FDA-registered laboratories to conduct assays of their products.

Following is a list of nutrients found in vitamin and mineral supplements and salient points regarding their biological need for adults.

Vitamin A

Studies show that 1800 IU of retinol (vitamin A) is needed a day to maintain adequate blood concentrations. An intake above this is considered necessary to produce liver storage. The RDA of 4000 IU for women and 5000 IU for men includes the factor of inefficient absorption by the body of the estimated portion of vitamin A obtained in carotene form. Biological need for vitamin A is about 3500 IU.

Vitamin D

The need for vitamin D decreases with age after cessation of skeletal growth to 200 IU after the age of 22. Children and pregnant women require 400 IU per day.

Vitamin E

Vitamin E is an antioxidant and may have properties that protect the body against environmental pollutants. It may protect the lungs from damage by air pollution. In the process, the vitamin itself is used up and needs to be replaced in order for it to continue its protection. Therefore, an amount above that which is recommended for normal maintenance may be desirable. If all of the tocopherols are included, the lesser tocopherols will aid the effectiveness of the potent alpha tocopherol. The vitamin should also be from a natural source. Although all other natural and synthetic vitamins are equally effective on the molecular level, studies show vitamin E is the exception, as the natural form has a more complete binding action within the cellular structure.

Vitamin C

Studies show that healthy adult males have a body ascorbate (vitamin C) pool of 1500 milligrams or more. A body pool of only 300 milligrams results in scurvy; at 600 milligrams psychological changes are evident. In studies of ascorbic acid metabolism and elimination rates, ingestion of 77.5 milligrams a day maintains a body ascorbate pool of 1490 to 1560 milligrams. Intake of 60 milligrams of C daily results in the saturation of leukocytes, or white blood cells. Above the amount needed for normal biological functioning, vitamin C is, like E, an antioxidant and may be effective in mitigating the effects of environmental pollutants that our bodies are exposed to daily in our food, water, and air. Therefore, an amount above that needed for normal maintenance may be desirable. Ingestion of above 100 milligrams of vitamin C at one time results in decreased efficiency of absorption and an increased rate of excretion of unmetabolized ascorbic acid.

Bioflavonoids

The proper ratio of the bioflavonoids to vitamin C is 1:10. Bioflavonoids are companions of vitamin C in many foods, especially citrus fruits. They aid in the absorption of vitamin C and assist it in many of its activities in the body. They are very important in strengthening the capillaries.

Vitamin B_1

Vitamin B_1 and vitamin B_2 are related to energy intake because they are a key in energy and carbohydrate metabolism. The minimum requirement for B_1 is between .33 and .35 milligrams per 1000 calories consumed. An intake of more than .5 milligrams per 1000 calories may be required to ensure tissue saturation. Certain red cell activities require .5 milligrams per 1000 calories. The RDA for B_1 of 1 to 1.6 milligrams is sufficient for the ingestion of 2000 to 3000 calories a day.

Vitamin B_2

Although urinary excretion of vitamin B_2 in diets containing up to .5 milligrams per 1000 calories is low, it rises sharply as dietary intake increases to .75 milligrams per 1000 calories. In studies relating to blood cell activity, B_2 intakes of .5 to .6 milligrams per 1000 calories established normalcy. The RDA for vitamin B_2 of 1.2 to 1.6 milligrams is sufficient for ingestion of about 2000 to 3000 calories a day.

Vitamin B_6

Vitamin B_6 requirement is complicated by the fact that high-protein diets require higher intakes of the vitamin. Optimum intake on a low-protein diet is 1.25 to 1.5 milligrams per day, increasing to 1.75 to 2 milligrams on a high-protein diet. RDA for vitamin B_6 is 2 to 2.2 milligrams a day.

Vitamin B_{12}

B_{12} is a group of cobalt-containing cobalamins. The vitamin has a long biological half-life because it is recycled from bile and other intestinal secretions. The daily loss of B_{12} is estimated at 2.6 micrograms, an amount that needs to be replaced. In studies of intakes of single oral doses of .5 micrograms or less, approximately 70 percent of B_{12} is absorbed by the body. This value decreases as the intestinal content of B_{12} increases. At 5 micrograms, 28 percent is absorbed; at 10 micrograms, 16 percent. At an intake of 3 micrograms twice a day, the body will absorb 2.64 micrograms total.

Folic acid and Biotin

Folic acid and biotin in foods are absorbed by the body at a 50 percent absorption rate, so their RDAs were increased to allow for this factor. 100 to 200 micrograms of folic acid per day is necessary to maintain tissue reserves; 150 micrograms of biotin is the actual bodily need.

Niacin

Niacin requirements are complicated by the fact that some niacin is obtained in the diet from the amino acid tryptophan. Sixty milligrams tryptophan provides around 1 milligram niacin. Studies suggest that 11.3 to 13.3 milligrams of niacin is necessary to prevent depletion of body stores.

Pantothenic acid, Choline, Inositol, PABA

The pantothenic acid requirement is between 10 and 15 milligrams a day. There are no studies available on the amount required by the body of choline and inositol. The average diet supplies between 400 and 900 milligrams of each nutrient. It is suggested that choline and inositol be taken in equal dosage amounts. There is no information on PABA requirement. PABA functions in the breakdown and utilization of proteins and in the formation of blood cells. It plays an important role in skin health, hair pigmentation, and the health of the intestines.

Calcium

Only 20 to 30 percent of the calcium from the food we eat is absorbed by the body. Of the 800 milligrams RDA for adults, the body will ultimately absorb 160 to 240 milligrams, which is the amount shown by balance studies to establish equilibrium in the body.

Phosphorus

Although the RDA for phosphorus is the same as for calcium, phosphorus is very plentiful in most diets, as it is contained in almost all foods. In contrast, calcium is in very few foods and has a very poor rate of absorption by the body. Consequently, most people are getting ample amounts of phosphorus and little calcium in their regular diets. Too much phosphorus upsets the calcium-phosphorus balance. The C:P ratio in the body varies from 2:1 in the bones to 1:1 in soft tissues.

Potassium

Ninety-nine milligrams is by law the highest amount allowed in a daily supplement.

Magnesium

The RDA for magnesium is 300 to 350 milligrams a day, because only about 50 to 75 percent of this amount is actually absorbed by the body from food. Actual bodily need is 150 to 300 milligrams.

Iron

The actual need for iron is 1 milligram for adult males and females and 1.8 milligrams for menstruating women. However, only 10 percent of iron is absorbed by our bodies from the food we eat, so to make sure the 1 milligram and 1.8 milligrams was ultimately absorbed, the RDA had to be set at 10 milligrams and 18 milligrams.

Zinc

The turnover of body zinc has been calculated from radioisotope studies to be 6 milligrams per day, an amount that needs to be replaced. The RDA for zinc is 15 milligrams, which takes into consideration that only about 40 percent (6 milligrams) will be absorbed from food by the body.

Iodine

The RDA of iodine is 150 micrograms; 50 to 75 micrograms daily prevents goiter in adults; conversely, excessive iodine intake has induced goiter, documented in Japan, where iodine-rich seaweed is habitually consumed. The mean dietary intake of iodine is estimated to be between 64 and 677 micrograms a day. Expected to receive the higher amounts are persons living in coastal areas with concentration of the mineral in the environment or persons consuming iodine-containing drugs.

Copper

Metabolic studies show that individuals consuming a varied diet established a mean copper requirement of

1.24 milligrams to produce balance in the body. Intakes of 3.9 milligrams and over result in copper accumulation. Approximately 10 to 30 percent of dietary copper is absorbed by the body. At this absorption rate, the RDA requirement of 2 to 3 milligrams is an actual bodily requirement of 200 to 900 micrograms.

Manganese

From 2.5 to 5 milligrams of manganese is recommended daily. Ingestion of dietary manganese of at least 2.5 milligrams a day has shown an equilibrium in the body. Manganese absorption by the body ranges from 3 up to 20 percent, leaving an actual bodily need of 75 micrograms to 1 milligram.

Chromium

As the predominant route of excretion of chromium is the urine, the minimal requirement for absorbable chromium can be estimated from the daily losses in urine. Studies have shown the minimum requirement to be 1 microgram. Adequate daily food intake is suggested to be between 50 and 200 micrograms. In other studies, 200 to 290 micrograms obtained from the diet produce near-equilibrium in the body. Because absorption of chromium from a varied diet is between .5 and 3 percent, this amount is equivalent to 1 to 9 micrograms actually absorbed.

Molybdenum, Nickel, Selenium, Silicon, and Vanadium

Studies indicate that these trace elements have essential functions in the body. However, there is a paucity of information on their requirements and their absorption rates by the body. Generally, minerals have a low percentage of absorption, so the actual bodily need of these trace elements may be relatively small.

Suggested recommendation for molybdenum is between 150 and 500 micrograms per day. Molybdenum is an essential part of two enzymes involved in iron mobilization and oxidation of fats. It is also a factor in copper metabolism.

From 50 to 200 micrograms is recommended for selenium. Studies show that a balance is maintained in men when 80 micrograms a day is ingested; for women it is 57 micrograms. Only about 55 percent of these amounts is actually absorbed by the body.

It is estimated that 300 to 500 micrograms of nickel is ingested daily by humans. In animal studies, 25 percent has been absorbed. Nickel is a factor in hormone, lipid, and membrane metabolism and an activator of some enzymes. The mineral may be involved in glucose metabolism. Significant amounts are found in DNA and RNA.

The requirement for silicon appears to be much higher than for the other trace elements, 9 to 14 milligrams per day, possibly because this mineral is found mainly in the fiber part of food and therefore little is actually absorbed by the body. Silicon is present in the connective tissues of the body such as tendons, cartilage, and blood vessels and may be essential for their integrity. It may work with calcium to make strong bones and therefore is an important factor in osteoporosis.

From 100 to 300 micrograms a day is recommended for vanadium. The absorption rate is not known. Vanadium is present in most body tissues and is important for iron metabolism and red cell growth. Children need the mineral for proper bone, cartilage, and tooth development.

PHYSICAL FORMS

Nearly all the nutrient supplements are available in many forms: tablet, capsule, liquid, powder, drops, or ointment. This variety allows people to choose a supplement form that best suits their needs.

The *tablet* is a compressed block of material available in a variety of potencies, especially higher ones. Once opened, all nutrients in this form should be stored in a cool, dark place (not in the refrigerator) because exposure to air will reduce potency. Tablets usually contain fillers and binders. For example, a 100-milligram tablet of a B vitamin will also contain about 200 milligrams of a filler to fill out the tablet. Tablets are also usually coated, most commonly with a sugar syrup or protein. Many people may have reactions to these additional ingredients, in which case changing brands may be desirable.

The *capsule* is a small container made of gelatin or other soluble materials. The ingredients inside the container can be either powder or liquid. Capsules may have a distinct advantage over tablets in that the likelihood that they will break down in the stomach is greatly enhanced. Tablets require tremendous pressure to bind all of the ingredients together. The result is a very hard substance which may not disintegrate in the stomach in persons with weakened digestive systems. Many people have weakened digestive systems, not only due to illness but as a result of the aging process. Most tablets are also coated, which may make them more difficult to dissolve. An advantage of the powder-filled capsule is that it can be opened and sprinkled on food or in beverages, a useful factor for those people who have difficulty swallowing. The liquid-filled capsule, as in vitamin E, has distinct advantages too. For example, a person suffering from a cold sore may pick up a capsule, insert a pin, gently squeeze, and apply the oil directly to the sore. The capsule will then seal itself, become airtight, and be ready for use again. The capsule is available in the same potencies as the tablet.

Nutrients in *liquid* form are easily taken and are especially good for children or elderly persons who find swallowing a tablet or capsule difficult. Vitamin C is available in liquid and may be the preferred form if one is suffering from a cold and finds swallowing a pill painful. The liquid is usually found in lower potencies and should be stored in the refrigerator. Once opened, a bottle of liquid nutrients rapidly loses potency.

Nutrients in *powdered* form can be sprinkled on foods and in beverages and are also easy for children or the elderly to consume. They are an excellent way to provide the essential amino acids. Powder should be kept in a dark place away from high humidity.

In some cases it may be desirable to obtain the nutrients in *drops* or *ointments*. For example, vitamin E ointment is recommended for treatment of burns to promote healing and reduce scarring.

Vitamins and minerals should be taken with meals unless otherwise directed by a physician. There are elements in food such as enzymes that will aid in full vitamin and mineral utilization.

The following table gives the various supplemental forms in which a nutrient may be found, together with its source. Supplemental forms are subject to change and may vary in different localities.

Nutrient	Form	Source	Explanation
VITAMINS			
Vitamin A	Retinol	Natural	From fish-liver oil.
	Carrot (oil)	Natural	Cannot be tolerated by persons suffering from gall-bladder problems and other digestive problems.
	Lemon grass	Natural	An herbal grass.
	Vitamin A palmitate	Natural	From fish-liver oil.
	Vitamin A palmitate	Synthetic	From fatty isomercital from lemon grass oil.
	Vitamin A acetate	Synthetic	Crystals formed from methonal.
Vitamin B complex	Brewer's yeast	Natural	Low-potency form.
Vitamin B_1 (thiamine)	Yeast, rice bran	Natural	Low potency.
	Thiamine hydrochloride	Synthetic	High potency.
	Thiamine mononitrate	Synthetic	High potency.
Vitamin B_2 (riboflavin)	Yeast, bran	Natural	Low potency.
	Riboflavin	Synthetic	High potency.
Niacin (B_3)	Yeast, bran	Natural	Low potency.
	Niacin, nicotinic acid	Synthetic	High potency. Will cause flushing or tingling sensation with high dosage.
	Niacinamide	Synthetic	High potency. Will not cause flushing or tingling sensation with high dosage.
Pantothenic acid (B_5)	Yeast, rice bran, royal bee jelly	Natural	Low potency.
	Calcium pantothenate	Synthetic	High potency.
Vitamin B_6 (pyridoxine)	Yeast or bran	Natural	Low potency.
	Pyridoxine hydrochloride	Synthetic	High potency.

Nutrient	Form	Source	Explanation
Vitamin B_{12}	Cobalamine concentrate	Natural	High-potency natural fermentation product.
	Cyanocobalamin	Natural	Low potency. From oily fish, liver, dairy products.
	Cyanocobalamin	Natural	High potency. Natural fermentation product.
	Hydroxocobalamin (B_{12b})		Believed to maintain high serum B_{12} levels longer than cyanocobalamin.
Biotin	Yeast, liver	Natural	Low potency.
	Biotin	Natural	High potency. From laboratory-grown cultures.
	D-biotin	Synthetic	High potency.
Choline	Soy oil, egg yolk, lecithin, liver, yeast	Natural	Low potency.
	Choline bitartrate	Synthetic	High potency.
	Choline chloride		
	Choline citrate		
Folic acid	Yeast, liver	Natural	Low potency.
	Folic acid	Synthetic	High potency.
Inositol	Soybeans, liver, yeast	Natural	Low potency.
	Corn	Natural	High potency.
Para-aminobenzoic acid (PABA)	Yeast, liver	Natural	Low potency.
	Para-aminobenzoic acid	Synthetic	High potency.
Pangamic acid (B_{15})	Apricot kernels, rice bran	Natural	Low potency.
	Pangamic acid	Synthetic	High potency.
	Calcium pangamate	Synthetic	High potency.
Vitamin C	Rose hips, acerola cherries, citrus fruits, green peppers	Natural	Low potency.
	Ascorbic acid	Synthetic	High potency.
	Calcium ascorbate	Synthetic	High potency. Nonacidic.
	Sodium ascorbate		
Vitamin D	D_3	Natural	High potency. From fish-liver oil or irradiation.
	D_2	Natural	High potency. From ultraviolet irradiation of ergosterol.
	Calciferol		
Vitamin E	Mixed tocopheryl	Natural	D-alpha and other tocopheryls that help alpha function better.
	d-alpha tocopherol	Natural	Low potency. From vegetable oils.
	d-alpha tocopheryl acetate	Co-natural	A natural derivative with synthetic products added.
	d-alpha tocopheryl succinate	Co-natural	A natural derivative with synthetic products added.
	dl-alpha tocopherol	Synthetic	Considered by some a more stable form.
	dl-alpha tocopheryl acetate	Synthetic	Considered by some a more stable form.
	dl-alpha tocopheryl succinate	Synthetic	Considered by some a more stable form.
Vitamin K	K_1	Natural	From chlorophyll of green plants.
	K_2	Natural	From fish meal or microorganism cultures.

Nutrient	Form	Source	Explanation
	K_3	Synthetic	
	Menadione		
Bioflavonoids (Vitamin P)	Rutin	Natural	Are factors that make vitamin C more effective. From citrus fruit rind.
	Hesperiden		
	Flavons		
	Bioflavonoids		
	Quercitin		
	Chalcone		
MINERALS			
Calcium	Calcium carbonate	Natural	From limestone.
	Calcium lactate	Natural	A salt of lactic acid from milk; easily absorbed; low potency.
	Calcium gluconate	Natural	A salt of gluconic acid from glucose; easily absorbed; one needs to take more to get equivalent potencies.
	Calcium oxide	Natural	
	Bone meal	Natural	Dried bones of cattle; type of calcium closest to calcium found in human bones and teeth; poorly absorbed; has high potency with other trace minerals.
	Dolomite	Natural	Calcium and magnesium; not to be used by elderly or persons with poor hydrochloric acid secretions.
	Di-cal phosphate	Co-natural	Bone meal or bone ash with additional 22% phosphorus.
	Eggshell calcium	Natural	Dried eggshell.
	Oyster-shell calcium	Natural	Natural calcium form with minimal phosphorus interference but with natural trace minerals.
	Liquid calcium	Natural	Good for person who has calcium-absorption problems.
Cobalt	—	—	Not available singly but in vitamin B_{12}.
Copper	Hemoglobin	Natural	Low potency.
	Chlorophyll		
	Copper carbonate	Natural	
	Copper gluconate	Synthetic	High potency.
	Copper sulfate	Synthetic	High potency.
Chromium	Yeast	Natural	
	Chromium carbonate	Natural	
Fluorine	—	—	Not available singly but in some complete-multimineral supplements.
Iodine	Sea kelp, seaweed	Natural	Includes trace minerals and other substances.
	Sea salt	Natural	Includes trace minerals and other substances.
	Potassium iodide	Synthetic	Table salt.
Iron	Desiccated liver	Natural	Low potency. Dried liver of cattle.
	Yeast, molasses, bone marrow	Natural	Low potency.
	Ferrous fumerate	Synthetic	High potency.
	Ferrous gluconate	Synthetic	High potency; more readily absorbed than ferrous fumerate.

Nutrient	Form	Source	Explanation
	Ferrous sulfate	Synthetic	High potency.
	Iron lactate	Synthetic	From iron and lactic acid.
	Iron oxide	Natural	
	Iron peptonate	Synthetic	From iron and beef proteins.
Magnesium	Liver, yeast	Natural	Low potency.
	Dolomite	Natural	Calcium and magnesium in natural (2:1) balance; not recommended for persons with poor hydrochloric acid secretions.
	Magnesium gluconate	Synthetic	High potency.
	Magnesium oxide	Natural	
	Magnesium palmitate	Synthetic	High potency.
	Magnesium sulfate	Synthetic	Epsom salts, calcium-free.
Manganese	Liver, yeast	Natural	Low potency.
	Manganese carbonate	Natural	
	Manganese gluconate	Synthetic	High potency.
Molybdenum	—	—	The mineral molybdenite—principal source.
Phosphorus	Bone meal	Natural	Contains additional calcium and other nutrients.
	Calcium phosphate	Synthetic	High potency.
	Potassium phosphate	Natural	
Potassium	Potassium gluconate	Synthetic	
	Potassium chloride	Synthetic	High potency.
	Potassium citrate	Natural	
Selenium	Yeast	Natural	From yeast cultures.
	Sodium selenite	Synthetic	
Silicon	Silica	Natural	From cereals and horsetail herb.
Sodium	Sodium chloride	Synthetic	Table salt.
Sulfur	—	—	Available in ointment form and in some complete-multimineral supplements.
Zinc	Liver, yeast	Natural	Low potency.
	Zinc citrate	Synthetic	From zinc carbonate and citric acid.
	Zinc gluconate	Synthetic	High potency. More readily absorbed than zinc sulfate.
	Zinc oxide	Natural	
	Zinc sulfate	Synthetic	
Protein	Meat or fish	Natural	Available in powder and tablet forms.
	Eggs or milk	Natural	Available in powder and tablet forms.
	Soybeans	Natural	Good source for vegetarians.
	Amino acid compounds	Natural	Available in tablet, liquid, and powder forms.
	Collagen	Natural	Available in liquid and tablet forms.
Unsaturated Fatty Acids (UFA)	Vegetable oils	Natural	Available in capsules.

REFERENCES

Ashmead, DeWayne. *Chelated Mineral Nutrition*. Huntington Beach, Calif.: Institute Publishers, 1981.

Callender, S., et al. Absorption of hemoglobin iron. *Brit. J. Haemat.*, Vol. 3, 1957, p. 186.

Chaitow, Leon. *Amino Acids in Therapy*. Wellingborough, Northamptonshire: Thorsons Publishers, Ltd., 1985.

Hallberg, L. and L. Solvell. Absorption of a single dose of iron in man. *Acta Med. Scand.*, Vol. 19, 1960, p. 358.

Hill, C. and G. Matrone. Chemical parameters in the study of in vivo and in vitro interactions of transition elements. *Fed. Proc.*, Vol. 29, 1970, p. 1474.

Kuhn, I., et al. Observations on the mechanism of iron absorption. *Amer. J. Clin. Nutr.*, Vol. 21, 1968, p. 1184.

Manis, J. and D. Schachter. Active transport of iron by intestine: Features of the two step mechanism. *Amer. J. Physiol.*, Vol. 203, 1962, p. 73.

Martinez-Torres, C. and M. Layrisse. Effects of amino acids on iron absorption from a staple vegetable food. *Blood*, Vol. 35, 1970, p. 669.

National Academy of Sciences, *Recommended Dietary Allowances*, 9th ed. Washington, D.C., 1980.

Pfieffer, Carl C. *Mental and Elemental Nutrients*. New Canaan, Conn.: Keats Publishing, 1975.

Skoryna, S. and D. Waldron-Edward, eds. *Intestinal Absorption of Metal Ions, Trace Elements and Radionuclides*. Oxford, England: Pergamon Press, 1971.

Turnball, A., et al. Iron absorption. IV. The absorption of hemoglobin iron. *J. Clin. Nutr.*, Vol. 41, 1962, p. 1897.

Underwood, Eric. *Trace Elements in Human and Animal Nutrition*. London, England: Academic Press, 1977.

Vohra, P., et al. Phytic-acid metal complexes. *Proc. Soc. Exp. Biol. Med.*, Vol. 120, 1965, p. 447.

APPROXIMATE NUTRIENT COMPOSITION OF THE BODY

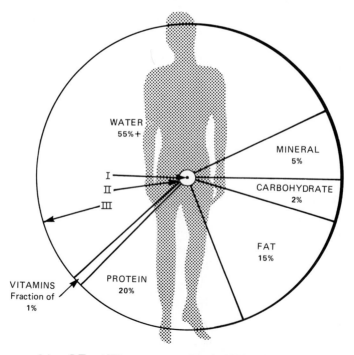

Spheres I, II, and III represent approximately 1,000 times the actual sizes of:

I = 1 microgram   II = 1 milligram   III = 1 gram

Ailments and Other Stressful Conditions

Good health is a product of heredity, environment, and nutrition. Nutritional deficiency, resulting in malnutrition or disease, is one of the major problems in modern society despite adequate food supply, primarily because of ignorance of good nutrition. A well-balanced diet, rich in all essential nutrients, is necessary to maintain a healthy body and mind.

Authorities have found that a number of diseases can appear when there is a deficiency of one or more nutrients. Most diseases caused by such deficiencies can be corrected when all essential nutrients are supplied. However, in some instances of severe deficiency, irreparable damage may be done.

The following pages list common ailments and stressful conditions that many authorities believe are related to nutrition. Common ailments are listed alphabetically by ailment together with explanations, including pertinent nutritional information regarding the nature of most of the ailments. These explanations are designed to give an understanding of the specific ailments.

The body member affected by each ailment is also identified. Nutrient listings for each ailment are given. These include those nutrients found by nutrition researchers to be beneficial in the treatment of the given ailment.

Nutrient quantities are given for some nutrients. They represent amounts of these nutrients which have been found by some researchers to be effective in the treatment of the ailment. All amounts are daily unless otherwise stated. When no quantity is listed, available research did not indicate an amount.

Note: These and the following quantity-of-nutrient listings do not constitute prescriptive amounts. They only represent research findings.

Many of the seemingly high doses result from clinical tests on ailing persons. These amounts would not necessarily be required, or even recommended, for a healthy person. Most dosages used in research are greater than those cited as daily allowances. We repeat:

These amounts are not prescriptive.

Individual tolerances to the nutrients may differ significantly. Each individual must determine, according to his own tolerances, the quantity of each nutrient that will be beneficial in the treatment of disease.

Factors influencing individual tolerances include a person's normal eating habits, previous amounts of vitamins ingested, height, weight, metabolic rate, reaction to stress, and environmental variances. Build up the dosages slowly: it took a long time for your body to become ill, so take your time in trying to heal it. If you wish to take large amounts of a nutrient, consult a physician.

AILMENTS

ABSCESS

An abscess is a localized infection with a collection of pus in any part of the body. An abscess may be located externally or internally and may be initiated by lowered resistance to infection, bacterial contamination, or injury. Symptoms of abscess include tenderness and swelling in the infected area, fever, and chills.

Antibiotics may be used to treat the infection, although in the case of a severe abscess, surgery may be necessary. Because the antibiotics used in treatment may interfere with the absorption of the B vitamins, supplementary B complex may be required. Fever increases the body's need for calories; vitamins A, C, and E; and extra fluids.

NUTRIENTS THAT MAY BE BENEFICIAL IN TREATMENT OF ABSCESS

Body Member	Nutrients	Quantity*
Body/Skin	Vitamin A	100,000 IU for 3 days
	Vitamin B complex	
	Vitamin C	
	Vitamin E	
	Water	

*See note, p. 222.

ACCIDENTS, SHOCK, AND SURGERY

Following injury, the body's need for all nutrients increases dramatically. The pituitary and adrenal glands release large quantities of hormones, resulting in the loss of body protein, and prevent formation of new protein needed for healing. (This can continue for a month or longer.) Soon the adrenals become ex-hausted from lack of pantothenic acid and vitamin B_2. Salt and potassium are depleted, causing partial intestinal and urinary paralysis. Bacteria in the intestine feed on stagnant food and gas begins to form. Vitamin C is rapidly depleted. A temporary deficiency of digestive enzymes and hydrochloric acid occurs.

Sufficient amounts of protein are vital for healing. Protein can be synthesized only when adequate amounts of vitamins and minerals are present. A lack of a single nutrient can delay healing. Vitamin C is vital for re-forming connective tissue. The speed of healing is directly proportional to the amount of vitamin C the body has available for its use. The vitamin is also involved in the forming of new blood vessels at the damaged area and in preventing hemorrhaging. It detoxifies the body of medications and harmful substances that may form.

Exhausted adrenals can be greatly helped by pantothenic acid. Vitamins B_2, C, and pantothenic acid can relieve patients who are unable to urinate. After any injury, 500 milligrams of vitamin C every two hours for several days aids in improvement and reinforces the body's defense of the stress that occurs from pain, x-rays, medications, intravenous feedings, and catherizations.[1]

Vitamin E helps the scarring process and also relieves the itching and pain as scar tissue contracts. It also protects the cells from destruction by decreasing their need for oxygen. Vitamin E helps to form new blood vessels at the site of injury and prevents the formation of blood clots. Proper blood clotting is a complex process and in addition to vitamin E requires many nutrients including calcium and vitamins C and K.

An injured person who is unconscious benefits substantially from an intravenous formula containing all nutrients. An adequate feeding given to unconscious patients results in healthy skin and hair and later to a quicker recovery. When poison has been swallowed, vitamin B_2, pantothenic acid, and large doses of vitamin C are recommended. Vitamin E and sufficient protein taken during the following days will also help the liver to detoxify the poison.[2]

Shock that is not treated quickly can result in irreversible damage and sometimes death. Undernourished persons are particularly vulnerable to shock. Vitamin C and most of the B vitamins are

[1]Davis, *Let's Get Well*, p. 263.
[2]Ibid., p. 269.

rapidly lost. Investigators studying shock report that when the cells of the body are damaged, their enzymes chemically change from being constructive to being destructive. They then release histamine, a primary shock-producing substance. Adequate vitamin C will prevent this transition. The vitamin will reverse shock occurring in many areas of medicine. Intravenous dosages of up to 120 grams of sodium ascorbate over a 3-hour period keep the body tissues saturated and successfully aid recovery. When shock has been brought on by severe hemorrhage, 3000 milligrams of vitamin C and 300 IU of vitamin E given as soon as possible can reduce the damage caused by an inadequate oxygen supply of the tissues.[3]

Preparation for surgery should begin at least a month in advance. Often if the body has been adequately supplied, intravenous feeding may be unnecessary following surgery. Sufficient protein, all vitamins and minerals, digestive enzymes, and acidophilus should be taken. Adelle Davis recommends that on the eve of surgery, the following be taken: 1000 milligrams vitamin C, 500 milligrams pantothenic acid, 20 milligrams vitamins B_2 and B_6, 1000 IU vitamin D, 300 IU vitamin E, and 500 milligrams calcium. Physicians have found that after surgery and in the following 24 hours, vitamin C is dramatically lost from the body. They recommend 10 grams of vitamin C before surgery, 10 grams in each tube feeding bottle after surgery, and 10 grams orally after fluids are discontinued.[4]

Convalescence requires a greater-than-normal amount of all nutrients. If supplements cannot be taken because of vomiting, vitamins stirred into creams can be absorbed through the skin. (Injections or surface application of vitamin B_6 may relieve the vomiting.)[5]

NUTRIENTS THAT MAY BE BENEFICIAL IN TREATMENT OF ACCIDENTS, SHOCK, AND SURGERY

Body Member	Nutrients	Quantity*
Blood/Circulatory system	Vitamin C	
	Vitamin E	
	Vitamin K	
	Calcium	

[3]Ibid., p. 265.
[4]Roger Williams & Dwight Kalita, eds., in *A Physician's Handbook on Orthomolecular Medicine*, p. 56.
[5]Davis, *Let's Get Well*, p. 268.

Body Member	Nutrients	Quantity*
Brain/Nervous system	Vitamin B complex	
	Vitamin C	3000 mg
	Vitamin E	300 IU
General	Protein	
	Digestive enzymes	
	Acidophilus	
	Vitamin B_2	20 mg
	Vitamin B_6	20 mg
	Folic acid	
	Pantothenic acid	500 mg
	Vitamin C	1000 mg–10 gm
	Vitamin D	1000 IU
	Calcium	500 mg
	Copper	
	Magnesium	
	Zinc	

*See note, p. 222.

ACNE

Acne is a common disorder of the oil glands in the skin characterized by the recurring formation of blackheads, whiteheads, and pimples. Acne occurs primarily on the face and sometimes on the back, shoulders, chest, and arms. The incidence of acne is greatest during puberty and adolescence, when hormones influencing the secretion of the oil glands are at their peak level of activity.

Psychological stress may be a significant factor in acne; therefore all nutrients needed to meet stress should be emphasized. Proper nutrition and skin cleanliness, together with adequate rest, exercise, fresh air, and sunlight, are helpful in the treatment of acne. Because the ultraviolet light of the sun contains actinic rays that sterilize the skin, use of a sunlamp when sunlight is unavailable, three times a week, may prevent bacterial infection and the resultant acne pimples.

Many authorities believe overindulgence in carbohydrates and foods with high fat content should be avoided. Candy, sweetened soft drinks, fried foods, and nuts should be avoided. An excess of oxalic acid found in chocolate, cocoa, spinach, and rhubarb may inhibit the body's absorption of calcium. Calcium helps maintain the acid-alkali balance of the blood necessary for a clear complexion.

Ingestion of too much salt has been shown to cause

acne. Improvement in 2 weeks and complete recovery in 2 months was observed in patients given a low-salt diet.

Vitamin A is especially beneficial for clear, healthy skin. Vitamin A acid, available by prescription, has been found to clear the skin in some people within 6 weeks.

The B-complex vitamins, especially riboflavin, pyridoxine, and pantothenic acid, help reduce facial oiliness and blackhead formation. Vitamin C aids in resisting the spread of acne infection, and vitamin D guards the body's store of calcium from excretion. Vitamin E has been found helpful in the prevention of scarring.[6]

Daily supplements of zinc have produced successful results in many people. Zinc is an efficient bacterial suppressor and a necessary element in the oil-producing glands of the skin. Many adolescents are deficient in zinc.

NUTRIENTS THAT MAY BE BENEFICIAL IN TREATMENT OF ACNE

Body Member	Nutrients	Quantity*
Skin	Vitamin A	50,000–100,000 IU daily for 1 month 10,000–25,000 IU
	Vitamin B complex	
	Vitamin B_2	5–15 mg
	Vitamin B_6	
	Niacin	100 mg three times daily
	Pantothenic acid	300 mg
	Vitamin C	1000 mg
	Vitamin D	
	Vitamin E	Also as ointment
	Unsaturated fatty acids	
	Calcium	
	Potassium	
	Sulfur	
	Zinc	30–100 mg

*See note, p. 222.

ADRENAL EXHAUSTION

Adrenal exhaustion is the progressive lessening of activity of the adrenal glands, which may eventually lead

[6]Davis, *Let's Get Well*, p. 161.

to complete functional failure. It is characterized by a low energy level in the morning which gradually rises, being highest late at night. The person retires but cannot fall asleep right away, then sleeps soundly but arises exhausted. Adrenal exhaustion is often categorized with insomnia.

The vitamins B_2, B_{12}, folic acid, and pantothenic acid with potassium and sodium stabilize the activity of the adrenal glands.

NUTRIENTS THAT MAY BE BENEFICIAL IN TREATMENT OF ADRENAL EXHAUSTION

Body Member	Nutrients	Quantity
Glands	Vitamin B complex	
	Vitamin B_2	
	Vitamin B_{12}	
	Folic acid	
	Pantothenic acid	
	Vitamin C	
	Vitamin E	
	Potassium	
	Sodium	
	Unsaturated fatty acids	

ALCOHOLISM

Alcoholism is a dependence on or addiction to alcohol. The body's outward reaction to alcohol suggests that it acts as a stimulant by producing aggressive social behavior such as loss of inhibitions, increased boldness, and sociability associated with drinking. In fact, alcohol is a depressant that acts to decrease the basic speed of all bodily functions, including muscle contractions, speed of reaction, digestion, and thinking processes.

Prolonged dependence upon this drug may result in severe problems in the pancreas and gastrointestinal tract as well as the emotional and mental problems associated with alcoholism. Severe deficiencies of many nutrients occur because the alcohol itself satisfies the body's caloric needs. (Alcohol contains about 70 calories per ounce.) Alcohol is a carbohydrate but contains no vitamins or minerals, which are needed for carbohydrate metabolism. The vitamins and minerals are then taken from other parts of the body, eventually leading to tissue depletion.

As the alcohol enters the bloodstream directly

through the walls of the stomach, it begins to act upon the central nervous system by changing the most basic mental functions and by destroying brain cells. Cells are destroyed by the withdrawal of necessary water from the tissues and cells. The liver works to neutralize the effects of alcohol upon the body by breaking down the composition of the alcohol. Under normal circumstances, especially if there is food in the stomach, the liver can effectively perform the function of breaking down the alcohol if not more than one drink per hour is consumed. However, when the liver is overworked, it must compensate by creating an increased tolerance for alcohol. After a time the liver compensates less rapidly, becomes fatty, and is less able to decompose the alcohol. As a result, the alcoholic develops a decreased tolerance for alcohol and less is needed to produce intoxication. As drinking continues over a period of time, the liver cells die and are replaced with scar tissue. This condition is known as cirrhosis of the liver.

Diet and nutrient supplements are very important in the treatment of alcoholism. Because of biochemical individuality, different nutritional approaches will be needed for different alcoholics.

Refined carbohydrates need to be eliminated from the diet. Rats placed on the typical American high-refined-carbohydrate diet eventually avoid the water bowl in favor of the bowl of whiskey.

In some cases, a strict diet adequate in calories and high in protein, which contains all the vitamins and minerals and especially high in B vitamins, reduced the alcoholic's desire to drink. Protein is necessary for tissue regeneration, particularly when cirrhosis of the liver occurs. Vitamin A is an anti-infective agent for upper respiratory infections such as tuberculosis and pneumonia which are common in alcoholics. The vitamin B complex is essential for the prevention and treatment of alcoholic neuritis, pellagra, and delirium tremens. Niacin and the amino acid glutamine have been shown to help to prevent the craving for alcohol. Vitamin C, which is often deficient in alcoholics, is needed to prevent scurvy. A zinc deficiency may occur, making the alcoholic more prone to cirrhosis of the liver and preventing vitamin K from being absorbed into the body. Iron is needed to correct the anemia that often develops. A magnesium deficiency can contribute to the occurrence of delirium tremens. A deficiency of potassium may also occur

in alcoholics, and supplements may be necessary. Choline aids in the decomposition of fat in the liver and helps maintain healthy kidneys jeopardized by heavy drinking.

Complications that can interfere with recovery are concurrent drug use, hypoglycemia, and perceptual distortions similar to those experienced by schizophrenics. Food allergy additions may also be a factor. Permanent brain damage may not respond to nutrient therapy.

NUTRIENTS THAT MAY BE BENEFICIAL IN TREATMENT OF ALCOHOLISM

Body Member	Nutrients	Quantity*
Brain/ Nervous system	Vitamin A	25,000 IU
	Vitamin B complex	
	Vitamin B$_1$	500–1500 mg 3 times daily
	Vitamin B$_2$	
	Vitamin B$_6$	100 mg–1 gm
	Vitamin B$_{12}$	
	Choline	
	Folic acid	5 mg
	Niacin	100 mg–6 gm
	Pangamic acid	
	Pantothenic acid	200–1000 mg
	Vitamin C	Up to 3–10 gm
	Vitamin D	1000 IU
	Vitamin E	Up to 1200 IU
	Vitamin K	
	Chromium	
	Iron	
	Magnesium	Up to 1000 mg
	Manganese	50 mg
	Zinc	150 mg
	Unsaturated fatty acids	
	Glutamine	1000 mg three times daily

*See note, p. 222.

ALLERGIES

An allergy is a sensitivity to some particular substance known as an allergen. The allergen may be harmless to some people but can cause a reaction in others. Almost any food may be an allergen to some people. The allergic reaction may be hay fever, asthma, hives, high blood pressure, abnormal fatigue, constipation, stomach ulcers, dizziness, headache, mental disorders, hyperactivity, or hypoglycemia. After eating, excessive tiredness, swelled stomach, palpitations, sweating, or mental fuzziness may be experienced.

Foods, as well as inhalants and chemicals, can cause a brain reaction mimicking typical psychological problems from the minor, such as listlessness, insomnia, and irritability, to more severe symptoms such as migraine headaches, depression, poor memory, violent outbursts, and hallucinations. Sometimes the brain sensitivity can be an allergy and an addiction at the same time. Allergic reactions can be brought on by eating a particular food, yet more severe reactions can result if the food is not eaten.

Allergens enter the body in numerous ways. They may be injected from drugs or vaccines; enter through the skin from cosmetics, insect bites or poison oak or ivy; they can be taken in by the mucous membranes of the nose from pollen or dust; or they can be absorbed through the intestinal tract from foods, bacteria, molds, or drugs.

Many allergens are transitory; the effects are felt at some times and not at others. A food may cause a reaction when a person is emotionally upset and yet no reaction is experienced when the mood is tranquil.

Susceptibility to an allergen depends on several factors including heredity (requiring unusually high amounts of one or more nutrients) and the condition of the body's immune system. Stress, poor diet, insufficient sleep, emotional traumas, and infections can predispose the body to allergic reactions. A healthy body can resist allergens, but a lack of any one nutrient can increase cell permeability, allowing easy entrance by foreign substances.

NUTRIENTS THAT MAY BE BENEFICIAL IN TREATMENT OF ALLERGIES

Body Member	Nutrients	Quantity*
General	Vitamin A	10,000–25,000 IU
	Vitamin B complex	
	Vitamin B_6	
	Vitamin B_{12}	
	Niacin	
	Pantothenic acid	100–200 mg
	Vitamin C	250 mg four times daily; up to 5000 mg
	Vitamin D	
	Vitamin E	Up to 800 IU
	Unsaturated fatty acids	
	Calcium	Up to 1000 mg
	Magnesium	
	Manganese	5 mg twice weekly for 10 weeks
	Potassium	

*See note, p. 222.

ANEMIA

A reduction of the amount of hemoglobin in the bloodstream and/or a reduction in the number of red blood cells themselves reduces the amount of oxygen available to all body cells. Carbon dioxide accumulates in the cells, causing decreased efficiency and lower rate of body processes. When the brain cells are deprived of oxygen, dizziness may result. Additional symptoms of anemia are general weakness, fatigue, paleness, brittle nails, loss of appetite, and abdominal pain.

Anemia often arises from recurrent infections and/or diseases involving the entire body. It can be caused by certain drugs that destroy vitamin E and other nutrients necessary for the health of the blood cells. Some insecticides damage bone marrow, often resulting in anemia and eventually death.

It may also be caused by inadequate intake or impaired absorption of nutrients or by excessive losses of blood through such conditions as heavy menstruation or peptic ulcer. It has been shown that excess amounts of vitamin K in the diet during pregnancy may cause anemia in newborn infants.

Iron, protein, copper, folic acid, and vitamins B_6, B_{12}, and C are all necessary for the formation of red blood cells. A deficiency in any of these nutrients can cause anemia, although iron-deficiency anemia is the most common form of the condition. Infants, adolescents, and women, particularly during pregnancy, are often deficient in iron and may require iron supplements.

Iron-deficiency anemia can occur even if the diet is rich in iron. A lack of vitamins B_1, B_2, niacin, pantothenic acid, or choline results in iron malabsorption. These nutrients are essential for the secretion of hydrochloric acid, which dissolves the iron before it is absorbed. Iron absorption can also be adversely affected by diahrrea, chronic use of laxatives, and malabsorption diseases such as sprue and celiac disease. Vitamin C aids in the absorption and retention of iron. Vitamin E may be needed to help maintain the health of red blood cells.

Pernicious anemia is a form of anemia resulting from a deficiency of vitamin B_{12}. It is a severe form of anemia in which there is a gradual reduction in the number of blood cells because the bone marrow fails to produce mature red blood cells. Pernicious anemia probably arises from an inheritable inability of the stomach to secrete a substance called the "intrinsic factor" which is necessary for the intestinal absorption of vitamin B_{12}.

Pernicious anemia occurs in both sexes. Its occurrence is rare in persons under the age of thirty, but susceptibility increases with age. Vegetarians are particularly susceptible to this type of anemia because sufficient vitamin B_{12} is found chiefly in animal proteins. In addition, the high levels of folic acid contained in vegetarian diets can mask a B_{12} deficiency.

Symptoms of pernicious anemia include weakness and gastrointestinal disturbances causing a sore tongue, slight yellowing of the skin, and tingling of extremities. In addition, disturbances of the nervous system, such as partial loss of coordination of the fingers, feet, and legs; some nerve deterioration; and disturbances of the digestive tract, such as diarrhea and loss of appetite, may occur.

Pernicious anemia may be fatal without treatment. Vitamin B_{12} injections together with a highly nutritious diet supplemented with large amounts of desiccated liver are the recommended treatment. Intake of the entire vitamin B complex will help maintain the health of the nervous system, although folic acid should not be taken in amounts exceeding 0.1 milligram daily. Folic acid has the effect of concealing the symptoms of pernicious anemia, allowing the unseen destruction of the nervous system to continue until irreparable damage is done. A diet rich in protein, calcium, vitamin C, vitamin E, and iron is recommended.

Sickle-cell anemia is characterized by red blood cells that become bent (sickled) and hard and clog the circulation system, depriving the body tissues of oxygen. It has been observed that these patients seem to have a high requirement for folic acid and have responded to ingestion of 5 milligrams or more of this vitamin per day.[7]

NUTRIENTS THAT MAY BE BENEFICIAL IN TREATMENT OF ANEMIA

Body Member	Nutrients	Quantity*
Blood/Circulatory system	Vitamin B complex	
	Vitamin B_1	50–100 mg
	Vitamin B_6	50–100 mg
	Vitamin B_{12}	20–100 mcg
	Folic acid	0.5–5 mg
	PABA	Up to 50 mg
	Pantothenic acid	Up to 100 mg
	Vitamin C	500 mg
	Vitamin E	Up to 1000 IU
	Calcium	
	Cobalt	
	Copper	
	Iron	10 mg
	Magnesium	
	Protein	

*See note, p. 222.

ARTERIOSCLEROSIS AND ATHEROSCLEROSIS

A thickening and hardening of the walls of the arteries is known as arteriosclerosis. Arteriosclerosis accurs in two forms. The first type of hardening is caused by a gradual deposit of calcium in the artery walls, resisting the flow of blood to the body cells. A second, more advanced type of hardening, called atherosclerosis, is due to the buildup of cholesterol or fatty deposits in the artery walls and contributes to the degeneration of the arteries involved. Atherosclerosis usually affects the aorta, heart, and brain arteries as well as the other blood vessels of the body and extremities.

Fat molecules are normally absorbed through the artery walls. When an excess of fatty material starts

[7]Ibid., p. 230.

to resist blood flow, fatty streaks begin to appear on the interior of the arteries. As more and more of this fat is introduced, the artery walls thicken and plaques of cholesterol narrow the arteries. The artery walls then lose their elasticity and become hard and brittle. Hemorrhages from small vessels located in the arterial wall beneath the plaques may cause the cholesterol deposits to break free from the wall, or a clot may form as blood passes over the rough edge of a plaque. The plaques, clots, or a combination of these may cause a total block in the vessel, resulting in death.

Partial blockage causing a limited blood supply can result in cataracts or coldness and pain in the extremities, sometimes leading to gangrene. Lack of sufficient blood to the brain causes confusion, senility, or strokes. Angina attacks occur when there is any restriction around the heart. A clot can form anywhere in the body and work its way to the brain or heart. Fatty deposits interfere with many diseases and delay complete recovery.

Symptoms of atherosclerosis are hypertension, cramping or paralysis of muscles, a sensation of heaviness or pressure in the chest, and pains that radiate from the chest to the left arm and shoulder. Factors that enhance the tendency to develop atherosclerosis are obesity, lack of exercise, hypertension, smoking, heredity, stress, and poor diet.

Stress uses up nutrients that are needed for fat utilization. Some physicians believe that stress alone may cause atherosclerosis regardless of blood fat levels. The greatest stress is placed where the arteries branch and curve; the faster the blood flow that occurs during stress, the more injury that occurs at these particular sites.

Persons with atherosclerosis that is considered hereditary may have an abnormally high genetic requirement for particular nutrients that properly metabolize fats. Too much sugar and refined carbohydrate consumption has been proved to be a major factor in atherosclerosis. Excess sugar and alcohol not utilized as energy by the body eventually turn into saturated fat.

Studies have shown that the amount of fats in the diet may not be the factor causing atherosclerosis, but rather how effectively the body metabolizes the fats. The amount of cholesterol consumed in the diet may not have any relation to serum cholesterol. If the body does not receive enough cholesterol for its needs, the liver begins to produce what is lacking.

Linoleic acid appears to be necessary for the utilization of saturated fats and cholesterol. Two other fatty acids are also essential but can be synthesized from linoleic acid as long as numerous vitamins and minerals are present to aid the conversion. Polyunsaturated oils are good sources of linoleic acid. However, they oxidize easily in the bloodstream, so taking vitamin E along with the oils is recommended. One of these fatty acids is also needed for the production of lecithin. Lecithin breaks down cholesterol and fats in the blood, allowing them to be effectively utilized by the cells of the body. Other nutrients vital for the production of lecithin are choline, inositol, vitamin B_6, and magnesium. The more saturated fats in the diet, the higher the need for linoleic acid and lecithin. Iodine taken with vitamin E has been shown to stimulate the thyroid gland, aiding in the metabolism of fats.

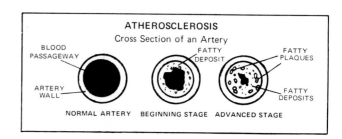

ATHEROSCLEROSIS
Cross Section of an Artery

NORMAL ARTERY   BEGINNING STAGE   ADVANCED STAGE

NUTRIENTS THAT MAY BE BENEFICIAL IN TREATMENT OF ARTERIOSCLEROSIS AND ATHEROSCLEROSIS

Body Member	Nutrients	Quantity*
Blood/Heart	Vitamin A	20,000–100,000 IU
	Vitamin B complex	
	Vitamin B_6	50 mg
	Vitamin B_{12}	
	Choline	500 mg
	Folic acid	
	Inositol	500 mg
	Niacin	100–500 mg under doctor's supervision
	Vitamin C	Up to 3000 mg

*See note, p. 222.

Body Member	Nutrients	Quantity*
	Vitamin E	600–1200 IU
	Bioflavonoids	300–600 mg
	Calcium	500 mg
	Chromium	
	Cobalt	
	Copper	
	Iodine	
	Iron	
	Magnesium	
	Manganese	
	Pectin	
	Phosphorus	
	Potassium	
	Selenium	
	Vanadium	
	Zinc	

*See note, p. 222.

ARTHRITIS

Arthritis results in inflammation and soreness of the joints. It has been suggested that arthritis is related to the body's immune system. Either the body is unable to produce enough antibodies to prevent viruses from entering the joints, or antibodies that are produced are unable to differentiate between viruses and healthy cells, thereby destroying both. Arthritis may also result from an allergy to certain foods.

Osteoarthritis and rheumatoid arthritis are the two main types of the disease. Osteoarthritis, usually found in elderly people, develops as a result of the continuous wearing away of the cartilage in a joint. Cartilage, which is a smooth, soft, pearly tissue, covers the ends of the bones at the joints. It provides a smooth surface for the bones to slide against, allowing easy movement of the joints. As a result of injury or years of use, cartilage becomes thin and may disappear. When enough cartilage has worn away, the rough surfaces of the bones rub together, causing pain and stiffness. Osteoarthritis usually affects the weight-bearing joints, such as the hips and knees. Symptoms of osteoarthritis include body stiffness and pain in the joints, especially during damp weather, in the morning, or after strenuous activity.

Rheumatoid arthritis affects the entire body instead of just one joint. Onset of the disease is often associated with physical or emotional stress; however, poor nutrition or bacterial infection may be just as likely a cause.

Rheumatoid arthritis destroys the cartilage and tissues in and around the joints and often the bone surfaces themselves. The body replaces the damaged tissue with scar tissue, causing the spaces between the joints to become narrow and fuse together. This causes the stiffening and crippling onset of the disease. Symptoms of rheumatoid arthritis include swelling and pain in the joints, fatigue, anemia, weight loss, and fever. These symptoms often disappear and recur at a later date.

Most rheumatoid arthritics have high serum copper and low iron levels, although the joints and lymph nodes have excess iron which may be responsible for the painful joints. The high copper levels may be the result of an inadequate supply of zinc, manganese, and sulfur in the diet.

A chelating agent, D-penicillamine, has been used for removal of the excess copper. The drug also removes zinc and possibly other trace minerals, so a trace element supplement excluding copper is taken along with this particular treatment.

Many nutritional cures for arthritis have been claimed, upon which research still continues. It is recommended that the arthritic have a well-balanced diet in order to provide his body with all the nutrients it needs for repair. If the arthritic is overweight he or she should lose weight in order to reduce the stress on weight-bearing joints.

Vitamin C is necessary to prevent the capillary walls in the joints from breaking down and causing bleeding, swelling, and pain. Folic acid, vitamin B_{12}, and iron may be helpful in treating the anemia that can accompany arthritis. The frequency of liver disorders in arthritic patients may deter the conversion of carotene into vitamin A. Difficulty in assimilating carbohydrates suggests vitamin B deficiency.

Superoxide dismutase (SOD) has been found to be effective by injection in relieving the stiffness, pain, and swollen joints in arthritis. SOD is a member of a group of enzymes found mainly in the fluids inside

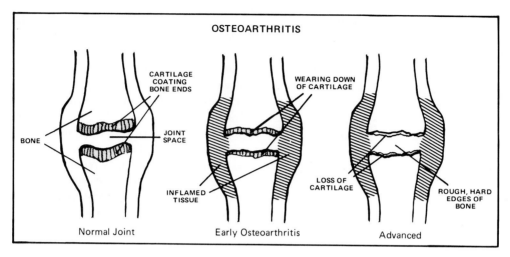

OSTEOARTHRITIS

CARTILAGE COATING BONE ENDS

BONE

JOINT SPACE

INFLAMED TISSUE

WEARING DOWN OF CARTILAGE

LOSS OF CARTILAGE

ROUGH, HARD EDGES OF BONE

Normal Joint   Early Osteoarthritis   Advanced

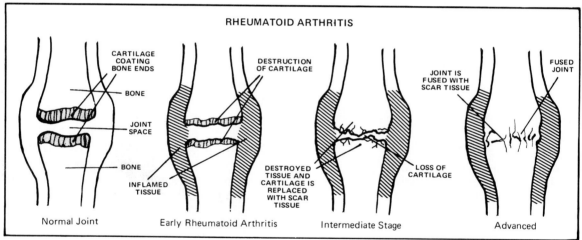

RHEUMATOID ARTHRITIS

CARTILAGE COATING BONE ENDS

BONE

JOINT SPACE

BONE

INFLAMED TISSUE

DESTRUCTION OF CARTILAGE

DESTROYED TISSUE AND CARTILAGE IS REPLACED WITH SCAR TISSUE

JOINT IS FUSED WITH SCAR TISSUE

LOSS OF CARTILAGE

FUSED JOINT

Normal Joint   Early Rheumatoid Arthritis   Intermediate Stage   Advanced

the cells. They protect the cells against damage caused by free radicals.

DMSO (dimethyl sulfoxide) is another radical scavenger that relieves the stiffness and pain. Its effects are enhanced when taken with other vitamins and minerals such as A, B complex, C, E, and zinc and selenium.

Cod-liver oil and royal bee jelly, rich in pantothenic acid, are reportedly helpful for arthritic persons.

Exercise is important in both the prevention and treatment of arthritis because unused joints tend to stiffen. Good posture is also important to prevent stiffness and crippling. Poor posture can cause body weight to be distributed unevenly, placing more stress on certain joints, thus resulting in unnecessary pain for the arthritic person.

NUTRIENTS THAT MAY BE BENEFICIAL IN TREATMENT OF ARTHRITIS

Body Member	Nutrients	Quantity*
Joints	Vitamin A	
	Vitamin B complex	
	Vitamin B$_2$	1000 mg under doctor's supervision
	Vitamin B$_6$	500 mg–2 gm
	Vitamin B$_{12}$	30–900 mcg per week
	Folic acid	5 mg
	Inositol	

*See note, p. 222.

Body Member	Nutrients	Quantity*
	Niacin	Up to 1000 mg under doctor's supervision
	PABA	2 gm
	Pantothenic acid	100 mg–1 gm
	Vitamin C	3000–5000 mg; children: 600 mg
	Vitamin D	
	Vitamin E	600–1000 IU
	Unsaturated fatty acids	
	Bioflavonoids	3000 mg
	Calcium	500 mg
	Copper	
	Iodine	
	Lecithin	
	Magnesium	500 mg
	Manganese	
	Phosphorus	
	Potassium	500 mg
	Selenium	
	Sulfur	200 mg
	Protein	
	Zinc	
	Cod-liver oil	1–2 tbsp

*See note, p. 222.

ASTHMA

Asthma is a chronic respiratory condition character-ized by difficulty in breathing, frequent coughing, and a feeling of suffocation. An attack of asthma is often precipitated by physical or emotional stress, respira-tory infections, air pollution, changes in temperature or humidity, and exposure to fumes such as those of gasoline or paint, as well as sulfur dioxide and sulfites. It may also be related to low blood sugar, disorders of the adrenal glands, or specific allergies.

Symptoms of asthma are tightness in the chest and difficulty in breathing usually accompanied by a wheez-ing or whistling sound. Violent coughing often occurs as the lungs attempt to expel mucus. An attack can last from several minutes to several days depending on individual situations and causative agents.

Skin tests are often given to pinpoint the patient's allergic tendencies. Common offenders are pollen, ani-mal hair, dust, and certain foods. Proper nutrition is necessary, and the asthmatic should eliminate from the diet those foods that may bring on an attack. A high fluid intake and the inhalation of steam may help to liquefy mucus and make it easier to expel it from the air passages. Vitamin A is necessary for general health of the lungs and, together with vitamin E, guards against visible and invisible air pollutants. The person should have a diet sufficient in the vitamin B complex to avoid deficiency symptoms of nervous-ness, which might bring on an asthma attack. The need for vitamin C is increased by stress and exposure to hot or cold weather, cigarette smoking, and indus-trial air pollution.

NUTRIENTS THAT MAY BE BENEFICIAL IN TREATMENT OF ASTHMA

Body Member	Nutrients	Quantity*
Lungs/ Respiratory system	Vitamin A	Up to 75,000 IU
	Vitamin B complex	
	Vitamin B_6	50 mg
	Vitamin B_{12}	30 mcg
	Choline	
	Inositol	
	Pangamic acid	
	Pantothenic acid	100 mg
	Vitamin C	600 mg
	Vitamin D	800–14,000 IU
	Vitamin E	600 IU; 32 IU for children
	Unsaturated fatty acids	
	Calcium	
	Manganese	5 mg twice daily for 10 weeks

*See note, p. 222.

AUTISM

Autism is an illness that involves the personality of children who do not react to their environment. The children do not learn to talk, or if they have learned they soon stop. They are withdrawn and do not respond to other people.

A research psychologist in San Diego, California, Dr. Bernard Rimland, has had positive results in treating autism with megavitamin therapy. In his study, 50 percent of the children tested improved significantly by showing a reduction in tantrums, increased alertness, improved speech, better sleep patterns, and greater sociability. The vitamins that were most prominent were niacin, pantothenic acid, B_6, and C. For the children not responding to the treatment, the doctor suggested an increase in the dosage of vitamin B_6. Improvement was then noted. Three percent of the children in the study got worse with the treatment, with noticeable side effects such as extreme sensitivity to noise and bed-wetting. Because B_6 in large quantities can deplete magnesium from a person with a marginal supply of the mineral, the children were given a magnesium supplement and the side effects disappeared. When the vitamin treatment was discontinued, a regression of the illness resulted.

Prevention magazine, October 1978, reports information on pangamic acid and autism that was related by Dr. Allan Cott, a New York psychiatrist, during an informal talk at the International Academy of Preventive Medicine. An autistic seven-year-old child, who had never spoken, was given 200 milligrams of pangamic acid daily. He seen began to use single words, then pairs. He began to play games, tried to dress himself, and became more gregarious. Another nonverbalizing and hyperactive child, after administration of pangamic acid, began to talk and was able, for the first time, to sit still. When the supplement was withdrawn, he reverted to hyperactivity, gaze aversion, fright, and hostility. The child began to improve 24 hours after the administration of pangamic acid was resumed. In 72 hours, there was full recovery. After nine months, the child began to answer questions and talk to himself.

It must be noted that not all autism stems from vitamin deficiency. Some behavioral problems result from diseases of the brain. Allergies may be a possibility. Lead, copper or aluminum intoxication can cause autism.

NUTRIENTS THAT MAY BE BENEFICIAL IN TREATMENT OF AUTISM

Body Member	Nutrients	Quantity*
General	Vitamin B complex	
	Vitamin B_1	
	Vitamin B_2	
	Vitamin B_6	Up to 450 mg
	Folic acid	
	Niacin	1–3 gm
	Pangamic acid	
	Pantothenic acid	200–600 mg
	Vitamin C	1–3 gm
	Vitamin E	
	Magnesium	
	Glutamic acid	

*See note, p. 222.

BACKACHE

Backache may be a symptom of a variety of disturbances in the muscles, tendons, ligaments, bones, or underlying organs. "Lumbago" is a general term frequently used to describe pain in the lower back.

A few of the many underlying causes of backache are arthritis, osteoporosis, infection and fever, tumor, peptic ulcer, emotional tension or stress, slipped disc or other spinal cord injury, and disorders of the urinary system. Muscle strain or sprain as a cause of backache is quite frequent and commonly results from excessive or improper physical exertion, incorrect posture, sleeping on soft beds, or incorrect lifting. Overweight, flat feet, and unequal leg length are other factors that may be responsible for back pain.

A backache that is accompanied by fever or headache should receive medical diagnosis.

The most painful back malady is the slipped disk. When a disk or its supporting ligaments become weakened, the disk slips out of alignment and presses against delicate spinal nerves, causing pain.

Back pain may be the result of localized tender spots of the muscles called trigger points. Some physicians inject these sore spots with procaine, killing the pain. An exercise program is then recommended. Trigger points and slipped disk can have many of the same symptoms, confusing diagnosis. Trigger points do not cause reflex or sensory loss, numbness, or weakness, which are common in disk injury.

If the skin itself is sensitive to touch, a condition called fibrositis may be indicated, which may be successfully treated by a pinching massage given regularly over a period of weeks or months.

Backache prevention includes exercise, good posture, proper lifting (by bending at the knees instead of the waist), and avoidance of unnecessary physical or emotional stress or strain.

Numerous treatments, varying according to the exact reason for the back pain, that have helped many people include chiropractic manipulation of the backbone, use of heat and cold penetration, injection of anesthetic-like compounds into the painful areas, application of radio-frequency beams that eliminate nerve pain surrounding a slipped disk, and acupuncture. Surgery seems to be necessary only in extreme circumstances.

Even in disk cases, exercises that retrain weak muscles can many times adequately improve the condition of the spinal column. Exercises to firm stomach muscles can relieve the strain of daily exertions placed on the lower back region. Many back pain sufferers do not have sufficient strength in their muscles to support their own weight. Again, proper exercise will strengthen and add resilience to weak muscles.

Certain nutrients are essential for maintaining a healthy back. Protein is necessary for firm supporting tissue. The B-complex vitamins, especially niacin, provide strength and health for nerve tissues. Vitamins C and D together with calcium are important in the development and maintenance of bones and nerve function.

NUTRIENTS THAT MAY BE BENEFICIAL IN TREATMENT OF BACKACHE

Body Member	Nutrients	Quantity*
Bones/Spine	Vitamin B complex	
	Niacin	
	Vitamin C	500–1500 mg
	Vitamin D	
	Vitamin E	50 IU
	Calcium	1–2 gm
	Magnesium	
	Manganese	
	Phosphorus	
	Zinc	
	Protein	

*See note, p. 222.

BALDNESS (ALOPECIA)

Baldness is the partial or complete loss of hair, most commonly in the scalp, resulting from heredity, hormonal factors, aging, or local or systematic diseases.

Stress, triggering a hormonal imbalance that overproduces androgen, a male hormone, can cause both male and female pattern baldness. Hair loss in women that occurs in cycles may be due to stress, diseases, surgery, childbirth, abortion, or it can occur after discontinuance of oral contraceptives. Certain medicines can cause hair loss in both men and women. They include antibiotics such as penicillin, sulfonamides, and mycin, the hyperthyroid drug carbimazole, and the anticoagulant heparin.

Male pattern baldness comprises 90 percent of hair loss cases. The hair usually starts to recede at the hairline, in a circle on the crown of the head, or at the back of the head. In male pattern baldness, hair follicles spend more time in a resting phase than in a growing cycle. However, hair continues to fall out. It is believed that the resting follicles can possibly be stimulated for regrowth.

Studies have shown that dihydrotestosterone, a hormone resulting from the metabolism of testosterone, causes the hair follicles to remain in the resting stage. Large amounts of a testosterone compound salve (as the cypionate) applied topically to the scalp can slow or even halt male pattern baldness by preventing the formation of dihydrotestosterone.

Inositol and PABA protect hair follicles, preventing hair loss and often premature graying. Biotin also may slow hair loss. It has been reported that cayenne pepper rubbed into the scalp has resulted in hair regrowth, possibly because of its stimulative effect on the cells.[8]

NUTRIENTS THAT MAY BE BENEFICIAL IN TREATMENT OF BALDNESS

Body Member	Nutrients	Quantity*
Hair/Scalp	Vitamin B complex	
	Vitamin B$_1$	
	Vitamin B$_2$	
	Vitamin B$_6$	50 mg
	Vitamin B$_{12}$	
	Biotin	
	Choline	500–1000 mg
	Folic acid	1 mg
	Inositol	500–1000 mg
	Niacin	50 mg

*See note, p. 222.

[8]Durk Pearson and Sandy Shaw, *Life Extension,* p. 218.

Body Member	Nutrients	Quantity*
	PABA	50 mg–3 gm
	Pantothenic acid	50 mg
	Vitamin C	1000 mg
	Vitamin E	Up to 1200 IU
	Bioflavonoids	50–100 mg
	Copper	
	Manganese	
	Potassium iodide	
	Zinc	

*See note, p. 222.

BEDSORES

A bedsore forms when pressure on a bony area of the body, such as the elbow, heel, or hip, cuts off the blood supply to that area. The affected area is thus deprived of essential nutrients, and therefore tissue is destroyed.

The most effective prevention for bedsores is relieving pressure on the vulnerable areas of the body by using protective padding, massaging the skin to stimulate circulation, and keeping the skin dry and clean. Treatment for bedsores includes a well-balanced diet high in protein, calories, and vitamins. In some cases, direct applications of vitamins C and E to the wound have been beneficial. Ointments containing vitamins A and D and sugar or honey are also often used in treating bedsores.

NUTRIENTS THAT MAY BE BENEFICIAL IN TREATMENT OF BEDSORES

Body Member	Nutrients	Quantity*
Skin	Vitamin A	
	Vitamin B complex	
	Vitamin B_2	5 mg daily
	Vitamin C	
	Vitamin D	
	Vitamin E	
	Copper	
	Zinc	
	Protein	

*See note, p. 222.

BELL'S PALSY (SEE ALSO "NEURITIS")

Bell's palsy is a type of paralysis characterized by distortion of the face due to a lesion of the facial nerve. It is accompanied by pain, weakness, and a sensation of pricking, tingling, or creeping on the skin, which may be a result of injury or irritation of a sensory nerve or nerve root.

NUTRIENTS THAT MAY BE BENEFICIAL IN TREATMENT OF BELL'S PALSY

Body Member	Nutrients	Quantity*
Brain/Nervous system	Vitamin B complex	
	Vitamin B_1	100–200 mg
	Vitamin C	
	Protein	

*See note, p. 222.

BERIBERI

Beriberi is a disease caused by a deficiency of thiamine. The disease seldom occurs outside the Far East, where the principal diet consists mainly of polished rise, which does not supply sufficient thiamine. Rare cases of beriberi in the United States are usually associated with stressful conditions, such as hypothyroidism, infections, pregnancy, lactation, and chronic alcoholism, which increase the body's need for thiamine.

Symptoms of beriberi in infants are convulsions; respiratory difficulties; and gastrointestinal problems, such as nausea, vomiting, constipation, diarrhea, and abdominal discomfort. Adult symptoms are fatigue, diarrhea, appetite and weight loss, disturbed nerve function causing paralysis and wasting of the limbs, edema, and heart failure.

The administration of thiamine will prevent and cure the disease. Because of the diarrhea that accompanies beriberi, the diet must be rich in all nutrients.

NUTRIENTS THAT MAY BE BENEFICIAL IN TREATMENT OF BERIBERI

Body Member	Nutrients	Quantity
General	Vitamin B complex	
	Vitamin B_1	
	Vitamin C	

BODY ODOR

Body odors are related to the internal health of the body. Certain nutrients appear to metabolically remove wastes in the body that cause odors. They include the minerals magnesium and zinc and vitamins B_6 and PABA.

NUTRIENTS THAT MAY BE BENEFICIAL IN TREATMENT OF BODY ODOR

Body Member	Nutrients	Quantity*
Glands	Vitamin B complex	
	Vitamin B_6	
	PABA	
	Magnesium	
	Zinc	20–40 mg
	Chlorophyll	

*See note, p. 222.

BONE ABNORMALITIES

Broken, inflamed, infected, decalcified, weak, or brittle bones require sufficient amounts of many nutrients to repair and heal properly.

Osteitis, osteomyelitis, and osteitis deformans, of which Paget's disease is a form, are bone inflammation diseases characterized by swelling, tenderness, pain, and often an infection.

Stress and often the immobilization of a part or all of the body increases the urinary loss of many nutrients. In osteitis deformans, stress causes a rapid loss of minerals from the bone and prevents the forming of new proteins so essential for building up the bone. Cortisone can cause a depletion of calcium from the bone.

Calcium is released from its storage areas in the bone and used for repair. Lack of adequate calcium in the diet will prevent this repair process because the calcium that is taken in will not be stored but will be used first by the soft tissues of the body. Slow healing is often an indication of low levels of calcium.

Magnesium and vitamin D are essential for the absorption of calcium. Bone repair depends on protein and all the nutrients needed for protein metabolism. Digestive enzymes and hydrochloric acid may be necessary to ensure sufficient digestion. Vitamin E can prevent stiffness and scarring. Vitamin C helps to heal and prevent infection.

NUTRIENTS THAT MAY BE BENEFICIAL IN TREATMENT OF BONE ABNORMALITIES

Body Member	Nutrients	Quantity
Bones	Vitamin A	
	Vitamin B complex	
	Pantothenic acid	
	Vitamin C	
	Vitamin D	
	Vitamin E	
	Calcium	
	Magnesium	
	Protein	
	Unsaturated fatty acids	

BRONCHITIS

Bronchitis is an inflammation of the tissues lining the air passage leading to the lungs. Chronic bronchitis can eventually lead to emphysema.

Factors that increase susceptibility to bronchitis are asthma and other respiratory diseases, air pollution, cigarette smoking, fatigue, chilling, and malnutrition. Food allergies may also be a cause.

Symptoms of bronchitis are a slight fever, back and muscle pain, and sore throat. A dry cough is followed by the coughing up of mucus as the inflammation becomes more severe.

Treatment for bronchitis includes rest, adequate fluid intake, and a well-balanced diet high in vitamins A and C. Vitamin A is essential to the health of the lung tissues; vitamin C helps fight infection and promotes healing. If the bronchitis victim is suffering from malnutrition, special attention should be paid to the adequate intake of protein and all other nutrients.

NUTRIENTS THAT MAY BE BENEFICIAL IN TREATMENT OF BRONCHITIS

Body Member	Nutrients	Quantity
Lungs/Respiratory system	Vitamin A	
	Vitamin C	
	Vitamin D	
	Vitamin E	

Body Member	Nutrients	Quantity
	Unsaturated fatty acids	
	Protein	
	Water	

BRUISES

A bruise is an injury that involves the rupture of small blood vessels, causing discoloration of underlying tissues without a break in the overlying skin. Bruises are frequently the result of falling or bumping into objects.

Factors that make one susceptible to bruising are overweight, anemia, and time of menstrual period. Frequent bruising without apparent cause may signal that the materials needed for clotting may not be present in the blood. Leukemia and excessive doses of anticlotting drugs can also cause frequent or large bruises.

Excessive bruising may indicate a lack of vitamin D, a natural blood-clotting agent. Also, vitamin C and bioflavonoid deficiencies may be characterized by a weakening of the small blood vessels, resulting in easier bruising. If the cause of bruising is anemia, there should be an increased intake of iron in the diet. If obesity appears to be a cause of bruising, a well-balanced reducing diet is indicated. Frequent bruising with no apparent cause, or a bruise that applies pressure to a neighboring portion of the body, requires medical attention.

DMSO, applied externally, may prevent the discoloration of bruises. DMSO acts as a scavenger of free radicals that are produced when blood vessels are damaged. The antioxidants; vitamins A, C, E, B_1, B_5, B_6; zinc; and selenium should be taken in conjunction with DMSO.

NUTRIENTS THAT MAY BE BENEFICIAL IN TREATMENT OF BRUISES

Body Member	Nutrients	Quantity
Blood/Circulatory system	Vitamin B complex	
	Folic acid	
	Vitamin C	
	Vitamin D	
	Vitamin K	
	Bioflavonoids	
	Iron	

BRUXISM (TOOTH-GRINDING)

Bruxism usually occurs during sleep and results in teeth that are loosened in their sockets, which causes tooth loss and gum recession. Two University of Alabama doctors believe that bruxism is a nutritional problem that can be helped with increased dosages of calcium and pantothenic acid.

Calcium is effective for treating involuntary movement of muscles, and pantothenic acid is important for maintaining proper motor coordination. Both nutrients are also antistress formulas. Another reported cause of bruxism, as expressed by a Swiss dental scientist, is a change in the central nervous system due to nervous tension or a conflict situation.

NUTRIENTS THAT MAY BE BENEFICIAL IN TREATMENT OF BRUXISM

Body Member	Nutrients	Quantity
General	Vitamin A	
	Vitamin B_1	
	Vitamin B_2	
	Vitamin B_6	
	Niacin	
	Pantothenic acid	
	Vitamin C	
	Vitamin E	
	Calcium	
	Iodine	
	Protein	

BURNS

A burn is a tissue injury caused by heat, electricity, radiation, or chemicals. There are three degrees of burn severity. A first-degree burn appears reddened, a second-degree burn includes blister formation, and a third-degree burn involves destruction of the entire thickness of skin and possibly of the underlying muscle.

Because of tissue destruction, massive losses of body fluids, proteins, sodium, potassium, and nitrogen can occur. Because large amounts of fluids are lost in extensive burns, the possibility of shock exists. Infection is another threat to the burn victim.

Immediate treatment measures for burns include cold applications to reduce pain and swelling and cleansing and covering of the burn to minimize the possibility of bacterial infection. Ointments, salves, or butter should not be applied to burns. They tend to promote infection and prevent circulation of air to the wound by retaining heat within the body. Treatment of chemical burns may include application of an antidote specific to the offending agent.

Diet is very important to burn victims, especially to those with extensive burns. The diet should be high in calories for energy and high in protein for tissue repair. Adequate intake of fluids in proportion to the amount of fluids lost is also essential. Vitamin C may be helpful for healing the wound, and the B vitamins are necessary to meet the body's increased metabolic demands. Intake of vitamin A, necessary for the health of the skin, should be increased, as well as intake of potassium. Some authorities indicate that vitamin E relieves pain and promotes healing in burns.[9]

Dr. Frederick Klenner of Reidsville, North Carolina, recommends that 30 to 100 grams of vitamin C be given intravenously to burn victims until healing has taken place. His studies have also shown that this treatment will supply the tissues with sufficient oxygen to make skin grafting unnecessary and can remove any smoke poisoning in fire victims.

NUTRIENTS THAT MAY BE BENEFICIAL IN TREATMENT OF BURNS

Body Member	Nutrients	Quantity*
Skin	Vitamin A	
	Vitamin B complex	
	Niacin	
	PABA	300 mg after each meal
	Pantothenic acid	
	Vitamin C	1000 mg
	Vitamin D	
	Vitamin E	200 IU after each meal; ointment
	Calcium	
	Iodine	
	Magnesium	
	Unsaturated fatty acids	

[9]Evan Shute, *The Heart and Vitamin E* (London: Shute Foundation for Medical Research, 1963), pp. 96–97.

Body Member / Nutrients	Quantity*
Potassium	
Zinc	
Protein	Up to 400 gm
Sodium	
Water	

*See note, p. 222.

BURSITIS

Bursitis arises from an inflammation of the liquid-filled sac, called a bursa, found within the joints, muscles, tendons, and bones, which helps to promote muscular movement and reduce friction. The affliction is commonly found in the hip or shoulder joints, elbows, or feet and is more commonly known as "frozen shoulder," "tennis elbow," or bunion.

Bursitis may be caused by stretched muscles, shoes that are too tight, injury such as a bump or bruise, or irritation from calcium deposits found in the bursa wall. It may also be the result of metabolic inefficiency caused by stress, which prevents proper absorption and utilization of food that is eaten.

Bursitis symptoms include swelling, tenderness, and agonizing pain in the affected area which frequently limits motion. Treatment involves removing the cause of the injury, clearing up any underlying infection, and possibly, surgically removing calcium deposits. Other measures include rest and immobilization of the affected part.

Vitamin E has also been found to be beneficial in the treatment of bursitis. The need for protein and vitamins A and C increases during infection, and extra amounts of these nutrients are required for bursitis victims.

NUTRIENTS THAT MAY BE BENEFICIAL IN TREATMENT OF BURSITIS

Body Member	Nutrients	Quantity*
Bones/ Muscles/ Joints	Vitamin A	
	Vitamin B complex	
	Vitamin B$_{12}$	1000 mcg daily for first 7–10 days; three times per week for next 2–3

*See note, p. 222.

Body Member	Nutrients	Quantity*
		weeks; one to two times per week for next 2–3 weeks
	Vitamin C	
	Vitamin E	
	Protein	

*See note, p. 222.

CANCER

Cancer cells appear as immature persistently dividing cells that do not fulfill their natural functions and invade surrounding tissue. These cells rob neighboring normal cells of their essential nutrients, causing a severe wasting away of the cancer patient. Cancer cells are capable of migrating and planting themselves in any part of the body, causing abnormal growths or tumors. Cancers are categorized according to the type of tissue from which they originate.

The importance of early detection in treatment of cancer cannot be overemphasized. This is the only chance for successful treatment of the disease. One must be always alert to the American Cancer Society's seven warning signs: unusual bleeding or discharge, appearance of a lump or swelling, hoarseness of cough, indigestion or difficulty in swallowing, change in bowel or bladder habits, a sore that does not heal, or a change in a wart or mole. Symptoms and their severity vary with the type and location of the cancer.

For the treatment of cancerous growths or tumors, surgery, radiation, and certain drugs have proved beneficial. Surgical operations remove the original growth and any secondary ones. Drugs, although unable to completely cure cancer, are used to reduce the growth or to delay the appearance of secondary growths. Radiation is often used to destroy cancer cells and to prevent them from spreading.

The ill side effects from radiation therapy, etc., such as vomiting and diarrhea, can be lessened or prevented by vitamins C, E, and the B complex. It is important to begin taking these vitamins several days before the treatment starts. The psychological stress of cancer greatly increases the need for vitamin C.[10]

[10]Davis, *Let's Get Well*, p. 300.

X-rays and other radiation treatments suppress the immune system and destroy vitamins A, C, E, K, B complex, and UFA; large amounts of vitamin E can protect vitamin A and the UFA. As malignant tissues are being destroyed, harmful by-products are made. The liver is able to neutralize these substances if adequate amounts of vitamins C, E, protein, and the amino acid methionine are present. Vitamin E can prevent radiation burns, relieve pain, and reduce scarring.

In animals, spontaneous cancers, especially of the thyroid, developed on iodine-deficient diets. Iodine deficiency has also been implicated in female breast cancer. Liver damage of any kind increases the susceptibility to cancer.

It is possible many trace minerals are necessary for cancer prevention. Additional amounts of copper given to animals in a laboratory test significantly retarded cancer development. In other studies, the inability to form antibodies and a poor resistance to infection were found to be caused by putrefactive bacteria inside the body. Proper maintenance of the intestinal flora may be a factor in cancer and can be accomplished by generous amounts of yogurt or acidophilus culture.

Further testing of animals show that the vitamins A, C, E, and B_1, the minerals selenium and zinc, and various amino acids have prevented development of cancers. They do this by stimulating the body's immune system and by acting as free radical scavengers. SOD (superoxide dismutase) has also been shown to destroy free radicals. Free radicals are chemicals produced by they body when exposed to harmful substances such as radiation, food and drink contaminants, rancid fats, and air pollution. They damage parts of the human cell, especially DNA and RNA, which in part direct the actions of each cell. Once this process is disturbed, cancer can develop.

It has been well established that persons who smoke or drink have a higher incidence of cancer. A chemical, acetaldehyde, found in cigarette smoke and made in the liver from alcohol, is known to be a carcinogen and a free radical producer. It also destroys cysteine, an antioxidant.

For the terminally ill cancer patient, the specific food needs depend on the location of the tumor. Generally, however, a high-protein, high-calorie diet is necessary to maintain and help restore normal cells. Iron is essential to the diet in order to prevent anemia, which is a frequent complication of cancer.

Vitamin K has been found to protect against certain cancer-causing substances.

NUTRIENTS THAT MAY BE BENEFICIAL IN TREATMENT OF CANCER

Body Member	Nutrients	Quantity*
General	Vitamin A	50,000 IU
	Vitamin B complex	
	Vitamin B_1	500 mg
	Vitamin B_2	100 mg
	Vitamin B_6	300 mg
	Niacin	100–300 mg
	Pangamic acid	50 mg twice daily
	Pantothenic acid	50–400 mg
	Choline	500–1000 mg
	Vitamin C	5–60 gm
	Vitamin D	
	Vitamin E	Up to 1200 IU
	Vitamin K	
	Chromium	
	Iodine	
	Iron	
	Magnesium	
	Molybdenum	
	Phosphorus	
	Potassium	
	Selenium	large doses
	Sulfur	
	Zinc	100 mg
	Protein	
	Unsaturated fatty acids	

*See note, p. 222.

CATARACTS

A leading cause of blindness, a cataract is a condition in which the lens of the eye, that part of the eye which focuses and allows us to see objects both near and far, becomes clouded or opaque. Cataracts may occur at any time in life but are usually associated with the degenerative changes that occur with age. Cataracts in young people are usually congenital but may be caused by a nutritional disorder or inflammatory condition in the eye. There is a high incidence of cataracts among diabetics.

Persons who drink large quantities of milk and do not efficiently utilize the milk sugar, galactose, can develop cataracts because the sugar increases the need for and causes a deficiency of riboflavin.

Stress and an inadequate diet often precipitate cataracts. Drugs and chemicals may also produce the disease. Improper deposition of calcium or cholesterol contributes to cataract formation by slowing circulation to the eyes.

Symptoms of cataracts include painless, progressive blurring and loss of vision, sensitivity to bright light, and the appearance of halos around lights. Surgical removal of the lens is necessary to restore normal vision and prevent blindness.[11]

Research has shown that a reduction of vitamin C and riboflavin in the lens of the eye may contribute to the development of cataracts. High blood sugar levels, as in diabetes, can cause cataract formation. Low levels of calcium in the blood can also cause cataracts. Maintaining an adequate intake of vitamin C, riboflavin, and calcium may be useful in preventing cataract formation.

In experiments, animal cataracts disappeared after the animals were given riboflavin, pantothenic acid, vitamin E, or the essential amino acids.

NUTRIENTS THAT MAY BE BENEFICIAL IN TREATMENT OF CATARACTS

Body Member	Nutrients	Quantity*
Eye	Vitamin A	100,000 IU
	Vitamin B complex	
	Vitamin B_2	
	Pantothenic acid	
	Vitamin C	500–15,000 mg
	Vitamin D	
	Vitamin E	400–600 IU
	Calcium	
	Selenium	
	Zinc	
	Protein	

*See note, p. 222.

[11]David Holvey, *The Merck Manual,* 12th ed. (Rahway, N.J.: Merck and Co., 1972), p. 1015.

CELIAC DISEASE

Celiac disease is an intestinal disorder caused by the intolerance of some individuals to gluten, a protein in wheat, rye, and barley. Ingestion of gluten irritates the intestinal lining, interfering with the absorption of nutrients and water.

It has been found that persons with celiac disease are extremely deficient in vitamin B_6. A lack of this vitamin causes diarrhea, vomiting, gas, and eczema.

It can also be triggered by intestinal infections or parasites and psychological stress. Protein deficiencies that occur on reducing diets or the excessive use of laxatives can alter the intestinal tract to the extent that absorption of gluten is impaired.

Symptoms of celiac disease are weight loss, diarrhea, gas, abdominal pain, and anemia. Malnutrition often accompanies this disorder because of the greatly reduced absorption of nutrients.

Celiac disease may be a factor in causing schizophrenia. The mental symptoms of celiac patients were greatly improved when they were placed on gluten-free diets.

Treatment for celiac disease includes eating a well-balanced, gluten-free diet that is high in calories and proteins and normal in fats. The diet excludes all cereal grains except rice and corn. Common nutrient deficiencies that occur with celiac disease and that should be corrected include deficiencies in calcium, vitamin B complex, and vitamins A, C, D, K, and E. Iron, folic acid, and vitamin B_{12} can be used to correct the anemia that usually accompanies celiac disease.

Adelle Davis believes that celiac patients may have an unusually high requirement for nutrients that are needed for gluten utilization. She recommends that the B vitamins be generously supplied, possibly resulting in the discontinuance of the gluten-free diet.

NUTRIENTS THAT MAY BE BENEFICIAL IN TREATMENT OF CELIAC DISEASE

Body Member	Nutrients	Quantity*
Intestine	Vitamin A	
	Vitamin B complex	
	Vitamin B_6	30 mg; 5 mg for infants
	Vitamin B_{12}	
	Folic acid	
	Vitamin C	
	Vitamin D	
	Vitamin E	
	Vitamin K	
	Calcium	
	Iron	
	Magnesium	
	Potassium	
	Proteins (no gluten)	

*See note, p. 222.

CHICKEN POX

Chicken pox is a highly contagious viral disease in which the chief symptom is generalized skin eruptions. One attack usually protects against the disease for life.

About 24 to 36 hours before the first series of eruptions, the patient may have a headache and a low fever. The rash appears as red bumps containing drops of clear fluid, usually on the face and trunk of the body. The fluid breaks out, forming a crust, and the eruptions continue in cycles for three or four days. Soothing lotions may be applied for relief of itching, and fingernails should be cut short to prevent scratching. The patient should be kept clean and should be frequently bathed with soap and water.

Fevers increase the body's need for calories and vitamins A and C. Extra protein is needed for the repair of tissues. The patient should be isolated for 10 to 14 days to prevent the spread of the infection.

Dr. Frederick Klenner dries up chicken pox with intravenous injections of up to 400 milligrams per kilogram of body weight of vitamin C given two or three times in a 24-hour period.

NUTRIENTS THAT MAY BE BENEFICIAL IN TREATMENT OF CHICKEN POX

Body Member	Nutrients	Quantity
Skin	Vitamin A	
	Vitamin C	
	Protein	

CHOLESTEROL LEVEL, HIGH

Cholesterol is a fatty substance manufactured by the liver. It is found only in animal fat; it is not contained in vegetable fat. Cholesterol is needed to form sex and adrenal hormones, vitamin D, and bile salts. It also has a vital function in the brain and nerves.

Cholesterol is manufactured from dietary saturated fats and refined carbohydrates. In addition, all cells in the body synthesize cholesterol; however, the liver and intestine are the major producers. Fatty tissues also produce a lot. This internally made cholesterol (about 1 to 2 gm daily) can collect in the arteries even in an individual who consumes no cholesterol.

Dietary cholesterol and fasting reduce the amount of cholesterol made by the body; high-fat diets increase the amount made. Saturated fats transport more cholesterol in the bloodstream than do unsaturated fats.

Some researchers believe that when cholesterol levels in the blood become abnormally high, fatty deposits composed of cholesterol and calcium tend to accumulate in the arteries, including those of the heart, increasing the susceptibility to heart attacks. Cholesterol deposits occur mostly in parts of the blood vessels which have been weakened by high blood pressure or undue strain.

Epidemiological studies reveal that the incidence of atherosclerosis is higher in countries where diets are high in saturated fats. However, vegetarians whose diet is low in saturated fats may develop atherosclerosis; but Eskimos, who eat large amounts of saturated fats, seldom develop the disease. This indicates there are other factors besides saturated fat that affect the cholesterol level of the blood, including stress, anxiety, cigarette smoking, overeating, lack of exercise, and high consumption of refined carbohydrates. Some people may not efficiently metabolize saturated fats. Other factors may include high blood pressure, diabetes, and gout.

Choline, vitamin B_{12}, biotin, lecithin, pangamic acid, methionine and possibly inositol are lipotropic substances—substances that must be present to prevent accumulation of fat in the liver. Since the liver regulates cholesterol, these vitamins may be essential. Deficiencies of magnesium, potassium, manganese, zinc, vanadium, chromium, or selenium, or of vitamins C, E, niacin, folic acid, or B_6 may also be significant.[12] Many of these nutrients are necessary for fat utilization.

Cholesterol in the blood must be kept in solution to prevent deposits from forming; lecithin seems to help the bile do this. Lecithin is contained in many fatty foods, but when these fats are hydrogenated, the lecithin is lost. Adequate supplies of unsaturated fatty acids (especially linoleic acid) and vitamin E seem to help control the cholesterol level of the blood and prevent atherosclerosis. Vitamin C aids in preventing the formation and deposition of cholesterol.

Several studies have confirmed the fact that pectin can limit the amount of cholesterol the body absorbs, thereby controlling the level of cholesterol accumulation in the bloodstream. Pectin is found in many fruits and berries, notably apples.

Garlic oil, bran, and yogurt or acidophilus have also proved beneficial.

NUTRIENTS THAT MAY BE BENEFICIAL IN TREATMENT OF HIGH CHOLESTEROL LEVEL

Body Member	Nutrients	Quantity*
Blood	Vitamin B complex	
	Vitamin B_6	
	Vitamin B_{12}	
	Biotin	
	Choline	
	Folic Acid	
	Inositol	
	PABA	
	Niacin	3–6 gm for 4 weeks 150–500 mg daily
	Pantothenic acid	
	Pangamic acid	120–300 mg for 10–30 days
	Vitamin C	500–1500 mg
	Vitamin D	
	Vitamin E	
	UFA	1–2 tbsp
	Bioflavonoids	

*See note, p. 222.

[12]Pfeiffer, *Mental and Elemental Nutrients,* p. 79.

Body Member	Nutrients	Quantity*
	Kelp	
	Lecithin	4–6 tbsp
		1–2 tbsp mainte-nance
	Calcium	
	Chromium	
	Magnesium	500 mg
	Manganese	
	Potassium	
	Selenium	
	Vanadium	
	Zinc	

*See note, p. 222.

CIRRHOSIS OF THE LIVER

Cirrhosis of the liver is a chronic disease characterized by degeneration and hardening of liver cells. Scarring of the liver tissue causes improper functioning and may result from alcoholism, malnutrition, viral hepatitis, or chronic inflammation or obstruction of certain ducts in the liver.

Early signs of the disease include fever, indigestion, diarrhea or constipation, and jaundice. Later symptoms include edema, anemia, and bleeding disorders characterized by the presence of spider-shaped bruises. A deficiency of the B complex and vitamins A, C, and K may also occur.

Optimal nutrition provides the key to recovery from the disease. A high-protein diet (1 gram of protein per kilogram of body weight, or approximately 75 to 100 grams of protein per day) is prescribed to promote regeneration of the liver cells. In the case of coma, however, protein should be restricted. A high-calorie (2500 to 3000 calories per day) and high-carbohydrate (300 to 400 grams per day) diet is needed to increase the storage of glycogen, to ensure that protein is used for regeneration, and to compensate for weight losses caused by fever. If nausea is present frequently, small meals are better tolerated than three large meals.

A common complication of cirrhosis is the failure of the liver to make vitamins available in an active form in the body. For this reason, the diet should be high in the B complex and vitamins A (not in the form of carotene), C, D, and K. If jaundice is present, special attention should be paid to the fat-soluble vitamins, A, D, E, and K, because some kinds of jaundice interfere with the absorption of these nutrients. If edema is present, sodium, which causes the body to retain water, should be restricted. All alcohol should be strictly avoided.

Alcohol greatly reduces the absorption of vitamin B_1 and other nutrients. A deficiency state can result, leading to liver injury despite an adequate diet. A B_1 deficiency produces confusion, memory loss, heart irregularities, and gastrointestinal problems. Damage to the liver from long-term excessive drinking is irreversible; however, further damage can be prevented by abstaining from alcohol, eating a nutritious diet, and taking vitamin and mineral supplements.

NUTRIENTS THAT MAY BE BENEFICIAL IN TREATMENT OF CIRRHOSIS OF THE LIVER

Body Member	Nutrients	Quantity*
Liver	Vitamin A	50,000 to 100,000 IU
	Vitamin B complex	
	Vitamin B_{12}	
	Choline	1–5 gm
	Inositol	
	Pangamic acid	
	Vitamin C	
	Vitamin D	
	Vitamin E	
	Unsaturated fatty acids	
	Vitamin K	
	Magnesium	
	Zinc	
	Carbohydrates	
	Protein	

*See note, p. 222.

COLDS

The common cold is a general inflammation of the mucous membranes of the respiratory passages caused by a variety of viruses. Colds are highly contagious.

On the average, Americans contact two or three colds per year.

The difficulty modern medicine has had in finding a cure for the common cold may lie in the fact that there are so many different types of viruses that cause colds. In addition, each new generation of viruses changes slightly in its chemical makeup. At the start of a cold, the body's immune system produces a chemical called an antibody which attacks the virus, preventing harm to healthy cells. For the body to effectively fight a virus, an antibody that exactly matches the virus must be produced. The body is just not able to produce antibodies that can copy all the slight variations of each new virus. Factors that lower the body's resistance to virus infection are fatigue, overexposure to cold, recent or present infections, allergic reactions, and inhalation of irritating dust or gas.

A small percentage of the population never have colds. It is believed that their body's immune system is high and able to resist infections.

The virus is spread about two days before the symptoms appear. Symptoms include nose and throat irritations, watery eyes, headaches, fever, chills, muscle aches, and temporary loss of smell and taste.

Prevention of colds includes adequate sleep and a well-balanced diet that reinforces the immune system. Treatment includes adequate fluid and protein intake to sustain the losses that occur with fever. Vitamin B$_6$ helps in the production of antibodies that defend the body against infection. Vitamin A is necessary to maintain the health of the mucous membrane of the respiratory passages. Some individuals have found that vitamin D is also helpful in the prevention of colds. UFA (unsaturated fatty acids) reduce the incidence and duration of colds.

Reports on the role of vitamin C in the treatment of the common cold are contradictory. However, many authorities claim that the intake of vitamin C in amounts from 1 to 2 grams daily is effective in preventing a cold.[13] Another source indicates that at the onset of a cold, vitamin C taken in amounts of 600 to 625 milligrams every 3 hours may be successful for treatment.[14] The amount of vitamin C recommended for the prevention and treatment of a cold varies from individual to individual.

[13]Guthrie, *Introductory Nutrition,* p. 225.
[14]"Summer Cold? Vitamin C . . . ," *Prevention,* July 1970, p. 49.

NUTRIENTS THAT MAY BE BENEFICIAL IN TREATMENT OF COMMON COLDS

Body Member	Nutrients	Quantity*
General	Vitamin A	50,000–150,000 IU for 1 month; then reduce to 25,000 IU
	Vitamin B complex	
	Vitamin B$_6$	100 mg
	Vitamin C	600–625 mg every 3 hours first 3 or 4 days, then 375–400 mg daily. Higher doses are also recommended.
	Vitamin D	
	Vitamin E	600 IU
	Unsaturated fatty acids	
	Bioflavonoids	200–600 mg
	Calcium	
	Zinc	
	Protein	
	Water	

*See note, p. 222.

COLITIS

Colitis is a disease in which the lining of part of the colon, or large intestine, is inflamed. There are several types of colitis, all of which are determined by the extent of the inflammation, the amount of the colon involved, and the degree of severity of the colitis symptoms. Enteritis is an inflammation of the small intestine or of the entire intestinal tract. Ileitis is an inflammation of the last section of the small intestine.

Although the cause of the disease is unknown, there is usually a correlation between colitis and depression or anxiety. The degree of a person's emotional stress will often indicate the severity of his colitis.

In early stages, colitis is characterized by abdominal cramps or pain, diarrhea, and the need to eliminate several times daily. These symptoms are accompanied by rectal bleeding as the condition becomes more severe. Instead of being absorbed by the body, water and minerals are rapidly expelled through the lower digestive tract, resulting in a loss of weight and, possibly, dehydration or anemia. Because of this rapid expulsion and decreased absorption of water and nutrients, the entire nutritional status of the colitis patient is in jeopardy.

A therapeutic diet for colitis should be high in protein and UFA (unsaturated fatty acids) to restore lost or worn-down tissues. Foods high in roughage, such as raw fruits and vegetables need not necessarily be avoided. Sometimes milk is not tolerated; therefore a calcium supplement may be necessary. Iron is necessary to deter the development of anemia and vitamin C to aid in the absorption of iron.

NUTRIENTS THAT MAY BE BENEFICIAL IN TREATMENT OF COLITIS

Body Member	Nutrients	Quantity*
Bowel/Intestine/Colon	Vitamin A	
	Vitamin B complex	
	Vitamin B_6	50 mg
	Folic acid	5 mg
	Pantothenic acid	
	Vitamin C	
	Vitamin E	
	Unsaturated fatty acids	
	Calcium	
	Iron	
	Magnesium	
	Phosphorus	
	Potassium	
	Zinc	
	Protein	

*See note, p. 222.

CONJUNCTIVITIS

Conjunctivitis is an inflammation of the mucous membrane that lines the eyelids and covers the white portion of the eye. Symptoms of conjunctivitis include redness, swelling, itching, and pus in the membrane. The condition may be caused by allergy, bacteria, virus, smoke, dust, or chemical irritants.

Deficiency of vitamin A, vitamin B_6, or riboflavin may cause conjunctivitis symptoms. The diet should be adequate in these vitamins to help prevent the condition. Certain forms of conjunctivitis are the result of a calcium deficiency. Vitamin D, magnesium, and phosphorus aid the absorption of calcium.

NUTRIENTS THAT MAY BE BENEFICIAL IN TREATMENT OF CONJUNCTIVITIS

Body Member	Nutrients	Quantity
Eye	Vitamin A	
	Vitamin B complex	
	Vitamin B_2	
	Vitamin B_6	
	Niacin	
	Vitamin C	
	Vitamin D	
	Calcium	
	Magnesium	
	Phosphorus	

CONSTIPATION

Constipation is a disorder causing decreased frequency of bowel movements, resulting in waste matter remaining in the colon and becoming dry and difficult to expel. Constipation may stem from a variety of causes. Insufficient muscle tone in the intestinal or abdominal wall due to a lack of exercise; repeated failure to heed the signal to eliminate; or excessive fatigue, nervousness, anxiety, stress, or excitement may result in constipation. A poor diet or a diet lacking in fluids or roughage can bring about constipation. The continued use of laxatives as a substitute for proper exercise, rest, and diet may result in dependency and merely perpetuate the problem.

The more fiber contained in the diet, from fruits, vegetables and whole grains, the softer and the larger the amount of feces will pass. Foods containing fats may be useful in the treatment of constipation because of their lubricating effect on the mucous walls of the colon. Other foods that may be helpful are garlic (the allicin in garlic stimulates the walls of the intestines), yogurt or acidophilus, and fruits—especially apples, papaya, pineapple, prunes, and figs.

**NUTRIENTS THAT MAY BE BENEFICIAL
IN TREATMENT OF CONSTIPATION**

Body Member	Nutrients	Quantity*
Intestine	Vitamin A	25,000 IU
	Vitamin B complex	
	Vitamin B$_1$	100 mg
	Vitamin B$_6$	
	Choline	500 mg
	Inositol	500 mg
	Niacin	
	Pantothenic acid	
	Vitamin C	1,000 mg
	Vitamin D	
	Vitamin E	
	Unsaturated fatty acids	
	Fiber	
	Calcium	
	Magnesium	
	Potassium	
	Zinc	
	Fats	
	Water	
	Acidophilus	

*See note, p. 222.

CRIB DEATH

Crib death is the number-one killer of children between the ages of one week and one year. Some of the children will show symptoms a day or so before death. These may include coughing, wheezing, vomiting, diarrhea, and poor appetite. They may exhibit restlessness or irritability or they may appear pale and listless. Progressively, the child will experience a bluish skin color, cold hands and feet, and difficulty in breathing. Internally, the lungs and respiratory tract become swollen and inflamed. Water and blood collect in the lungs and the tubes connecting the lungs to the bloodstream become spastic.

Through her own studies, Dr. Joan L. Caddell, a pediatric cardiologist, believes the cause of crib death is a magnesium deficiency. A borderline yet critical deficiency of the mineral in the mother during preg-

nancy, and secondarily in the infant's diet, may precipitate crib death.[15]

Most crib deaths occur between the second and fourth months, the time of most rapid growth. Rapid growth depletes magnesium. A magnesium deficiency also is a factor in the release of histamine. Histamine is a substance that increases the permeability of the capillaries, allowing nutrients and oxygen to leak out and collect in sites such as the lungs.[16]

Dr. Frederick Klenner suggests that adequate daily intake of vitamin C will prevent crib death attributed to suffocation, of which the symptoms may be as slight as congested nasal passages.[17] He has also treated infants of crib syndrome, a less acute condition, with calcium gluconate and massive injections of vitamin C. He attributes crib syndrome to a possible brain trauma at birth. The symptoms are similar to those of a cold. He states that adequate amounts of vitamin C taken by the mother during pregnancy could prevent this condition. Researchers and physicians have also linked the pregnant mother's cigarette smoking and a deficiency of vitamins B$_1$ and E to infant crib death.

**NUTRIENTS THAT MAY BE BENEFICIAL
IN TREATMENT OF CRIB DEATH**

Body Member	Nutrients	Quantity
Lungs/Respiratory system	Vitamin B$_1$	
	Vitamin C	
	Vitamin E	
	Calcium	
	Magnesium	
	Selenium	

CRIME AND DELINQUENCY

Studies from many correctional institutions across the country prove that poor nutrition is directly related to the behavior and personality patterns of offenders in the criminal justice system. Anything that affects

---

[15] Prevention Magazine Staff, *The Encyclopeida of Common Diseases,* p. 382.

[16] Ibid., p. 381.

[17] Roger Williams and Dwight Kalita, eds., *Physicians' Handbook on Orthomolecular Medicine,* p. 51.

the body also affects the brain, and certain centers in the brain control behavior.

Repeated studies have shown that 80 to 85 percent of criminal offenders have hypoglycemia, with the usual symptoms of dizziness, cold sweats, nervousness, and fatigue. Hypoglycemia results from a diet too high in refined carbohydrates and often in caffeine. Sugar consumption in excess can cause behavorial problems such as depression, hyperactivity, and antisocial behavior.

Many offenders have been found to be deficient in vitamin B_1. A lack of this vitamin can result in irritability, anger, and aggressiveness. Refined carbohydrates lack vitamin B_1. The more carbohydrates eaten, the more vitamin B_1 is needed. Unrefined foods contain sufficient B_1 for the body; refined foods do not.

Allergic reactions to particular foods and food additives have also been found to be a factor in criminal behavior. Allergies can cause pressure on certain nerves in the brain, activating aggression. The symptoms may range from mild irritation to severe psychosis.

A change to unrefined foods plus vitamin and mineral supplementation can effectively reduce re-arrests and improve behavior, morale, mood, and self-motivation.

NUTRIENTS THAT MAY BE BENEFICIAL IN TREATMENT OF CRIME AND DELINQUENCY

Body Member	Nutrients	Quantity
General	Vitamin B complex	
	Vitamin B_1	150–300 mg until normal B_1 blood level is reached
	Vitamin B_6	
	Niacin	
	Vitamin C	
	Zinc	

CROUP

Croup encompasses a variety of conditions in which there is a high-pitched cough and difficulty in breathing. Fever may or may not accompany the disorder. Croup usually affects children under the age of five.

Conditions that may bring on the symptoms of croup are virus, diphtheria, a foreign body in the throat, and swelling due to a throat infection.

Croup may vary greatly in severity depending upon its cause. Any underlying infections should be treated, and any obstruction in the throat should be removed. The breathing of warm moist air from a humidifier often brings relief from cough.

Nutritional treatment for croup involves a well-balanced diet high in protein to promote the growth and repair of tissues. If fever is present, the need for vitamins A and C is increased. Increased fluid intake is also essential, especially when croup occurs in very small children or infants.

NUTRIENTS THAT MAY BE BENEFICIAL IN TREATMENT OF CROUP

Body Member	Nutrients	Quantity
Lungs/Respiratory system	Vitamin A	
	Vitamin C	
	Protein	

CYSTIC FIBROSIS

Cystic fibrosis is a hereditary disease affecting certain glands in the body, such as the gallbladder, pancreas, and sweat glands. The disease usually begins during infancy, though symptoms may manifest themselves later in life.

The greatest danger at the onset of the disease is malnutrition due to an underproduction of digestive juices. As a result, all foods, especially fats, are poorly digested and absorbed, and a deficiency in all nutrients, particularly in the fat-soluble vitamins, occurs. In addition, the sweat glands produce an unusually salty perspiration, draining the body of salt and making the patient susceptible to heat exhaustion. The mucous glands in the lungs, which normally aid in moistening the air passages, produce a thick mucus that blocks the passages and promotes the growth of harmful bacteria.

Treatment for the malnutrition that occurs with cystic fibrosis may include medication to compensate for the lack of digestive juices. The recommended diet is 25 percent higher than normal in calories, the majority being in protein, which is easier to digest than fats, and starches, which are nutritionally better than sugars. The intake of fluids and salt should be increased, particularly during hot weather. Because of the poor absorption of nutrients, additional vitamins—A, the B complex, C, D, E, and K—should be included in the diet.

A New Zealand physician, Dr. Robert B. Elliot, who based his treatment on the fact that persons afflicted with cystic fibrosis have abnormally low blood levels of linoleic acid, gave periodic infusions of soy oil, which contains a large amount of linoleic acid, to several groups of children. Oral supplementation was not effective. The results showed at least one of the characteristic biochemical abnormalities of the disease improved in all children tested.

At the University of Pennsylvania School of Medicine and the Wistar Institute, researchers gave 13 children afflicted with cystic fibrosis dietary supplements of corn oil, vitamin E (to prevent oxidation), and pancreatic enzymes. After a year on the diet, all the children gained weight, grew taller, and seemed healthier and happier. In individual cases, the supplements relieved symptoms such as diarrhea, sodium loss, and general problems associated with poor nutrition. Running and walking exercises were also part of the program. Regular exercise helped the patients to keep their lungs clear of mucus and may be a factor in slowing the deterioration of lung function.

NUTRIENTS THAT MAY BE BENEFICIAL IN TREATMENT OF CYSTIC FIBROSIS

Body Member	Nutrients	Quantity*
Glands	Vitamin A	
	Vitamin B complex	
	Vitamin B$_2$	
	Vitamin B$_6$	
	Pantothenic acid	
	Vitamin C	
	Vitamin D	
	Vitamin E	300–1500 mg
	Vitamin K	
	Copper	
	Selenium	
	Sodium (salt)	
	Zinc	
	Protein	
	Lecithin	
	Acidophilus	

*See note, p. 222.

CYSTITIS (BLADDER INFECTION)

Cystitis is an inflammation of the urinary bladder. It is most frequently caused by bacteria that ascend from the urinary opening, but it may also be caused by infected urine sent from the kidneys to the bladder. Cystitis most frequently occurs in females.

Symptoms of cystitis are pain in the lower abdomen and back and frequent, urgent, and painful urination in which the urine may contain blood or pus. Fever may possibly accompany these symptoms. Treatment for cystitis includes increasing the fluid intake and maintaining a well-balanced diet. Vitamin B complex helps to maintain the muscle tone in the gastrointestinal tract and liver. Vitamin C helps ward off and clear up the infection. Vitamin E maintains proper functioning of the liver.

NUTRIENTS THAT MAY BE BENEFICIAL IN TREATMENT OF CYSTITIS

Body Member	Nutrients	Quantity*
Bladder	Vitamin A	25,000–50,000 IU
	Vitamin B complex	
	Vitamin B$_6$	
	Pantothenic acid	
	Vitamin C	5000–10,000 mg
	Vitamin D	
	Vitamin E	600 IU
	Zinc	
	Fluids (water)	

*See note, p. 222.

DANDRUFF

Dandruff may simply be dry flakes that brush off the hair or it may be more serious, a condition called seborrheic dermatitis. This latter type results from sebaceous glands that have become overactive. Emotional traumas, illness, or hormonal imbalance can aggravate and worsen seborrheic dermatitis.

Dandruff can lead to hair loss and possibly baldness. Studies have shown that it results from an inadequate diet and an inefficient carbohydrate metabolism. Sugar often triggers dandruff.

It can substantially be controlled by a diet of unrefined carbohydrates and B vitamin supplements, along with a shampoo designed to control dandruff. The antioxidants, vitamins C and E, and selenium are also helpful.

NUTRIENTS THAT MAY BE BENEFICIAL IN TREATMENT OF DANDRUFF

Body Member	Nutrients	Quantity
Skin/Scalp	Vitamin A	
	Vitamin B complex	
	Vitamin B_6	
	Vitamin C	
	Vitamin E	
	Unsaturated fatty acids	
	Selenium	
	Zinc	

DEPRESSION (SEE "MENTAL ILLNESS")

DERMATITIS

Dermatitis is an inflammatory, usually recurring, skin reaction. It can be caused by contact with an irritating agent that is ingested or found in the environment. Dermatitis may be associated with hereditary allergic tendencies and may be aggravated by emotional stress and fatigue.

One type of dermatitis is eczema. Eczema is a type of skin eruption characterized by tiny blisters that weep and crust. Chronic forms are characterized by scaling, flaking, and eventual thickening and color changes of the skin. Itching is almost always present.

If the irritating agent is a food item, it should be eliminated from the diet. Deficiency of any of the B vitamins can cause dermatitis, and these vitamins should, therefore, be present in the diet in adequate amounts. Linoleic acid (unsaturated fat) and vitamin B_6 have been found to cure infants who have dermatitis caused by a fat-free diet.[18] Vitamin A is also essential for maintaining healthy skin tissue. A protein deficiency can cause chronic eczema.

[18]Krause and Hunscher, *Food, Nutrition and Diet Theapy,* p. 56.

NUTRIENTS THAT MAY BE BENEFICIAL IN TREATMENT OF DERMATITIS

Body Member	Nutrients	Quantity*
Skin	Vitamin A	50,000–75,000 IU for 2 to 3 months; then reduce to 25,000 IU
	Vitamin B complex	
	Vitamin B_2	
	Vitamin B_6	
	Biotin	
	Niacin	300 mg
	Vitamin D	
	Unsaturated fatty acids	
	Potassium	
	Sulfur (ointment form)	
	Zinc	
	Protein	

*See note, p. 222.

DIABETES

Diabetes is a metabolic disorder characterized by decreased ability, or complete inability, of the body to utilize carbohydrates. Carbohydrates are normally broken down within the body in the form of glucose, the body's main energy source. Insulin, a hormone produced in the pancreas, is essential for the conversion of this glucose into energy. In the diabetic there is insufficient production of insulin, and therefore glucose cannot be converted to energy but instead accumulates in the blood, resulting in symptoms ranging in severity from mental confusion to coma.

The major symptoms of diabetes are excessive thirst, frequent urination, increased appetitie, and loss of weight. Other symptoms, though less characteristic of the disease, are muscle cramps, impaired vision, itching of the skin, and poorly healing wounds.

The tendency to develop diabetes frequently seems to be hereditary. Other conditions that contribute to its development are pregnancy, surgery, physical or emotional stress, and obesity. Weight control through proper nutrition is an important factor in the prevention of diabetes.

Methods of medical treatment for diabetes are used in conjunction with a specific diet. In mild cases of the disease, diabetes can be regulated by diet alone. In more severe cases, regulation of the diet is accompanied by oral medication or injections to increase the pancreatic output of insulin. Exercise is a factor in diabetes treatment because it determines insulin needs.

Certain nutrients—vitamins B_1, B_2, B_{12}, pantothenic acid, C, protein, and potassium—and small frequent meals each containing some carbohydrate can stimulate insulin production within the body. The time involved in stimulating natural insulin production will vary with individuals. This will have the same effect as insulin dosage, so symptoms of insulin shock must be watched and dosages reduced as necessary.

Unless a diabetic is overweight, his caloric intake may remain the same but his calorie sources must be regulated. Since the diabetic cannot properly utilize carbohydrates, their intake must be greatly restricted. Concentrated sources of carbohydrates, such as cakes, cookies, and candy, should be avoided. The diabetic may be allowed some fruits and vegetables because their carbohydrate content is not as great as that of sweets. However, depending upon the individual diet, fruits and vegetables that have the greatest carbohydrate content may have to be avoided also. High-complex carbohydrates, such as whole grains and beans, may be permitted. The diabetic diet needs to be higher than normal in protein.

Generally, a well-balanced diet rich in vitamins and minerals is one of the most important factors in the control of diabetes. Some authorities find that the diabetic is unable to convert carotene into vitamin A, while others deny such findings. It is advisable, however, for the diabetic to ingest at least the Recommended Dietary Allowance of vitamin A from a non-carotene source, such as fish-liver oil.[19] Because the diabetic, especially when on insulin therapy, loses vitamin C more readily than does the nondiabetic, daily supplementation of vitamin C is necessary. The minerals zinc, chromium, and manganese have been associated with the treatment of diabetes.

Diabetic retinitis, a hemorrhaging of the eye, is often a complication of diabetes. It is apparently brought on by stress and can be prevented with substantial

[19]Normal Jollife, ed. *Clinical Nutrition,* 2d ed. (New York: Harper Bros., 1962), p. 489.

amounts of protein and the vitamin B complex, B_{12}, C, and pantothenic acid.

NUTRIENTS THAT MAY BE BENEFICIAL IN TREATMENT OF DIABETES

Body Member	Nutrients	Quantity*
Blood/ Circulatory system	Vitamin A	10,000–25,000 IU
	Vitamin B complex	
	Vitamin B_1	10 mg
	Vitamin B_2	10 mg
	Vitamin B_6	500–1000 mg
	Vitamin B_{12}	25 mcg minimum
	Inositol	2–6 gm
	Niacin	Up to 100 mg
	Pantothenic acid	
	Pangamic acid	
	Vitamin C	1000–4000 mg
	Vitamin D	400 IU
	Vitamin E	400–1200 IU
	Unsaturated fatty acids	2 tbsp
	Calcium	
	Chromium	150–200 mcg
	Iron	
	Magnesium	500 mg
	Manganese	Up to 50 mg
	Potassium	300 mg
	Zinc	100–150 mg
	Protein	
	Lecithin	3 tbsp

*See note, p. 222.

DIARRHEA

Diarrhea is a condition causing frequent elimination of stools abnormally watery in nature. The condition is fairly common and can exist alone or as a symptom of other diseases. Diarrhea is accompanied by increased thirst, abdominal cramps and bloating, intestinal rumbling, and loss of appetite.

Because of the decreased appetite associated with diarrhea and rapid expulsion of food through the lower digestive tract, an individual with diarrhea does not properly absorb nutrients and can therefore develop nutrient deficiencies. In addition, the change in consistency of the stool causes the body to lose a great amount of water, a loss that can cause dehydration as well as the loss of minerals and water-soluble vitamins.

The most frequent cause of diarrhea is the presence in the colon of bacteria foreign to the intestinal tract. Bacteria may come from poisoned, poorly refrigerated, undercooked, or partially rancid food. Radiation therapy or antibiotics can destroy friendly bacteria in the intestines. Emotional stress, such as anxiety, is another major cause of diarrhea. Diarrhea can also be brought about by food allergies, the prolonged use of laxatives, or a diet that is overly abundant in roughage, which increases the movement of food through the intestines. Milk, food additives, and unripe fruits are other causes.

The diet of the diarrhea patient need not be low in bulk but rich in protein, carbohydrates, oils, vitamins, and minerals to compensate for the loss of all nutrients that occurs with the condition. Digestive enzymes should be taken with meals to aid digestion. The diet should be supplemented with the water-soluble B-complex vitamins and vitamin C as well as with sodium, magnesium, and potassium, which are bound closely to water and which the body always loses when it becomes dehydrated. An adequate fluid intake is the most essential aspect of the treatment for diarrhea, to replace the water that is lost in the stools, thereby preventing dehydration.

NUTRIENTS THAT MAY BE BENEFICIAL IN TREATMENT OF DIARRHEA

Body Member	Nutrients	Quantity*
Bowel	Vitamin A	25,000 IU
	Vitamin B complex	
	Vitamin B$_1$	200 mg reduced to 50 mg after 2 weeks
	Vitamin B$_2$	10 mg
	Vitamin B$_6$	50–100 mg
	Folic acid	
	Niacin	100 mg three times daily reduced to 100 mg daily after 2 weeks
	Pantothenic acid	100 mg
	Vitamin C	1000–3000 mg

Body Member	Nutrients	Quantity*
Cells	Unsaturated fatty acids	
	Calcium	2 gm
	Chlorine	
	Iron	
	Magnesium	500 mg
	Potassium	
	Sodium	
	Fiber	
	Protein	
	Acidophilus	

*See note, p. 222.

DEAFNESS

Sound travels through three different sections of the ear. The outer ear passes incoming sound waves to the eardrum, located in the middle ear. The middle ear transfers these sounds through three tiny bones that vibrate a fluid in the cochlea, which is located in the inner ear. The cochlea has tiny hairs protruding from its walls that relay the sound vibrations as electrical impulses to the brain. The brain then interprets these impulses as sound.

The quality of hearing is dependent upon the condition of the eighth cranial nerve, located in the inner ear, where sound is transferred to the brain. Conductive deafness and perceptive (or nerve) deafness are two common types of hearing damage.

Conductive deafness is caused by an obstruction that prevents the transmission of sounds to the inner ear. Sounds may still be sent but distinguishing them is difficult. Otosclerosis, wax accumulation (cerumen), boils on the ear canal, and ear drum damage are causes of this type of deafness.

Perceptive deafness occurs in the inner ear and the neural pathways to the brain. Examples of this type of deafness are gradual hearing loss due to aging (presbycusis), congenital problems, Ménière's syndrome, and damage from drugs, excessive noise, or infectious diseases such as mastoiditis. A deficiency of the B vitamins in the diet may be a very important factor in perceptive deafness.

In otosclerosis, the tiny bones in the middle ear become hard and overgrown, interfering with sound transmission. Once the disease occurs, surgery appears to be the only alternative. However, vitamin A (by injection) has been shown to improve this condition in humans; and in animals, a lack of the vitamin to cause it.

Earwax, or cerumen, is a naturally occurring substance, a secretion forming from sebaceous and sweat glands that are located in the outer section of the ear canal. The wax is made up of water, fats, and lecithin, and functions as a lubricant and trap of such particles as bacteria and dust. Its importance should not be underestimated; for example, dust on the eardrum would distort sound, and without lubrication, infections could become serious and even life-threatening. Cerumen is excreted by the motions of the jaws while eating and talking; it eventually falls out during sleep. Symptoms of impacted cerumen include tinnitus (a ringing in the ears), earache, reflex cough, dizziness, an echo sensation, and disturbances in behavior seen especially in mental patients. If the wax is left too long in the ear, it can become a medium for bacterial and fungal growth. Two major causes of impacted earwax are refined foods, which need little chewing action, and air pollution. Excessive pollutants build up on the wax, increasing the susceptibility to infection and causing difficult expulsion.

Presbycusis is associated with the aging process. It is gradual and often not noticed for years. The higher tones are lost first; eventually understanding conversation becomes difficult. Because this disease is one of the results of aging, nutrients involved in slowing the aging process, vitamins B and C for example, are important in its prevention. At a hearing clinic in Alabama, hard-of-hearing patients improved markedly when given yeast and liver (sources of the B complex), vitamin C, and glutamic acid.

Exposure to 85 decibels or more for prolonged times can result in ear damage. Excessive noise contracts the tiny blood vessels in the ear, and repeated exposure progressively increases the time required for them to return to normal, eventually resulting in injury, possibly permanent. Normal conversation registers at 60 decibels, a loud motorcycle at 110, and rock music amplified to its peak registers at 120 decibels. Noise level is too loud if a person needs to shout to be heard by someone standing a few feet away.

Excessive fat in the diet appears to collect in the blood vessels of the ear, causing obstruction. Controlled experiments have been conducted between persons who consumed a high-fat diet and others on a low-fat diet. The patients on the low-fat diet experienced better hearing. In other studies, many patients with hearing loss and ear problem symptoms had elevated cholesterol levels, abnormal glucose tolerance (diabetes), and were overweight. Their hearing was significantly improved by reducing dietary fats and refined foods and losing weight.

NUTRIENTS THAT MAY BE BENEFICIAL IN TREATMENT OF DEAFNESS

Body Member	Nutrients	Quantity
Ear	Vitamin A	
	Vitamin B complex	
	Vitamin C	
	Vitamin E	
	Zinc	
	Glutamic acid	

DIVERTICULITIS

Diverticulitis is the inflammation of the small sacs (diverticula), or out-pouchings, that may be found along the small or large intestine (colon). When empty, the diverticula remain dormant and without complication. However, when food particles get trapped in the sacs and are digested by the bacteria normally present in the colon for this purpose, the digested food particles become stagnant, a situation that leads to inflammation and infection. Diverticulitis may be hereditary, or it may accompany old age, when the muscles of the colon are weakened from years of use.

As diverticulitis becomes more severe, the infection can spread out of the sacs to the rest of the colon and to other organs of the abdomen. In very severe cases, the disease can result in perforation of the wall of the colon, causing severe bleeding for which immediate surgical attention is necessary.

Diverticulitis can manifest itself in a short but severe attack or in a long-term, less severe problem. Symptoms of the disease include cramps and pain in the lower abdomen accompanying bowel movements, abdominal bloating, and the frequent urge to eliminate followed by constipation. If infection ensues, fever can develop.

The most effective prevention for diverticulitis is to avoid constipation. One of the best ways to accomplish this is by a marked increase in fluid intake, which helps to prevent dehydration of intestinal material. A diet high in roughage will prevent further accumulation of food in the diverticula.

Because some of the B vitamins are manufactured by the intestinal bacteria, a deficiency may occur if these bacteria are destroyed by the infection. It is therefore necessary that the diet provide adequate amounts of the B vitamins, especially folic acid. Acidophilus will destroy putrefactive bacteria in the colon and aid in the growth of beneficial bacteria and the manufacture of B vitamins.

NUTRIENTS THAT MAY BE BENEFICIAL IN TREATMENT OF DIVERTICULIS

Body Member	Nutrients	Quantity*
Intestine	Vitamin B complex	
	Folic acid	
	Vitamin C	
	All minerals	
	Fiber	
	Water	
	Acidophilus	

*See note, p. 222.

DIZZINESS/VERTIGO

Dizziness is characterized by a sensation of giddiness, unsteadiness, or lightheadedness. The terms "vertigo" and "dizziness" are often used interchangeably, but true vertigo is a sensation of spinning or a feeling that the floors are sinking or rising. True vertigo is usually accompanied by nausea, vomiting, perspiration, and headache.

Dizziness and vertigo both may be caused by infections of or injuries to the inner ear, which normally helps to maintain the body's sense of balance. A physical injury such as a concussion or skull fracture may injure the inner ear; in this type of injury, dizziness may occur long after the injury is supposedly healed. Brain tumors, anemia, high or low blood pressure, lack of oxygen or glucose in the blood, psychological stress, or nutritional deficiencies may be other causes of vertigo.

A deficiency of vitamin B_6 or niacin may cause dizziness. Including these B-complex vitamins in the diet may prevent and alleviate the sensation.

NUTRIENTS THAT MAY BE BENEFICIAL IN TREATMENT OF DIZZINESS/VERTIGO

Body Member	Nutrients	Quantity
Brain/Nervous system	Vitamin B complex	
	Vitamin B_1	
	Vitamin B_2	
	Vitamin B_6	
	Vitamin B_{12}	
	Choline	
	Inositol	
	Niacin	
	Vitamin C	
	Vitamin E	
	Calcium	

DRUG ABUSE OR DEPENDENCY

The use or abuse of drugs, whether illegal or legal, resulting in dependency over a prolonged period may have several detrimental effects on the general state of health of an individual. Research shows that most drugs have definite side effects, including severe depletion of essential nutrients stored in the body.

Continued use of illegal drugs, such as narcotics, stimulants, barbiturates, and hallucinogens, may result in dependency and severe mental and physical deterioration. Prolonged use may result in damage to the cells, chromosome damage, male sterility, and increased risks of cancer.

Of nearly as great a concern is the problem of indiscriminate use of legal drugs, both prescription and patent medicines. The classic example is the common aspirin tablet. Although many people consider average doses of aspirin completely harmless, researchers invariably discover that when taken in daily doses such as those used to relieve the pain of arthritis, aspirin causes irritation to the stomach lining and varying amounts of internal bleeding. This bleeding may be extensive enough to cause slight anemia. Aspirin-induced irritation of the stomach and accompanying internal bleeding may be very dangerous to ulcer sufferers. There may also be instances of severe allergic reactions to aspirin itself.

Especially dangerous is the habitual use of combinations of drugs such as sleeping pills to go to sleep, stimulants to wake up in the morning, and alcohol to calm down in the midafternoon. A person following such a daily pattern may be just as "hooked" on drugs as any recognized addict. In fact, the taking of such substances as alcohol and sleeping pills (barbiturates) together may so severely depress the body functions as to cause death.

It should be stressed that drugs may produce dietary deficiencies by destroying nutrients, preventing their absorption, and increasing their excretion. Also, many drugs depress the appetite; therefore people who become reliant upon drugs tend to eat inadequately, thus depriving themselves of the essential nutrients necessary for good health. See "Nutrients That Function Together" (p. 108) for information on nutrient antagonists.

Large doses of vitamin C (from 25 to 85 grams daily for 4 days, then reduced to 10 grams) have been successfully used to cure heroin, methadone, and barbiturate addiction. Heroin use increases body acid and causes the depletion of potassium and calcium; sodium bicarbonate to neutralize the acid and potassium bicarbonate and calcium carbonate have eased and eliminated the withdrawal from heroin.

EAR INFECTION

An ear infection can occur in any of the three sections within the ear. The outer ear is that section which is visible, plus the ear canal, a skin-lined tube that ends at a disk known as the eardrum. The middle ear is composed of three small bones that lie on the inward side of the eardrum. These bones connect with the inner ear, which changes sound waves into nerve impulses and sends them to the brain.

Infection in the outer ear is usually caused by swimming in contaminated water or by damage to the wall of the ear canal. A symptom of the infection is severe pain, possibly accompanied by fever.

Infection in the middle ear is most frequently due to the spread of bacteria to the ear from infection in the nose and throat. Symptoms include earache, a

feeling of fullness in the ear, diminished hearing, and fever.

Infection in the inner ear usually arises from meningitis or from the spread of a middle-ear infection. Symptoms include loss of hearing, dizziness, nausea, vomiting, and fever. Severe ear infections may result in permanent scarring and partial or total loss of hearing.

Medical treatment for ear infection involves rest, warmth applied to the ear, antibiotics, and surgical draining of the infected area. Nutritionally, the body's needs for vitamins A and C are increased during a fever. A well-balanced diet adequate in protein is necessary to help the body fight infection and repair damaged tissue.

**NUTRIENTS THAT MAY BE BENEFICIAL
IN TREATMENT OF EAR INFECTION**

Body Member	Nutrients	Quantity*
Ear	Vitamin A	50,000 IU
	Vitamin B complex	
	Vitamin C	
	Protein	
	Acidophilus	

*See note, p. 222.

ECZEMA

Eczema is a skin condition characterized by inflammatory itching and the formation of scales. Sometimes eczema is related to an allergic reaction. Vitamins A and C together with the B-complex vitamins are helpful in the prevention and healing of eczema.

**NUTRIENTS THAT MAY BE BENEFICIAL
IN TREATMENT OF ECZEMA**

Body Member	Nutrients	Quantity*
Skin	Vitamin A	50,000–75,000 IU for 2 to 3 months; 25,000 IU for next few months if condition does not clear up
	Vitamin B complex	

*See note, p. 222.

Body Member	Nutrients	Quantity*
	Vitamin B$_2$	15 mg
	Vitamin B$_6$	25–50 mg and mixed in ointment
	Biotin	
	Choline	
	Inositol	
	PABA	
	Vitamin C	Up to 1,000 mg
	Vitamin D	800 IU
	Unsaturated fatty acids	1–3 tbsp
	Magnesium	
	Sulfur	Ointment
	Zinc	
	Primrose oil	

*See note, p. 222.

EDEMA (FLUID RETENTION)

Edema is a condition in which excess fluid is retained by the body, either localized in one area or generalized throughout the body. This retention of fluids appears as swelling. Swelling is most often seen in the hands, in the feet, or around the eyes, but it may be located in any area of the body.

Disorders that can cause edema are poor kidney functioning, congestive heart failure, protein or thiamine deficiency, varicose veins, phlebitis, or sodium retention. Other factors that may cause edema are standing for long periods of time, pregnancy, premenstrual tension, the use of oral contraceptives, injury to an area of the body (such as a sprain), or allergic reactions (such as an insect bite). Edema is often indicative of adrenal exhaustion.

If edema is the result of protein or thiamine deficiency, correction of the deficiency is essential. Sodium, as found in table salt, is often restricted in diets of individuals who are prone to edema, because excess sodium causes the body to retain water. Individuals who are prone to edema should try to promote good circulation by elevating the legs while at rest, exercising regularly, avoiding restrictive clothing, and refraining from crossing the legs.

An increase in vitamin B$_6$ intake reduces fluid retention. Diets sufficient in pantothenic acid, calcium, and vitamin D increase salt excretion; whereas a high-carbohydrate diet retains salt and water in the tissues.

NUTRIENTS THAT MAY BE BENEFICIAL IN TREATMENT OF EDEMA

Body Member	Nutrients	Quantity*
General	Vitamin B complex	
	Vitamin B$_1$	
	Vitamin B$_6$	50–200 mg
	Pantothenic acid	
	Vitamin C	2000–5000 mg
	Vitamin D	
	Vitamin E	
	Calcium	
	Copper	
	Potassium	
	Protein	
	Low sodium	

*See note, p. 222.

EMPHYSEMA

Emphysema is characterized by abnormal swelling and destruction of the tiny air sacs of the lungs. These sacs become thin and stretch, thus losing their elasticity. This results in an accumulation of used air in the lungs and leads to a decreased ability to utilize fresh air.

Factors that may contribute to the onset of emphysema are exposure to air pollution, various dusts, cigarette smoking, bronchitis, asthma, or other respiratory diseases. Symptoms of the condition include wheezing, shortness of breath and difficulty in breathing, and coughing often accompanied by mucus. Weight loss occurs as the condition progresses, and the victim may develop a characteristic "barrel chest."

Vitamins A and C provide some protection against emphysema by helping to maintain healthy tissues in the respiratory passage. The vitamin B complex and protein are necessary to strengthen the deteriorating tissue. Since the emphysema victim suffers from a lack of oxygen, many authorities suggest that vitamin E may be beneficial. Vitamin E also acts as an antioxidant, preventing the oxidation of vitamin A and the unsaturated fatty acids.

**NUTRIENTS THAT MAY BE BENEFICIAL
IN TREATMENT OF EMPHYSEMA**

Body Member	Nutrients	Quantity*
Lungs/ Respiratory system	Vitamin A	50,000 IU
	Vitamin B complex	
	Folic acid	
	Pangamic acid	50 mg three times daily
	Vitamin C	3000–5000 mg
	Vitamin D	
	Vitamin E	Up to 1600 IU
	Protein	

*See note, p. 222.

ENVIRONMENTAL POLLUTION

Our bodies are being continually exposed to pollutants—pollutants in the food we eat, the water we drink, and the air we breathe. The human system has evolved metabolic processes that can effectively assimilate toxins that are injested periodically. However, when chronic or continual exposure occurs or when new substances are encountered that the system cannot detoxify, adverse reactions can manifest. Chronic effects are muted, often invisible, and not immediately experienced. They can result in cancer that may be latent for 10 to 30 years; metabolic and genetic changes that affect growth, health, behavior, and resistance to disease; teratogenicity (formation of birth defects), following the translocation of an agent across the placental membrane to the fetus; or premature death from a delayed response to a cumulative toxin.

Certain nutrients are particularly effective in lessening the adverse effects of many pollutants. Protection from ozone, an oxidizing chemical found in city air and green countrysides, can be obtained from vitamins A, E, and PABA.

Lead is found in the air, in dust particles, and in drinking water from lead water pipes. Lead suppresses the body's immune system and interferes with the actions of the free radical scavengers. Vitamin C removes lead from bone and the brain. Experiments have shown that susceptibility to lead accumulation in the body correlates with the nutritional status of the individual. In animals, lead absorption is greatly diminished when dietary calcium is adequate.

Polynuclear aromatic hydrocarbons (PAH) are carcinogenic compounds that are formed from the burning of organic substances such as wood, coal, oil, and tobacco. The antioxidants—vitamins B_1, C, and E, calcium pantothenic, cysteine (an amino acid), selenium, and zinc—protect the body from damage by these hydrocarbons.

Radioactive metals that are released from coal-burning power plants as fly ash concentrate in the bones and remain for life, creating free radicals in the body. Free radical scavengers such as vitamins A, C, E, and the enzyme superoxide dismutase (SOD) can offer protection. Strontium 90 is a product of nuclear reactions. Chemically resembling calcium, it can replace the mineral in the body if sufficient calcium is not present, thereby releasing radiation throughout the body. Strontium 90 also inhibits certain actions of vitamin D.

Cigarette smoke prevents the cilia, hairlike projections, from expelling pollutants out of the lungs. Smoke adversely affects the immune system. The nonsmoker who breathes in the smoke is an involuntary victim of this pollutant. Nutrients that build up the immune system and protect against free radical reactions such as vitamins A, C, and E and the minerals selenium and zinc, can help ward off some of the deleterious effects of cigarette smoke.

Carbon monoxide is a component of cigarette smoke as well as of the air in traffic areas. This chemical inhibits the oxygen-carrying capacity of the blood to the brain. Carbon monoxide poisoning is not readily diagnosed. Symptoms are headache, dizziness, irritability, nausea, and decreased mental alertness; loss of consciousness and death result from excessive doses. The pollutant has the same density as air and therefore stays at the surface level of city streets. Heavy exercise near city streets and eating at sidewalk restaurants can subject an individual to added levels. A high-protein diet including vitamin E and the sulfur-containing amino acids such as cysteine, can effectively reduce the toxicity of carbon monoxide.

Cadmium, found in refined foods, coffee, tea, cigarette smoke, and the air as a result of automobile exhaust, can cause hypertension and heart disease. The metal depletes the body of zinc and iron. Chlorine, used as a water disinfectant, is an oxidizing agent and destroys vitamins C and E. Hexavalent chromium, an air, water, and cigarette smoke pollutant, produces gastrointestinal hemorrhage and possibly cancer. Vitamin C is able to convert this toxic form of chromium into the innocuous form, trivalent chromium. Copper is found in drinking water as a result of industrial waste leachate and corroded plumbing. It is also sometimes added to the water supply for algae control. Excessive copper causes irritation of the gastrointestinal tract and mental disorders; zinc function is impaired; and molybdenum, manganese, and magnesium are depleted. Vitamin C aids in the stabilization of the trace metals.

Nitrates and nitrites, used to prevent bacterial growth in meat, can combine with amines, forming carcinogenic nitrosamines. Vitamin C in adequate doses can prevent this transformation.

Selenium and vitamin C effectively protect against mercury poisoning.

NUTRIENTS THAT MAY BE BENEFICIAL IN TREATMENT OF ENVIRONMENTAL POLLUTION

Body Member	Nutrients	Quantity
General	Vitamin A	
	Vitamin B complex	
	Vitamin B$_1$	
	Vitamin B$_6$	
	Niacin	
	PABA	
	Pantothenic acid	
	Vitamin C	
	Vitamin E	
	Calcium	
	Selenium	
	Zinc	
	Protein	
	SOD	

EPILEPSY

Epilepsy is a disease characterized by seizures. There are two forms of seizures. A sensory seizure involves only a change in sensation or a loss of consciousness, while a convulsive seizure (convulsion) involves abnormal muscular behavior. Epileptic seizures are caused by an electrical disturbance in the nerve cells in one section of the brain and may be the result of such factors as head injury or infection, rabies, tetanus, meningitis, rickets, lead poisoning, malnutrition, hypoglycemia, or fever.

Epilepsy occurs in both sexes and at all ages. An individual may experience only one seizure in his lifetime or several seizures per day. Factors that may precipitate a seizure are fatigue, overeating or overdrinking, emotional tension or excitement, fever, new environmental stresses, or menstruation.

The epileptic should maintain a well-balanced diet and should avoid taking in excessive amounts of food or fluid at one time, because these may bring on an attack. Alcoholic beverages should also be avoided. Regular exercise and rest should be encouraged. If the proper nutrients are given, anticonvulsant drugs can often be discontinued.

Dr. Yukio Tanaka of St. Mary's Hospital in Montreal, Canada, through recent research has demonstrated a link between manganese deficiency and convulsions in humans. He also states that pregnant women with a deficiency of manganese may give birth to epileptic children. Pregnant rats maintained on a low-manganese diet delivered young with poorly coordinated movements and a susceptibility to convulsions.

Excellent results have been obtained by the administration of vitamin B$_6$. If there are no results from this vitamin, its poor absorption may be the reason. When large doses of B$_6$ are given alone, the other B vitamins should accompany it, especially vitamins B$_2$ and pantothenic acid, so further harm is not done. A lack of vitamin B$_6$ and magnesium is closely associated with convulsions, which may often be prevented by an adequate supply of these nutrients in the diet. Sensitivity to noise, irritability, twitching, and perhaps bed-wetting and tremors are early warning signs of epilepsy.

NUTRIENTS THAT MAY BE BENEFICIAL IN TREATMENT OF EPILEPSY

Body Member	Nutrients	Quantity*
Brain/ Nervous system	Vitamin A	10,000 IU
	Vitamin B complex	
	Vitamin B$_6$	100 mg; under doctor's supervision, up to 300 mg

*See note, p. 222.

Body Member	Nutrients	Quantity*
	Vitamin B$_{12}$	25 mcg
	Folic acid	0.5 mg
	Niacin	50 mg
	Pangamic acid	50 mg twice daily
	Pantothenic acid	50 mg twice daily
	Vitamin C	2000 mg
	Vitamin D	1000 IU
	Vitamin E	Begin dosage at 300 IU; increase up to 2000 IU
	Calcium	1000 mg
	Magnesium	800 mg; 500 mg for children
	Manganese	

*See note, p. 222.

EYE DISORDERS

Many eye defects or abnormalities can be traced to faulty nutrition; and many could be prevented. The good health of the mother during pregnancy is essential so that the fetus is properly fed with all nutrients. Other factors that may cause eye problems are tooth infections (because of common nerves and blood vessels) and oral contraceptives. One of the side effects of the pill is the possible formation of blood clots that occur most often in small blood vessels such as those found in the eye. Vitamins A, B complex, C, and E and protein are especially important for good eye health.

A lack of vitamin A, even a slight deficiency, can cause easy tiring of the eyes, sensitivity to light variations, dry eyelids, susceptibility to eye infections, and possible ulcerations and irreversible blindness.

Insufficient B-complex vitamins results in paralyzed eye muscles, itching, burning, light sensitivity, bloodshot eyes, and watering eyes. Vitamin B$_2$, specifically, has corrected eye symptoms such as color disturbance, inability to see part of an image or printed page, halos around lights or objects, and spots floating in front of the eyes.

Vitamin C and rutin are necessary to prevent or clear up infections. They also help prevent capillary fragility and tissue hemorrhaging; in addition, vitamins

B$_2$, niacin, and E may be beneficial for retinal hemorrhage.

Studies have shown that vitamin E can improve eyesight. Protruding eyes are a sign of vitamin E deficiency. Supplements of vitamin E have resulted in decreased severity and duration in the acute stage of retrolental fibroplasia. In combination with vitamins A or C, vitamin E may relieve cases of eye conditions that do not respond to any single vitamin. Arteriosclerosis of the eye has been reversed with the use of vitamins C and E.[20] A deficiency of vitamin E is possibly a factor in detached retina. Use of vitamin E has also relieved weak eye muscles, crossed eyes, blurred vision, and double vision; taking the B complex may also be helpful.

Sufficient protein, essential for the health of the lens, is necessary for healing and preventing infections, retinitis, and myopia.

Amblyopia is a dimness of sight. Vitamin B$_1$ is used to correct it.

Bitot's spots are characterized by white, foamy, elevated, and sharply outlined patches on the white of the eyes, caused by a deficiency of vitamin A and protein.

Corneal ulcers can result in scar tissue, causing permanent damage if not properly treated. They may be healed by vitamins B$_2$, B$_6$, pantothenic acid, and C, and protein.

Eyestrain occurs when the eyes have been abused by using them excessively in improper light. Too little light, glaring light and reflections, shadows on work areas, and flickering light such as that from some fluorescent tubes cause the eyes to make numerous unnecessary adjustments that may lead to eyestrain. Eyestrain may also be a result of uncorrected eyesight; eyes should be checked regularly by an eye specialist for any corrections or adjustments that should be made. Frequent relaxation of the eyes, especially by changing the range of focus by looking up and away from your work toward a distant object, may alleviate strain caused by improper light and headaches caused by nervous tension. Adequate intake of the vitamins necessary for eye health is helpful.

Nearsightedness often results from stress. Tension can appear when there is an undersupply or poor absorption of calcium. Adolescents are particularly sus-

[20]Shute, *Health Preserver*, p. 91.

ceptible to this eye disorder because of the stress of growth, allergies, and often an inadequate diet. Symptoms of nearsightedness are eyestrain, squinting, dizziness, fatigue, headaches, and possibly low blood pressure. The disorder may be prevented or alleviated with vitamins B_2, C, D, E, and pantothenic acid, calcium, protein, and the unsaturated fatty acids.

Night blindness is the inability to see well in dim or dark light. The major cause of night blindness is deficiency of vitamin A. Vitamin A is necessary for the formation of visual purple, the substance in the eyes which enables them to adjust from bright light to darkness. Other causes of night blindness are fatigue, emotional disturbances, or hereditary factors. Adequate intake of vitamin A will protect against night blindness. Riboflavin, niacin, thiamine, and zinc have been reported to relieve night blindness when vitamin A has not produced a response, and attention should therefore be paid to ensure their adequate intake.[21]

Retinitis pigmentosa is a gradual degeneration of the retina, resulting in blindness. The early stages are characterized by night blindness and other vitamin A–deficient disorders. It appears that persons with this disorder absorb vitamin A very poorly. Improvement has been accomplished by vitamin A injections and by water-based vitamin A, unsaturated fatty acids, bile tablets, lecithin, and vitamin E, all taken daily.

**NUTRIENTS THAT MAY BE BENEFICIAL
IN TREATMENT OF EYE DISORDERS**

Body Member	Nutrients	Quantity
Eye	Vitamin A	
	Vitamin B complex	
	Vitamin B_1	
	Vitamin B_2	
	Vitamin B_6	
	Niacin	
	Pantothenic acid	
	Vitamin C	
	Bioflavonoids	
	Vitamin D	
	Vitamin E	
	Calcium	
	Magnesium	

[21]Krause and Hunscher, *Food, Nutrition and Diet Therapy,* p. 497.

Body Member	Nutrients	Quantity
	Zinc	
	Protein	
	Lecithin	
	Unsaturated fatty acids	

FATIGUE

Fatigue is a feeling of physical and mental weariness which may be caused by a variety of conditions, such as anemia, physical exertion, nutrient deficiency, weight loss, obesity, boredom or emotional tension, or almost any disease process. In addition to a feeling of weariness, symptoms of fatigue include headache, backache, irritability, and indigestion.

Adequate rest, exercise, and a well-balanced diet can prevent fatigue. Reducing to a normal weight is necessary when overweight is present.

A mild deficiency of magnesium can result in chronic fatigue. A diet insufficient in potassium causes muscular weakness, irritability, and a tired feeling. Deficiencies of the vitamin B complex, vitamins C and D, or iron may cause fatigue and therefore should be corrected.

**NUTRIENTS THAT MAY BE BENEFICIAL
IN TREATMENT OF FATIGUE**

Body Member	Nutrients	Quantity
General	Vitamin A	
	Vitamin B complex	
	Folic acid	
	Vitamin C	
	Vitamin D	
	Iron	
	Magnesium	
	Manganese	
	Potassium	
	Fiber	

FEVER

Fever is the elevation of body temperature above normal. Normal temperature varies from individual to individual, although normal is generally considered to be within the range of 97° to 99°F. When the body temperature is raised not more than 5°, the rise does not completely interfere with bodily functions. However, when fever reaches 106°F, convulsions are common, and if fever should reach 108°F, irreversible brain damage frequently results.

Fever accompanies a wide variety of diseases ranging from mild to severe and can be considered a warning that something is wrong within the body. Symptoms associated with fever include flushed face, headache, nausea, body aches, little or no appetite, and occasionally, diarrhea or vomiting. The skin may be either hot and dry or warm to the touch with some degree of perspiring. Perspiration is the natural result of the body's attempt to lower its temperature.

Because fever increases the body's use of energy, the caloric needs are greatly increased and intake should be adjusted accordingly. Additional protein is needed to replace and rebuild the damaged body tissue and to form antibodies, substances manufactured by the body to fight infection. A high fluid intake is necessary to compensate for the loss that occurs with fever. Sodium and potassium are lost when fluid is lost; therefore their replacement is also necessary during fever. The increased energy expenditure that occurs during fever increases metabolism; because vitamin A, the B complex, and vitamin C are involved in the process of metabolism, deficiencies of these nutrients may arise also. The vitamin B complex especially should be increased during an extended fever since these vitamins may stimulate the appetite. Additional calcium may also be required because of its decreased absorption during fever.

NUTRIENTS THAT MAY BE BENEFICIAL IN TREATMENT OF FEVER

Body Member	Nutrients	Quantity
General/Head	Vitamin A	
	Vitamin B complex	
	Vitamin B$_1$	
	Vitamin C	
	Vitamin D	
	Calcium	
	Phosphorus	
	Potassium	
	Sodium	
	Protein	

FLATULENCE (INTESTINAL GAS)

Flatulence is the most common digestive disturbance. Most people have some gas; however, if the gas begins to cause discomfort, it may be an indication of a more complex problem.

Two causes of flatulence are swallowed air and gases liberated by putrefactive bacteria that are living on undigested food. Both often occur simultaneously. Excessive swallowing of air can occur while eating or drinking, eating too fast, or eating when anxious or upset. The air passes into the stomach and becomes trapped in the intestines where it expands and stretches nerve endings, causing discomfort. Eating too much food overwhelms the digestive enzymes. The undigested food becomes a breeding ground for putrefactive bacteria which form gas. Efficient digestion depends upon hydrochloric acid, bile, and other digestive secretions and enzymes.

Other causes of flatulence are milk products (because of a deficiency of lactase, an enzyme necessary for lactose absorption), beans (because several of their sugars cannot be split by intestinal enzymes), and certain vegetables and fruits such as cucumbers, cabbage, and apples; whole grains may also be a problem for some people. The high fiber in these foods remains undigested, fermenting in the intestine. Fried foods and the concentrated sugars of dried fruits can cause gas. (The sugars can be diluted by boiling or soaking the dried fruits.) If no reason can be found for digestive disturbances, psychological problems may be the factor.

Pantothenic acid has been shown to relieve intestinal gas and distension when there is no physical cause. The B vitamin aids in bowel motility and efficient digestion. Without pantothenic acid, acetylcholine cannot be produced. This chemical transmits messages to nerves that control the motor and secretory activities of the intestine. Gas pains were relieved in postoperative patients and prevented in others when they were given 250 mg of pantothenic acid daily.

Fermented foods such as yogurt and buttermilk aid in the digestion of high-fiber and other foods by increasing friendly bacteria in the colon. They are also well tolerated by persons who have a lactase deficiency. Other foods that may be helpful are lemon juice and cider vinegar. Carminative herbs stimulate digestion by increasing gastric juices, decreasing the amount of putrefactive bacteria, and stimulating intestinal motility. These include garlic, anise, fennel, and caraway. Exercise stimulates intestinal peristalsis and helps break down large gas bubbles.

**NUTRIENTS THAT MAY BE BENEFICIAL
IN TREATMENT OF FLATULENCE**

Body Member	Nutrients	Quantity
Intestine/Stomach	Vitamin B complex	
	Pantothenic acid	
	Digestive enzymes	
	Hydrochloric acid	
	Bile	
	Acidophilus	

FLU

The term "flu" can refer to two different conditions. Stomach flu, or gastroenteritis, is the inflammation of the lining of the stomach. The inflammation has a variety of causes, such as food poisoning, certain viruses, alcohol intoxication, sensitivity to drugs, and allergies. Influenza, also called the flu, is an acute viral infection of the respiratory tract. It is highly contagious and easily spread by sneezing and coughing.

Symptoms of gastroenteritis include diarrhea, vomiting, possible fever, chills, and abdominal cramps that vary in severity, but recovery is usually within one or two days. Treatment for stomach flu includes bed rest and abstention from food until the stomach can tolerate it. A regular well-balanced diet should then be introduced as soon as possible. Repeated vomiting and diarrhea can cause potassium and fluid loss, which should be corrected as soon as possible. If fever is present, intake of vitamins A and C should be increased.

Symptoms of influenza include chills, high fever, sore throat, headache, abdominal pain, hoarseness, cough, enlarged lymph nodes, aching of the back and limbs, and frequent vomiting and diarrhea. Serious complications, such as pneumonia, sinus infections, and ear infections, can develop.

Influenza vaccines are available which help the body become immune to the virus. Many doctors recommend that elderly persons, pregnant women, and persons with heart, kidney, or lung disease have these vaccinations. The protection from respiratory infection is greatly enhanced when vitamin C is taken along with the vaccine.

There is no specific treatment for influenza other than to treat its symptoms and try to prevent complications. The fever that usually accompanies influenza requires additional calories in several small feedings and additonal vitamin B complex to metabolize these calories. Protein is neded for repair of tissue destroyed by fever. Infections accompanied by fever also increase the need for vitamin A and C. Vitamin A is especially important in influenza for the health of the lining of the throat. Increased fluid intake is also important in the event of fever. Antibodies depend on adequate dietary iron for their production process.

Russian pharmacologists are using garlic oil as an antibiotic against flu. Studies have shown that the allicin in garlic destroys harmful bacteria in the body without interfering with the body's natural bacteria. Use of garlic products that have the allicin removed may not be effective.

**NUTRIENTS THAT MAY BE BENEFICIAL IN
TREATMENT OF FLU**

Body Member	Nutrients	Quantity*
Lungs/Respiratory tract	Vitamin A	
	Vitamin B complex	
	Vitamin B_1	50–200 mg
	Vitamin B_2	10 mg
	Vitamin B_6	50–100 mg
	Vitamin C	300 mg–3 gm
	Niacin	50–100 mg
	Pantothenic acid	25–300 mg
	Potassium	
	Protein	

*See note, p. 222.

FRACTURE (BROKEN BONE)

A fracture is any break in a bone. When the bone breaks but the skin remains intact, the fracture is called "closed" or "simple." When the bone breaks through the skin, an opening for bacteria is created and the fracture is called "open" or "compound."

Most fractures occur as the result of an accident, but some occur because of tumors, osteoporosis, or deficiencies of vitamin D or calcium. Fracture symptoms include limb deformities, limited limb functioning, shortening of the limb in fractures of long bones, pain, a grating sensation if the broken bone ends rub against each other, and swelling and discoloration of the skin overlying the fracture area.

First aid treatment for fractures should include covering any wound and immobilizing or splinting the broken part in the position it was found. Medical treatment involves replacing the bone pieces into their normal position.

In the healing process, a bridge of tissue composed largely of protein fibers grows across the ends of the broken bones. Calcium and phosphorus then deposit among these protein fibers to form a new bone. The diet must therefore be high in protein and adequate in calcium and phosphorus. However, calcium intake should not be unusually high because a high calcium intake may promote kidney stone formation during the immobile period while the cast is on. Vitamin D intake must be adequate because it is essential for the absorption of calcium and phosphorus. Potassium is required for cell formation, vitamin C is necessary for the maintenance and development of bones, and vitamin A helps to increase the rate of bone growth. The diet should be high in calories to provide the energy necessary for new bone cell formation.

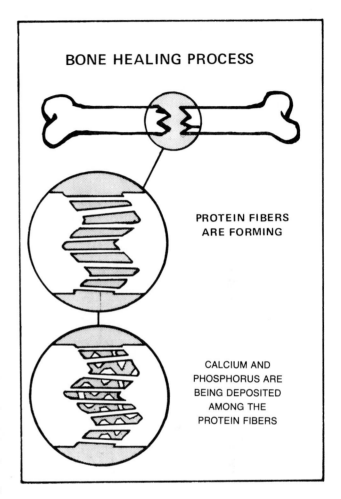

BONE HEALING PROCESS

PROTEIN FIBERS ARE FORMING

CALCIUM AND PHOSPHORUS ARE BEING DEPOSITED AMONG THE PROTEIN FIBERS

NUTRIENTS THAT MAY BE BENEFICIAL IN TREATMENT OF FRACTURE

Body Member	Nutrients	Quantity*
Bones	Vitamin A	
	Pantothenic acid	
	Vitamin C	
	Vitamin D	
	Calcium	
	Magnesium	500 mg
	Phosphorus	
	Potassium	
	Protein	160 gm
	Silicon	

*See note, p. 222.

GALLBLADDER DISORDERS

The gallbladder is a small pear-shaped sack that hangs between the lobes of the liver and contains bile. Bile is necessary for the digestion of fats. As fat-containing foods enter the small intestine, the gallbladder empties its bile, and simultaneously the liver begins to produce more bile.

Too little protein or too much refined carbohydrate in the diet prevents adequate bile production. Consequently fats remain in large undigested particles and the fat-soluble vitamins, A, D, E, and K, are left unabsorbed. Part of the undigested fats combine with calcium and iron, preventing their absorption and creating hard stools, resulting in constipation. Eventually this condition can cause anemia and porous, easily fractured bones. Undigested fats also melt and coat protein and carbohydrate foods, preventing them from enzyme digestion and absorption. Intestinal bacteria thrive on all the undigested food and cause the release of gas in the intestines.

An inflamed gallbladder can be caused by drugs, chemicals, or bacteria. The liver should be supplied with complete proteins and the B, C, and E vitamins to aid detoxification.

A diet supplying sufficient B vitamins aids the emptying of the gallbladder. Though a low-fat diet may be temporarily adhered to before and after surgery, such a diet should generally be avoided by persons with gallbladder diseases because it does not supply sufficient amounts of the necessary nutrients, which could result in other serious deficiency states.

NUTRIENTS THAT MAY BE BENEFICIAL IN TREATMENT OF GALLBLADDER DISORDERS

Body Member	Nutrients	Quantity
Gallbladder	Vitamin A	
	Vitamin B complex	
	Vitamin C	
	Vitamin D	
	Vitamin E	
	Lecithin	
	Bile	
	Acidophilus	

GALLSTONES

Gallstones develop when deposits of cholesterol or calcium combine with bile. Bile is a secretion produced by the liver to emulsify fats so that they can be digested. Most of the bile manufactured by the liver is stored in the gallbladder until the small intestine calls for it when fat has been ingested. However, some bile travels directly from the liver to the small intestine. Gallstones may form in the passages between liver and gallbladder, between liver and intestine, or in the gallbladder itself. Gallstones are more frequently found in diabetics, obese persons, elderly people, and females, especially those who have had children.

Gallstone formation begins to appear when cholesterol crystalizes out of solution and forms stones. Nearly half of all gallstone patients are without symptoms. It is when a stone obstructs any of the bile passages that symptoms occur. These symptoms characteristically include nausea, vomiting, and severe right upper abdominal pain that may radiate to the right shoulder or back. The symptoms commonly occur a few hours after eating a heavy meal of fatty or fried foods. If the stone totally obstructs one of the bile passages, jaundice (a yellowish cast to the skin and eyeballs), dark urine, clay-colored stools, and itching of the skin may also occur.

Gallstones can be prevented and sometimes dissolved by reducing saturated fats and excess carbohydrates in the diet (carbohydrates in excess change into saturated fats), and by taking adequate amounts of the vitamins A, B complex, and E. Chenodeoxycholic acid, a substance particularly abundant in goose liver and goose bile, has been used medically to dissolve gallstones.

A diet deficient in vitamin C and high in cholesterol has been shown to cause the development of gallstones. The vitamin is necessary for the conversion of cholesterol into bile acids.

Lecithin reduces cholesterol levels; the B vitamins increase the body's production of lecithin and also stimulate the emptying of the gallbladder.

In studies, bran added to the diet has lowered the cholesterol concentration of the bile.

NUTRIENTS THAT MAY BE BENEFICIAL IN TREATMENT OF GALLSTONES

Body Member	Nutrients	Quantity
Gallbladder	Vitamin A	
	Vitamin B complex	
	Vitamin C	
	Vitamin D	
	Vitamin E	
	Vitamin K	
	Lecithin	
	Bran	

GASTRITIS

Gastritis is a disease in which the mucous lining of the stomach becomes irritated and inflamed. If gastritis is prolonged, the stomach walls become very thin, secreting almost entirely mucus and very little digestive acid. In this condition the stomach is unable to produce the intrinsic factor, a substance necessary for the absorption of vitamin B_{12}, which the body needs for the formation of red blood cells. Thus the gastritis patient is in danger of developing pernicious anemia.

Symptoms of gastritis include dyspepsia, or indigestion, vomiting, headache, coated tongue, and abnormal increase or decrease in appetite. Diarrhea and abdominal cramps also may occur.

The cause of gastritis appears to be overindulgence in alcohol, coffee, or highly seasoned or fried foods, all of which increase the activity of the stomach, thereby irritating it more. Eating rancid foods can cause bacterial infection, which may cause gastritis. Recurring cases of gastritis may be the result of ulcers or of the buildup of poisonous body wastes due to such diseases as chronic uremia or cirrhosis of the liver. Any condition causing stress can bring on the symptoms of gastritis. The ailment has been experimentally induced by the same deficiencies that result in ulcers.

In treating gastritis, fried foods and highly seasoned foods should be avoided. Alcohol, coffee, aspirin, and other substances that irritate the stomach lining must be eliminated. Frequent small meals are easier for the stomach to digest than fewer large meals. If gastritis is severe, iron supplements and injections of vitamin B_{12} may be helpful for preventing pernicious anemia.

**NUTRIENTS THAT MAY BE BENEFICIAL
IN TREATMENT OF GASTRITIS**

Body Member	Nutrients	Quantity
Stomach	Vitamin A	
	Vitamin B complex	
	Vitamin B_6	
	Vitamin B_{12}	
	Folic acid	
	Inositol	
	Pantothenic acid	
	Vitamin C	
	Vitamin D	
	Vitamin E	
	Calcium	
	Lecithin	
	Linoleic acid	
	Iron	

GLAUCOMA

Glaucoma is characterized by an increase in pressure of the fluid within the eyeball and a hardening of the surface of the eyeball. The cause of glaucoma is currently unknown, but usually it occurs after age forty and it may be due to tumor, trauma, infection, and in one type, heredity. Glaucoma is often associated with anxiety and stress, allergy, or hormone disorders. Symptoms include eye discomfort or pain, especially in the morning, blurred vision, halos around lights, inability to adjust to a darkened room, and loss of vision at the sides. Early detection of glaucoma can substantially reduce the incidence of blindness resulting from it.

Glaucoma cannot be cured, but it can be controlled through the use of prescribed eye drops. The diet of those affected should be rich in vitamin A, essential for eye-tissue health. If the symptoms of anxiety are related to a deficiency of the B vitamins, then correction of this deficiency would decrease the susceptibility of an individual to glaucoma. Alcohol, tobacco, coffee, and tea should be avoided.

Glaucoma is often an indication of adrenal exhaustion; therefore, nutrients necessary for the adrenals should be taken. The nutrients that meet the demands of stress should also be emphasized. Italian physicians have significantly reduced the intraocular pressure in the eyes of glaucoma patients by administering large doses of vitamin C (500 milligrams per 2.2 pounds of body weight).

**NUTRIENTS THAT MAY BE BENEFICIAL
IN TREATMENT OF GLAUCOMA**

Body Member	Nutrients	Quantity*
Eye	Vitamin A	25,000 IU
	Vitamin B complex	
	Vitamin B_2	
	Choline	Up to 2 gm
	Inositol	
	Vitamin C	7 gm five times daily
	Vitamin D	
	Bioflavonoids	

*See note, p. 222.

GOITER

A goiter is an enlargement of the thyroid gland. The thyroid gland is located at the base of the neck. It secretes a fluid, the hormone thyroxine, which is made from iodine and tyrosine, an amino acid. The thyroid, through the thyroxine hormone, regulates metabolism, or the burning of food, growth, and body temperature and influences mental and emotional balance; it is also a factor in the function of the reproductive system.

Thyroid disorders are caused by an inadequate intake of iodine, resulting in insufficient thyroxine production, or a disorder elsewhere in the body that requires more thyroxine than the gland can manufacture. Goiter may be caused by a lack of iodine in the diet, inflammation of the thyroid gland due to infection, or under- or overproduction of thyroxine by the thyroid gland.

Symptoms of goiter are a swelling at the base of the neck, hoarseness, change in the rate of metabolism, and in extreme cases, difficulty in swallowing and breathing. Treatment of goiter varies with the cause. If goiter is due to an iodine deficiency, increasing the intake of iodine will prevent further enlargement of the gland and, in some cases, reduce its size. Vitamin A is necessary for the proper metabolism of iodine; this vitamin is also important for the functioning of the pituitary gland, which secretes a substance that regulates the thyroid. Tyrosine cannot be used without vitamins B_6 and C. Vitamin E increases the absorption of iodine. The use of iodized salt has helped to eliminate goiter in many places where iodine does not occur naturally in foods.

Kelp is an excellent source of iodine, low in sodium, and is better retained by the body than potassium iodide.

NUTRIENTS THAT MAY BE BENEFICIAL IN TREATMENT OF GOITER

Body Member	Nutrients	Quantity
Thyroid	Vitamin A	
	Vitamin B complex	
	Vitamin B_6	
	Choline	
	Vitamin C	
	Vitamin E	
	Calcium	
	Iodine	
	Protein	

GOUT

Gout is a metabolic disturbance characterized by an excess of uric acid in the blood and deposits of uric acid salts in the tissue around the joints, especially in the fingers and the toes. It can also occur in the heel, knee, hand, ear, or any joint in the body. Gout results when certain crystals are formed as an end product of improper protein metabolism. These crystals are deposited in a joint, forming a bump or growth that irritates the joint, causing it to become inflamed; thus an attack of gout occurs.

Gout often appears to be hereditary. However, factors such as obesity, increasing age, and improper diet increase an individual's susceptibility to gout. Alcohol, a large meal, or any physical or emotional stress also may bring on an attack of gout.

Emphasis should be placed on including adequate intake of fluids to prevent the buildup of the gout-producing crystals in the kidneys. A gradual weight-reduction program for overweight individuals will help prevent gout attacks, but a rapid weight loss may bring on attacks, due to the stressful effect on the body.

The diet most often recommended for gout restricts purines, substances from which uric acid is formed. This diet is very low in the B vitamins and vitamin E. Some investigators believe that the amount of uric acid in foods is too small to cause gout and that the cause really lies in the inefficient breakdown of proteins by the body. However, if a low-purine diet is preferred, generous amounts of all vitamins and minerals, especially the B-complex vitamins and vitamin E, should be taken.

Pantothenic acid is necessary for the conversion of uric acid into the harmless compounds, urea and ammonia. Many gout patients are deficient in this B vitamin, resulting in uric acid accumulation. Stress rapidly depletes pantothenic acid as well as other B vitamins. A lack of vitamin E allows excessive formation of uric acid. A diet of incomplete proteins or one too high or too low in isolated amino acids can also produce too much uric acid. Fruits, vegetables, and juices aid uric acid excretion.

**NUTRIENTS THAT MAY BE BENEFICIAL
IN TREATMENT OF GOUT**

Body Member	Nutrient	Quantity*
Joints	Vitamin A	
	Vitamin B complex	
	Vitamin B₁	
	Pantothenic acid	
	Vitamin C	Up to 5000 mg
	Vitamin E	
	Calcium	
	Iron	
	Magnesium	
	Phosphorus	
	Potassium	
	Complete protein	
	Acidophilus	

*See note, p. 222.

HAIR PROBLEMS

Healthy hair is dependent upon blood circulation and quality, which in turn are dependent upon nutrition. Partial lack of any nutrient can cause hair problems. A well-balanced diet is important to maintaining healthy hair, although hereditary graying and balding cannot be completely prevented by nutritional means.

Hair is composed primarily of protein. A deficiency of protein in diet can result in a temporary change of hair color and texture, resulting in dull, thin, dry hair. If the protein deficiency is corrected, the hair will return to its normal condition.

A deficiency of vitamin A may cause hair to become dull, dry and lusterless and eventually to fall out. However, an excess of vitamin A may cause similar problems.

Hair loss occurs during stress or when the diet is inadequate in the B vitamins—especially B_6, biotin, inositol, and folic acid—or in magnesium, sulfur, or zinc. An underactive thyroid causes the hair to fall out. Excess copper results in hair loss in women who take oral contraceptives and in women in the last months of pregnancy (hair growth will return after

birth). Intoxication by heavy metals such as mercury, lead, and cadmium causes hair loss.

Graying hair can indicate a deficiency of nutrients in other parts of the body. A return of normal hair color has been accomplished by supplements of copper, folic acid, pantothenic acid, and/or PABA; 5 milligrams of folic acid and 300 milligrams of PABA and pantothenic acid along with the B complex have been shown to prevent the loss of and to restore hair color in some persons.

Good hygiene is also important for healthy hair. This includes brushing the hair properly and washing it with a mild shampoo. Exposure to wind and sun may cause brittle, broken hair.

**NUTRIENTS THAT MAY BE BENEFICIAL
IN TREATMENT OF HAIR PROBLEMS**

Body Member	Nutrients	Quantity
Hair	Vitamin A	
	Vitamin B complex	
	Vitamin B₆	
	Biotin	
	Folic acid	
	Inositol	
	PABA	
	Pantothenic acid	
	Vitamin C	
	Copper	
	Iodine	
	Magnesium	
	Sulfur	
	Zinc	
	Protein	

HALITOSIS

Halitosis is an unpleasant odor of the breath. It may be caused by improper diet, poor mouth hygiene, nose or throat infections, extensive teeth or gum decay, excessive smoking, or the presence of bacteria that are foreign to the mouth.

Diabetes or nervous tension may be the cause of bad breath. Other sources are chemicals that may be present in the body such as arsenic, lead, bismuth, and methane. Most often, however, bad breath can be attributed to putrefactive bacteria living on undigested food, which release gas through expelled air. All nutrients necessary for efficient digestion are essential, as well as digestive enzymes. Improving the intestinal bacteria by eating yogurt is also helpful.

Other treatments for halitosis involve proper mouth hygiene, including regular tooth brushing. Often the use of dental floss is recommended. A carefully balanced diet is essential for the prevention of halitosis. Avoiding excessive consumption of carbohydrates may help prevent tooth decay that can cause bad breath. Vitamin C is needed to prevent scurvy, which can cause the gums to bleed and become infected. Vitamin A is necessary for the overall development and health of the gums and teeth.

NUTRIENTS THAT MAY BE BENEFICIAL IN TREATMENT OF HALITOSIS

Body Member	Nutrients	Quantity*
Mouth	Vitamin A	
	Vitamin B complex	
	Vitamin B$_6$	50 mg
	Niacin	
	PABA	
	Vitamin C	1000 mg or more
	Magnesium	
	Zinc	
	Digestive enzymes	
	Acidophilus	
	Chlorophyll	

*See note, p. 222.

HAY FEVER (ALLERGIC RHINITIS)

Hay fever is a reaction of the mucous membranes of the eyes, nose, and air passages to seasonal pollens and dust, feathers, animal hair, and other irritants. Reacting to the irritant, large numbers of antibodies are produced to attack the allergen; however, these antibodies also release histamine, which makes the capillaries more permeable to fluid accumulation, resulting in swelling and irritation.

Hay-fever symptoms include itching in the eyes, nose, and throat, a clear, watery discharge from the nose and eyes, frequent sneezing, and nervous irritability. Alcoholic beverages and stressful situations may precipitate an attack of hay fever.

The most effective treatment for hay fever is to avoid the irritant. Vitamin A is essential for the general health of the respiratory system. Some authorities believe that vitamin C in doses of 200 or more milligrams daily can relieve hay-fever symptoms.[22]

Dr. Mitsuo Kamimura, of the department of dermatology at the Sapporo Medical College in Japan, has tested the antihistamine effect of vitamin E on both animals and humans. His studies reveal that the vitamin prevents the symptoms of allergies, is more effective if given before symptoms begin than after the fact, and applied topically, can reduce itching and redness. He believes the vitamin decreases the permeability of the capillaries and depresses the release of histamine.

NUTRIENTS THAT MAY BE BENEFICIAL IN TREATMENT OF HAY FEVER

Body Member	Nutrients	Quantity*
Lungs/Respiratory system	Vitamin A	50,000 IU for 4 months
	Vitamin B complex	
	Vitamin C	100–1000 mg
	Vitamin E	300 IU

*See note, p. 222.

HEADACHE

A headache is a pain or ache in any portion of the head. It is a symptom rather than a disease in itself. Most commonly, headaches fall into one of three categories: tension headaches, resulting from a contraction of the neck, scalp, or forehead muscles; vascular headaches, caused by uneven dilation rates of the blood vessels in the brain; and sinus headaches, caused by inflamed mucous membranes of the nose. Sinus headaches are often brought on by changes in the weather, onset of menstruation, or a head cold.

There are many possible causes of headache such as diseases of the eye, nose, or throat, trauma to the head, air pollution, drugs, alcohol, tobacco, fever, generalized body infections, disturbances of the digestive tract and circulatory system, brain disorders, anemia, low blood sugar, niacin or pantothenic acid deficiency,

[22]Guthrie, *Introductory Nutrition,* p. 225.

an overdose of vitamin A, allergies, salt, excessive carbohydrates, allergenic foods, oral contraceptives or other sources of estrogen, improper bite, bruxism, the chewing of gum, food additives such as nitrites in meats, stuffy rooms (caused by an electrical imbalance of the ion count of the air), and premenstruation (possibly a result of water retention in the brain tissues, which can be relieved by vitamin B_6).

A migraine is a particular type of headache caused by the alternating constriction and dilation of the blood vessels in the brain. It is often hereditary. There are two types of migraine: classic migraine, which is preceded by lightheadedness, flashing lights, and supersensitivity to noise; and common migraine, accompanied by nausea, a general feeling of ill-being, and sometimes depression and irritability. The face may be pale, swollen, and sweaty. A migraine attack may last for hours or days.

Cluster headaches, a variant of the migraine, are sudden and severe, usually located on one side of the face or head, producing sweating and tearing. Vigorous exercise or the inhalation of pure oxygen has alleviated the pain in many individuals. Many persons with this type of headache have unusually high copper levels in the body, which can be lowered by zinc supplements.

Treatment for headache depends upon the underlying cause. Repeated headaches may be a symptom of a serious disorder and therefore deserve attention, or they may be the result of stress. Learning better ways of coping with stress and relieving nervous tension is often the most effective treatment for headaches and migraine. Acupuncture has been shown to be effective in preventing or lessening the severity of headache in many people. Massage, a hot bath, moist heat, or cold packs can help tension headaches. To alleviate sinus headaches, the inflamed, congested membranes of the nose can be drained by using steam humidifiers or warm packs applied over the eyes and cheekbones. Acupressure has also helped some individuals.

Vitamin therapy may take a period of time, from 6 months to 2 years in some people, before headache symptoms disappear or diminish substantially. Special attention should be paid to preventing deficiencies of iron, niacin, and pantothenic acid. Vitamin A may also prove helpful to some headache victims. The B complex, especially niacin, is a very important factor in maintaining normal dilation of the blood vessels. Acidophilus is helpful for establishing the friendly intestinal bacteria from which the body produces the B vitamins. Niacin, calcium (taken in the morning), zinc, magnesium, and sometimes potassium and tryptophan (an amino acid), along with relaxation, may help the pain of migraine.

NUTRIENTS THAT MAY BE BENEFICIAL IN TREATMENT OF HEADACHE

Body Member	Nutrients	Quantity*
Head	Vitamin A	
	Vitamin B complex	
	Vitamin B_1	
	Vitamin B_2	10 mg per meal
	Vitamin B_6	50 mg
	Niacin	100 mg three times daily
	Pangamic acid	100 mg
	Pantothenic acid	100 mg
	Vitamin C	Up to 4 gm
	Vitamin D	
	Vitamin E	Up to 1200 IU
	Calcium	500 mg
	Iron	
	Magnesium	
	Potassium	
	Zinc	
	Tryptophan	2–4 gm
	Acidophilus	

*See note, p. 222.

HEART DISEASE

The heart is the chief organ of the circulatory system; it is the most delicate and yet the most durable because it is made of the toughest muscle fibers of the body. The heart is a very efficient pump, but over a million Americans die of heart disease each year.

The arteries supplying the heart with blood are formed around the heart like a crown, or corona, thus called coronary arteries. If the circulation in these arteries has been decreased to such an extent that little oxygen reaches the heart, pain results, called *angina*. Attacks are brought on by a heavy meal, unaccustomed physical exertion, stress, emotional tension, or exposure to cold. The frequency and duration of attacks vary and may range from several attacks per day to one attack every few years.

The pain varies greatly in severity from a mild pressure to an intolerable agony. It usually starts in the upper chest or throat and radiates to the left shoulder and down the left arm. The patient is pale, sweaty, and very apprehensive. These symptoms are similar to those of a heart attack but can be differentiated in that the pain lasts only for minutes and can be relieved by rest. However, if the blood supply is insufficient enough, angina pectoris can progress to a heart attack.

If atherosclerosis has impaired circulation to the point where a coronary artery becomes completely plugged and no oxygen reaches the heart, a heart attack known as a *coronary occlusion* results. Fatty deposits take years to build up on the artery walls; however, a blood clot, formed quickly in persons with atherosclerosis at any stage (including children), can clog an artery and cut off oxygen supply, causing a heart attack called a *coronary thrombosis*. Symptoms may begin anytime. The most frequent complaint is an excruciating pain, usually starting in the lower chest or upper abdomen. The pain often spreads to the neck and shoulders, down the arms, especially to the left side, and possibly to the back. The pain increases in severity and is not relieved by rest or nitroglycerin, a medication often prescribed for patients with mild angina pectoris. The pain causes the patient to appear very restless and anxious. In 15 percent of heart attack cases, however, no pain is experienced and the attack is known as a "silent coronary."[23]

Additional heart attack symptoms include perspiration and pale skin, a decrease in blood pressure, weak and rapid pulse, and, possibly, nausea and vomiting. A moderate fever usually appears 24 to 48 hours after the onset of the attack.

Immediate medical attention is necessary and can best be obtained at a coronary care unit in a hospital setting. Usually the patient will be given an electrocardiogram, or EKG, a test designed to detect changes in heart function or damage to some part of the heart. But often this test will not show the heart damage until hours or days after the attack. A blood test is

[23]Lillian Brunner, et al., *Medical Surgical Nursing* (New York: J. B. Lippincott Co., 1959).

also often done to help detect if a myocardial infarction, or heart attack, has occurred.

During the first three weeks of treatment, the patient runs a great risk of suffering further irregularities in heart function. The immediate effort in treatment is for the patient to obtain rest, to decrease the workload of the heart. Pain medication and oxygen therapy are often applied. Because the workload of the heart increases after meals, the diet during the first few days often consists of six small feedings low in sodium. Cold fluids should be avoided because they may trigger irregularities in heart function. Protein intake must be adequate to replace protein lost in damaged heart cells. By six weeks the healing is almost complete and increased amounts of activity can be tolerated.

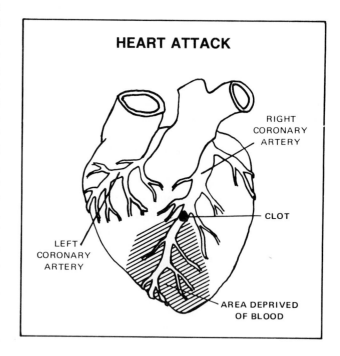

A heart that is weakened or damaged by diseases such as rheumatic fever, heart attack, hypothyroidism, arteriosclerosis, or beriberi is unable to properly pump the blood through the body. This inefficient circulation, which leads to congestion of many organs with blood and other tissue fluids, is *congestive heart failure.* Early symptoms of congestive heart failure are abnormal fatigue and shortness of breath following work or exercise. Swelling, particularly in the ankles and feet, is a further symptom. Congestion of the abdominal organs causes nausea, lack of appetite, and gas. Fluid in the lungs impairs breathing and in some cases causes a persistent cough.

A damaged heart requires special dietary attention. Poor appetite, inefficient digestion, and excessive nutrient loss from the body after heart failure can result in a state of malnutrition. A nutritionally balanced diet is important for efficient operation of the heart. Protein foods, fresh vegetables and fruits, and whole grains should be substituted for high intake of refined starches, sweets, and hydrogenated fats. Protein is essential to the strength of all muscles, including the heart. An overconsumption of fat is believed to be detrimental because it may weaken arteries, reduce their elasticity, and clog them with cholesterol.

Supplementary intake of vitamin E is needed as an oxygen conserver to keep oxygen in the blood. The vitamin strengthens the heart muscle, at times acts as a diuretic to rid the body of excess fluid, decreases elevated blood pressure, has similar actions as digitalis, and may be as effective as anticoagulant drugs in preventing clots. (Vitamin E temporarily raises blood pressure, so heart patients should begin with low doses, perhaps 100 IU daily. Its use may be hazardous in individuals with rheumatic heart disease.) Vitamin E, through interaction with unsaturated fatty acids, also allows for the reduction of cholesterol. This will prevent the metabolic imbalance that causes cholesterol to collect in the arteries. (Increased oil consumption should be followed by increased vitamin E.)

A deficient operation of the thyroid gland may be involved in some cases of faulty fat metabolism. Vitamins A, C, and B complex and the minerals zinc and selenium are necessary for the maintenance of arterial health and repair and protection against atherosclerosis. Chromium assists the metabolism of blood fats, and superoxide dismutase (SOD) possibly aids the restoration of the heart tissue. Copper levels appear to be extremely low in persons who develop an aneurysm (a bubble), leading to a rupture of the artery and death. Copper is important for vessel strength and elasticity.

A pulse rate of about 70 beats per minute for men and 80 beats per minute for women is best for the heart. A pulse rate of 100 is usually considered abnormally high, although there are variations in normal rates. To lower a pulse rate, reduce the intake of food, avoid emotional stress, and curtail use of drugs, alcoholic drinks, and tobacco products. It should be remembered that substances to which one is allergic will raise the pulse rate and thus produce further stress on the heart.

Overweight can be a contributing factor to both high pulse rate and high blood pressure; excess pounds greatly tax the heart and the circulatory system in general. A properly balanced diet will lead to reduction of pounds without the adverse symptoms experienced when eating only one or two foods as is common in many fad diets.

Stress may raise blood pressure as well as pulse rate. Fluctuations of blood pressure against artery walls contribute to arterial injury and hardening. Exercise is an excellent way to deal with stress and improve muscle tone of the heart and entire body. Unless otherwise advised by your physician, begin walking for ten minutes a day and gradually increase up to one hour. Walking should be at a brisk pace but must be begun slowly. Strenuous exercise (work or recreation) to which one is not accustomed should be avoided because the heart may not be able to meet the unusual requirements made upon it.

NUTRIENTS THAT MAY BE BENEFICIAL IN TREATMENT OF HEART DISEASE

Body Member	Nutrients	Quantity*
Heart/Blood/ Circulatory system	Vitamin A	
	Vitamin B complex	
	Vitamin B$_1$	
	Vitamin B$_6$	100 mg
	Choline	
	Folic acid	
	Inositol	
	Niacin	100 mg–3 gm
	Pantothenic acid	
	Vitamin C	1–3 gm
	Vitamin D	
	Vitamin E	300–1200 IU
	Calcium	1000 mg
	Chromium	
	Copper	
	Iodine	
	Magnesium	500 mg or more

*See note, p. 222.

Body Member	Nutrients	Quantity*
	Manganese	
	Phosphorus	
	Potassium	regulated carefully
	Selenium	
	Zinc	
	Protein	
	Unsaturated fatty acids	
	Lecithin	
	RNA	
	Digestive enzymes	

*See note, p. 222.

HEMOPHILIA

Hemophilia is a hereditary blood disease characterized by a prolonged coagulation time. The blood fails to clot, and abnormal bleeding occurs. Hemophilia is a sex-linked hereditary trait, transmitted by normal females carrying the recessive gene. This disease occurs almost exclusively in males. There is no known cure for hemophilia. Transfusion of fresh whole blood or plasma is required in emergencies to provide the necessary coagulation factors.

Anemia is common and has been successfully corrected with vitamins C and E. Vitamin E, if taken continuously, may shorten the clotting time and prevent hemorrhaging in hemophiliacs.

NUTRIENTS THAT MAY BE BENEFICIAL IN TREATMENT OF HEMOPHILIA

Body Member	Nutrients	Quantity
Blood/Circulatory system	Niacin	
	Vitamin C	
	Bioflavonoids	
	Vitamin E	
	Calcium	
	Acidophilus	

HEMORRHOIDS (PILES)

Hemorrhoids are ruptured or distended veins located around the anus. The most common cause of hemor-rhoids is strain on the abdominal muscles due to factors such as heavy or improper lifting, pregnancy, overweight, constipation, or an extremely sedentary life. The flow of blood through the vessels of the anus is particularly sensitive to the pressure and strain of pregnancy and constipation. The blood collects in these vessels and the pressure against the weakest sections causes tiny bulges or piles. They may itch, tear, and bleed, causing pain.

Treatment for severe hemorrhoids may involve surgical removal. Breathing normally under any type of strain will eliminate abdominal pressure. The bioflavonoids strengthen the capillaries. Vitamin E can prevent and dissolve blood clots. Ointments containing vitamins A and D or E or vitamin E suppositories can lubricate and relieve pain. Preventive measures include an improved diet containing fiber, fluids, and exercise, and cleanliness.

NUTRIENTS THAT MAY BE BENEFICIAL IN TREATMENT OF HEMORRHOIDS

Body Member	Nutrients	Quantity*
Intestine	Vitamin A	25,000 IU
	Vitamin B complex	
	Vitamin B$_6$	25 mg after each meal
	Vitamin C	1000–2000 mg
	Vitamin E	600 IU, also as suppository
	Bioflavonoids	
	Calcium	
	Fluids	
	Fiber	

*See note, p. 222.

HEPATITIS

Hepatitis is an inflammation of the liver caused by infection or toxic agents. It begins with flulike symptoms of fever, weakness, drowsiness, abdominal discomfort, and headache, possibly accompanied by jaundice. Soon extreme fatigue and loss of appetite occur. The liver is unable to eliminate the poisons, allowing them to build up in the system; and it cannot store and process certain nutrients that are vital for the body.

There are two types of viral hepatitis: infectious hepatitis (hepatitis A and hepatitus non A, non B) is caused by the ingestion of contaminated shellfish (prevented by cooking for at least 6 minutes), contaminated water, or inhalation of airborne germs from infected persons, or by injections, or body secretions; serum hepatitis (hepatitis B) is more serious and sometimes fatal. It is contracted from contaminated blood transfusions, injections using unsterilized needles, or from contaminated chemicals taken into the system by injection.

Recovery from hepatitis involves abstention from alcohol, a diet adequate in all nutrients and rest. A high-protein and/or a high carbohydrate diet, unsaturated fatty acids, fluids, and vitamins B complex, C, and E should be continued long after recovery because sensitivity to toxic materials may persist.

NUTRIENTS THAT MAY BE BENEFICIAL IN TREATMENT OF HEPATITIS

Body Member	Nutrients	Quantity*
General/Liver	Vitamin A	
	Vitamin B complex	
	Vitamin B_6	
	Pangamic acid	
	Pantothenic acid	
	Vitamin C	10 gm
	Vitamin E	
	Unsaturated fatty acids	
	Protein	
	Zinc	
	Fluids	

*See note, p. 222.

HERPES SIMPLEX I and II

Herpes Simplex I (HSV I) and Herpes Simplex II (HSV II) are two of five types of human herpes simplex viruses. (The other three cause chicken pox, mononucleosis, and shingles.) The virus moves into healthy cells, reprogramming them to work for the virus. It will remain in some form in the body for life; however, with time the body eventually becomes more efficient in suppressing it.

Most of the time, the virus will remain dormant and will not be contagious. However, the virus will become active when the body's immune system is weakened, whether from stress, disease, or an environmentally related factor.

Other than being basically inconvenient, the virus can become serious in two situations. If it is transmitted to the eyes, blindness can result; therefore it is important that the hands be washed after contact with the lesions. Second, pregnant women who have HSV II need to take special precautions upon delivery; if the virus is active at the time, a caesarean will have to be performed.

Recognizing the symptoms that indicate that the virus is becoming active is very important in preventing exposure to other persons. During the early warning signs, the virus is active beneath the skin and is just as contagious as when the lesions actually appear. Once the blisters form, they will last for about 1 to 5 days. They will then rupture and form a scab, the final stage. At this healing stage the virus is probably not contagious because it has run its course and is gone.

HSV I results in cold sores on the mouth, eyes, or nose. It is mainly contracted by kissing or sharing a utensil containing moist saliva of the infected person. The early warning sign that an outbreak is about to occur is a numbing or tingling sensation around the mouth, which may last for a day or two before the blister appears. Within about 48 hours the blister ruptures and begins to heal.

HSV II is sexually transmitted. The lesions of HSV II that occur in men are usually located on the penis, scrotum, or, rarely, inside the urinary tube. The early warning signs are an itching or numb feeling on the penis. The testicles and groin area may be tender. Fatigue and an ill feeling may be experienced.

The early warning signs of HSV II in women are similar to those in men. The area around the outside of the vagina begins to itch or tingle; the upper inner thighs become tender, and headaches, fever, or a sick feeling may occur. Most women have the infection inside the vagina as well, with the symptoms of irritation and a watery discharge. The blisters will appear on the inner or outer lips of the vagina, around the clitoris, or around the anal area.

Outbreaks of herpes can be prevented or greatly limited in frequency and duration by following certain guidelines. The treatment basically involves strengthening the immune system, which will not only prevent herpes activation but will also raise the body to a higher state of health, resulting in a better defense against other diseases. Stress is the most-recognized link with herpes outbreaks. Stress lowers the resistance to disease and decreases immune system activity. Therefore stress management is of utmost importance. Stress can not only have a psychological cause but can also result from fatigue and lack of adequate sleep, menstruation, sunburn, fever, drugs, alcohol, caffeine, inadequate diet, refined carbohydrates, sugar, and tap water. Many of these factors cause stress on the body by depleting it of essential nutrients or loading it with harmful substances.

The best efforts should be made to obtain an adequate, nutritious diet and remove any stressful situation that could precipitate a virus outbreak in the individual. Certain supplements have been shown to have a direct effect on the virus: lysine, an amino acid; vitamins B complex, C, and E; and the mineral zinc. Topical treatments that may aid the healing of lesions are vitamin E oil (applied at the beginning of symptoms through the last stage), providone-iodine solution (obtained at drugstores), a cream containing lithium (available at health-food stores), and ice (applied for 1½ to 2 hours).

NUTRIENTS THAT MAY BE BENEFICIAL IN TREATMENT OF HERPES SIMPLEX I AND II

Body Member	Nutrients	Quantity
General	Vitamin B complex	50 mg
	Vitamin C	1–10 gm
	Vitamin E	400–1200 IU
	Zinc	20–50 mg
	Lysine	400 mg; during outbreak 400 mg three times daily

HYPERACTIVITY

Hyperactivity is a disorder of certain mechanisms in the central nervous system. The hyperactive child is generally characterized as being fidgety, aggressive, impulsive, easily frustrated, unable to concentrate, clumsy; he or she sleeps poorly and has poor school grades despite an average or above-average IQ. The disorder may be a result of boredom or feelings of insecurity. Some hyperactive children are reasonably quiet, but most have varying degrees of muscle incoordination.

A diet containing refined carbohydrates has been found to cause increased hyperactivity. Food additives commonly cause adverse responses; the hyperactive child does not have the natural bodily defenses necessary to ward them off. These substances may be very small in size but a susceptible individual can get a reaction from an infinitesimal molecular amount. Lead and heavy metal accumulation in the body also appear to affect behavior.

Large doses of vitamins B_1, B_2, niacin, pantothenic acid, folic acid, and choline, and the minerals zinc, magnesium, and manganese have successfully treated the underlying causes of hyperactivity and adjusted the chemical imbalance of the brain. A minimum of 3 to 6 months is requried before substantial results are manifest; however, a general slowing of the hyperactivity and increased concentration may initially be observed. The diet of a hyperactive child should consist of well-balanced meals of unrefined foods and foods free of chemical additives, including colorings. Vitamin C can aid the body in removing heavy metals.

The quantities below have been used in a clinical setting for children of 35 to 45 pounds. (For a child less than 35 pounds, quantities were adjusted as follows: 1 gm niacin, vitamin C in 500 mg doses twice a day increased to one 2 gm dose a day if tolerated, B_6 and pnathothenic acid at 100 mg twice a day increased to 200 mg twice a day. For a child 45 pounds plus, vitamin C and niacin were gradually increased to 3 gm a day.)

NUTRIENTS THAT MAY BE BENEFICIAL IN TREATMENT OF HYPERACTIVITY

Body Member	Nutrients	Quantity*
Brain/Nervous System	Vitamin B_1	
	Vitamin B_2	
	Vitamin B_6	200–400 mg
	Vitamin B_{12}	

*See note, p. 222.

Body Member	Nutrients	Quantity*
	Choline	
	Folic acid	
	Niacin	1–2 gm
	Panthothenic acid	200–600 mg
	Vitamin C	1–3 gm
	Vitamin E	
	Calcium	
	Magnesium	
	Manganese	
	Zinc	
	L-glutamine	
	Lecithin	

*See note, p. 222.

HYPERTENSION (HIGH BLOOD PRESSURE)

Hypertension is an abnormal elevation of blood pressure. The cause is generally unknown, but hypertension often accompanies arteriosclerosis or kidney diseases. Blood pressure is the force exerted by the blood against the walls of the blood vessels. The pressure can temporarily rise after physical activity or emotional tension but after a period of relaxation will return to normal. An abnormal condition arises when the pressure does not return to normal and remains high. This is called essential hypertension, meaning independent of local cause, or disease without apparent cause. If this condition persists, it can cause heart and kidney diseases or stroke.

In approximately 10 percent of the cases of hypertension, the cause can be found in a physical disorder such as a kidney infection, an obstruction of an artery of the kidney, a disorder of the adrenals, or a constriction of the aorta of the heart. Hypertension of these origins can usually be corrected. However, exact reasons for hypertension in most people may be difficult to find.

Atherosclerosis can cause hypertension because the blood has great difficulty in passing through arteries that are plugged with fatty substances; consequently the blood pressure becomes high. Stress can cause the disease because tension causes the arterial walls to contract and become smaller. Other factors associated with the onset of hypertension are heredity, obesity, high salt intake, cigarette smoking, excessive use of stimulants such as coffee, tea, or drugs, and use of oral contraceptives.

Symptoms of hypertension may be nonexistent, or they may include headache, nervousness, insomnia, nosebleeds, blurred vision, edema, shortness of breath, dizziness, ringing in the ears, and eventually hemorrhaging in the eyes.

Stress is an important factor to be considered in hypertension. Many people drive themselves too hard and consequently become hypertensive. These people must learn to avoid stressful conditions by changing their lifestyle. They should take regular, unhurried meals, try to avoid worry, allow themselves plenty of leisure time, take vacations, and generally use moderation in all things. If their occupation involves excessive emotional and physical stress, they may have to consider changing it or adjusting it to make it less stressful. Steps should be taken to alleviate the prolonged stress of unexpressed emotions. Some people, because of their personality characteristics, overreact to emotional situations, causing more-frequent and longer-lasting elevations of the blood pressure. If this is not corrected, sustained hypertension could result.

Sodium is a primary cause of hypertension because it causes fluid retention, which adds additional stress to the heart and circulatory system. Increasing the potassium, calcium, and vitamin D intake will cause the body to excrete more sodium. Vitamin C can help to maintain the health of the blood vessels that are strained by the greater pressure placed on them by hypertension.

Regular exercise is essential in preventing high blood pressure because it keeps the circulatory system healthy. Promoting a tranquil outlook on life is of primary importance in reducing and preventing hypertension.

NUTRIENTS THAT MAY BE BENEFICIAL IN TREATMENT OF HYPERTENSION

Body Member	Nutrients	Quantity*
Blood/ Circulatory system/ Heart	Vitamin B complex	
	Choline	
	Inositol	

*See note, p. 222.

Body Member	Nutrients	Quantity*
	Niacin	
	Pangamic acid	
	Pantothenic acid	
	Vitamin C	1000–3000 mg
	Vitamin D	
	Vitamin E	100–600 IU
	Bioflavonoids	100–300 mg
	Calcium	800 mg three times daily
	Lecithin	
	Magnesium	500 mg
	Potassium	
	Protein	
	Fiber	
	Garlic	

*See note, p. 222.

NUTRIENTS THAT MAY BE BENEFICIAL IN TREATMENT OF HYPERTHYROIDISM

Body Member	Nutrients	Quantity*
Gland, thyroid	Vitamin A	100,000 IU
	Vitamin B complex	
	Choline	
	Folic acid	
	Inositol	
	Vitamin C	
	Vitamin E	1000 IU
	Calcium	
	Iodine	4–6 mg
	Magnesium	
	Carbohydrates	
	Protein	

*See note, p. 222.

HYPERTHYROIDISM

Hyperthyroidism is overproduction of hormones by the thyroid glands. Symptoms of the condition are nervousness, irritability, fatigue, weakness, loss of weight, goiter, insomnia, fluctuating moods, tremor of the hands, easy perspiring, intolerance of heat, and rapid pulse. Hyperthyroidism can be caused by hereditary factors, emotional stress, or other unknown factors.

The excess production of thyroid hormones speeds up all body processes. As a result, all nutrients in the body are used up at a greater rate. The diet should therefore be increased in all nutrients. If weight loss has been great, additional protein may be necessary to replace muscle tissue that may have been lost. Particular attention should be paid to the adequate intake of the vitamin B complex because it is needed for the metabolism of the extra carbohydrates and protein. Coffee and tea containing caffeine should be avoided because caffeine increases the metabolic rate, thereby resulting in more calories being expended. Nicotine and the initial effects of alcohol also increase the metabolic rate and should be avoided.

HYPOGLYCEMIA (LOW BLOOD SUGAR)

Hypoglycemia is an abnormally low level of glucose, or sugar, in the blood. There are three general types of hypoglycemia. Two of them are rare organic forms involving the pancreas: tumors of the pancreas and enlargement of the island of Langerhans. The most common form is called functional hypoglycemia (FH) and is caused by an inadequate diet that is too high in refined carbohydrates or that results in impaired absorption and assimilation of food ingested. An over-consumption of carbohydrates causes the blood sugar level to rise rapidly, stimulating the pancreas to secrete an excess of insulin. This excess insulin removes too much sugar from the blood, resulting in an abnormally low blood sugar level.

Heredity may be the susceptibility factor but the disease is precipitated most often by an inadequate diet. In some people, hypoglycemia can contribute to other illnesses such as epilepsy, allergies, asthma, ulcers, arthritis, impotence, and mental disorders. Functional hypoglycemia is often found in persons with such disorders as schizophrenia, alcoholism, drug addiction, juvenile delinquency, hyperactivity, and obesity.

Symptoms of FH are episodic and have a direct relationship to the time and type of meal that was last eaten. Symptoms include fatigue, weakness in legs, swollen feet, tightness in chest, constant hunger, eyeache, migraine, pains in various part of the body, nervous habits, mental disturbances, and insomnia. Rapid fluctuations in blood sugar level give rise to many bizarre symptoms that may suggest mental disorder; however, a glucose tolerance test will ascertain the amount of sugar in the blood at a given time. FH may be subclinical, meaning that the symptoms are subtle and difficult to diagnose; the patient may have a low but acceptable blood sugar level that does not drop until the last hours of a prolonged test.

The therapeutic diet for hypoglycemia is high in protein, low in carbohydrates, and moderate in fat. (A diet high in unrefined complex carbohydrates, with low to moderate protein, has also been used successfully.) The diet may be supplemented with high-protein between-meal snacks. Heavily sugared foods should be avoided, and foods with high natural sugar content should be restricted. Carbohydrates should include only those that are slowly absorbed, such as fruits, vegetables, and whole-grain products, so that the change in the blood sugar level will be gradual. Caffeine, alcohol, tobacco, and other simulants should be avoided because they are capable of precipitating an attack of hypoglycemia. Vitamin and mineral supplementation is necessary to supply tissues that are markedly depleted. Digestive enzymes may be needed to ensure proper absorption of food.

NUTRIENTS THAT MAY BE BENEFICIAL IN TREATMENT OF HYPOGLYCEMIA

Body Member	Nutrients	Quantity*
Blood/ Circulatory System	Vitamin A	up to 75,000 IU
	Vitamin B complex	
	Vitamin B_1	30 mg
	Vitamin B_2	30 mg
	Vitamin B_6	60 mg
	Vitamin B_{12}	25–50 mcg; injections may be necessary
	Biotin	
	Choline	900 mg
	Folic acid	2.5 mg
	Inositol	270 mg
	Niacin	300–450 mg
	PABA	
	Pantothenic acid	100–300 mg
	Vitamin C	2–5 gm
	Bioflavonoids	1 gm
	Vitamin E	300 IU
	Calcium	
	Chromium	
	Copper	
	Iron	
	Magnesium	
	Manganese	
	Phosphorus	
	Potassium	
	Zinc	
	Methionine	
	Protein	
	Digestive enzymes	

*See note, p. 222.

HYPOTENSION (LOW BLOOD PRESSURE)

The blood vessel walls of a person with hypotension are usually very relaxed and possibly flabby or stretched. Few nutrients or little oxygen can reach body tissues from vessels in this condition. The disease is often accompanied by hypoglycemia, hypothyroidism, or anemia. Symptoms of low blood pressure are fatigue, lack of endurance, sensitivity to heat and cold, development of a rapid pulse on exertion, and little interest in sex. The individual requires more sleep than normal persons and often wakes up tired.

Systolic blood pressure as low as 100 or 80 may be considered healthy as long as that has always been normal for that person. However, if the systolic pressure has suddenly dropped to that level or if an individual has any of the above symptoms, hypotension may be the cause.

Mild deficiencies of calories, protein, or vitamins C and B complex (especially pantothenic acid) have produced low blood pressure. Adrenal exhaustion is commonly associated with the disease.

The diet should be sufficient in all nutrients, with emphasis on complete proteins, and the vitamins B complex, C, and E. Since excessive amounts of salt may be excreted because of an undersupply of pantothenic acid, salty foods should be eaten daily until the pressure has reached normal.

NUTRIENTS THAT MAY BE BENEFICIAL IN TREATMENT OF HYPOTENSION

Body Member	Nutrients	Quantity
Blood/Circulatory system	Vitamin A	
	Vitamin B complex	
	Vitamin B_1	
	Pantothenic acid	
	Vitamin C	
	Vitamin D	
	Vitamin E	
	Manganese	
	Protein	

HYPOTHYROIDISM

Hypothyroidism is the underproduction of hormones by the thyroid gland, resulting in lowered cellular metabolism. The brain cells are affected and intellectual capacity is lowered and impaired. For the newborn baby, this may mean mental retardation unless the hormone is quickly supplied. If an adult has additional forms of stress such as infection or surgery, a coma may result. In the elderly, hypothyroidism is often mistaken for senility, exhibiting similar symptoms of depression, poor memory, and mental confusion. The condition may be hereditary, or it may result from a deficiency of iodine.

The illness develops slowly, and early symptoms such as fatigue, lack of zest, and sensitivity to cold may be attributed to other sources, such as stress. Symptoms of hypothyroidism are fatigue, decreased appetite, dull, dry hair and skin, constipation, lack of mental and physical vigor, sleeplessness, slurred speech, clumsiness, and numbness and tingling in the hands and feet. A low thyroid level may cause night blindness and even deafness. Men may become impotent and have a low sperm count. Women's sex drive is lowered; they may not ovulate; and menstruation may be excessive or irregular.

An adequate diet supplying all nutrients at an optimal level is essential. Treatment for hypothyroidism may include administration of thyroid hormone. Organic iodine, such as that found in kelp, may be

better retained in the body and less likely to be readily excreted than potassium iodide.

NUTRIENTS THAT MAY BE BENEFICIAL IN TREATMENT OF HYPOTHYROIDISM

Body Member	Nutrients	Quantity
Gland, thyroid	Vitamin B complex	
	Vitamin B_6	
	Choline	
	Vitamin C	
	Vitamin E	300 IU
	Iodine	4 mg or 1 tsp kelp
	Protein	

INDIGESTION (DYSPEPSIA)

Dyspepsia is imperfect or incomplete digestion, manifesting itself in a sensation of fullness or discomfort in the abdomen accompanied by pain or cramps, heartburn, nausea, and large amounts of gas in the intestines. Dyspepsia may be a symptom of a disorder in the stomach or small or large intestine, or it may be a complaint in itself. If indigestion occurs frequently and with no recognizable cause, medical investigation is advised.

The digestive tract is similar to a tube that begins at the mouth and extends through the body to the rectum. As food is chewed, it mixes with saliva, a composition of mucus and digestive enzymes. After being swallowed, the food moves through the esophagus and into the stomach. Glands in the stomach walls secrete hydrochloric acid, digestive enzymes, and the hormone gastrin. These substances are essential in digesting the food. When the food becomes semiliquid, called chyme, it moves into the small intestine, where more digestive enzymes are secreted for further breakdown of the food and nutrients are absorbed. The chyme then passes into the large intestine, where some absorption of nutrients takes place. The remaining solid matter is excreted as waste.

Usually dyspepia is the result of psychological stresses, anxiety, worry, or disappointment disturbing the nervous mechanism that controls the contractions of stomach and intestinal muscles. Other causes are overeating or eating too rapidly; improper diet, such as a diet overabundant in carbohydrates at the expense of other nutrients; or overconsumption of stimulants such as coffee, tea, or alcohol. Smoking before or during a meal or swallowing too much air with meals, as in periods of nervousness or anxiety, can also bring about indigestion.

Too little hydrochloric acid impairs the absorption of several vitamins and minerals and the digestion of protein. Insufficient amounts of hydrochloric acid can be brought about by a lack of vitamins A and B complex and low protein intake. This condition also results in a decreased amount of digestive enzymes and impaired stomach movements necessary to mix the food with the enzymes.

Heartburn, or acid or sour stomach, usually is caused by eating too fast or when exhausted or emotionally upset. Swallowing air during meals, especially easy when anxious, can result in heartburn. The air warms to body temperature, expands, and is belched with enough force to push stomach acid into the esophagus where it irritates membrane tissues, causing discomfort. Antacids and alkalizers are possibly more destructive than helpful. They neutralize all the acid in the stomach, preventing efficient digestion and thus interfering with vitamin and mineral absorption.

In treating dyspepsia, the diet should be nutritionally well balanced. The individual should eat slowly and avoid eating when overtired or upset. Hydrochloric acid tablets and digestive enzymes may be helpful. Papaya contains enzymes that can break down protein and other foods in the stomach. Peppermint has a soothing effect on the digestive tract and stimulates digestive secretion.

INFECTIONS

Infections are the starting point of many illnesses and often are not serious enough for medical attention. However, they can result in a wide variety of serious illnesses including swollen glands or tonsils, sore throat, colds, hay fever, encephalitis, and virus pneumonia. White blood cells, lymph cells, and antibodies mobilize to prevent any bacteria, virus, or toxin from entering the body. An adequate diet is essential for the maintenance and reinforcement of these defenses.

Stress rapidly depletes the body of many nutrients including the B complex and C vitamins. These nutrients are vital for the formation of antibodies. In addition, vitamin C directly destroys bacteria, viruses, and toxins. It aids the adrenal glands in stimulating the production of antibodies and white blood cells. Vitamin A is also important in this production and in preventing and clearing up infections of the skin, cornea of the eye, and the mucous membranes that line all body cavities. The blood vitamin A drops very low during infections and often much is lost in the urine. Cortisone and other drugs given for infections can deplete the body of this vitamin. If antibiotics are taken, acidophilus is a necessary supplement to replace the intestinal bacteria that are destroyed. The body's natural defenses are made of protein, and therefore recovery from any infection will be prevented unless sufficient amounts of complete protein are obtained.

If an individual is too ill to eat, acidosis may develop, causing irritability, headaches, and nausea. Ingesting small amounts of complex carbohydrates, such as fruit, fruit juice, or any food containing starch or natural sugar, every few hours may alleviate this condition.

NUTRIENTS THAT MAY BE BENEFICIAL IN TREATMENT OF INDIGESTION

Body Member	Nutrients	Quantity*
Stomach	Vitamin B complex	
	Vitamin B$_1$	50 mg
	Vitamin B$_6$	50 mg
	Folic acid	
	Niacin	100 mg
	Pantothenic acid	
	Hydrochloric acid	
	Digestive enzymes	
	Acidophilus	

*See note, p. 222.

NUTRIENTS THAT MAY BE BENEFICIAL IN TREATMENT OF INFECTIONS

Body Member	Nutrients	Quantity*
General	Vitamin A	
	Vitamin B complex	
	Vitamin B$_6$	10–30 mg
	Pantothenic acid	100–300 mg
	Vitamin C	2–3 gm
	Protein	
	Acidophilus	

*See note, p. 222.

INSOMNIA (SLEEPLESSNESS)

Insomnia is a difficulty in falling asleep, in staying asleep, or in sleeping soundly. The need for sleep varies from person to person, but in general it tends to decline as one grows older.

The majority of cases of insomnia are caused by mental disturbances such as depression, an obsessive-compulsive personality, or schizophrenic tendencies. Other causes are anxiety, tension, physical pain, or discomfort. Insomnia may originate from the environment, diet, medical problems, or faulty digestion, resulting in deficiencies of vitamins, minerals, and enzymes. Medical problems include hyper- or hypothyroidism, asthma, heart disorders, ulcers, migraine headaches, arthritis, diabetes, kidney disease, and epilepsy. Many foods in the diet are stimulating, including caffeine and salt (which stimulates the adrenal glands in the same way caffeine does). Salt also can lead to high blood pressure, a disease that can make sleep difficult. Environmentally, heat, cold, humidity, noise, or a too hard or too soft bed can interfere with sleep.

Insomnia perpetuates itself, in that thinking about the inability to sleep creates further tension in the mind and body. Only by relaxing and ceasing to worry about insomnia can a person resume sleeping and thus relieve his anxiety and tension. In learning to change his patterns of thought associated with sleep, the insomniac must establish a new bedtime routine, which might include such muscle and mind relaxers as leisurely walks, warm baths, massages, hot milk, soft music, or quiet meditation. Camomile tea has been shown in tests to have a soothing action on the nerves and body.

The well-nourished person who enjoys good health and a feeling of well-being probably will be less troubled by insomnia than one who subsists on a diet deficient in some essential nutrients. Deficiencies in the B vitamins, particularly B_6 and pantothenic acid, have resulted in insomnia. In some cases, vitamin B_{12} has been helpful in treating anxiety in insomniacs. Vitamin C, protein, calcium, magnesium, and potassium can also calm the nerves and promote sleep.

The amino acid tryptophan (found in milk as well as in other foods) is converted to serotonin in the body; increased serotonin levels generally induce sleep and prevent waking during the night. Vitamins B_6 and

C are necessary for the conversion of tryptophan to serotonin. Sleeping pills or barbiturates should be used only as a last resort because they may produce dependence and other serious side effects.

NUTRIENTS THAT MAY BE BENEFICIAL IN TREATMENT OF INSOMNIA

Body Member	Nutrients	Quantity*
Brain/Nervous system	Vitamin B complex	
	Bitamin B_6	10–100 mg
	Vitamin B_{12}	25 mg
	Inositol	1–10 gm
	Niacin	100 mg–2 gm
	Pantothenic acid	100 mg
	Vitamin C	1 gm
	Vitamin D	2000 IU
	Vitamin E	400 IU
	Calcium	2 gm
	Magnesium	250 mg
	Phosphorus	
	Potassium	
	Tryptophan	2 gm

*See note, p. 222.

INTESTINAL PARASITES

There are several types of parasitic worms which can live in human intestines, the most common being pinworms, tapeworms, hookworms, and roundworms. Worms irritate the intestinal lining and therefore cause poor absorption of nutrients. Signs of worms often include diarrhea, hunger pains, appetite loss, weight loss, and anemia. Diagnosis can be made by examining the stools or, occasionally, by inducing the vomiting of worms. The extent of the intestinal damage is then determined by the type of worm, the size of the worm, and the number of worms present.

Pinworms are the most common parasitic worm in the United States. The chief symptom of this small, threadlike worm is rectal itching, especially at night. Pinworms are transmitted when eggs, which lodge under the fingernails when a person scratches, contaminate food. Personal hygiene is most important for the control of pinworms.

Tapeworms can be contracted from eating insufficiently cooked meats, especially beef, pork, and fish. The most common tapeworm in the United States, beef tapeworm, grows to a length of 15 to 20 feet in the intestines.

Hookworms are often found in the soil or sand in moderate climates. They can enter the body by boring holes in the skin of the bare feet or can enter by mouth if food contaminated by dirty hands is eaten.

Roundworms are most common in children. These worms can leave the intestines and settle in different areas of the body, causing diseases such as pneumonia, jaundice, or periodontitis.

Animals that have been given diets deficient in protein and vitamins A and some of the B complex have become infested with several types of parasites, including trichinae (from undercooked pork), and trichomonas, which grows in the lungs, intestines, or around the vagina. When the diet was improved, the parasites gradually died.

A diet high in refined carbohydrates, supplying few nutrients, increases a person's susceptibility to infestation. When a person is afflicted with parasites, the body's supply of all nutrients is depleted to the point that supplementation of all nutrients is necessary to restore normal health. Nutrients of special importance are vitamin A; the B complex, especially thiamine, riboflavin, B_6, B_{12}, and pantothenic acid; vitamins C, D, and K; and calcium, iron, and protein. Acidophilus is especially helpful for amebic dysentery and possibly for all intestinal infestations. Sufficient stomach acid destroys parasites contained in food.

NUTRIENTS THAT MAY BE BENEFICIAL IN TREATMENT OF INTESTINAL PARASITES

Body Member	Nutrients	Quantity
Body/Intestine	Vitamin A	
	Vitamin B_1	
	Vitamin B_2	
	Vitamin B complex	
	Vitamin B_6	
	Vitamin B_{12}	
	Pantothenic acid	
	Vitamin D	
	Vitamin K	
	Calcium	
	Iron	
	Potassium	
	Sulfur (ointment form)	
	Protein	
	Unsaturated fatty acids	
	Hydrochloric acid	
	Acidophilus	

JAUNDICE

Jaundice is a condition in which the skin, whites of the eyes, and urine become abnormally yellow because of the presence of pigments from worn-out red blood cells. Normally these cells are excreted in bile as waste products; however, in jaundice they accumulate in the blood and are deposited in the tissues.

The disease can be caused by a condition that prevents the bile from entering the intestines: surgical trauma, swelling or spasms of the bile duct, or obstruction of the duct by a stone, cyst, or cancer.

Anemia can often result in jaundice; severe liver damage or cirrhosis can also occur as a result of jaundice. Jaundice may indicate blood, kidney, or liver disorders; a doctor should be consulted in cases of jaundice.

The diet should be high in nutrients that build up the red blood cells, especially the B vitamins, C, E, magnesium, and protein. Tissue relaxants such as vitamins B_6, magnesium, and calcium can alleviate muscular spasms of the bile duct.

NUTRIENTS THAT MAY BE BENEFICIAL IN TREATMENT OF JAUNDICE

Body Member	Nutrients	Quantity*
Blood	Vitamin A	
	Vitamin B complex	
	Vitamin B_6	50–100 mg
	Vitamin C	1000–1500 mg every 3 hours in acute conditions, given even during fasting. In chronic conditions, 3000–5000 mg daily
	Vitamin D	

*See note, p. 222.

Body Member	Nutrients	Quantity*
	Vitamin E	600 IU
	Choline	
	Folic acid	1–5 mg
	Niacin	
	Pantothenic acid	100 mg
	Calcium	
	Lecithin	3–4 tbsp
	Magnesium	
	Phosphorus	
	Protein	
	Unsaturated fatty acids	

*See note, p. 222.

KIDNEY DISEASES

Kidney diseases are given various names according to the part of the organ most seriously damaged. Bright's disease refers to several types of kidney damage including nephritis, which most often affects children (see Nephritis), and nephrosis, which is less acute and affects older persons. Symptoms, which appear gradually, include puffiness around the eyes, frequent urination, headaches, and a high blood cholesterol.

Inability to control urination, called bed-wetting, may be due to a magnesium deficiency; inability to pass urine may be caused by a potassium, vitamin B_2, or pantothenic acid deficiency.

The diet of anyone with kidney disease should be adequate for repair and should meet the needs of stress, to prevent irreparable damage from occurring.

A potassium deficiency can be created by excessive salt intake, cortisone therapy, or diuretics that are often prescribed for kidney diseases. Diuretics also cause the loss of other water-soluble nutrients, such as vitamins B complex and C and magnesium. Stress, medications, and diuretics cause such a great loss of vitamin C that hemorrhaging can result, a condition that can also be caused by a choline or vitamin E deficiency.

When urine formation is greatly inhibited, urea, a by-product of food breakdown, becomes too concentrated and can become toxic. A low-protein diet (but at least 40 grams) has been recommended to prevent this condition. Vitamin B_6 can stabilize urea levels. Vitamin C has been shown to increase urine produc-

tion, although it is impaired by a diet too high in salt. Vitamin A increases urine output. Vitamin E acts as a diuretic. To prevent a salt deficiency, 500 milligrams of sodium should be obtained daily.

NUTRIENTS THAT MAY BE BENEFICIAL IN TREATMENT OF KIDNEY DISEASES

Body Member	Nutrients	Quantity
Kidney	Vitamin A	
	Vitamin B complex	
	Vitamin C	
	Bioflavonoids	
	Vitamin E	
	Potassium	

KIDNEY STONES (RENAL CALCULI)

Kidney stones are abnormal accumulations of mineral salts, which form in the kidney but may lodge anywhere in the urinary tract. They can be the size of sand or gravel or as large as bird eggs. Often removed surgically, they can reappear if the diet is not improved. The stones are composed primarily of calcium phosphate or oxalate. They form most rapidly in urine that is alkaline as opposed to acid.

A deficiency of magnesium leads to the increase of urine alkalinity, most often resulting in the formation of calcium phosphate stones.

A deficiency of vitamin B_6 greatly increases the oxalic acid content of the urine and also allows increased alkalinity, leading to calcium oxalate stones. Only about 2 percent of the oxalic acid taken in the diet is absorbed and subsequently excreted. Most of this substance is made inside the body from an improperly utilized amino acid, glycine. The cause of this inefficient utilization is a deficiency of vitamin B_6.

Conditions that influence greater body loss of calcium (which if not kept in solution will result in stones) are a deficiency of vitamin D, which is necessary for calcium absorption; stress, which draws out minerals from the bones, increasing calcium excretion; and a diet too low in protein, which produces the albumin essential for calcium retention.

Stone formation may also be due to overactivity of the parathyroid gland, which causes an elevated level of calcium in the blood. Additional conditions that increase the risk of kidney stone formation are dehydration, prolonged periods of bed rest, infections, and rarely, overingestion of vitamin D and calcium.

Symptoms of kidney stones include pain originating in the middle back which radiates around the abdomen toward the genitalia, increased urination that may contain blood or pus, nausea, and vomiting. Irritation by the stone may induce an infection in the urinary tract, giving rise to fever, chills, and general discomfort.

Adelle Davis has reported that existing stones can be dissolved by a diet high in calcium, protein, and vitamin A plus foods containing all other essential nutrients.[24]

Too little potassium, common in refined-food diets, too much salt, and not enough fruits and vegetables make the urine too alkaline, eventually preventing minerals from being held in solution and causing them to deposit as stones.

Because a very small percentage of the body's oxalic acid actually comes from oxalic-acid-containing foods (stones are still formed on an oxalic-acid-free diet), these foods need not necessarily be restricted. Persons whose diets are deficient in vitamin A tend toward kidney stone formation, so an adequate supply of this vitamin should be included in the diet. To ensure the proper absorption of vitamin B_6, adequate amounts of magnesium and vitamin B_2 are required.

Sometimes stones are composed of uric acid (a diet recommended for gout is helpful) or cystine, an amino acid. Intake of citrus fruits and vegetables produces an alkaline urine, which keeps uric acid and cystine in solution. Persons with cystine stones should limit their protein to 70 grams per day.

NUTRIENTS THAT MAY BE BENEFICIAL IN TREATMENT OF KIDNEY STONES

Body Member	Nutrients	Quantity*
Kidney	Vitamin A	
	Vitamin B_2	
	Vitamin B_6	50 mg
	Vitamin C	
	Vitamin E	
	Magnesium	250–500 mg

*See note, p. 222.

[24]Davis, *Let's Get Well*, p. 203.

KWASHIORKOR

Kwashiorkor is a severe malnutritional disease caused by a diet which supplies adequate calories through its carbohydrate content but which is seriously lacking protein. Kwashiorkor commonly develops in children who are between the ages of one and five and who are weaned from milk to a diet of primarily starches and sugars.

Symptoms of kwashiorkor include changes in the skin and hair, retarded growth, diarrhea, loss of appetite, nervous irritability, and edema. Severe infections and many vitamin deficiencies often accompany kwashiorkor.

The initial treatment for the disease is aimed at correcting the protein deficiency. Because of the patient's poor ability to tolerate fat, a skim-milk formula is often used in treatment. Gradually, additional foods are added until the patient progresses to a well-balanced diet. Vitamin deficiencies, if they exist, must be corrected.

NUTRIENTS THAT MAY BE BENEFICIAL IN TREATMENT OF KWASHIORKOR

Body Member	Nutrients	Quantity
Body	Vitamin A	
	Folic acid	
	Vitamin C	
	Vitamin D	
	Vitamin E	
	Chromium	
	Copper	
	Iron	
	Magnesium	
	Selenium	
	Protein	

LEG CRAMP, "CHARLEY HORSE"

A leg cramp is an involuntary contraction, or spasm, of a muscle in the leg or foot. Cramps most commonly occur at night, when the limbs are cool, particularly after a day of unusual exertion, and more frequently in the elderly, the young, and persons with arteriosclerosis. These cramps seem to be caused by unnatural positions which impair the blood supply to the lower extremities, causing the muscles to abnormally contract, thus bringing about cramps. A cramp usually lasts only a few seconds or minutes. If a cramp occurs while a person is walking, it may be a signal of seriously impaired circulation, but a cramp that occurs while a person is resting does not indicate this severity. Patients most susceptible to repeated leg cramps are those with advanced arteriosclerosis.

Leg cramps may signify a variety of nutritional deficiencies. The most common is lack of calcium, which is necessary for normal muscle contraction. Other deficiencies indicated are thiamine, pantothenic acid, biotin, and magnesium. Occasionally a sodium loss, such as occurs in heavy perspiration or diarrhea, may result in muscle cramps. A vitamin C deficiency also can be responsible for pains in the muscles and joints. Prevention and treatment for leg cramps should include an adequate diet containing sufficient amounts of these nutrients.

A "charley horse" is a pulled and bruised muscle that results in soreness and stiffness. It is usually caused by a blow or a forceful stretch of the leg during athletic activity. A person who has suffered a charley horse should have a high intake of protein to rebuild damaged tissues.

NUTRIENTS THAT MAY BE BENEFICIAL IN TREATMENT OF LEG CRAMP

Body Member	Nutrients	Quantity*
Leg	Vitamin B complex	
	Vitamin B1	
	Vitamin B_2	
	Biotin	
	Pantothenic acid	100 mg
	Vitamin C	
	Vitamin D	
	Vitamin E	400–1000 IU
	Calcium	
	Magnesium	800 mg
	Phosphorus	
	Sodium	
	Protein	
	Unsaturated fatty acids	

*See note, p. 222.

LEUKEMIA

Leukemia is a fatal blood disease characterized by an overproduction of white blood cells. There are two basic types of leukemia: acute leukemia usually occurs in children and young adults, and chronic leukemia is usually found only in adults.

Acute leukemia is marked by a sudden onset of symptoms. In chronic leukemia, symptoms develop more slowly. Symptoms of the disease include bleeding from the gums, nose, stomach, and rectum and abnormally easy, excessive bruising of the skin. Pain in the upper abdomen, anemia, fever, and increased susceptibility to infection are further leukemia symptoms.

The cause of leukemia is unknown. However, some theories suggest that excessive exposure to radiation, x-rays, or chemical pollution may cause the disease. Animals deficient in vitamin E develop excessive white blood cells and abnormal bone marrow.

A well-balanced diet containing all vitamins is helpful in maintaining strength in the leukemia victim, and possibly extends their lifetime. Supplementing the diet with vitamin B complex and iron may aid in the treatment of the anemia that accompanies the disease. Vitamin C may be helpful in fighting the infections that are often associated with leukemia.

The use of folic acid is controversial because sometimes it can accelerate the development of leukemia and at other times it has been shown to improve the general well-being of the patient without affecting the disease. Folic acid antagonists, which are often given as part of the treatment, can cause a severe depletion of the vitamin and possibly do more damage to the cell than would the cancer. If an antagonist is used, the diet should be supplied with sufficient vitamins B complex, C, and E, and complete proteins to aid the liver in detoxification and alleviate the side effects of the drug.

NUTRIENTS THAT MAY BE BENEFICIAL IN TREATMENT OF LEUKEMIA

Body Member	Nutrients	Quantity
Blood	Vitamin B complex	
	Vitamin B_{12}	
	Folic acid	
	Vitamin C	

Body Member	Nutrients	Quantity
	Vitamin E	100 IU six times daily
	Bioflavonoids	
	Copper	
	Iron	
	Zinc	

LIVER DISORDERS

The liver, located under the diaphragm just above the stomach, is the largest organ of the body. Countless chemical reactions take place in the liver every day, including the synthesis of amino acids, protein breakdown, sugar conversion and storage, as well as the storage of some vitamins and minerals. It also produces lecithin, cholesterol, enzymes, and bile and detoxifies harmful substances such as pesticides, food additives, and environmental pollutants. Liver damage can result from chronic alcoholism, social drinking, overweight, drug or chemical ingestion, or improper diet.

Slight liver injury may go largely unnoticed, producing vague symptoms such as digestive disturbances and fatigue. Long before actual damage is detected, the liver may have degenerated cells; accumulated fat and scar tissue; and greatly reduced enzymes and bile, resulting in poor food utilization. Starch is neither formed nor stored, causing chronic fatigue and overweight; lecithin is not properly synthesized; and fats are inefficiently used. When the liver cannot synthesize certain enzymes needed to inactivate various hormones, such conditions as water retention, hypoglycemia, hyperthyroidism, and excessive male or female hormones in the opposite sex can result.

A deficiency of the B vitamins, C, E, and certain amino acids limits enzyme synthesis. A severe vitamin C, E, and protein deficiency may result in massive cell death and hemorrhaging of the liver. Liver damage in animals has occurred when they are fed diets high in refined carbohydrates, high in saturated fats, or low in magnesium, calcium, and the sulfur-containing amino acids.

The liver can usually regenerate if the diet is adequate, supplying all essential nutrients including complete proteins and vitamins B complex, C, and E.

Vitamins A, C, E, and choline aid the liver in detoxifying harmful drugs and chemicals. Vitamin B_6, magnesium, acidophilus, digestive enzymes, and lecithin can prevent the accumulation and formation of ammonia, which results from a damaged liver's inability to properly break down proteins.

In some cases of liver disease, liquid accumulates in the abdomen, a condition called ascites. The liver does not produce enzymes needed to inactivate a urine-controlling hormone and insufficient urine is formed.

Ascites can be helped by an adequate diet and 2 tablespoons of brewer's yeast after each meal.

NUTRIENTS THAT MAY BE BENEFICIAL IN TREATMENT OF LIVER DISORDERS

Body Member	Nutrients	Quantity
Liver	Vitamin A	
	Vitamin B complex	
	Vitamin B_1	
	Vitamin B_2	
	Vitamin B_6	
	Choline	
	Niacin	
	Pantothenic acid	
	Vitamin C	
	Vitamin E	
	Calcium	
	Magnesium	
	Protein	
	Lecithin	
	Acidophilus	
	Hydrochloric acid	
	Digestive enzymes	

MEASLES

The two main varieties of measles are German measles and common measles. German measles is usually a mild illness with a rapid recovery period, alarming only to pregnant women. If a woman contracts German measles during the early months of her pregnancy, malformation such as heart defects, deafness, mental retardation, and blindness of the newborn commonly occur.

Symptoms of German measles may include fever, headache, and stiff joints, although most people seldom complain of any symptoms. A rash that lasts for about three days appears on the arms, chest, and forehead.

Since German measles is a virus that must run its course, there is little that can be done medically for its treatment. One attack of or vaccination for the disease will usually produce lifelong immunity against German measles. Lotions may be applied to the rash to relieve itching, and the patient should stay away from other people to avoid spreading the disease. A well-balanced diet rich in all nutrients is recommended.

Common measles is a highly contagious disease spread by droplets from the nose, throat, and mouth. The first symptoms of common measles are fever, cough, and inflammation of the eyes. Within 24 to 48 hours, small red spots with white centers appear on the inside of the cheeks. A rash which is first seen on the side of the neck and which then spreads to the rest of the body usually appears 3 to 5 days after the onset of the first symptoms. As the rash spreads, fever goes down. Common measles may have many serious complications, such as pneumonia, encephalitis, and injury to the nervous system.

The patient should be isolated in a well-ventilated room, which should be darkened if the patient is sensitive to light. Fevers increase the body's need for calories and vitamins A and C. Although the patient may not desire food for the first few days, he or she should be encouraged, but not forced, to eat. Frequent small meals and special foods may be beneficial. Increased fluid intake in any form, such as water, fruit juices, or milk, is essential to the measles patient.

NUTRIENTS THAT MAY BE BENEFICIAL IN TREATMENT OF MEASLES

Body Member	Nutrients	Quantity
General/Skin	Vitamin A	
	Vitamin C	1 gm every two hours for 2 days, none for the next 2 days, 1 gm every 2 hours for 4 days
	Vitamin E	
	Protein	

MÉNIÈRE'S SYNDROME

Ménière's syndrome is a disease of the inner ear characterized by recurrent attacks of deafness, tinnitus, vertigo, nausea, vomiting, sound distortion, and a feeling of pressure in the inner ear.

Conditions in the inner ear that may cause the disease are hemorrhage, fluid imbalance, or a spasm of a blood vessel subsequently leading to vasodilation and an increased flow of blood. Allergies, eye or mental strain, stress, alcohol, tobacco, or an inadequate diet—especially a deficiency of the B vitamins—can precipitate Ménière attacks. Ménière patients have been found to be chronically deficient of the B vitamins, possibly due to defective utilization of the vitamin. Gallbladder disease occurs in these patients at twice the rate of the general population.

Nicotinic acid, or niacin, because of its vasodilator action, has been shown to be effective in controlling Ménière's syndrome that is caused by vasodilation.

Because attacks often follow an illness in which antibiotics are given, adequate intake of all nutrients is recommended; acidophilus aids in the restoration of beneficial intestinal bacteria and also in the manufacture of the B vitamins. Reducing dietary salt may be helpful.

NUTRIENTS THAT MAY BE BENEFICIAL IN TREATMENT OF MÉNIÈRE'S SYNDROME

Body Member	Nutrients	Quantity*
Ear	Vitamin B complex	
	Vitamin B_1	10–25 mg four times daily for 2 weeks
	Vitamin B_2	10–25 mg four times daily for 2 weeks
	Vitamin B_6	
	Niacin	100–250 mg four times daily for 2 weeks
	Vitamin E	
	Calcium	
	Unsaturated fatty acids	

*See note, p. 222.

MENINGITIS

Meningitis occurs when the three layers of membranes lying between the skull and the brain become infected by bacteria, viruses, or fungi. These infecting organisms are commonly spread via the bloodstream from acute infections of the nose and throat.

Meningitis is more commonly found in children than in adults. Symptoms include headache, stiff neck, high fever, chills, nausea, vomiting, changes in temperament, and drowsiness, which may develop into a coma.

Medical attention for meningitis should be sought promptly. The drug selected for treatment of the disease depends on the type of infecting organism. During the fever, the body's needs for vitamin A and C are increased. Large doses of vitamin C have been used successfully because of its antibacterial actions. The vitamin works more efficiently if sufficient calcium is also taken.

A well-balanced diet adequate in protein is necessary to help the body ward off infection and repair damaged tissue.

NUTRIENTS THAT MAY BE BENEFICIAL IN TREATMENT OF MENINGITIS

Body Member	Nutrients	Quantity
Brain	Vitamin A	
	Vitamin C	
	Vitamin D	
	Calcium	
	Protein	

MENTAL ILLNESS

Only slight changes in the molecular amounts of numerous chemicals can bring on changes in the brain affecting behavior, mood, and perception. Medical professionals have found that using megavitamin therapy for many psychological disorders has doubled the recovery rate and, for instance, eliminated the suicidal tendencies of schizophrenics.

Mental illness as a physical disease can result from low brain concentrations of vitamins B_1, B_6, B_{12}, niacin, pantothenic acid, folic acid, vitamin C, and various minerals and amino acids.

A vitamin B_1 deficiency results in loss of appetite, depression, irritability, confusion, loss of memory, inability to concentrate, fear, and sensitivity to noise. Manifestations of a niacin deficiency include anxiety, depression, fatigue, insomnia, and headache; as the illness progresses, failing vision, hallucinations, vertigo, and a salty taste are experienced. Vitamin B_6 is essential for the metabolism of all amino acids and for a strong immune system. Low levels of vitamin B_{12} create poor concentration, depression, agitation, and hallucinations. Persons deficient in pantothenic acid become easily upset, irritable, depressed, tense, dizzy, and numb. Folic acid levels have been found to be low in a large percentage of psychiatric patients. Vitamin C is necessary for folic acid conversion, and deficiencies of C can cause listlessness and increased susceptibility to stress of the blood vessels. Insufficient amounts of the minerals can cause muscle weakness, fatigue, indifference, apathy, hyperactivity, poor equilibrium, and uncoordinated movements. Inadequate amounts of complete proteins, resulting in an imbalance of the amino acids, can cause depression, apathy, irritability, and the desire to be left alone; uric acid levels may rise, a condition that has been associated with self-mutilating behavior in children.

In a study of over 200 mentally ill persons with wide-ranging psychological disorders, they responded to two basic treatments. (The disturbances worsened under psychological stress.) Type I persons, metabolically characterized by slow oxidation of carbohydrates and certain amino acids and slow utilization of fats, improved with the following daily supplements: 30 milligrams each of vitamins B_1, B_2, and B_6; 75 milligrams each of niacin and PABA, 900 milligrams vitamin C, 7500 units vitamin D, 900 milligrams potassium citrate, 300 milligrams magnesium chloride, 0.6 milligrams copper gluconate, 30 milligrams manganese oxide, and 200 milligrams iron. Type II persons, metabolically characterized by fast oxidation of carbohydrates and certain amino acids and a slightly higher than normal oxidation of fats and other amino acids, improved with: 50,000 units vitamin A; 200 units vitamin E; 20 micrograms vitamin B_{12}; 400 milligrams niacinamide; 100 milligrams each of pantothenic acid, vitamin C, choline, and bioflavonoids; 180 milligrams inositol; 660 milligrams calcium; 500 milligrams phosphorus; 0.45 milligrams iodine; and 20 milligrams zinc sulphate.[25]

In contrast to vitamin deficiencies that require the usual therapeutic doses, vitamin dependencies are an indication of a genetic disturbance that involves only one reaction catalyzed by a vitamin. The dependency responds only to very large doses of the particular vitamin.

Indoor pollution can be a cause of mental disturbances, dependent upon individual susceptibility to the buildup of cumulative exposures. Sources include odors and fumes from gas appliances (especially the gas stove), the combustion products of gas, oil, or coal, insecticides, refrigerants, plastics, hair sprays, paint, and disinfectants. Symptomatic reactions range from mental confusion and physical and/or mental fatigue to depression and advanced psychotic states.

When various other treatments have produced unsatisfactory results, mental disorders including schizophrenia have responded to fasting and its detoxifying process. Abstention from food also relieves the brain of allergens. In a study of schizophrenia, over 90 percent of the patients reacted neurologically to common foods; and environmental substances, including wheat, and corn products, milk, tobacco, and petroleum products and their combustion by-products.[26] Alcohol and sugar often induce and aggravate allergies. Allergic reactions range from the mild, such as weakness, dizziness, anxiety, and depression, to severe psychotic symptoms, such as catatonia, paranoid delusions, and hallucinations. At the same time, offender foods can be addictive; they are often a favorite food and are eaten for relief of the allergic reaction, creating a vicious cycle. Certain vitamins appear to have antiallergy properties, controlling reactions if the offending substance is removed. These include vitamin C (large doses are necessary), and vitamins A, D, B_6, pantothenic acid, niacin, and pangamic acid.

Some psychiatric disorders may be genetically transmitted and many adults developing schizophrenia were hyperactive and/or had learning disabilities as children. Children with *learning disabilities* exhibit hyperactivity, sleep difficulties, poor attention span, and often hypoglycemia. Many of these children are fed inadequate diets high in salt, refined carbohydrates, and processed foods with artificial colors and flavors. They often have high body levels of lead and copper and low levels of zinc, potassium, and manganese.

A large percentage of these children can be helped by taking high dosages of vitamins and minerals. The following has been used in clinical studies: 1 to 3 grams each of niacin and vitamin C, 50 to 60 milligrams pantothenic acid, 50 to 400 milligrams vitamin B_6, 300 to 600 units vitamin E, 250 to 500 milligrams calcium, 100 to 500 milligrams magnesium, and 8 to 15 milligrams lecithin granules plus a high-protein, low-carbohydrate diet and digestive enzymes.[27] Attention should also be made to avoid any food causing an allergic reaction.

A deficiency of certain neurotransmitters, chemicals in the brain that transmit signals from one nerve cell to another, can cause *depression*. These include norepinephrine and serotonin. The immune system of depressed persons is usually very low and therefore is ineffectively responding to diseases, including cancer. The amino acids, tyrosine or L-phenylalanine, given in doses of 500 to 1000 milligrams daily for 2 weeks, has been shown to alleviate depression in many persons.[28] These amino acids are natural precursor of certain neurotransmitters. (In large doses, phenylalanine can cause a rise in blood pressure, so persons with high blood pressure should start with a low dosage and gradually increase the amount.) Vitamins C and B_6 (200–1500 mg) are necessary for the conversion process of both phenylalanine and tyrosine. The B vitamins, choline, (up to 3 gm/day) and lecithin (up to 80 gm/day) increase acetylcholine levels in the brain. (These compounds should not be used for persons in the depressive phase of manic-depression because the depression may increase.) Pantothenic acid is required for the conversion. Additional nutrients that have been shown to be helpful are the B complex, ½ to 4 gm/day niacin, 14 mg/day folic acid (not to be used by persons with high levels of blood histamine), vitamin B_{12}, pangamic acid, 150 mg/day zinc, 50 mg/day manganese, and 1–8 gm/day of the amino acid tryptophan.[29]

There are claimed to be three general categories of *schizophrenia*. Histapenics, comprising approxi-

[25]Williams and Kalita, eds., *Physician's Handbook on Orthomolecular Medicine*, p. 188.
[26]Ibid., p. 140.
[27]Ibid., p. 189.
[28]Pearson and Shaw, *Life Extension*, p. 185.
[29]Atkins, *Dr. Atkins' Nutrition Breakthrough*, p. 88.

mately 50 percent of schizophrenics, have abnormally low blood and brain histamine and high serum copper levels. Symptoms include overstimulation and disperception of the senses, time, body, self, and of others. They have frequent hallucinations and often report seeing and being tyrannized by spirits. Histapenic children are hyperactive, generally appear healthy, and have a high pain threshold. These patients have been successfully treated with the administration of 3 gm vitamin C, 3 gm niacin, 2 mg folic acid, 200 mg B_6, B_{12} (weekly injections were recommended), 200 IU vitamin E, and 100 mg rutin. Niacin, folic acid, and B_{12} raise the blood histamine level. Niacin may precipitate an attack of gout, so doses of the vitamin were increased gradually.

Lithium may be needed in severe cases. For the hyperactive histapenic child, in addition to the vitamins, sufficient amounts of rutin or Deaner (a prescription drug) can be used to replace Ritalin and the amphetamines.

Histadelic persons, 20 percent of the schizophrenics, have abnormally high levels of blood histamine. Symptoms include suicidal depression, obsessive rumination, contact loss with reality, blank-mindedness, and often severe headaches. Calcium (1 gm calcium lactate) reduces histamine levels and aids in the prevention of headaches. Methionine, an amino acid, detoxifies histamine. Zinc and manganese are used as treatment because many histadelics show a deficiency; niacin (200 mg) and vitamin E (200 IU) are also included. Lithium treatment may be necessary.

The third type of schizophrenics, about 30 to 40 percent, are called pyroluric. The mauve factor (kryptopyrrole) found in their urine depletes the body of zinc and vitamin B_6, which may result in abnormal EEGs. The pyrrole combines with B_6 and zinc, producing a combined deficiency. Patients have many of the classical symptoms of schizophrenia, but they have better insight and affect. They may be unable to remember dreams or to experience the loss of dreaming; they may have white spots on the fingernails, a sweetish breath odor, sensitivity to sun, inability to tan, stretch marks, irregular menstruation and possibly tremors, spasms, and amnesia. Doses of zinc and possibly manganese and up to 1½ gm of B_6 taken each morning and evening has been shown to effect a positive response, with complete social rehabilitation.

Except for certain sub-types of schizophrenias, the following daily treatments, have been used and clinical improvements observed: 20 mg–1 gm B_1, 20 mg B_2, 1–4 gm niacin, 75–200 mg B_6, 15 mg pantothenic acid, 3–4 gm C, 600–1200 IU E. If patients respond poorly, insufficient absorption may be the causative factor making parenteral injections an alternative.

There are many illnesses that mimic schizophrenia, including brain syphilis, porphyria (an abnormal blood pigment), homocysteinuria (secretion of an abnormal amino acid), thyroid deficiency, pellagra (a niacin deficiency), amphetamine psychosis, a vitamin B_{12}–folic acid deficiency, and cerebral allergies.

Dr. Henry Turkel of Detroit, Michigan, believes that *mental retardation* of Down's syndrome (Mongolism) may be due to an accumulation of metabolite by-products that cause water retention, calcification, and interference in the assimilation of nutrients and the elimination of wastes. He has used enzymes, hormones, vitamins, and minerals to cleanse the blood and tissues of Down's patients, resulting in the improvement in their appearance and in physical and mental performance.[30]

In Russia, pangamic acid has been used to improve the respiration of the brain, which is required for proper brain function. In addition, niacin and vitamin C are necessary for tissue respiration. Large doses of vitamin B_6, manganese, and zinc can possibly result in normal functioning of some retarded persons.[31] Mental retardation has also been treated with 10–20 mg/day of glutamic acid or glutamine, resulting in improvement in personality and increased intelligence.

The disease may possibly be aggrevated by too-high levels of body lead, and there is evidence that deficiencies of vitamins B_{12} and niacin may be responsible.

Anxiety neurosis may be genetic or it may result from a defective metabolism of lactate production or adrenal secretion. Neurotic patients may need more calcium or vitamin C than normal. They are often helped by a hypoglycemic diet, particularly if they exhibit the symptoms of depression, anxiety, fatigue, irritability, or hypochondria. Other nutrients that are beneficial for anxiety include the B complex, inositol, niacin, pantothenic acid, magnesium, and the amino acid tryptophan, taken in divided doses after meals.

[30]Williams and Kalita, eds., *Physician's Handbook on Orthomolecular Medicine,* p. 190.

[31]Ibid.

Nutrient deficiencies or allergic reactions result in a lowered immunological defense system, laying fertile ground for the growth of harmful organisms that quickly multiply and become toxic. Infectious organisms in brain cultures and bacterial infections in the urine have been consistently found in a majority of schizophrenics. To improve this condition, allergy-provoking substances need to be avoided; vitamin B_6 and pantothenic acid are necessary for the formation of antibodies, aided by vitamin B_2, zinc, manganese, and magnesium, building up the immune system. Vitamin C detoxifies bacteria and viruses, and vitamin A also suppresses certain bacteria.

The diet of persons showing signs of mental disturbances should be improved, eliminating all processed foods and foods containing sugar and white flour. Standard medications such as tranquilizers and antidepressants can usually be lowered as the patient begins to recover, resulting in fewer side effects and toxicities.

Drug medications given to psychiatric patients may have several adverse affects on nutrient therapy. For example, L-Dopa induces a vitamin B_6 deficiency (side effects of the drug can be offset by niacin); Dilantin is a folic acid antagonist; penicillamine, used to chelate copper out of the body in schizophrenics, also chelates zinc and vitamin B_6, causing a deficiency.

MONONUCLEOSIS

Mononucleosis is an infectious disease, believed to be caused by a virus. It affects primarily the lymph tissues or glands that are located in the neck, armpits, and groin. The lymph glands remove many microscopic materials such as bacteria and viruses, thus helping to prevent the infection from spreading throughout the body. Symptoms of mononucleosis include sore throat, fever, chills, swollen glands, and fatigue. The disease can be transmitted through communal drinking utensils, kissing, and possibly blood transfusions. In one study, persons who had a particular antigen in their blood to fight the virus were immune to mono.

Adequate rest, exercise, and nutrition are essential for the maintenance of general health and the prevention of mononucleosis. Protein is needed to stimulate the formation of antibodies, substances produced by the body to help protect it against other infections

that may accompany or follow mononucleosis. Potassium and vitamin C supplements may be needed to compensate for the loss that occurs during fever. Vitamin A is needed for the health of the tissue lining of the throat. If there is a deficiency of thiamine, riboflavin, or biotin, supplementing these nutrients in the diet may be helpful in preventing fatigue and headaches.

NUTRIENTS THAT MAY BE BENEFICIAL IN TREATMENT OF MONONUCLEOSIS

Body Member	Nutrients	Quantity
Blood	Vitamin A	
	Vitamin B complex	
	Vitamin B_1	
	Vitamin B_2	
	Vitamin B_6	
	Biotin	
	Choline	
	Pantothenic acid	
	Vitamin C	
	Potassium	
	Protein	

MOUTH AND TONGUE DISORDERS

A deficiency of the B vitamins in particular can manifest in various abnormalities of the mouth, gums, and tongue. A sore mouth is one of the first indications of a B_6 deficiency; a lack of folic acid causes the development of ulcerated lips and sore mouth, throat, and esophagus. The mouth, throat, esophagus, tongue, and gums become sore from insufficient niacin. The gums become puffy, tender, and bleed easily as a result of inadequate vitamin C. The oral membranes become susceptible to canker sores when vitamins C and niacin are undersupplied.

The tongue of a healthy person is smooth and an even red color. Geographic tongue occurs from a prolonged deficiency of the B vitamins; the taste buds clump together and create fissures and ridges. Inadequate B_2 can discolor the tongue turning it purplish, and insufficient niacin can color it bright red; a smooth shiny tongue indicates a B_{12} or folic acid deficiency. An enlarged beefy-looking tongue can result from a lack of pantothenic acid. If putrefactive bacteria is allowed to grow in the intestinal tract, the condition can be reflected as a coated tongue. Including acidophilus in the diet will aid the growth of beneficial bacteria as well as create a medium for the manufacture of the B vitamins.

NUTRIENTS THAT MAY BE BENEFICIAL IN TREATMENT OF MOUTH AND TONGUE DISORDERS

Body Member	Nutrients	Quantity
Mouth	Vitamin B complex	
	Vitamin C	
	Acidophilus	

MULTIPLE SCLEROSIS

Multiple sclerosis is a chronic disease that causes the deterioration of the protective covering of the nerves in the brain and spinal cord, resulting in the hardening of various parts of the nervous system and the development of scars or lesions on the disturbed nerves. The cause of the disease is unknown, although it has been seen to follow malnutrition, emotional stress, and infections.

Autopsy studies have shown a great deficiency of lecithin in the brain and the myelin sheath that covers the nerves. The small amounts of lecithin that were present were abnormal, containing saturated instead of unsaturated fatty acids. Nutrients that are necessary for the manufacture of lecithin are probably needed by the MS patient, including vitamins B_6, choline, inositol, the essential fatty acids, and magnesium. Also of special interest is the fact that a deficiency of magnesium in normal persons results in muscle spasms, weakness, twitching, and inability to control the bladder, all characteristics of MS.

Pregnant women deficient in linolenic acid can pass the same defect to the fetus, making the brain and spinal cord susceptible to the destruction of the sheaths around their nerve fibers. The defect may not manifest until the child is fifteen or sixteen years old, when the brain has fully developed.

An inherited need for vitamin D may lead to MS. The vitamin is vital for the proper development of the nervous system, and poorly constructed neural tissues may break down in later years. Calcium is depen-

dent on vitamin D for its ultilization. Long-term sufferers of MS cannot benefit from the vitamin; however, in the young patient starting to exhibit symptoms, it may possibly slow or even stop the progress of the disease.

Multiple sclerosis usually occurs in persons between the ages of twenty-five and forty. The disease progresses slowly and may disappear for periods of time but returns intermittently, usually in a more severe form. Symptoms of the disease include visual and speech disturbances, dizziness, bowel and bladder disorders, weakness, lack of coordination, paralysis, loss of balance, and emotional instability.

Dr. Frederick Klenner of Reidsville, North Carolina, uses massive doses of the B vitamins as well as other nutrients, including minerals, unsaturated fatty acids, and amino acids, to treat MS.

Vitamin B_{12} has been used to increase stability in standing and walking in some cases of the disease.[32]

The seed oils, especially safflower, sunflower, corn, soybean, and primrose (all rich in linolenic acid), are a source of the unsaturated fatty acids, which are important for the development and integrity of the brain and spinal cord. Daily supplements of 2 tablespoons of seed oil have been reported to reduce the severity and increase the period of remission in MS persons.

A diet rich in seed oils, fish, vegetables, fruits, whole grains, and vitamin and mineral supplements (minerals preferably in the orotate form) and very limited in saturated fats, sugar, and processed foods is extremely beneficial for the MS patient. Allergies to particular foods should be taken into consideration and the offending food eliminated from the diet; gluten in wheat is a common offender. Adequate rest and exercise are especially important for the MS patient, to relieve fatigue. Constipation can be alleviated by drinking adequate amounts of water and following a diet high in unrefined roughage foods.

Alcohol and smoking should be avoided. Alcohol interferes with unsaturated fatty acid conversion, increases the saturated-fat blood count, destroys various B vitamins, and worsens MS symptoms. Smoking adversely affects a diet high in unsaturated fatty acids, lowers blood levels of vitamin C, and temporarily worsens MS symptoms.

A neurologist at the University of Oregon Health

[32]Prevention Magazine Staff, *Complete Book of Vitamins*, p. 257.

Sciences Center in Portland has been successfully treating MS patients with a daily high-potency vitamin supplement and minerals and a controlled diet. High-fat foods are eliminated and replaced with foods containing unsaturated fatty acids. Foods such as packaged cake mixes, cheeses, pastries, and other processed items are also not consumed, because they contain hidden or unknown quantities of saturated fat. The doctor also advises his patients to eat whole-grain breads and cereals and to take wheat germ or vitamin E to keep the unsaturated oils from being oxidized once inside the body. Observed results of the patients have been a reduction in relapses, more energy, the ability to continue walking and working, and an increase in life expectancy. Also, when the treatment was started in the early stages of the disease with little evident disability, 90 to 95 percent of the cases remained unchanged or improved during the following 20 years.[33]

NUTRIENTS THAT MAY BE BENEFICIAL IN TREATMENT OF MULTIPLE SCLEROSIS

Body Member	Nutrients	Quantity*
Brain/Nervous system	Vitamin B complex	
	Vitamin B_1	100 mg
	Vitamin B_2	150 mg
	Vitamin B_6	100–200 mg
	Vitamin B_{12}	
	Choline	700–1400 mg
	Niacin	100 mg
	Pangamic acid	
	Pantothenic acid	100 mg
	Vitamin C	Up to 1000 mg
	Vitamin E	Up to 1800 IU
	Calcium	
	Copper	
	Iron	
	Magnesium	
	Manganese	
	Selenium	
	Zinc	
	Protein	

[33]Roy Swank, *The Multiple Sclerosis Diet Book* (New York: Doubleday, 1977).

Body Member	Nutrients	Quantity*
	Unsaturated fatty acids	2 tbsp
	Lecithin	3 tbsp or more
	Primrose oil	2 capsules three times daily

*See note, p. 222.

MUSCLE WEAKNESS

Strong and normally functioning muscles are reflected in an individual's carriage and grace of movement. Weak muscles can be seen in every age group, from the wobbly neck of the infant to the stoop of all ages. Muscle tone that is under par interferes with blood circulation, lymph flow, and digestion and often causes constipation. Weak muscles of the internal organs result in their sagging, interfering with their particular functions.

Muscles are largely made up of protein and essential fatty acids; however, almost every nutrient is involved in their contraction, relaxation, and repair. For example, potassium, very low in diets of high fats and refined foods, is necessary for the contraction of every muscle in the body. Besides a poor diet, a potassium deficiency can be brought on by stress, diarrhea, kidney damage, diuretics, or cortisone therapy. The results of insufficient amounts of the mineral are fatigue, gas distention, spasms or twisting of the bowel, constipation, and possibly inability to pass urine.

Vitamin E is essential for the formation of the nuclei of muscle cells and of enzymes that are needed for muscular contractions. A deficiency of the vitamin increases the need for oxygen in the muscles, interferes with the metabolism of certain amino acids, and causes the loss of phosphorus in the urine and the B vitamins by rancidity. In addition, too much calcium is left to settle in muscle tissue. Pregnant women often have difficult deliveries because of the lack of enzymes needed for muscle contraction. A deficiency can also be suspected if a child cannot sit up well at three months old.

NUTRIENTS THAT MAY BE BENEFICIAL IN TREATMENT OF MUSCLE WEAKNESS

Body Member	Nutrient	Quantity
Muscle	Vitamin E	
	Manganese	
	Potassium	
	Zinc	
	Unsaturated fatty acids	
	Protein	
	All essential nutrients	

MUSCULAR DYSTROPHY

There are five major and three less common types of muscular dystrophy, each with its own pathology; one form may affect persons at a specific age, another involves the degeneration of a specific muscle area in the body. Some forms may stop progressing, but so far none have gone into complete remission. The disease is currently considered to be largely hereditary except for one type that occurs in adults around the ages of forty or fifty.

In dystrophic tissue, the oxygen requirement is tremendously increased, many enzymes necessary for muscle function are greatly reduced, and the essential fatty acids that form the structural part of the muscle are destroyed. The cell membrane becomes increasingly permeable, allowing nutrients to leak out into the blood. Eventually the muscles are replaced by scar tissue.

Some time before muscular dystrophy can be detected, amino acids and a substance called creatine are lost in the urine. This indicates that muscle tissue is breaking down. If the degeneration has not advanced too far, the administration of vitamin E has prevented further progression. It is speculated that the hereditary factor of the disease may be an abnormally high genetic requirement for vitamin E, which is essential for the formation of the nucleus of every cell.

The major symptom is great weakness in the legs and back, so that the patient has trouble walking. The weakness gradually progresses throughout the muscles of the body, creating partial, then total, paralysis.

In animal studies, dystrophy has been produced from a deficiency of protein and vitamins A, B_6, E, and choline. Vitamin E and choline, found primarily in the germ of cereals, are easily deficient in diets of refined foods because of their removal during the refining process. (They are not replaced as are some nutrients.) Chlorine in drinking water and rancid fats also destroy vitamin E.

The diet of a person with muscular dystrophy (and for the pregnant woman as well) should be adequate in all essential nutrients including complete proteins and vegetable oils. In the early stages, muscular wasting may be arrested and remissions prolonged. In others, the disease may not worsen and often improvements, including muscle strength, can be observed without complete recovery.

NUTRIENTS THAT MAY BE BENEFICIAL IN TREATMENT OF MUSCULAR DYSTROPHY

Body Member	Nutrients	Quantity
Muscles	Vitamin A	
	Vitamin B complex	
	Vitamin B_6	
	Vitamin B_{12}	
	Choline	
	Niacin	
	Pantothenic acid	
	Vitamin C	
	Vitamin E	
	Potassium	
	Protein	
	Unsaturated fatty acids	

MYASTHENIA GRAVIS

Myasthenia gravis affects muscles in any part of the body but most often the muscles of the face and neck. In the disease, there is an underproduction of acetylcholine, a compound that transmits nerve impulses to the muscles. It is characterized by exhaustion and progressive paralysis. Symptoms include double vision, drooping eyelids, choking, and difficulty in breathing, swallowing, and talking (imperfect articulation, stammering, and stuttering).

Recovery from this ailment has occurred in many cases if the diet is adequate. Many nutrients are needed for the production of acetylcholine, including the vitamin B complex, protein, and potassium. Vitamin E aids the utilization of acetylcholine; if the vitamin is undersupplied, acetylcholine is destroyed by oxygen. Manganese is a component of certain enzymes that are involved in muscle contraction.

NUTRIENTS THAT MAY BE BENEFICIAL IN TREATMENT OF MYASTHENIA GRAVIS

Body Member	Nutrients	Quantity
Muscles	Vitamin B complex	
	Vitamin B_1	
	Vitamin B_2	
	Vitamin B_6	
	Vitamin B_{12}	
	Choline	
	Folic acid	
	Inositol	
	Pantothenic acid	
	Vitamin C	
	Vitamin E	
	Magnesium	
	Manganese	
	Potassium	
	Sodium—for a short period	
	Protein	
	Lecithin	

NAIL PROBLEMS

Nails are composed almost entirely of protein. Abnormal or unhealthy nails may be the result of a local injury, a glandular deficiency such as hypothyroidism, or a deficiency of certain nutrients.

A protein deficiency can cause opaque white bands to appear on the nails or cause them to become dry, brittle, and very thin. Insufficient amounts of complete proteins and/or vitamin A slow down the rate of nail growth (which is also affected by various drugs). A shortage of vitamin A or calcium in the diet may also cause dryness and brittleness. A lack of the B vitamins causes nails to become fragile, with horizontal or vertical ridges appearing. The B complex is also

a factor in fungus infestation found underneath the nails. Frequent hangnails usually indicate an inadequate intake of vitamins C and folic acid and protein. An iron deficiency can disturb the growth of the nails, causing dryness, brittleness, thinning, flattening, and eventually the appearance of moon-shaped nails. White spots can be caused by a zinc deficiency.

Any nail abnormality indicates that the diet is not adequate; a well-balanced diet supplying all essential nutrients is recommended.

NUTRIENTS THAT MAY BE BENEFICIAL IN TREATMENT OF NAIL PROBLEMS

Body Member	Nutrients	Quantity
Nails	Vitamin A	
	Vitamin B complex	
	Folic acid	
	Vitamin C	
	Calcium	
	Iron	
	Zinc	
	Protein	

NAUSEA AND VOMITING

Nausea and vomiting can indicate the presence of many diseases including an infected appendix, low blood sugar, or food poisoning. If the symptoms persist, a physician should be consulted.

Both illnesses have been produced by a deficiency of magnesium or vitamin B_6. If caused by vitamin B_6, butterflies and burning stomach pain, bloating, abdominal soreness and cramps, and the passing of gas both orally and rectally will accompany the sickness.

Vitamin B_6 has been successfully used to alleviate the nausea and vomiting of pregnancy and radiation and motion (car, sea, air) sickness. Vomiting babies may also be helped by magnesium and yeast or wheat germ (vitamin B_6 sources).

NUTRIENTS THAT MAY BE BENEFICIAL IN TREATMENT OF NAUSEA AND VOMITING

Body Member	Nutrients	Quantity
Stomach	Vitamin B complex	
	Vitamin B_6	
	Magnesium	

NEPHRITIS (KIDNEY INFECTION)

Nephritis is the inflammation of one or both of the kidneys. The most common form of nephritis, pyelonephritis, occurs among females, especially during childhood or pregnancy. It is caused by bacteria from the stools being introduced into the urinary opening by wiping in a forward direction. The bacteria then travel to the bladder and finally to the kidney. Another form of nephritis, glomerulonephritis, occurs as a reaction to an infection elsewhere in the body, such as an infection in the throat. The disease can also be caused by drugs, particularly those containing aspirin and other painkillers. Environmental pollutants such as bichloride of mercury, other heavy metals, and carbon tetrachloride can adversely affect the kidneys.

Symptoms of nephritis may be nonexistent, or they may include blood and/or albumin in the urine, fatigue, lower back or abdominal pain, fever, chills, edema, nausea and vomiting, loss of appetite, and frequent urge to urinate. Anemia and high blood pressure may accompany severe nephritis.

Nephritis has been produced in animals deficient in choline. The capillaries are damaged and severe hemorrhages occur; urine formation is decreased and circulation is inhibited. Insufficient vitamin E can result in tubules plugged with dead cells, decreasing the amount of urine that can pass.

Medical treatment of nephritis includes antibiotics, bed rest, and increased fluid intake. Kidney function has markedly improved when vitamin A has been taken. Vitamin E protects the kidneys from toxic substances, prevents scarring, and increases the flow of urine. Zinc supplements will replace the zinc removed from the urine by albumen. Because cortisone is often given for nephritis, nutrients that increase the body's natural production of cortisone, including the B complex, pantothenic acid, vitamin C, and complete protein, are recommended.

NUTRIENTS THAT MAY BE BENEFICIAL IN TREATMENT OF NEPHRITIS

Body Member	Nutrients	Quantity*
Kidney	Vitamin A	50,000–75,000 IU
	Vitamin B complex	
	Vitamin B$_2$	25 mg
	Vitamin B$_{12}$	
	Choline	1000 mg
	Folic acid	
	Inositol	
	Pantothenic acid	
	Vitamin C	
	Vitamin E	300–600 IU
	Calcium	250 mg
	Iron	
	Magnesium	
	Water	
	Protein	
	Lecithin	

*See note, p. 222.

NEURITIS

Neuritis is the inflammation or deterioration of a nerve or group of nerves. Symptoms of neuritis vary with its cause. Some symptoms are pain, tenderness, tingling and loss of the sensation of touch in the affected nerve area, redness and swelling of the affected areas, and in severe cases, convulsions.

Causes of neuritis include injury to a nerve, such as in a direct blow or a nearby bone fracture; infection involving a nerve; diseases such as diabetes, gout, and leukemia; poisons such as mercury, lead, or methyl alcohol; and dietary deficiency of the vitamin B complex, especially thiamine. A thiamine deficiency results in the impairment of nerve tissue so that it cannot properly utilize carbohydrates for energy. Sometimes neuritis may be purely mechanical, caused by pressure on the nerves when sleeping in a cramped position or possibly from a too soft mattress.

Treatment for neuritis also varies with the cause. If neuritis is caused by poisons, exposure to them should be ended, and if it is caused by a specific disease or trauma, treatment should be given. When a thiamine of vitamin B complex deficiency is responsible, administration of these vitamins will result in recovery within 3 to 4 days. Adequate intake of the B vitamins is necessary even when a deficiency does not exist, since they are needed for the general health of nerve tissue.

A well-balanced diet is important to the individual

with neuritis for the maintenance and repair of muscles and nerves. If infection is present, protein, calorie, and fluid intake should be increased.

NUTRIENTS THAT MAY BE BENEFICIAL IN TREATMENT OF NEURITIS

Body Member	Nutrients	Quantity*
Nervous system	Vitamin B complex	
	Vitamin B_1	
	Vitamin B_2	
	Vitamin B_6	100–300 mg
	Vitamin B_{12}	
	Niacin	
	Pantothenic acid	
	Calcium	
	Magnesium	
	Protein	

*See note, p. 222.

OSTEOPOROSIS (BRITTLE BONES)

Osteoporosis is a reduction in the total mass of bone, with the remaining bone being fragile or "brittle." Symptoms of the disorder include increased incidence of fractures, pains in the hip and back, and reduced height. Osteoporosis is primarily a disease of the aged, usually beginning at about age fifty.

A major cause of osteoporosis is an inadequate intake of calcium over a period of years. Other causes are inability to absorb sufficient calcium through the intestine, calcium-phosphorus imbalance, lack of exercise, or lack of certain hormones.

A diet that is adequate in protein, calcium, magnesium, phosphorus, vitamin C, and vitamin D is the best prevention and treatment for osteoporosis. Trace amounts of fluorides from foods or drinking water also protect against bone decomposition. Some form of physical activity is also recommended.

NUTRIENTS THAT MAY BE BENEFICIAL IN TREATMENT OF OSTEOPOROSIS

Body Member	Nutrients	Quantity*
Bones	Vitamin B_{12}	30–900 mcg
	Vitamin C	Up to 1000 mg
	Vitamin D	Up to 5000 IU
	Vitamin E	600 IU
	Calcium	1–2 gm
	Copper	
	Fluoride	
	Magnesium	500–1000 mg
	Phosphorus	
	Protein	

*See note, p. 222.

OVERWEIGHT AND OBESITY

Overweight and obesity are one of the major nutritional problems in America today. Statistics show that people of average weight (see the "Desirable Height and Weight Chart," p. 310) have a longer lifespan, have more energy, and usually feel better than those people who are overweight. Overweight and obesity precipitate such conditions as heart disease, kidney trouble, diabetes, high blood pressure, malnutrition, complications of pregnancy, and psychological problems. Glandular malfunctions, malnutrition, emotional tension, boredom, habit, and love of food are some causes of overweight.

It is very likely that malnutrition is the main cause of overweight. When there is inadequate intake of all essential nutrients, fat is not readily or efficiently burned. Fat is burned only if sufficient energy is produced. Energy production depends upon almost every known nutrient. The B vitamins are important for energy production. Fat is burned at a greatly reduced rate if pantothenic acid and protein are undersupplied. Vitamin B_6 is necessary for the energy conversion of stored fat. It is also a factor in the utilization of protein and fat. Proteins are needed for the proper functioning of many energy-producing enzymes. Protein itself cannot be effectively used without many other nutrients, including choline and vitamin B_6. Sufficient vitamin E doubles fat utilization. Lecithin aids the cells to burn fat; any deficiency of the nutrients necessary for lecithin production, specifically choline and inositol, results in poor fat utilization.

Liver damage is common in overweight persons. When the liver is injured, sufficient amounts of energy-producing enzymes are unable to be synthesized. A diet including complete proteins, the vitamins B complex, choline, B_{12}, C, and E and lecithin aid the restoration of the liver.

Some individuals who experience an uncontrollable hunger may have damaged brain cells in the hypothalamus, the area that regulates the desire to eat. This damage can occur from certain food, or foods or environmental substances to which the person is allergic. Certain medications such as tranquilizers, viral infections, nutritional deficiencies, or other brain injuries can also adversely affect these cells. Other persons may have the desire for a specific food to which they have an allergic addiction. If they do not obtain this food, they experience typical withdrawal reactions. In both situations, a diet high in all essential nutrients and avoidance of the offending substance can gradually result in weight reduction.

Calories and exercise are essential considerations in losing weight. Fat is metabolically formed in the body when more food energy or calories are consumed than the body is able to use. One pound of fatty tissue is equal to 3500 calories. When the number of calories used during the day exceeds the amount consumed, the body oxidizes its supplies of fat to produce energy, and thereby a reduction of body weight results. A daily decrease of 1000 calories results in approximately 2 pounds of weight loss per week. Calories may be burned up by the basal metabolism, which includes normal body functions such as breathing and digestion. All activity, such as walking, talking, working, or playing baseball, uses up additional energy and calories. For example, one hour of average office work probably used up only 10 to 15 calories, whereas moderate housework may require 70 calories per hour more than basal metabolism requirements. Brisk walking uses up about 110 calories per hour; driving a car uses about 40. Strenuous exercise and hard physical labor may require more than 400 calories per hour.

Research appears to indicate that it is not entirely the amount of food eaten that adds weight but the kind of food eaten. Unrefined foods contain all nutrients that are necessary for efficient energy production. Refined foods, however, not only lack most of these nutrients but tremendously increase the body's requirement for them.

In order to lose weight safely, a person must set up a sensible long-range diet plan that includes all the essential nutrients and minerals. Diets that lack or greatly reduce one or another of the nutrients, notably carbohydrates, can possibly be injurious to the body by inducing an abnormal metabolic state that could cause innumerable complications leading to permanent cellular damage. Carbohydrates should be chosen from the best nutritional sources, such as whole-grain products and fruits that contain essential nutrients. Fat intake should come primarily from sources of unsaturated fatty acids and from such animal fats as butter and whole milk, which are good sources of fat-soluble vitamins. Excess fat is hard to metabolize and can upset liver and kidney functions. In general, losing weight is a matter of consciously curbing the amount of food eaten, regulating the types of food eaten, and increasing daily activity.

NUTRIENTS THAT MAY BE BENEFICIAL IN TREATMENT OF OVERWEIGHT AND OBESITY

Body Member	Nutrients	Quantity*
	Vitamin B complex	
	Vitamin B_2	
	Vitamin B_6	Up to 100 mg
	Vitamin B_{12}	
	Choline	
	Folic acid	
	Inositol	500 mg
	Pantothenic acid	
	Vitamin C	Up to 1000 mg
	Vitamin E	Up to 600 IU
	Calcium	500–1000 mg
	Magnesium	250–500 mg
	Phosphorus	
	Protein	
	Lecithin	
	Unsaturated fatty acids	

*See note, p. 222.

PANCREATITIS

Pancreatitis is an inflammation of the pancreas, a long slender organ that secretes insulin and digestive enzymes. When the inflammation is mild, the small duct that leads from the pancreas to the small intestine becomes swollen, and digestive enzymes are not able to pass through. When the pancreas is severely inflamed, it is no longer able to produce these enzymes, greatly interfering with digestion and causing many nutrients to remain unabsorbed.

The illness is difficult to treat because so many nutrients needed for healing are lost as a result of poor absorption. Much gas is formed and often hemorrhages in the pancreas, the kidney, and the eyes occur. Pancreatic cells that are damaged are replaced by scar tissue that eventually becomes calcified. Persons with the disease store abnormally high amounts of iron, a characteristic of a B_6 deficiency.

Pancreatitis has been brought about by stress, an inadequate diet, a deficiency of vitamin B_6 or protein, various drugs and chemicals, and also as a result of cortisone therapy. The diet of a person who has pancreatitis should be made adequate in all nutrients. Digestive enzymes are essential with every meal; if gas still forms, more enzymes are needed. Oils may be eaten, but solid fats should be avoided. Yogurt or acidophilus milk, which is mostly predigested, is recommended.

NUTRIENTS THAT MAY BE BENEFICIAL IN TREATMENT OF PANCREATITIS

Body Member	Nutrients	Quantity*
Pancreas	Vitamin B complex	
	Vitamin B_6	60 mg
	Vitamin E	300 IU
	Digestive enzymes	
	Lecithin	
	Acidophilus	

*See note, p. 222.

PARKINSON'S DISEASE

Parkinson's disease, also called shaking palsy or paralysis agitans, is a slowly progressive disease of the nervous system in which an essential type of nerve cell is destroyed. The cause of the disease is unknown, but symptoms begin when there is an imbalance of two chemicals in the brain, dopamine and acetylcholine. These substances transfer messages between nerve cells that control muscle function. In Parkinsonism, the amount of dopamine is diminished, the imbalance is created, and nerve signals become confused.

Symptoms of Parkinson's disease include muscular rigidity and cramping, involuntary tremors that include a characteristic pill-rolling movement of the thumb and forefinger as they rub against each other, impaired speech, a staring facial expression, drooling, and a short, shuffling gait. Despite these symptoms, sensation and mental activity are not impaired. There is often a loss of appetite and some weight loss, giving rise to the possibility of malnutrition developing. Chronic constipation may complicate the condition.

There is no cure for the disease, although drugs may be used to alleviate the symptoms. L-Dopa, a drug most often used to reestablish balance with acetylcholine, has many side effects. Vitamin C may help to alleviate these reactions. The B vitamins, especially B_6, tend to diminish the effectiveness of L-Dopa. However, Adelle Davis, in her book *Let's Get Well*, reported that vitamin B_6, given along with the other B vitamins and magnesium, has resulted in progressive improvement. Patients begin to feel stronger, walk with a steadier gait, have better bladder control, a greater sense of well-being, better mental alertness, and a decrease in muscular cramps, trembling, and rigidity. Zinc may also be needed to make sure the B_6 does not interfere with the effect of the drug L-Dopa. Sometimes improvement is not noticed in persons who have had a severe case of the disease for several years.

Modification of the diet and treatment of the constipation may also be helpful. Frequent small meals will increase the patient's nutrient and caloric levels, thus preventing malnutrition. A marked increase in fluid intake is also necessary because the normal secretions of the intestines may be lessened by some of the prescribed drugs. High-residue food will assist in alleviating constipation.

NUTRIENTS THAT MAY BE BENEFICIAL IN TREATMENT OF PARKINSON'S DISEASE

Body Member	Nutrients	Quantity*
Brain/Nervous system	Vitamin B complex	
	Vitamin B_2	Up to 100 mg
	Vitamin B_6	10–200 mg
	Niacin	
	Vitamin C	Up to 1000 mg
	Vitamin E	600 IU

*See note, p. 222.

Body Member	Nutrients	Quantity*
	Calcium	
	Magnesium	500 mg
	Glutamic acid	
	Protein	

*See note, p. 222.

PELLAGRA

Pellagra is a disease caused by a deficiency of the B vitamins, particularly riboflavin, niacin, and thiamine. The disease occurs frequently in populations whose diets consist mainly of corn. Although the disease is seldom found in the United States, its rare occurrence affects persons with gastrointestinal disturbances or chronic alcoholism.

Symptoms of pellagra are diarrhea, loss of appetite and weight, reddened and swollen tongue, weakness, depression, and anxiety. Itchy dermatitis on the hands and neck is a prominent characteristic of the disease.

A diet that is adequate in the B vitamins and protein will prevent pellagra. A diet rich in the B vitamins niacin, thiamine, riboflavin, folic acid, and vitamin B_{12} will cure the disease.

NUTRIENTS THAT MAY BE BENEFICIAL IN TREATMENT OF PELLAGRA

Body Member	Nutrients	Quantity
Skin	Vitamin B complex	
	Vitamin B_1	
	Vitamin B_2	
	Vitamin B_{12}	
	Folic acid	
	Niacin	
	Protein	
	Tryptophan	

PERNICIOUS ANEMIA

Pernicious anemia is a form of anemia resulting from a deficiency of vitamin B_{12}. It is a severe form of anemia in which there is a gradual reduction in the number of blood cells because the bone marrow fails to produce mature red blood cells. Pernicious anemia probably arises from an inheritable inability of the stomach to secrete a substance called the "intrinsic factor," which is necessary for the intestinal absorption of vitamin B_{12}.

Pernicious anemia occurs in both sexes. Its occurrence is rare in persons under the age of thirty, but susceptibility increases with age. Symptoms of pernicious anemia include weakness and gastrointestinal disturbances causing a sore tongue, slight yellowing of the skin, and tingling of extremities. In addition, disturbances of the nervous system, such as partial loss of coordination of the fingers, feet, and legs; some nerve deterioration; and disturbances of the digestive tract, such as diarrhea and loss of appetite, may occur.

Pernicious anemia may be fatal without treatment. Vitamin B_{12} injections together with a highly nutritious diet supplemented with large amounts of desiccated liver are the recommended treatment. Intake of the entire vitamin B complex will help maintain the health of the nervous system, although folic acid should not be taken in amounts exceeding 0.1 milligram daily. Folic acid has the effect of concealing the symptoms of pernicious anemia, allowing the unseen destruction of the nervous system to continue until irreparable damage is done. A diet rich in protein, calcium, vitamin C, vitamin E, and iron is recommended. If iron, vitamin C, and hydrocloric acid are taken with each meal to ensure absorption, the production of the intrinsic factor may be stimulated enough so that persons with a mild case of the disease can decrease the doses of vitamin B_{12}.

NUTRIENTS THAT MAY BE BENEFICIAL IN TREATMENT OF PERNICIOUS ANEMIA

Body Member	Nutrients	Quantity*
Blood/ Circulatory system	Vitamin B complex	
	Vitamin B_6	50–100 mg
	Vitamin B_{12}	50–100 mcg in injections
	Folic acid	
	Vitamin C	
	Vitamin E	
	Calcium	
	Cobalt	
	Protein	

*See note, p. 222.

PHLEBITIS

Phlebitis, the inflammation of a vein wall, is usually found in the legs and can be a complication of varicose veins. Symptoms of phlebitis include reddening and cordlike swelling of the vein, increased pulse rate, slight fever, and pain accompanying movement of the afflicted area.

A complication that may occur in individuals with phlebitis is thrombophlebitis, the formation of a clot in the inflamed vein. If this clot should break loose from the vein wall and lodge in a blood vessel that supplies some vital area with blood, serious and possibly fatal damage may occur. In some cases, the use of oral contraceptives has been related to the occurrence of thrombophlebitis.

Factors that seem to encourage the onset of phlebitis are operations, especially in the lower abdomen, childbirth, and infections resulting from injuries to veins. Phlebitis can be prevented by the treatment of varicose veins so that inflammation does not set in. Infections in the legs or feet, especially fungus infections of the toes, should be given immediate attention as a safeguard against phlebitis. Regular exercise is a further preventive measure.

Supplementing the diet with niacin, part of the vitamin B complex, may be useful to help prevent clot formation. Vitamin C can help strengthen the blood vessel walls. Some research indicates that vitamin E may dilate blood vessels, thus discouraging the formation of varicose veins and phlebitis.

NUTRIENTS THAT MAY BE BENEFICIAL IN TREATMENT OF PHLEBITIS

Body Member	Nutrients	Quantity*
Blood/Circulatory system/Legs	Vitamin B complex	
	Niacin	
	Pantothenic acid	100 mg
	Vitamin C	5–25 gm
	Vitamin E	200–600 IU

*See note, p. 222.

PNEUMONIA

Pneumonia is an ailment in which the tiny air sacs in the lungs become inflamed and filled with mucus

and pus. The primary causes of pneumonia are bacteria, viruses, chemical irritants, and allergies. Factors that contribute to the onset of pneumonia are colds, alcoholism, malnutrition, and foreign matter in the respiratory passages. Symptoms of the disease vary from mild to severe, but they usually include sharp pains in the chest, fever and chills, fatigue, rapid respiration, and cough.

Vitamin A is necessary for maintaining the health of the lining of the respiratory passages. A deficiency of the vitamin increases susceptibility to respiratory infections, which in turn can lead to pneumonia. Since protein loss accompanies high fever and because protein is necessary for the repair of body tissue, its intake should be increased during pneumonia. Water and fluid intake should be increased to prevent dehydration that can result from fever and perspiration. Vitamin C intake is required to fight infection. Because deficiency of the vitamin B complex usually occurs with pneumonia, an increased intake is necessary. Some research shows a correlation between vitamin E deficiency and lung disease.

NUTRIENTS THAT MAY BE BENEFICIAL IN TREATMENT OF PNEUMONIA

Body Member	Nutrients	Quantity*
Lungs/ Respiratory system	Vitamin A	
	Vitamin B complex	
	Vitamin C	500 mg every 90 minutes
	Vitamin D	
	Vitamin E	
	Vitamin K	
	Bioflavonoids	
	Protein	

*See note, p. 222.

POLIO

Polio is a virus infection of the spinal cord which destroys the nerves controlling muscular movement, resulting in paralysis of certain mucles. There are two stages of this disease: the infectious stage, when the virus is active, and the noninfectious, or recovery, stage. Symptoms of the infectious stage include fever, nausea, diarrhea, headache, and irritability.

During the infectious stage, the diet of the polio patient should be high in protein and potassium to replace that which is lost because of the rapid tissue destruction. Caloric intake should also be increased because of the increased energy expenditure during fever, and additional B vitamins are necessary to help metabolize the additional calories. Fever creates the need for additional sodium because of the loss that occurs with perspiration. Fluid intake should also be increased during fever to compensate for loss and to dilute toxic substances produced by the virus. Fever and the accompanying increase in metabolism also increase the need for vitamins A and C.

Dr. Frederick Klenner of Reidsville, North Carolina, has used massive amounts of vitamin C (injections) in treating polio. Calcium should accompany vitamin C treatment because it increases the effectiveness.

NUTRIENTS THAT MAY BE BENEFICIAL IN TREATMENT OF POLIO

Body Member	Nutrients	Quantity
Brain/Nervous system	Vitamin A	
	Vitamin B complex	
	Vitamin C	
	Calcium	
	Magnesium	
	Potassium	
	Sodium	
	Protein	

PROSTATITIS

Prostatitis is the inflammation of the prostate, a male sex gland. The usual cause of prostatitis in young men is a bacterial infection from another area of the body which has invaded the prostate. Prostatic enlargement, which is usually found in older males, is often due to gradual enlargement over a period of several years.

Symptoms of acute prostatitis are pain between the scrotum and rectum, fever, frequent urination accompanied by a burning sensation, and blood or pus in the urine. Symptoms of long-term prostatitis are frequent and burning urination, lower back pain, and

premature ejaculation, or loss of potency. As prostatitis becomes more advanced, urination becomes increasingly difficult.

Treatment for prostatitis involves increasing the fluid intake to meet the increased needs during infection and to stimulate urine flow, thus preventing retention of urine. Urinary retention can result in cystitis and possibly in a kidney infection. Increased protein and calories are needed during fever and infection, to replace lost body tissues and energy. A well-balanced diet rich in vitamin A, the B complex, and vitamin C is also important during fever and infection. Adding pollen to the diet has resulted in substantial improvement for many people. The reason is not exactly known, but it may be due to the magnesium, zinc, unsaturated fatty acid, and sex hormone content of the pollen. Some sources advocate the avoidance of alcoholic beverages, spicy foods, and exposure to very cold weather if prostatitis is present.[34]

NUTRIENTS THAT MAY BE BENEFICIAL IN TREATMENT OF PROSTATITIS

Body Member	Nutrients	Quantity*
Gland, prostate	Vitamin A	
	Vitamin B complex	
	Vitamin B$_6$	
	Vitamin C	100–5000 mg
	Vitamin E	600 IU
	Magnesium	
	Zinc	
	Unsaturated fatty acids	2 T.
	Protein	
	Water	

*See note, p. 222.

PRURITUS ANI

Pruritus ani is a form of contact dermatitis characterized by an itching or burning of the rectum. This area is covered and often moist, which are good conditions for germ and fungi growth. Moisture in the rectal area is often present because its sweat glands are connected to the sexual glandular system. These sweat glands are highly responsive to emotion or sexual

[34]Robert E. Rothenberg, *Health in the Later Years,* rev. ed. (New York: Signet Books, 1972), p. 499.

excitation and a large amount of perspiration is released. This moisture, high in protein and carbohydrates, is a favorable environment for bacterial growth. The moisture can also cause the release of dyes from clothing worn in this region, which can aggravate the condition.

Pruritus ani has been associated with a deficiency of vitamins A and B complex and iron. Diabetic persons often have this rash because of the high sugar content of the skin; sugar is another good breeding ground for fungal growth.

The diet should be adequate in the B vitamins, vitamin A, and iron. Acidophilus may be helpful. Excessive amounts of citrus juices should possibly be avoided. The area should be kept as dry as possible and clean hygiene habits followed.

NUTRIENTS THAT MAY BE BENEFICIAL IN TREATMENT OF PRURITUS ANI

Body Member	Nutrients	Quantity
Rectum	Vitamin A	
	Vitamin B complex	
	Iron	
	Acidophilus	

PSORIASIS

Psoriasis, a recurring disease, is characterized by eruptions on the skin of red circular patches of all sizes covered with dry, silvery scales. The patches enlarge slowly, forming more extensive patches. Psoriasis appears mainly on the legs, arms, scalp, ears, and lower back. It appears that psoriasis may result from a faulty utilization of fats.

Exposure to sunlight or ultraviolet light reduces the scaling and redness of psoriasis. A reduction in animal protein and fat intake can be useful for treating psoriasis. Vitamin A, the B complex, vitamin C, and vitamin D, all of which play a part in skin health, have been found to be useful in treating some cases of the disease. Some researchers have also found vitamin E to be effective in healing psoriasis.[35]

[35]Prevention Magazine Staff, *Complete Book of Vitamins*, p. 389.

NUTRIENTS THAT MAY BE BENEFICIAL IN TREATMENT OF PSORIASIS

Body Member	Nutrients	Quantity*
Skin	Vitamin A	Up to 100,000 IU during first week; reduce to 25,000 IU for 3 months; repeat; ointment in the acid form
	Vitamin B complex	
	Vitamin B_2	
	Vitamin B_6	100–200 mg
	Vitamin B_{12}	
	Folic acid	
	Pantothenic acid	
	Vitamin C	Up to 3000 mg
	Vitamin D	
	Vitamin E	Up to 1600 IU
	Bioflavonoids	
	Magnesium	
	Sulfur	Ointment
	Zinc	
	Lecithin	3 tbsp
	Unsaturated fatty acids	

*See note, p. 222.

PYORRHEA (SORE GUMS)

Pyorrhea is an infectious disease of the gums and tooth sockets characterized by the formation of pus and usually by loosening of the teeth. Gum disorders such as puffiness, tenderness, soreness, and bleeding are often related to vitamin C and bioflavonoid deficiencies that cause increased capillary fragility. Sore gums may also indicate a niacin deficiency. All nutrients that fight infection and rebuild bones should be emphasized.

NUTRIENTS THAT MAY BE BENEFICIAL IN TREATMENT OF PYORRHEA

Body Member	Nutrients	Quantity*
Teeth/Gums	Vitamin A	
	Vitamin B complex	
	Vitamin B$_1$	
	Vitamin B$_2$	
	Vitamin B$_6$	
	Biotin	
	Folic acid	
	Niacin	300 mg
	Pantothenic acid	
	Vitamin C	1–3 gm
	Vitamin D	
	Bioflavonoids	300 mg
	Calcium	
	Magnesium	
	Manganese	
	Zinc	
	Protein	

*See note, p. 222.

RHEUMATIC FEVER

Rheumatic fever is an infection, caused by streptococcal bacteria in the body, which occurs most frequently in children between the ages of four and eighteen. It affects one or more of the following body members: joints (arthritis), brain (chorea), heart (carius), tissues (nodules), and skin (erythema marginatum). Residual heart disease is a possible complication.

A salt-restricted diet containing all essential nutrients, together with a planned exercise program to relieve joint pain, is recommended. Bioflavonoids have been found valuable for treating and preventing rheumatic fever.

NUTRIENTS THAT MAY BE BENEFICIAL IN TREATMENT OF RHEUMATIC FEVER

Body Member	Nutrients	Quantity*
General	Vitamin A	
	Vitamin B complex	
	Vitamin B$_2$	

Body Member	Nutrients	Quantity*
	Vitamin B$_6$	
	Pantothenic acid	100 mg
	Pangamic acid	
	Vitamin C	1–10 gm
	Vitamin D	
	Vitamin E	100–600 IU
	Bioflavonoids	
	Zinc	
	Protein	

*See note, p. 222.

RHEUMATISM

Rheumatism is a general term referring to acute and chronic conditions characterized by stiffness of muscles and pain in the joints. Rheumatism includes such conditions as arthritis and bursitis, as well as other diseases.

NUTRIENTS THAT MAY BE BENEFICIAL IN TREATMENT OF RHEUMATISM

Body Member	Nutrients	Quantity
Muscles/Joints	Vitamin A	25,000 IU
	Vitamin B complex	
	Vitamin B$_6$	50–100 mg
	Pangamic acid	
	Pantothenic acid	50–250 mg
	Vitamin C	500 mg or more
	Vitamin D	1200–2500 IU
	Vitamin E	100–600 IU
	Bioflavonoids	
	Calcium	
	Phosphorus	
	Potassium	
	Zinc	
	Protein	
	Hydrochloric acid	
	Digestive enzymes	

RICKETS AND OSTEOMALACIA

Rickets is primarily a childhood disease of malnutrition in which there is a deficiency of vitamin D, calcium, and/or phosphorus. The chief symptom of rickets is an inability of the bones to retain calcium. This causes them to become soft, which results in deformities when the bones are called upon to support weight that they are too weak to support. Such deformities include bowlegs, knock-knees, protruding breastbone, narrowed rib cage, and bony beads along the ribs. Other symptoms of rickets include tetany and easily decaying teeth. However, weight gain and growth are generally normal in children with rickets.

The adult form of rickets is known as osteomalacia. It is most likely to occur at times of bodily stress such as pregnancy or during breast-feeding. Its causes may be a kidney defect or disease, a deficiency of calcium or phosphorus, or an inability to use vitamin D. It may occur in persons who get little sunshine or in those on diets so low in fats that inadequate bile is made and vitamin D is not absorbed.

In addition to the symptoms of rickets, aching of joints and generalized weakness occur. Vitamin D, calcium, and phosphorus work together to form strong bones; if one of these nutrients is missing, the result is rickets or osteomalacia. Vitamin D is needed for proper absorption and use of calcium and phosphorus, which hardens the bones. A deficiency of vitamin C can make the bones less able to retain calcium and phosphorus. Therefore the diet must be adequate in vitamin C, calcium, and phosphorus. To stimulate bile flow, oils should be used instead of solid fats; lecithin and digestive enzymes should also be included.

NUTRIENTS THAT MAY BE BENEFICIAL IN TREATMENT OF RICKETS AND OSTEOMALACIA

Body Member	Nutrients	Quantity
Bones	Vitamin A	
	Vitamin C	
	Vitamin D	
	Calcium	
	Magnesium	
	Phosphorus	
	Lecithin	
	Unsaturated fatty acids	
	Hydrochloric acid	
	Digestive enzymes	

RHINITIS

Rhinitis is the inflammation of the nasal mucosa, causing nasal congestion with increased secretion of mucus.

No specific treatment is known; general measures include rest, adequate fluid intake, and a well-balanced diet. Vitamin A and vitamin C have been used successfully in the treatment of rhinitis. Sulfonamides and antibiotics are of no value and should not be administered.

NUTRIENTS THAT MAY BE BENEFICIAL IN TREATMENT OF RHINITIS

Body Member	Nutrients	Quantity*
Mucous membrane	Vitamin A	
	Vitamin C	Up to 1 gm
	Protein	

*See note, p. 222.

SCIATICA

Sciatica refers to severely painful spasms along the sciatic nerve of the leg. This nerve runs from the back of the thigh, down the inside of the leg, to the ankle. Among the possible causes of sciatica are trauma or inflammation of the nerve itself, sprained joints in the lower back, rupture of a disk between the spinal bones, or neuritis.

Treatment for sciatica includes rest and hot, wet applications to the affected leg for the relief of pain and inflammation. The vitamin B complex is essential for the health of nerve tissue.

NUTRIENTS THAT MAY BE BENEFICIAL IN TREATMENT OF SCIATICA

Body Member	Nutrients	Quantity*
Leg/Nervous system	Vitamin B complex	
	Vitamin B$_1$	25 mg/cc (injections)
	Vitamin B$_{12}$	Injection
	Vitamin D	
	Vitamin E	

*See note, p. 222.

SCURVY

Scurvy is a malnutrition disease caused by a diet that is deficient in vitamin C. Symptoms of adult scurvy include swelling and bleeding of the gums, tenderness of joints and muscles, rough, dry, discolored skin, poor healing of wounds, and increased susceptibility to bruising and infection. Because vitamin C facilitates the absorption of iron, scurvy may be complicated by anemia.

An infant with scurvy experiences joint pain that causes him to assume a position called the "scrobutic pose," in which he is comfortable only when lying on his back with his knees partially bent and his thighs turned outward. The vitamin C deficiency makes the infant's bones less capable of retaining calcium and phosphorus, causing them to become weak and eventually brittle.

Scurvy responds dramatically, usually in 2 or 3 days' time, to the daily administration of 100 to 200 milligrams of vitamin C. In treating complications such as anemia and bone changes, a well-balanced diet high in protein, iron, calcium, vitamin D, and magnesium is also necessary to promote tissue repair.

NUTRIENTS THAT MAY BE BENEFICIAL IN TREATMENT OF SCURVY

Body Member	Nutrients	Quantity*
General	Vitamin A	
	Vitamin B complex	
	Folic acid	
	Vitamin C	300–1000 mg
	Vitamin D	
	Bioflavonoids	
	Calcium	
	Iron	
	Magnesium	
	Protein	

*See note, p. 222.

SHINGLES (HERPES ZOSTER)

Shingles (herpes zoster) is an infection caused by a virus of the nerve endings in the skin. The disease is characterized by blister and crust formation and severe pain along the involved nerve, which may last for several weeks. The infection commonly occurs on the chest or abdomen, although it may occur on the face around the eyes.

The B vitamins are necessary for the proper functioning of the nerves. Intramuscular injections of thiamine hydrochloride and vitamin B_{12} have successfully been used in the treatment of herpes zoster. Vitamins A and C help promote healing of the skin lesions characteristic of the disease. Massive doses of vitamin C can limit the infection of shingles. Calcium and magnesium are important for the transmission of nerve impulses and protection of sensitive nerve endings. Vitamin E ointment rubbed in the nerve root for 10 minutes followed by 10 minutes of heat several times a day has been shown to produce excellent results.[36]

NUTRIENTS THAT MAY BE BENEFICIAL IN TREATMENT OF SHINGLES

Body Member	Nutrients	Quantity*
Skin	Vitamin A	
	Vitamin B complex	
	Vitamin B_1	200–300 mg
	Vitamin B_6	
	Vitamin B_{12}	500 mcg (injections)
	Vitamin C	
	Vitamin D	
	Calcium	
	Magnesium	
	Protein	

*See note, p. 222.

SINUSITIS

Sinusitis is the inflammation of one or more of the sinus cavities, or passages. Sinusitis usually occurs in the nasal sinuses, which are located in the bones surrounding the eyes and nose. Symptoms of the inflammation include nasal congestion and discharge, fatigue, headache, earache, pain around the eyes, mild fever, cough, and an increased susceptibility to infection.

Sinusitis may be the result of a cold, sore throat, tonsilitis, or poor mouth hygiene. Recent studies indicate that a deficiency of vitamin A, which helps maintain the health of the mucous membrane of the nose and throat, may cause the condition. Smoking, damp weather, or the ingestion of spicy foods or alcohol may aggravate sinusitis.

Adequate intake of vitamin A may be useful in the

[36]Shute, Dr. Wilfrid E., *Health Preserver*, p. 99.

treatment of sinusitis, especially if a deficiency exists. Vitamin C can help fight the infections that may occur with this condition, and protein will help restore damaged sinus tissues. Potassium, calcium, vitamin A, and zinc, which is necessary for vitamin A mobilization from the liver, aid the work of the cilia. (Cilia are tiny little "fingers" in the nasal passages that help the expulsion of mucus.)

NUTRIENTS THAT MAY BE BENEFICIAL IN TREATMENT OF SINUSITIS

Body Member	Nutrients	Quantity
Sinuses	Vitamin A	
	Vitamin B complex	
	Vitamin C	
	Vitamin E	
	Calcium	
	Potassium	
	Zinc	
	Protein	

SKIN PROBLEMS

Bites, stings, and poisons adversely affect many people, especially those who are allergic to bites. More people die of bee stings than from poisonous insects. Persons with these known allergies should carry vitamin C with them and if bitten, take large amounts of the vitamin immediately and frequently thereafter.

Dr. Frederick Klenner has successfully used large doses of vitamin C, 4 grams every few hours, to treat the bites of black widow spiders, highland moccasins and rattlesnakes. His patients made complete recoveries in as short a time as 38 hours. He recommends calcium be taken with the vitamin because it increases the effectiveness of the treatment and decreases the sensitivity to pain. A reaction to poison oak or ivy can be alleviated by taking large quantities of calcium and vitamin C. Following any bite, sting, or poison, pantothenic acid should be increased and vitamin E applied topically to reduce the pain.

A *boil, or furuncle,* is an infected nodule on the skin with a central core of pus surrounded by inflamed and swollen tissue. A boil forms when skin tissue is weakened by chafing, lowered resistance due to disease,

or inadequate nutrition. Boil symptoms include itching, mild pain, and localized swelling.

Proper hygiene is essential for the treatment of boils. The infected areas should be washed several times daily and swabbed with antiseptic. Hot compresses can relieve pain and promote healing. The person should receive adequate rest and pay special attention to eating a well-balanced diet. Vitamins A, C, and E are necessary for health of the skin. Vitamin A can also be applied locally. Sufficient zinc in the diet, 30 milligrams per day, may actually prevent boils from occurring. *Canker sores* are shallow open sores found anywhere on the mouth. They are usually located on the mucous membrane inside the lips and cheeks, and are often hard to distinguish from cold sores or herpes simplex I. A canker sore is identified by a sensation of burning and tingling and a slight swelling of the mucous membrane. The sore, a white center surrounded by a red border, is tender to pressure and is painful when acids or spicy foods are eaten. The sore lasts from 4 to 20 days and heals spontaneously, leaving no scar. The specific cause of canker sores is unknown, although they appear to be brought on by anxiety, other emotional stress, or sensitivity to various foods and substances that produce allergic-type reactions.

Because stress is the most common instigator, the B complex taken in large doses often reduces the active time of the sores. Oral doses (50 mg) and topical application of zinc have successfully prevented or shortened the duration of canker sores; magnesium and vitamins B_1 and B_2 were also included in several of the tests. Other studies have shown that many canker sore patients are likely to be deficient in iron, folic acid, and vitamin B_{12}. The sores have cleared quickly when acidophilus tablets or yogurt is eaten several times a day.

Vitamins A and D are necessary for maintaining the condition of mouth tissue and may also be applied locally. The B complex helps in the general condition of the skin, tongue, and digestive system. A well-balanced diet that provides adequate amounts of these vitamins protects against the formation of canker sores.

A *carbuncle* is a painful localized infection producing pus-filled areas in the deeper layers of the skin tissues under the skin. It commonly appears as a group of boils but is usually more painful, deeper, and slower-healing than an ordinary boil. Carbuncles are formed when bacteria enter lesions in the skin, causing infection. Symptoms of carbuncles include fever and chills, fatigue, and weight loss. Treatment for carbuncles demands proper hygiene, including frequent washing of the infected area with soap and water, and application of an antiseptic. Hot compresses can relieve pain and promote healing. Bed rest is beneficial, and a well-balanced diet is essential. Vitamins A, D, and C are necessary for health of the skin. If a fever is present, vitamin E may reduce scarring. Calorie and nutrient levels should be increased. Vitamin A or E may be applied locally.

Dry skin can result from a deficiency of vitamins A, C, or B complex. Because the oils of the skin are largely unsaturated, the unsaturated fatty acids are needed for moist skin. Vitamin A is necessary for natural skin growth and repair, and pantothenic acid is required for the synthesis of the fats and oils essential for proper skin function. Na-PCA, the skin's natural moisturizer which decreases with age, is available as a spray or cream for topical application.

Fungus infestations can refer to athlete's foot, ringworm (appearing on any part of the body), infestations on or around the genitals and anus or around the mouth (causing thrush), or inflammations on the fingers or under the fingernails. The most common cause of these infestations is the destruction of beneficial bacteria by antibiotics, drugs, or radiation, resulting in the takeover by undesirable fungi. Besides being taken as a drug, antibiotics often are found in the food supply because antibiotic supplements are given to animals as treatment for diseases and also as a feed additive. Persons with any type of fungal infestation should establish an adequate diet including generous amounts of the A, B, and C vitamins, raw fruits, vegetables, whole grains, and yogurt or acidophilus.

Ichthyosis resembles fish skin in appearance (*ichthus* is Greek for fish) and is characterized by widespread patches of dry skin that turn dark and scaly. Physicians in Egypt have discovered that niacin completely clears the disease after a period of treatment. Niacin should be accompanied by the other B vitamins. In other cases, vitamins A (150,000–200,000 IU daily) and C (up to 10 gm daily) have cleared up the skin with no signs of vitamin A toxicity.

Impetigo is a skin disease caused by bacterial infection. The disease occurs primarily in children, especially in those who are undernourished. Impetigo is characterized by pus-filled skin lesions located mainly on the face and hands. These lesions rupture and form a honey-yellow crust over the infected area. The disease is spread by scratching the lesions and contaminating other skin areas with the fingers. Strict hygiene is essential to prevent spread of the infection to other parts of the body or to other people. Neglected impetigo in adults may result in boils, ulcers, or other complications. Vitamin A is necessary for the health of skin tissue and, vitamins C, D, and E may be helpful in aiding the skin in its recovery from impetigo. The disease often disappears after topical application of vitamins A and E.

Itching skin often arises from an iron deficiency, especially if there is no other disease present. Numbness and tingling sometimes accompany the itching, indicating slight nerve dysfunction.

Lip problems, including sore lips, whistle marks, and cracks at the corners of the mouth, usually indicate a vitamin B complex deficiency—specifically vitamins B_2, B_6, folic acid, or pantothenic acid. Unsaturated fatty acids may also be undersupplied. When adequate amounts of these nutrients are taken, the conditions should disappear quite easily, although whistle marks may take some time.

Lupus erythematosus primarily affects the connective tissue. The disease is characterized by anemia, joint stiffness, and signs of adrenal exhaustion. Large doses of the B complex and all essential nutrients—especially vitamin E (900–2000 IU) and pantothenic acid–(900 mg–15 gm) have been reported to result in complete recovery with no recurrence unless the vitamins were discontinued.[37] 50 mg manganese taken morning and evening is also recommended.

Oily skin (and hair) has been produced in persons only slightly deficient in vitamin B_2. Doses of 15 milligrams daily have cleared up the condition; the entire B complex may be beneficial.

Pigmentation of the skin commonly appears as spots or across the forehead, sometimes coinciding with the stress of pregnancy and then referred to as pregnancy cap. The skin of affected individuals may become deeply pigmented. The disease is connected with an inadequate diet; vitamins A, B complex, C, D, and E are needed. The discoloration has disappeared after

[37]Davis, *Let's Get Well*, p. 292.

folid acid (5 mg), pantothenic acid, and/or niacin (100 mg) were taken with each meal. Pigmentation may be due to high copper levels. Zinc will cause the secretion of copper from the body.

Prickly heat is a rash consisting of tiny inflamed pimples that itch, sometimes quite severely. Research has suggested that the disease occurs when the sweat glands no longer function in a particular part of the body, probably because of fatigue. The rash develops wherever there is excessive sweating, such as the inside of the thighs or under a tight diaper on a baby. Cornstarch is effective as an allaying compound. Studies have shown that vitamin C (1 gm daily) can prevent or cure prickly heat. It apparently has a connection with the enzyme systems that relate to the sweat glands.

Purpura is characterized by spontaneous bruising or bleeding and tiny bumps in the skin and mucous membranes. The disease has been considered rare but is now seen more frequently, especially in women. Researchers believe it may be due to the heavy use of estrogen, both in oral contraceptives and as a treatment during menopause. Estrogen (as well as other drugs, chemicals, and infections) destroys vitamin E, which is essential for capillary integrity. Doses of the vitamin (400–600 IU daily) have been shown to prevent or result in recovery from the disease.

Scars have been prevented and removed by vitamin E. For example, an excessive amount of scar tissue called a keloid, which causes pain and itching, has been relieved by 1200 IU of vitamin E taken daily. The vitamin (200–300 IU daily) has removed scars from the fingers and palms in a condition called Dupuytren's contracture; the same amount has corrected Peyronie's disease, which is characterized by abnormal scar tissue on the penis that causes pain on erection and impotence. The vitamin is effective when taken orally as well as applied topically. Sufficient zinc in the diet can prevent keloids.

Stretch marks can appear on teenagers and males as well as previously overweight persons and pregnant women. These marks can be prevented and sometimes removed by vitamin E (up to 600 IU daily), the B complex, pantothenic acid (up to 300 mg/day) and an adequate intake of zinc and vitamin C.

Ulcers of the skin heal more rapidly when vitamin E (400 IU daily) is taken and also applied topically. All nutrients are necessary to stimulate healing of the sore, including vitamins C, pantothenic acid, folic acid, and the UNS fatty acids.

Vitiligo is a condition in which the skin is unable to manufacture a pigment, melanin, in certain areas, resulting in light patches of skin marked by a dark border. An adequately nutritious diet is especially important in the disease, and it has been helped with supplements of hydrochloric acid and digestive enzymes that assure proper absorption. The B complex, pantothenic acid (150–300 mg/day), PABA (100–1000 mg/day)—all also applied topically—and vitamins B_6 and C, zinc, and manganese have all aided in the improvement and cure of this condition. Injections of the vitamins along with the tablets may be necessary.

Warts are possibly of viral origin and occur when the body's immune system is low. 25,000–50,000 IU of vitamin A have caused warts to disappear. Vitamin E (500 IU), taken orally and also applied topically, is additionally beneficial.

Wrinkles and the loss of elasticity result from a damaged mechanism called cross-linking, in which proteins are bonded together, preventing them from functioning properly. The skin appears to be particularly susceptible to damage, and alcohol, tobacco, and sunlight are major offenders. Cross-linking can be slowed down or prevented by taking the antioxidants such as vitamins A, B_1, C, and E, and zinc and selenium.

STRESS

Stress is any physical or emotional strain on the body or mind. Physical stress occurs when an external or natural change or force acts upon the body. Extreme heat or cold, overwork, injuries, malnutrition, and exposure to drugs and poisons are examples of physical stress. Emotional stress may be a result of fear, hate, love, anger, tension, grief, joy, frustration, and/or anxiety. Physical and emotional stress can overlap, as in special body conditions such as pregnancy, adolescence, and aging. During these times, body metabolism is increased or lowered, changing the body's physical functions, which, in turn, affect the person's mental and emotional outlook on life. A certain amount of stress is useful as a motivating factor, but when it occurs in excess or is of the wrong kind, the effect can be detrimental.

The metabolic response of the body to either physical or emotional stress is to produce more adrenal hormones. These adrenal hormones are secreted by glands that lie above the kidneys. When released into the blood, these hormones prepare the body for action by increasing blood pressure and heartbeat and by making extra energy available. These body responses are useful when physical action is needed, but in our modern civilization there is usually little physical outlet for them, and the body must react to stress by channeling the body's responses inward to one of the organ systems, such as the digestive, circulatory, or nervous system. When this happens, the system reacts adversely, and conditions such as ulcers, hypertension, backache, atherosclerosis, allergic reactions, asthma, fatigue, and insomnia often develop.

Anxiety, a fearful or distressful feeling, is responsible for the stress of many individuals. Anything that threatens a person's body, job, loved ones, or values may cause anxiety. If the person cannot cope with the situation, stress on the body is increased, resulting in many of the disorders associated with stress. Change in attitude or life-style may be necessary to eliminate the needless strain and allow the body to resume normal functioning.

The increase in the production of adrenal hormones which occurs with stress increases the metabolism of protein, fats, and carbohydrates, producing instant energy for the body to use. As a result of this increased metabolism, there is also an increased excretion of protein, potassium, and phosphorus and a decreased storage of calcium. Many of the disorders related to stress are not a direct result of the stress itself but a result of nutrient deficiencies caused by increased metabolic rate during periods of stress. For example, vitamin C is utilized by the adrenal gland during stressful conditions, and any stress that is sufficiently severe or prolonged will cause a depletion of vitamin C in the tissues.

People experiencing stress need to maintain a nutritious, well-balanced diet with special emphasis on replacing the nutrients that may be depleted during stress.

NUTRIENTS THAT MAY BE BENEFICIAL IN TREATMENT OF STRESS

Body Member	Nutrients	Quantity
General	Vitamin A	
	Vitamin B complex	
	Vitamin B$_1$	
	Vitamin B$_2$	
	Vitamin B$_6$	
	Vitamin B$_{12}$	
	Biotin	
	Choline	
	Folic Acid	
	Inositol	
	Niacin	
	PABA	
	Vitamin C	
	Vitamin D	
	Vitamin E	
	Calcium	
	Chromium	
	Copper	
	Iodine	
	Iron	
	Magnesium	
	Manganese	
	Phosphorus	
	Potassium	
	Selenium	
	Zinc	
	Carbohydrate	
	Fat	
	Protein	

STROKE

A stroke, or cerebrovascular accident, occurs when the blood supply of an area of brain cells is cut off for a long period of time, resulting in the death of the deprived cells due to lack of oxygen and nutrients essential for the proper function of the brain. The blood vessels may be blocked by atherosclerosis, clotting, or hemorrhaging. The process is similar to that of a heart attack, the difference being cell death in the brain during a stroke.

Typical symptoms include impaired memory and attention span, tingling or lack of feeling in limbs, a feeling of heaviness in the limbs, and loss of movement. Symptoms are often restricted to one side of the body, as seen in the frequent right- or left-sided paralysis. Strokes may be so small that they are not even noticed or so severe as to be fatal. It is difficult to tell the extent of injury or cell death at the time the stroke occurs, and the long-term outlook therefore depends upon the area and extent of the brain damage. Physical and speech therapy are often helpful in rehabilitating the patient.

Predisposing factors are prolonged high blood pressure, atherosclerosis, diabetes, old age, obesity, and cigarette smoking. Preventive dietary measures include restricting sodium intake to reduce high blood pressure and reducing cholesterol intake to prevent further cholesterol buildup in blood vessels.

The diet should be well balanced, with special emphasis on B vitamins and vitamin C because they are needed for general health of the blood vessels. Vitamin E can be of help to prevent clots, reducing the need for oxygen. Reduction of overweight by sensible dieting is of the utmost importance. Whole grains, fruits, vegetables, and complete proteins should be emphasized. All nutrients should meet the demands of stress and should lower blood cholesterol.

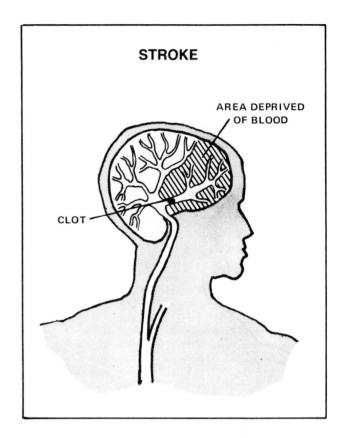

STROKE

AREA DEPRIVED OF BLOOD

CLOT

NUTRIENTS THAT MAY BE BENEFICIAL IN TREATMENT OF STROKE

Body Member	Nutrients	Quantity*
Blood	Vitamin B complex Choline	
	Inositol	
	Vitamin C	
	Vitamin E	300 IU, gradually increasing to 600 IU
	Bioflavonoids	
	Potassium	
	Selenium	
	Zinc	
	Protein	
	Lecithin	

*See note, p. 222.

SUNBURN

Sunburn is caused by excessive exposure to ultraviolet rays, which actually burn up surface skin and later the lower cells. The amount of exposure to ultraviolet rays which causes burning depends basically on four things: the individual, place, time, and atmospheric conditions.

Caution should be used in exposing oneself to the sun for extended periods of time between 10:00 A.M. and 2:00 P.M., when most of the ultraviolet rays are present. Reflections from water, metal, sand, or snow may double the amount of rays one absorbs.

Burns may be classified in three degrees. First-degree sunburn causes reddening of the skin and possibly slight fever. Second-degree sunburn causes reddening of the skin accompanied by water blisters. Third-degree sunburn causes lower cell damage and the release of fluid, resulting in eruptions and breaks in the skin where bacteria and infection can enter.

Cold water soaking or cold water compresses, together with additional intake of vitamins A, C, and E, are recommended for treatment of sunburn.

NUTRIENTS THAT MAY BE BENEFICIAL IN TREATMENT OF SUNBURN

Body Member	Nutrients	Quantity*
Skin	Vitamin A	
	Vitamin B complex	
	Vitamin B_6	
	PABA	1000 mg plus ointment
	Vitamin C	
	Vitamin E	
	Calcium	
	Zinc	

*See note, p. 222.

SWOLLEN GLANDS

Swollen glands is a term commonly used to describe enlargement of the lymph nodes, or glands of the neck, on both sides of the throat. Technically, however, it can also describe enlargement of any of the lymph glands, such as those located in the armpit or groin. The enlargement of lymph glands is usually a signal of an infection in the area, because the lymph glands function to filter out microscopic material, such as bacteria, in order to prevent the spread of infection.

Symptoms include enlarged or swollen glands that may be hard or soft. These symptoms may be accompanied by heat, tenderness, and reddening of the overlying skin, and fever.

Swollen glands may simply indicate a localized infection or may be a symptom of a more serious disease. Swollen gland conditions may occur with such disorders as mononucleosis, measles, chicken pox, leukemia, cancer, tuberculosis, and syphilis.

Treatment includes maintaining a well-balanced diet and fighting the particular infection that is causing the lymph node enlargement. In general, infection requires an increased intake of protein, fluids, and calories. If the infection is accompanied by fever, the diet should be rich in vitamins A and C and B complex.

NUTRIENTS THAT MAY BE BENEFICIAL IN TREATMENT OF SWOLLEN GLANDS

Body Member	Nutrients	Quantity
Glands/Lymph nodes	Vitamin A	
	Vitamin B complex	
	Vitamin B_6	
	Pantothenic acid	
	Vitamin C	
	Protein	
	Water	

TICS, TREMORS, AND TWITCHES

Tics, tremors, and twitches are often caused by an imbalance of minerals, an excess of lead in the body, an allergic reaction to food or chemicals, or by drugs and medication. The most common cause is a deficiency of potassium and/or magnesium. These minerals are essential for the conduction of nerve impulses that pass to a muscle and control its movement. Sometimes the B complex vitamins, necessary for the health of the nervous system, are found to be deficient, and when B complex is taken, symptoms disappear. If an excess of lead is found, calcium or zinc can effectively leach the toxic metal out of the body.

NUTRIENTS THAT MAY BE BENEFICIAL IN TREATMENT OF TICS, TREMORS, AND TWITCHES

Body Member	Nutrients
Muscle/Nervous system	Vitamin B complex
	Vitamin B_6
	Vitamin B_{12}
	Niacin
	Magnesium
	Potassium

TONSILITIS

Tonsilitis is an inflammation of the tonsils, which are glands of lymph tissue located on either side of the entrance to the throat. Tonsilitis may be caused by virus infections when the body's resistance is lowered or by an improper diet that is high in carbohydrates and low in protein and other nutrients.

Symptoms of tonsilitis include pain, redness and swelling in the back of the mouth, difficulty in swallowing, hoarseness, and coughing. Headache, earache, fever and chills, nausea and vomiting, nasal obstruction and discharge, and enlarged lymph nodes throughout the body are additional symptoms of tonsilitis.

In cases of severe tonsil infection, surgical removal may be necessary. The most effective means of prevention for tonsilitis is maintaining a well-balanced diet that is adequate in protein, vitamins, and minerals. The regular intake of vitamin C may help prevent tonsilitis.

NUTRIENTS THAT MAY BE BENEFICIAL IN TREATMENT OF TONSILITIS

Body Member	Nutrients	Quantity
Glands, tonsil	Vitamin A	
	Vitamin B complex	
	Vitamin B_2	
	Vitamin B_6	
	Folic acid	
	Pantothenic acid	
	Vitamin C	
	Vitamin D	
	Vitamin E	
	Protein	

TOOTH AND GUM DISORDERS

Cavities (dental caries) are the primary dental problem in the United States. Most cavities are caused by persistent eating of refined sugars and starches, which mix with saliva to form an acid that erodes tooth enamel. One can control cavities by avoiding refined-carbohydrate foods, eating a nutritionally balanced diet, and properly cleansing the mouth, including brushing both teeth and gums and cleansing between the teeth with dental floss following meals and snacks.

Although cavities are the major dental disease, a condition known as priodontitis accounts for the loss of more teeth than do cavities. Periodontitis, an inflammation of the gums and the bones that surround and support the teeth, can accompany mouth and upper respiratory infections, or it may be caused by poor fillings, poorly fitting dentures, improper cleansing of teeth and gums, or inadequate diet. Periodontitis begins as a condition known as gingivitis, in which the gums redden, swell, and tend to bleed. If not treated, gingivitis can lead to pyorrhea (see p. 194), characterized by further gum inflammation accompanied by a continuous discharge of pus, gum recession, and loosening of teeth.

Although all vitamins and minerals are essential for the proper formation and continued health of the teeth, an adequate vitamin C intake is especially helpful for the prevention of gingivitis and pyorrhea, while a deficiency of it causes teeth to loosen and break down. Vitamin A seems to control the development and general health of the gums; a lack of this vitamin often results in gum infection. Vitamin A is also necessary for the formation and maintenance of tooth development in children. Minerals important for healthy teeth are sodium, potassium, calcium, phosphorus, iron, and magnesium.

A varied diet of fresh fruits, green leafy vegetables, meat, and whole-grain bread will provide the teeth and gums with needed exercise and supply the body with vitamins and minerals essential for dental health.

NUTRIENTS THAT MAY BE BENEFICIAL IN TREATMENT OF TOOTH AND GUM DISORDERS

Body Member	Nutrients	Quantity*
Teeth/ Gums	Vitamin A	
	Vitamin B_6	
	Niacin	
	Vitamin C	Up to 10 gm
	Vitamin D	
	Bioflavonoids	
	Calcium	1100 mg
	Copper	
	Fluorine	
	Iron	
	Magnesium	
	Manganese	
	Phosphorus	
	Potassium	
	Sodium	
	Zinc	
	Protein	
	Unsaturated fatty acids	1–2 tbsp

*See note, p. 222.

TUBERCULOSIS

Tuberculosis is a contagious disease caused by bacterial infection. A person normally has some defense against the bacteria, but when the body is weakened or run-down, its susceptibility to infection is increased. Tuberculosis usually affects the lungs, but it may also involve other organs and tissues.

Many tuberculosis patients may exhibit mild symptoms from which they recover completely. This usually means that the body has successfully controlled the bacteria. Mild symptoms of the disease include fatigue and appetite and weight loss. As the disease becomes more severe, symptoms include fever, increased perspiration, and rapid loss of weight and strength. Coughing up blood is often the first indication of a severe form of the disease.

A tuberculosis patient should be isolated in a hospital for treatment during the contagious state. Antibiotics, adequate rest, and proper diet comprise the most effective therapy for tuberculosis. Supplementation with vitamin A is necessary because the patient is less able to convert carotene to vitamin A. Vitamin C may also be deficient in the tuberculosis patient; thus additional intake may be necessary. Extra vitamin D is needed for the absorption of additional calcium, which the patient needs in order to form a case, or wall, around the invading bacteria. If the patient is losing blood, increased iron intake is required to rebuild the red blood cells. A diet high in protein and the necessary vitamins and minerals will help a person maintain his or her ideal weight and thus help prevent tuberculosis from recurring.

NUTRIENTS THAT MAY BE BENEFICIAL IN TREATMENT OF TUBERCULOSIS

Body Member	Nutrients	Quantity*
Lungs/ Respiratory system	Vitamin A	10,000–40,000 IU
	Vitamin B complex	
	Vitamin B$_6$	2 mg six times daily
	Vitamin B$_{12}$	50 mcg six times daily
	Niacin	
	Pantothenic acid	
	Vitamin C	500 mg six times daily
	Vitamin D	
	Calcium	
	Iron	
	Phosphorus	
	Zinc	
	Manganese	
	Protein	

*See note, p. 222.

ULCER

At the onset of stress, the body's defense of the lining of the stomach is damaged; the stomach is unable to secrete sufficient mucus to protect against the strong acid essential for digestion, and an ulcer results. Gastric ulcers occur in the stomach; peptic ulcers refer to those in the intestines; and duodenal ulcers are found in the duodenum, a short tube through which the stomach empties. A hemorrhaging ulcer occurs when the ulcer has penetrated a blood vessel, causing it to bleed. Symptoms of an ulcer vary and can include stomach pain, low back pain, headaches, choking sensations, and itching.

Studies have shown that the ulcerated stomach processes almost all foods impartially and that what aggravates an ulcer is the anxiety state of the individual before eating. The ulcer patient should make all efforts to eliminate the source of stress. Because a deficiency of almost any nutrient can cause the development of ulcers, the diet should be well balanced, meet all the demands of stress, and promote healing.

Foods should be chosen according to physical reactions; if a certain food causes discomfort, then the food should not be eaten. Meals should be small and frequent because greater quantities of stomach acids are released during larger meals. Coffee, alcohol, and strong tea increase the amount of stomach acid and should be avoided. The herb comfrey has been known for centuries to have a healing affect on ulcers.

NUTRIENTS THAT MAY BE BENEFICIAL IN TREATMENT OF ULCER

Body Member	Nutrients	Quantity*
Stomach	Vitamin A	25,000–50,000 IU
	Vitamin B complex	

*See note, p. 222.

Body Member	Nutrients	Quantity*
	Vitamin B$_2$	5 mg three times daily
	Vitamin B$_6$	
	Vitamin B$_{12}$	
	Choline	
	Folic acid	
	Pantothenic acid	50–100 mg three times daily
	Vitamin C	
	Vitamin D	
	Vitamin E	600–1,200 IU
	Vitamin K	
	Bioflavonoids	
	Calcium	
	Iron	
	Manganese	
	Zinc	
	Protein	
	Acidophilus	
	Unsaturated fatty acids	
	Aloe vera	

*See note, p. 222.

Symptoms that may accompany underweight are weakness, fatigue, sensitivity to cold, hunger, dizziness, and loss of ambition. Underweight may be caused by poor eating habits, a nervous condition, overactivity, illness, heredity problems, or poorly functioning digestion and absorption processes.

Underweight can be corrected by removal of the underlying causes and improvement of the diet. The diet should be well balanced, consisting of whole unrefined foods, many of which should be high-calorie such as cheeses, salad oils, butter, nuts, and seeds. Extra protein is needed to rebuild tissues. Frequent smaller feedings may be of help in weight gain. Exercise is important during weight gain, so that muscles, rather than fat, are formed. For the same reason, weight should not be gained at the rate of more than a pound or two per week. Any vitamin deficiencies should be corrected as quickly as possible.

NUTRIENTS THAT MAY BE BENEFICIAL IN TREATMENT OF UNDERWEIGHT

Body Member	Nutrients	Quantity
Body	Vitamin B complex	
	Protein	
	Unsaturated fatty acids	
	Digestive enzymes	

UNDERWEIGHT

Underweight develops when more calories are utilized by the body than are consumed. Underweight without a lack of nutrients may or may not be serious, depending upon the degree of underweight. The thin person is probably less apt to suffer from heart diseases and certain other ailments and will live longer than a person who is overweight. Malnutrition occurs when an individual is deficient in the nutrients necessary for life. Individuals with this problem are very susceptible to infections, lack nutrient reserves for times of stress, and are easily fatigued. When underweight and malnutrition are severe, there is starvation, the body's stores of nutrients and fats are depleted, and muscle tissue is broken down to provide energy for bodily functions.

VAGINITIS

Vaginitis is an inflammation of the vagina, usually caused by bacterial or yeast infection, excessive douching, vitamin B deficiency,[38] or intestinal worms. Symptoms of vaginitis include a burning or itching sensation and an abnormal vaginal discharge that is white or yellow. Vaginitis is common in pregnant or diabetic women and in women using antibiotics or oral contraceptives.

Adequate rest, a healthful diet, and meticulous personal hygiene are important for the treatment of vaginitis. Cotton underwear is sometimes recommended because it allows for free circulation of air. Vaginal

[38]Davis, *Let's Get Well,* p. 308.

itching may be prevented by the intake of vitamin A and the B complex if a deficiency is present.

NUTRIENTS THAT MAY BE BENEFICIAL IN TREATMENT OF VAGINITIS

Body Member	Nutrients	Quantity*
Reproductive system	Vitamin A	25,000–50,000 IU
	Vitamin B complex	
	Vitamin B$_2$	6 mg
	Vitamin B$_6$	
	Vitamin D	
	Vitamin E	Also as suppository
	Protein	
	Acidophilus	

*See note, p. 222.

VARICOSE VEINS

Varicose veins are veins that have become enlarged, twisted, and swollen. They may be located anywhere in the body, but they are most commonly found in the legs.

Factors that inhibit blood circulation, such as obesity, certain hereditary conditions, tight clothing, crossing of legs, and a sedentary occupation, can increase susceptibility to varicose veins. A pregnant woman or a woman who has had several pregnancies is usually more prone to varicose veins than are most other women, because pregnancy causes increased pressure on the legs.

It is essential that individuals who must sit for extended periods of time receive adequate exercise. Elevating the legs while resting is another preventive measure.

Adequate amounts of the B vitamins and vitamin C are necessary in the diet for the maintenance of strong blood vessels. Some research has indicated that vitamin E can dilate blood vessels and improve circulation, thus perhaps reducing the susceptibility to varicose veins.[39]

[39]Prevention Magazine Staff, *Complete Book of Vitamins*, p. 352.

NUTRIENTS THAT MAY BE BENEFICIAL IN TREATMENT OF VARICOSE VEINS

Body Member	Nutrients	Quantity*
Leg	Vitamin B complex	
	Vitamin C	Up to 3000 mg
	Vitamin E	600–1000 IU
	Bioflavonoids	300–500 mg
	Protein	
	Unsaturated fatty acids	
	Lecithin	

*See note, p. 222.

VENEREAL DISEASE

Venereal disease is usually acquired through intimate contact with the sexual organs of an afflicted individual. The most frequent vehicle of the disease is the act of sexual intercourse or intimacy associated with sexual intercourse. Gonorrhea and syphilis are the two most common types of venereal disease.

Gonorrhea is transmitted through sexual intimacy or from the mother to the newborn infant as it passes through an infected birth canal. Within 3 to 14 days after contact, males experience burning, pain, and discharge of pus upon urination. Complications of gonorrhea in males may include prostatitis and testes infection. Females may have increased urinary frequency and a yellowish discharge from the vagina, but there are usually no immediate symptoms until the infection has included all of the reproductive organs of the pelvic region. Complications of gonorrhea may result in sterility in both sexes.

Syphilis is also most commonly spread through sexual intimacy, but it may also be received through a break in the skin that has come in contact with a chancre, or open sore, fresh blood, semen, or a vaginal discharge from an infected individual. Syphilis can also be transmitted from the mother to the fetus via the bloodstream during pregnancy.

There are three distinct stages of syphilis. First, a chancre appears 10 to 28 days after contact at the point where the infecting organism entered the body, but it disappears in 2 to 5 weeks. Other possible symptoms of this stage include fever, weight loss, and anemia.

Six weeks to six months after appearance of the chancre, the second stage begins. It is characterized by skin rashes, hair loss, warts near the mouth or anus, fever, headache, sore throat, and possibly bone pain. The next one to several years may be without symptoms.

During the third stage the disease is no longer contagious. In this stage the organisms settle in specific body organs and destroy them. Commonly, the circulatory system and nervous system are attacked, often resulting in death.

Treatment for venereal disease includes massive injections of antibiotics, usually penicillin, to rid the body of the venereal organism. Early treatment is essential to prevent complicating tissue damage. To prevent the spread of venereal disease, an afflicted person should abstain from sexual intercourse and intimacy until the disease has been cured. In addition to obtaining medical treatment, an afflicted person should maintain a well-balanced diet high in protein to help repair the tissue damage that has occurred.

NUTRIENTS THAT MAY BE BENEFICIAL IN TREATMENT OF VENEREAL DISEASE

Body Member	Nutrients	Quantity
General	Vitamin B complex	
	Protein	
	Acidophilus	

NOTE: Quantities shown are not prescriptive; some are extremely high and represent therapeutic test dosages. Individual needs and tolerances will vary according to body size, metabolism, age, diet, and ailment. Consult a physician who is familiar with nutritional therapy.

NORMAL LIFE CYCLE

PREGNANCY

Pregnancy is a stressful condition involving numerous physical and mental changes in the mother's body as the fetus develops. The tissues in the breasts and uterus increase, the blood supply increases, there is a frequent urge to urinate, there is slight nausea in the morning or even later in the day, the menstrual period is absent, and the need for sleep and fluids is increased. Because of these changes, all nutritional needs of the mother increase in preparation for the newborn baby.

A woman who has maintained a nutritionally balanced diet throughout her life has the best possible chance of bearing a healthy child. The conditions of the fetus during the prenatal period can help the child develop, or prevent him or her from ever achieving full genetic potential.

During pregnancy, nutritional needs are increased, and the condition of the mother and her child could be greatly improved by dietary supplementation. All known nutrients must be supplied to the expectant mother.

Recent evidence suggests that the fetus competes with the mother for available nutrients and that if the mother does not eat properly, the child will suffer the consequences, which could be severe and permanent. The pregnant woman need not be on a severely restricting diet; she should be free to gain weight—within reason, of course—on good, wholesome food containing all vital nutrients.

Doctors have found that edema in well-nourished, nontoxemic pregnant women may actually be protective for mother and fetus; therefore, low-salt diets and diuretics should be taken carefully. The attending obstetrician should be consulted to differentiate between benign physiological edema and pathological edema.

Miscarriage can result from infections, nutrient deficiency, too-low caloric or protein intake, oral antibiotics, and hazardous chemicals in the environment. Studies have shown that women susceptible to miscarriage may be able to carry to full term if sufficient amounts of vitamin C are taken, (500 mg–4 gm increasing to as much as 10–15 gm at the end of pregnancy); along with bioflavonoids to increase the vitamin's effectiveness.[40] Vitamin E (up to 200 IU with each meal) and folic acid have been shown to be helpful in preventing miscarriages.[41]

Toxemia, characterized by sudden weight gain, headache, and high blood pressure, occurs in the late months of pregnancy and can result in the death of

[40]Prevention Magazine Staff, *The Encyclopedia of Common Diseases,* p. 1026.
[41]Davis, Adelle & Marshall Mandell, M.D., *Let's Have Healthy Children,* p. 43.

the newborn baby. The illness may be attributed to the overuse of diuretics or poor nutrition. Laboratory animals developed a condition similar to toxemia when fed diets deficient in magnesium, B_6, choline, and protein.

Birth defects can be a disease of heredity, but they are just as likely to result from fetus-damaging drugs; environmental pollutants; viral, parasitic, or bacterial infections; and poor nutrition. Poor diets lacking in any vitamin, mineral, or enzyme for the mother will deprive the fetus of necessary building materials. Any shortage can result in a stillbirth; a premature infant of low birth weight; a baby with brain damage, including impaired intelligence and psychological disturbances; or a baby with weak immunity to infections. Ingestion by the mother of nicotine, alcohol, chemical food additives, and drugs can interfere with the fetal enzyme system and growth factors. Any interference with the B-complex metabolism in the fetus will produce deformities or abnormalities. Iodine deficiency during pregnancy may cause mental retardation.

Oral antibiotics can destroy the B vitamins and vitamin K. Lack of vitamin K can cause hemorrhaging in the placenta. Hemorrhaging, which is due to capillary fragility, can also be caused by a deficiency of vitamin C and the bioflavonoids. Nervousness, insomnia, and muscle cramps may be a sign of calcium, magnesium, or vitamin B_6 deficiency.

Protein, calcium, and iron are especially important to the development of bones, soft tissues, and blood of the body. Protein of both animal origin (meat, eggs, cheese, milk, fish, etc.) and plant origin (whole-grain cereals, nuts, peas, beans, soybeans, lentils, etc.) should be included in the diet because the body can make the fullest use of these products in combination. Protein is also needed to provide for the 20 percent increase in blood volume during pregnancy. An adequate supply of vitamin D is needed to ensure proper absorption and utilization of calcium and phosphorus. Additional iron is essential to prevent anemia in both mother and baby and to guard the mother against excessive blood loss during birth. Adequate iron also guards against miscarriage and fetal malformation. Vitamin C, vitamin K, and the bioflavonoids are necessary to strengthen blood vessels and to prevent excessive bleeding. In late pregnancy and postdelivery, thiamine requirements are greatly increased. In addition, the pregnant woman should take special care to ensure adequate intake of the vitamin B complex, protein,

and calcium, which help to normalize emotional states that occur frequently during pregnancy.

Nausea and morning sickness due to nervous conditions will probably respond to additional intake of B vitamins. Vitamin B_6, specifically; 25 mg with each meal for nausea and 250 mg or more daily for vomiting. Vitamin B_6 has been found to be effective in regulating fluid retention associated with the development of toxemia. The nutrients vitamin C and E are known to have diuretic actions.

Because calcium, with vitamin D to assure proper absorption, is known to decrease sensitivity to pain, the mineral may ease the pain of labor. Taking 2000 mg between the beginning of labor and the time of arrival at the hospital has resulted in easier deliveries for many women. Vitamin E also has desensitizing properties and increases the elasticity and expandability of the vaginal tissues. Zinc may help to ease the difficulties of birth; and keeping the muscles strong with sufficient protein, magnesium, potassium, unsaturated fatty acids, and vitamin E can make delivery easier and shorter.

The end results of proper prenatal nutrition are a more comfortable pregnancy, an easier delivery, a healthier baby, and a greater chance of successfully nursing the baby.

BREAST-FEEDING

Lactation is the secretion and yielding of milk by the mammary gland. Preparation for lactation begins during early pregnancy, when the increased production of the hormones estrogen and progesterone leads to the storage of maternal energy in the form of fat. After the baby is born, changes occur in the ductless glandular system of the mother's body which initiate the secretion of milk.

The higher the mother's intake of vitamins, minerals, protein, and unsaturated fatty acids, the more these nutrients will appear in her milk. The nursing mother needs to take at least 6000 IU of vitamin A and up to 300 mg of vitamin C. Protein needs are greatly increased; vitamin K can be supplied by yogurt, cabbage, or spinach; sufficient vitamin E and iron (in the organic form to prevent destruction of vitamin E) is needed. The average breast milk contains insufficient amounts of the B vitamins, so particular attention should be made to include them. If adequate calcium is not provided in the mother's diet, the mineral will be leached out of her bones to supply the milk. Calcium requirements are higher during lactation than at any other time; magnesium and vitamin D ensure proper absorption of calcium. Consumption of refined flours and sugars increases the saturated-fat content of breast milk; therefore whole-grain foods and natural carbohydrates are recommended.

Minor fluctuations in milk supply occur in many women. Feeding more frequently can often increase milk production. However, if after a few days supply is still low, other factors may be the cause, such as low thyroid hormone secretion, high fever, fatigue or anxiety in the mother, excessive cigarette or marjuana smoking, pregnancy, birth control pills (which can also have a harmful effect on the milk and baby), and general anesthetics. Breast stimulation is decreased if the baby is given a pacifier or fed unnecessary liquids or solids.

If the baby is sick or has an immature sucking reflex, the sucking will not be enough to sufficiently stimulate the breast. Babies with malformations of the nose, mouth, lips, or tongue, premature or brain damaged babies, and those with heart defects or lung problems may be weak nursers. But they can still be nursed with time and patience and if small frequent feedings are given. Sometimes a baby will be weakened by infections of the urinary or respiratory tract or nervous system, which can be remedied by proper treatment. Nasal congestion caused by an allergy or respiratory infection will make it difficult for the infant to breathe and nurse at the same time. Mild salt-water nose drops and gentle removal of mucus with a nasal syringe, together with proper treatment of the underlying problem, can help relieve the condition. Jaundiced babies often do not nurse well and should be treated for the illness while maintaining the feedings. Other ailments that need special treatment and can interfere with the infant's obtaining full benefit of the nutrients in breast milk include hypoglycemia, diabetes, and malabsorption diseases such as cystic fibrosis and celiac disease.

To maintain adequate milk supply, both breasts should be given to the child during each feeding. The mother should feed the baby frequently, drink lots of liquids—water, juice, milk, and soup—to replace fluids used in making milk, eat healthful foods, and relax before and during nursing.

INFANCY AND CHILDHOOD

The period of life from birth to maturity is one of intense growth and development. Heredity, environment, and nutrition are the major determinants of a child's growth potential. Nutrition, however, is the single most important factor in determining the healthy growth and development of a child.

Foods supply the chemicals necessary for forming all tissues, especially muscles, bones, blood, and teeth, and also for repairing tissues. Children need extra calories to provide energy for this growth and for the increased activity and metabolic rate in youth. Children require the same nutrients as adults for good nutrition, however, often in greater proportions. See the "Nutrient Allowance Chart" on p. 311 for children's Recommended Dietary Allowances.

Colic may be an end result of the pregnant mother's poor diet, making an infant more susceptible to deficiencies and illnesses. An overanxious, tense mother can upset an infant, interfering with digestion and eventually resulting in colic. Other causes may be a lack of B vitamins, B_6, pantothenic acid, potassium, magnesium, or calcium. When digestion is incomplete, bacteria grows on the undigested food, producing gas, distension, and gas or colic pain; the B vitamins are essential for proper digestion. A deficiency of magnesium, calcium, potassium, or B_6 can cause intestinal cramping or colic. One or more of those nutrients given in supplemental form plus a small amount of powdered digestive enzymes and yogurt or acidophilus may help to alleviate a colic condition. Colic may also be caused by copper and/or lead in the tap water used to feed the baby.

Diaper rash can be caused by a deficiency of unsaturated fatty acids or the fat-soluble vitamins—A, D, E, or K. The diet of a child with the rash should be made adequate in all nutrients. Vitamin A or E applied topically to the inflamed area can reduce pain and bring improvement in a shorter period of time. A more severe form of diaper rash called thrush is caused by a fungus and is common among bottle-fed babies. It appears to be caused by a vitamin A deficiency and often follows antibiotic therapy, which destroys the intestinal bacteria. Intake of the B vitamins (25 milligrams of each), vitamin C (100–1000 milligrams), and yogurt will help clear up the condition. If it is severe, vitamin A supplements (10,000–20,000 IU) may be necessary.

Vaccines, although invaluable at certain times, can have detrimental effects on the child's nutrient resources. Vitamin C, the B vitamins, and the intestinal bacteria where vitamins B and K are manufactured are particularily susceptible to destruction. At these times, an adequate diet and supplements of vitamins C and B and yogurt or acidophilus are recommended.

ADOLESCENCE

Adolescence is a period when profound physiological and emotional changes occur within a young person, signifying the onset of puberty and continuing until maturation.

The physical development and rapid growth associated with adolescence make this a time when good nutrition is vitally important for the building of a strong, healthy body. The need for calories, protein, and other body-building elements increases during this period. Adolescents need protein, calcium, phosphorus, and vitamin D for proper bone formation. Protein is especially important for the development of new tissues and contains the amino acids vital for growth.

MENSTRUATION

Menstruation is the cyclical process that continuously prepares the uterus for pregnancy; it starts at puberty and continues through menopause. Menstruation occurs on an average of every 28 days except during pregnancy and lactation. It is characterized by a passing of the blood-rich uterine lining, lasting approximately 4 or 5 days. However, individuals may differ in time between periods and duration of menstrual flow.

Women whose general health and resistance are good are apt to have less premenstrual tension or cramping than those women suffering from poor nutrition and lack of physical exercise. Symptoms of premenstrual tension include abdominal bloating, weight gain, breast tenderness, irritability, headache, depression, and, possibly, edema of the legs.

Studies have shown that approximately ten days before menstruation, the blood calcium and zinc drops

steadily and progessively while the blood copper rises. The results can be premenstrual tension, nervousness, headaches, insomnia, and depression. The decreased calcium and zinc acts as a stress on the body, causing weight gain and lowering resistance to allergies and infections. When cramping occurs, calcium taken every hour generally brings relief. More calcium is retained when magnesium and vitamin D are adequate. Complete proteins and vitamins B complex and C are also needed. Cramps that don't respond to calcium may be relieved with vitamin B_6, niacin, and/or potassium and magnesium. Vitamin B_6 can also regulate the water balance of premenstruation.

The loss of blood which occurs during menstruation causes a loss of iron. The diet should be adequate in iron and iodine to replace loss, plus vitamin C to aid in iron absorption. The vitamin B complex, especially vitamin B_6 and folic acid, may relieve some of the tension associated with menstruation. Vitamin A may relieve general symptoms associated with premenstrual tension. Noticeable improvement in menstruation has been observed in persons taking 200–1000 mg daily doses of vitamin C.

Irregular or cessation of menstrual flow often indicates a state of general malnutrition. The B vitamins and vitamin E may be particularly helpful in correcting the condition. Menstrual cycles of a young girl that do not begin until age fourteen or even seventeen, or cycles that have started at thirteen but are irregular for up to a year, may indicate a deficiency of zinc. To establish regular cycles, taking vitamin B_6 along with zinc is recommended.

Excessive menstruation may be a sign of uterine cancer and a physician should be consulted. Other causes may be a vitamin E deficiency, an underactive thyroid (helped by iodine, protein, and vitamin E), or liver damage.

MENOPAUSE

Menopause is the period in a woman's life marked by glandular changes that denote the end of her menstrual cycle and reproductive years. Menopause usually results from a decreased production of the female sex hormones when a woman is between the ages of forty-two and fifty-two.

Poor diet, lack of exercise, and emotional stress may

exaggerate the symptoms and discomfort of menopause. Some women experience severe nervous symptoms and become irritable, overly excitable, or depressed. They may have headaches, abdominal pains, rushes of blood to the head and upper body known as "hot flashes," backaches, leg cramps, nosebleeds, frequent bruises, varicose veins, and even ulcers. Some women find themselves extremely fatigued or experiencing insomnia.

Usually within a period of months or a year or two, the body readjusts and the symptoms disappear. Although the menstrual periods cease, a woman's normal sexual needs remain after menopause, and she does not need to experience rapid aging.

If long-term nutrient deficiencies have left the body unprepared for the stress of menopause, and particularily if symptoms are severe, all nutrients needed for a stressful situation and for stimulating the adrenals should be taken. (See Stress and Adrenal Exhaustion.)

The vitamin E requirement (up to 1200 IU daily) is exceptionally high during menopause, and supplements have relieved night sweats, hot flashes, backaches, fatigue, nervousness, insomnia, dizziness, shortness of breath, and heart palpitations in many persons. If estrogen is taken, the need for the vitamin increases further.

As estrogen made from the ovaries gradually decreases, the adrenal glands start to make both estrogens and androgens and take over many actions of the ovarian hormones. As the output of estrogen decreases, calcium is less well absorbed and urinary losses are greater. A deficiency of calcium can cause nervousness, irritability, insomnia, headaches, and depression. Vitamin D and magnesium are needed for proper calcium absorption: 2 gm calcium, 1000 IU vitamin D and 1 gm magnesium daily have been used effectively in a clinical setting.

Vitamins A, B complex, C, and zinc are important for skin maintenance. The B complex, especially pantothenic acid and PABA, relieves nervous irritability. Vitamin C together with bioflavonoids increases capillary strength. The calcium-phosphorus balance should be carefully maintained during the mature years, and an increase in protein with reduction of carbohydrates is generally recommended. The herb don quai has reportedly been beneficial in relieving some of the symptoms of menopause.

SEX

A satisfying sex life requires a healthy body, which depends on sound nutrition, exercise, and sufficient rest. For the most part, sexual function is controlled by the endocrine glands, which secrete specific hormones. In order to function properly and produce sufficient hormones, these glands have certain nutritional needs. The pituitary gland has both direct and indirect effects on sexual and reproductive functions. Its hormones need the B complex vitamins, pantothenic acid, niacin, vitamin E, and zinc. Any deficiency of the pituitary causes underdeveloped sex organs, early menopause in women, and impotence in men. The adrenal glands produce a small but significant amount of sex hormone. These glands need vitamin A, the B vitamins, pantothenic acid, vitamin B_1, niacin, vitamins C and E, and the unsaturated fatty acids. Adrenal exhaustion can result in little strength or desire for sex. An inadequately supplied thyroid can also cause a lack of desire or strength for sex. Iodine, the B vitamins, vitamin B_1, and vitamin E are essential for the production of its hormone, thyroxine.

The male sex gland, the testis, is composed of two glands; one secretes testosterone and the other produces sperm. Women also secrete some testosterone. (Testosterone increases sexual desire in both sexes.) Vitamins A, C, E, and folic acid work with testosterone to produce sperm and other male characteristics such as a deep voice and facial hair. The nutrient content of sperm includes calcium, magnesium, zinc, sulfur, and vitmins B_{12}, C, and inositol. A deficiency of vitamin E causes a degeneration of the testicles; too-low levels of zinc result in immovable, useless, and infertile sperm. In male laboratory animals, a manganese deficiency causes loss of sex drive, lack of semen, and degeneration of the seminal tubules; a lack of selenium results in infertility. Testosterone levels proportionately decrease with the amount of marijuana smoked.

The female sex glands, the ovaries, secrete two hormones, estrogens and progesterones. The B vitamins, folic acid, niacin, vitamin E, and zinc are necessary for the functioning of these hormones. Insufficient estrogen causes, among other conditions, delayed sexual maturation and lack of development or shrinkage of the breasts and genitals.

The sex hormones are made from cholesterol. Cholesterol-containing foods need not be limited as long as the body has sufficient amounts of the other nutrients needed to properly metabolize the cholesterol. These include the vitamins B complex, C, and E, magnesium, manganese, zinc, and lecithin. Refined and processed foods are greatly lacking in these nutrients; in their absence cholesterol is unable to enter the cells and remains in the blood, eventually forming plaques.

Impotence, the male's inability to achieve erection of the penis, has been related to a magnesium or a combined zinc and vitamin B_6 deficiency. Other factors associated with impotence are emotional problems, physical illnesses such as diabetes, and the intake of drugs and alcohol. (Frigidity is the female counterpart of impotence.) Although levels of testosterone decrease with age, this does not cause erectile impotence because the penis requires only minimal amounts of the hormone for successful operation.

Infertility or sterility can occur in the male or female and is often the result of a zinc deficiency. Studies have shown that the higher the blood histamine level in men, the quicker the ejaculation. Men too low in histamine cannot achieve ejaculation. Women with too-low histamine are unable to achieve orgasm; the B vitamins niacin and folic acid raise blood histamine. Calcium and the amino acid methionine lower blood histamine; therefore they are helpful for men who ejaculate prematurely.

Sexual desire and performance can be adversely affected by numerous things including drugs, alcohol, cigarette smoking, caffeine, some common medicines such as certain tranquilizers, antihypertensives, and anticholinergics, and the birth control pill. The most common oral contraceptives are composed of two synthetic hormones, estrogen and progestin. The pill has been shown to interfere with carbohydrate and fat metabolism and to destroy certain nutrients, including several B vitamins and vitamins C and E. It increases copper and iron levels and decreases zinc levels. The pill may also aggravate schizophrenia, cause migraine headaches, and increase the rise of hypertension and the formation of blood clots. Women who smoke, are above age 35, and have type A blood should not use the contraceptive pill because blood clots can occur.

AGING

Aging is a natural biological process; however, predisposition to premature aging or death may be caused by an improper diet and bad habits. As people age, the immune system, which protects the body from bacteria, viruses, and diseases of all kinds, begins to break down. The immune system is made up of the thymus gland, the spleen, lymph nodes and ducts, white blood cells, bone marrow (where white cells are made), antibodies, complement, and interferon. The thymus gland, located behind the breastbone, instructs certain white blood cells, called T-cells, what and when to attack. These T-cells in turn control other white blood cells that make antibodies. When the thymus gland no longer directs efficiently, harmful substances such as bacteria, viruses, and cancer cells are not attacked but are left free to invade body tissues. Sometimes directions from the thymus are so confused that some of the body's own cells attack the body itself, a process that is thought to cause diseases such as arthritis and multiple sclerosis. Scientific studies have shown that the thymus gland can increase in size and its functional capacity improve with certain nutrients, including vitamins A, C, and E, the minerals zinc and selenium, and one of the amino acids, cysteine.

Enzymes called proteases can stimulate certain immune system cells. These enzymes are found in raw pineapple and papaya. They can also aid in the destruction of hard bonds that form in the body, a process called cross-linking that results in such conditions as hard, inflexible arteries and wrinkled skin. Cross-linking at the molecular level causes the body to become stiff and less agile; large molecules such as collagen, a protein in connective tissue, become welded together by cross-links. The master and copy instructors of all cell functions, the nucleic acids DNA and RNA, can also be cross-linked, in which case they do not function properly and abnormal cells results. These abnormal cells can cause aging as well as many other conditions, including cancer.

Cross-linking can be caused by a chemical, acetaldehyde, found in cigarette smoke and smog and made in the liver from alcohol; and by free radicals, destructive entities that are created by radiation and the oxidation of fats and are a product of normal metabolism. Free radicals damage proteins, fats, and DNA and

RNA. They cause the visible brownish pigment accumulation in the skin called age spots. Damage from free radicals and cross-linking can be greatly reduced by taking antioxidant nutrients such as vitamins A, C, E, B_1, B_5, B_6, and the bioflavonoids, the minerals zinc and selenium, and cysteine, an amino acid. (When taking the B vitamins, it is best to take them as part of the entire complex, as they have an interacting relationship. The same applies to the amino acids; it is preferable to obtain them from foods containing complete proteins.)

The function of the brain depends on chemicals called neurotransmitters, which are made from certain nutrients. These chemicals enable brain cells to communicate with each other and relay messages. As aging progresses, fewer neurotransmitters are produced and the ability to respond to their messages is reduced. Acetylcholine is a neurotransmitter which affects the emotions of sex and plays a role in memory and learning. Low acetylcholine levels can cause forgetfulness, inability to concentrate, sleeplessness, and poor muscle coordination. Mucous membranes become dry and susceptible to irritation and infection. The brain makes acetylcholine from choline, found in fish for example, and lecithin. Pantothenic acid is required for this conversion process. Another neurotransmitter affecting sex, memory, and learning is norepinephrine (NE). Too-low levels of NE in the brain can also cause depression. NE is made from phenylalanine and tyrosine, amino acids found in protein foods such as meat, eggs, and cheese.

A deficiency of serotonin, a neurotransmitter that has a calming effect, results in numerous sleep disorders, such as the inability to fall or stay asleep, and is often observed in older persons. Tryptophan, an amino acid, is used by the brain to make serotonin. The amino acid can be found in relatively large amounts in milk and bananas.

Aging also affects RNA synthesis; less RNA is produced, leaving little for memory storage. RNA supplements can be taken, although during its metabolism RNA forms uric acid and can precipitate gout attacks in those persons who are susceptible to the disease. Vitamin B_{12}, however, is an alternative because it stimulates RNA synthesis. Fish contains relatively large quantities of RNA.

Preventive nutrition is the best defense against mental and physical aging. The diet should include natural unprocessed foods which contain all essential nutrients. Additional supplementation may be advisable. Alcohol, preferably in the form of wine and beer, should be consumed in moderation, if at all. Cigarette smoking has many hazards, from destruction of vitamin C to the creation of free radicals and lung cancer. Moderate exercise is stimulating to all the body organs and systems. If one is predisposed to genetic disorders, proper nutrition and care may reduce or relieve many of the attendant symptoms.

Herbs

In meadows, prairies, and wildwoods, people for centuries have been collecting herbs to use as medicine. Vast amounts of information have been collected and tested; much of this information had never been written down, but had been passed on verbally instead. A disadvantage of most archaic theory is that it is permeated with magic, superstition, and dogma that is, for all practical purposes, irrelevant. Many Renaissance herbalists recorded information from ancient herbalists such as Pliny or Dioscorides without testing the ancients' claims, thus preserving statements that were to cast a suspicious light over the rest of the Renaissance findings about herbs.

In the *Journal of the Florida Medical Association,* August 1967, Drs. Max Michael, Jr., and Mark V. Barrow wrote, "It cannot be denied that folk remedies have yielded potent therapeutic weapons when one remembers the instances of digitalis and other drugs. That most of the remedies of the past and most of the present are without scientific foundation is probable. That there are traces of some compounds in many of the folk remedies which have appropriate pharmaceutical effects is also known. Before one closes his mind to all folk remedies and looks on them with derision, he must reckon with the fact that some indeed may be efficacious."[1]

Walter Lewis, professor of biology at Washington University in St. Louis, Missouri, states that the approach to research since the synthetic era, with little regard for past data, ". . . has served to delay the application of many potential benefits. For example, it is unfortunate that man's first cosmopolitan tranquilizer derived from rauvolfia did not come into general use until 1952, despite the long history of its use in Ayurvedic medicine in India, or that cromolyn, the miraculous prophylactic drug for asthma, has only recently been introduced, though its use in the form of ammi seeds was part of Bedouin folk medicine for centuries."[2]

Pharmaceutical companies have begun to search for plants that can cope with the diseases that are associated with our modern life-style. Stress, coronary disease, ulcers, rheumatism, and other ailments have already yielded to the power of plants. Even antitumor properties have been found in several species.[3]

There may be a word of caution to the chemist who first isolates the beneficial substance and leaves the rest of the root, bark, stem, leaf, or flower behind. This purified chemical may act favorably on a particular part of the body, but may also have deleterious effects on other parts of the body. Side effects may

[1]Max Michael, Jr., and Mark V. Barrow, *Journal of the Florida Medical Association,* vol. 54, no. 8, pp. 778–84, August 1967.

[2]Walter H. Lewis, *Medical Botany* (New York: John Wiley & Sons, 1977), p. vii.

[3]Michael, *Medical Botany,* pp. 127–32.

include rashes, dizziness, fainting, palpitations, blurred vision, diarrhea, or depression. The constituents of the plant that were discarded in the laboratory may have an inherent balancing or modifying mechanism that exerts control over the active principle. Both digitalis and rauvolfia have recently been shown to be of greater benefit when the whole part of the plant involved was taken.

The exact reason for the positive effect that herbs exert on the human body is not always known. It is evident, however, that the nutrients stored within the plants' cellular structure are in forms that are easily metabolized by the gastric juices, enzymes, and hormones of the body. The therapeutic action of herbs comes from *alkaloids,* organic nitrogenous compounds that cause certain chemical reactions within the body. Herbs also contain minerals, vitamins, and salts that help the body to resist disease, strengthen tissues, and improve the nervous system. They also contain glycosides, which are important sugars for the proper functioning of the heart and bloodstream. Tannins present in herbs aid recovery from illness by preventing passage of harmful bacteria. Plant mucilage can assist in the proper functioning of the intestines.

In order to receive the beneficial effects that can be obtained from herbs, the herbs must be consumed regularly for long periods of time, sometimes indefinitely. There are exceptions, such as golden seal, which if taken too long can retrogress the illness. Herbs should be kept in air-tight containers away from heat, light, and dampness to prevent deterioration of their active ingredients.

One very important note: Case histories of different allergies reveal the vast differences among individual metabolisms. If an herb does not agree with you or if you feel adverse effects, discontinue using the herb and find one that does agree with you. Herbs can be potent. Practice moderation. Adverse side effects are possible with many herbs when they are taken in overdoses. THE INFORMATION IN THIS SECTION IS NOT INTENDED TO REPLACE THE SERVICES OF PHYSICIANS.

Following is a summary of some of the most common herbs. There are hundreds of herbs available, about which information can be found in the many books written exclusively about this subject. Herbs can be obtained from health-food stores, from herbal- ists who are listed in the Yellow Pages, from homeopathic pharmacies, and from some food markets.

ALFALFA (*Medicago sativa*)

Medicinal Use

Mild laxative, tonic, stomachic, diuretic.

Comments

Centuries ago, the Arabs used alfalfa as feed for their horses, because they claimed that it made the animals swift and strong. They then tried the herb themselves and became so convinced of its benefits to their health and strength that they named the grass "Al-Fal-Fa," which means "Father of All Foods."

The roots of the alfalfa plant burrow deep into the earth to reach minerals that are inaccessible to most other plants. Alfalfa contains vitamins A, E, K, B, and D. It is high in protein and contains phosphorus, iron, potassium, chlorine, sodium, silicon, magnesium, and other trace elements. Alfalfa has eight enzymes known to promote chemical reactions that enable food to be assimilated properly within the body.

Alfalfa has been effective for aiding stomach ailments, gas pains, ulcerous conditions, dropsy, and pain and stiffness of arthritis. It may eliminate retained water, help cure peptic ulcers, and help in treating recuperative cases of narcotic and alcohol addiction and also in treating cases of overweight.

Alfalfa herb tea is said to possess no unfriendly components and may be given to children and adults of all ages. It is good for nursing mothers and for others who wish to abstain from beverages that contain caffeine. The tea is especially pleasant when it is combined with a mint-flavored herb.

ANGELICA (*Angelica archangelica*)

Medicinal Use

Aromatic, stimulant, carminative, diuretic, diaphoretic, emmenagogue, tonic, expectorant, stomachic.

Comments

Is is thought by many that angelica derived its botanical name, *Angelica archangelica,* from its blooming date, May 8, which used to be the day of Michael the Archangel. In eighteenth-century Europe, giving a bouquet of angelica to one who was dearly loved meant "you are my inspiration."

Angelica has been used as a remedy for stomach problems such as sour stomach, heartburn, gas or colic, and for colds, coughs, shortness of breath, and fever. It may be good for sluggish liver and spleen, rheumatism, and nervous headache. It is useful for ulcers (taken internally and tea-dropped externally), because it restores normal tissues. Because of its unique ability to clear tiny passages, angelica has been used to relieve dimness of vision and of hearing by placing drops of the tea into the eyes and ears. Large doses may have a positive effect on blood pressure, heart action, and respiration. In Eurasia, angelica is considered a tonic to improve well-being and mental harmony. In England, the plant juice has been placed into carious teeth, and the oil has been used in dental preparations. Angelica salve applied externally is beneficial as a skin lotion and for relief of rheumatic pains. A decoction can be applied to the skin for itching and wounds. As a compress it is helpful for gout. Angelica has a tendency to increase the sugar in the urine, so those with diabetes or with diabetic tendencies should avoid it.

The dried leaf stalks of angelica are often preserved with sugar, thus forming a confection (also known as angelica) that is used in sweetmeats and cake decorations. The hollow stems of the plant can be added to stewed apples or rhubarb. In Iceland, both stems and roots are eaten raw with butter. The Norwegians make a bread with the roots, and in Lapland the stalks are regarded as a delicacy. As a bath additive, it is soothing to the nerves.

CHAMOMILE (*Anthemis nobilis*)

Medicinal Use

Stomachic, antispasmodic, tonic, emmenagogue, stimulant, tonic, aromatic, anodyne, vermifuge.

Comments

Chamomile is widely known for its applelike fragrance and flavor. It derives its name from the Greek *kamai* (on the ground) and *melon* (apple), for "ground apple."

Chamomile may relieve upset stomachs, colds, bronchitis, bladder troubles, dropsy, and jaundice. Intermittent and typhoid fever may be broken in the early stages through ingestion of the tea. It is helpful in regulating the menstrual cycle, rheumatic pains, headaches, and hysteria. It has been traditionally used as a sleep inducer and mild sedative. In Italy, a million cups of chamomile are drunk each day, and an Italian company now markets it under the slogan "cup of serenity." It is effective for colic in infants and is a good remedy for a child's fever and restlessness. The tea can be used as a wash for sore or weak eyes and for open sores and wounds, as a gargle, and as a poultice for pains and swellings. A chamomile poultice is helpful in preventing gangrene. When sponged over the body and left to dry, the tea acts as an insect repellant.

The dried leaves and flowers have for centuries been used as a hair rinse for blond hair, as an additive for baths, and as a scent among linen.

COMFREY (*Symphytum officinale*)

Medicinal Use

Demulcent, astringent, pectoral, vulnerary, mucilagineous, anodyne, emollient, hemostatic, refrigerant.

Comments

Comfrey is high in calcium, potassium, phosphorus, and other trace minerals. It contains protein and vitamins. The leaves are rich in vitamins A and C. It is a good source of the amino acid lysine, which is usually lacking in diets that contain no animal products. It is also one of the few vegetable sources of vitamin B_{12}. Chemical analysis has shown that comfrey contains the healing agent allantoin, which is known to promote granulation and formation of epithelial cells, thus increasing the speed at which nature can heal a wound, internal irritation, or broken bone. B_1, B_2, niacin, pantothenic acid, D, E, and choline are other vitamins found in the comfrey plant. Comfrey is recommended for all pulmonary complaints and hemoptysis. It is helpful for coughs; consumption; ulceration or soreness of the kidneys, stomach, or bowels; bloody urine; rheumatic pains; digestive disorders; and eczema and other skin disorders. It is useful for scrofula, anemia, dysentery, diarrhea, leucorrhea, colitis, gall and liver diseases, and hemorrhoids. Comfrey cleanses the entire system of impurities. In some parts of Ireland, it is eaten as a cure for defective circulation and used to strengthen the blood.

Bruises, sores, ulcerous wounds, and broken bones can be dressed externally with a poultice made from comfrey, which is also useful for boils and carbuncles. A little Vaseline may first be applied to avoid irritation from the prickly leaves. Fomentations or poultices can be used for any kind of inflammatory swelling. Comfrey ointment can be used for scratches, sores, itches, burns, and rashes. Fomentations relieve sore breasts and headache. A decoction makes a good gargle and mouthwash for throat inflammations, hoarseness, and bleeding gums. Dried comfrey can be ground and added to bread and muffins. It also tones the skin when it is added to the bath.

DANDELION (*Taraxacum officinale*)

Medicinal Use

Diuretic, tonic, slight aperient, hepatic, depurative, stomachic, cholagogue.

Comments

Dandelion has a high vitamin and mineral content. It is very useful for treating kidney and liver disorders, and helpful with jaundice, skin diseases, scrofula, and loss of appetite. It is useful for treating dropsy, fever, inflammation of the bowels, infectious hepatitis, edema resulting from liver problems, rheumatism, gout, and stiff joints. Dandelion increases the activity of the liver, pancreas, and spleen. Based on a compilation by Dr. Norman Farnsworth, professor of pharmacognosy at the University of Illinois in Chicago, dandelion has been shown to contain insulin substitutes that are needed by diabetics. The Chinese use a dandelion poultice for snake bites. The milky juice can be applied daily to warts.

Young dandelion leaves can be used in salads. The larger leaves can be cooked as a vegetable. Dandelion wine is made from the flowers, and the roots are dried and ground to make a coffee substitute.

EUCALYPTUS (*Eucalyptus globulus*)

Medicinal Use

Antiseptic, antispasmodic, stimulant, expectorant, aromatic.

Comments

The leaves and oil from this tree are an extremely potent but safe antiseptic, which results from the antimicrobial properties of one of their constituents, eucalyptol. An infusion is good for scarlet, typhoid, and intermittent fevers; and for indigestion. It is soothing to inflamed mucous membranes; thus it is a relief for asthma and croup. The oil may be applied locally for ulcers, growths, wounds, sores, neuralgic or rheumatic pains, pyorrhea, and burns. When inhaled, eucalyptus is valuable for treating asthma, diphtheria, sore throat, and stuffy nose. A solution of 1 teaspoon of oil to 1 cup of warm water may be rubbed into the skin as an effective insect repellent. The oil may be taken internally in small doses only. Excessive doses of eucalyptus may produce digestive disturbances, nausea, vomiting, diarrhea, kidney irritation, muscular weakness, and related effects.

Eucalyptus is a major ingredient in many commercial medicines such as cough and sore throat lozenges, nasal sprays, and chest rubs. A facial steam that is made with the leaves or oil in a pot of boiling water, and inhaled with a towel placed over the head, is effective for relieving congestion. This same water can be poured on sauna rocks. Eucalyptus tea or oil can also be put into the bath.

GINSENG (*Panax quinquefolium*)

Medicinal Use

Tonic, stimulant, demulcent, stomachic, anodyne, sedative, slight laxative, diaphoretic, carminative, alterative.

Comments

The Chinese have used ginseng for over 5000 years. They composed the name "ginseng" from two words meaning "man-plant." Often the roots resemble the shape of a man, sometimes in detail. It was given the botanical name *Panax,* which means "all-healing" and is related to the word "panacea."

Ginseng strengthens the heart and nervous system. It builds up general mental and physical vitality and resistance to disease by strengthening and stimulating the endocrine glands that control all basic physiological processes, including the metabolism of minerals and vitamins. Dr. Keijiro Takagi, dean of the faculty of pharmaceutical sciences at the University of Tokyo, stated that "with the use of ginseng there is a significant anti-fatigue reaction in mice. We also learned that ginseng aids in the acceleration and acquisition of learning."[4] In a Chinese study, high blood sugar levels in animals were lowered with ginseng, and it was found to be effective for counteracting the deficiency of vitamins B_1 and B_2. Soviet researchers report that ginseng normalizes the level of arterial pressure and is effective in the treatment of both hypotension and hypertension.

Ginseng may be effective for treating colds, coughs, rheumatism, neuralgia, gout, diabetes, anemia, insomnia, stress, headache, backache, and double vision. Women find it helpful for normalizing menstruation and easing childbirth. It is believed to rejuvenate the entire system, to increase sexual energies, and to contain compounds that may exhibit antitumor value. In an experimental study in Eastern Europe, ginseng was used effectively as a mouthwash against periodontal disease, which is a progressive destruction of the supporting structures of the teeth. Ginseng's value is mainly as a preventative. It must be taken over a long period of time to stimulate rejuvenation and virility.

GOLDEN SEAL (*Hydrastis canadensis*)

Medicinal Use

Tonic, laxative, alterative, detergent, aperient, diuretic, antiseptic, astringent, deobstruent, antiperiodic.

[4]Dian Buchman, "Ginseng: An Oriental Panacea," *The Herbalist,* June 1977, p. 30.

Comments

Golden seal was one of the favorite herbs of the Cherokee Indians of North America. The name "golden seal" was given to the herb because of the seallike scars on the golden-yellow root. It has a very positive effect on the mucous membranes and body tissues. It is excellent for all catarrh conditions, whether of the throat, nose, bronchial passages, intestines, stomach, or bladder. It is a tonic for spinal nerves and is helpful for treating spinal meningitis. It is helpful with indigestion, biliousness, and liver disorders. It increases the secretion of bile and gastric juices. Golden seal is useful for treating typhoid fever, gonorrhea, leucorrhea, and syphilis. It is helpful with mouth sores, ulcerations of the stomach and bowels, dysentery, and diarrhea. Golden seal shows experimental activity that is useful for diabetics. Small doses taken frequently will help to relieve nausea during pregnancy. It is an excellent nontoxic substitute for quinine. A douche that is made with an infusion of golden seal will soothe inflammations of the vagina and uterus. Golden seal will help to alleviate pyorrhea and sore gums when the teeth and gums are brushed with the tea. An infusion, cooled, can be applied to an inflamed eye.

An external wash is effective for skin diseases and sores. Sprinkle the powdered root on after washing with the tea. The powder may also be snuffed up the nostrils for nasal congestion or catarrh.

Golden seal should not be taken in large amounts during pregnancy. Persons with hypoglycemia and severe hypertension should avoid using it internally. It also has a tendency to retrogress an illness after use for too long a time.

HAWTHORN (*Crataegus oxyacantha*)

Medicinal Use

Tonic, antispasmodic, sedative, vasodilator.

Comments

A yellow substance from the hawthorn was isolated by Ullsperger (*Pharmazie,* 1951, p. 141), who found that it caused the dilation of the coronary vessels. Fasshauer reported (*Deutsche Med. Wchnschr.,* vol.

76, p. 211, 1951)[5] that 100 heart patients who required continual therapy were given the liquid extract of hawthorn. The results were generally beneficial. Marked improvement was shown in patients with mitral stenosis and heart diseases of old age. For other patients who used hawthorn, digitalis could be either temporarily discontinued or considerably reduced. Scientific investigation has also found hawthorn to be helpful for insomnia, for alleviating irregular heart rhythm, and for a variety of other heart ailments, including angina pectoris. It has been used to treat high blood pressure when taken over a period of time, arteriosclerosis, inflammation of the heart muscle (myocarditis), arthritis, and rheumatism. It may be effective for alleviating nervous conditions and stress from daily pressure. Although hawthorn is nontoxic, large doses can cause dizziness.

LICORICE (*Glycyrrhiza glabra*)

Medicinal Use

Demulcent, pectoral, emollient, expectorant, laxative, diuretic.

Comments

Archeologists have found great quantities of licorice stored among other treasures in the 3000-year-old tomb of King Tut-Ankh-Amen of Egypt. The practice of placing this herb in the tombs was instituted to enable the spirit of the deceased person to make a sweet drink in the next world.

Licorice has been used for centuries as a confection, and because of its saponin content, it is an effective soother of various internal pains. It is helpful for alleviating such ailments as inflamed stomach, bronchitis, sore throat, coughs, irritations of the bowel and kidney, and indigestion. In Denmark, experiments have shown licorice to be very effective for treating duodenal and peptic ulcers. It also contains a female hormone that has estrogenic action. Southern Europeans drink large amounts of licorice water, because they believe it to be a blood purifier. The Romans thought so highly of its medicinal value that it was included

in the rations of the Roman legions. The licorice root has a substance known as glycyrrhizin, which is fifty times sweeter than sugar cane. Despite this fact, it alleviates rather than increases thirst.

Licorice can be added to other, less pleasant-tasting herbs to make them more palatable. Licorice root sticks can be sucked on by persons who wish to stop smoking. Excessive licorice intake can lead to cardiac dysfunction and hypertension.

PEPPERMINT (*Mentha piperita*)

Medicinal Use

Stimulant, stomachic, carminative, aromatic, vermifuge, anodyne, antispasmodic, cholagogue, tonic.

Comments

According to the Greek philosopher-scientist Theophrastus, 300 B.C., the botanical name *mentha* was derived from Greek mythology. Mintho was a beautiful nymph who was loved by Pluto, god of the underworld. Persephone, who had been abducted by Pluto to reign with him over his domain, became jealous of Mintho and changed her into a fragrant and lowly plant, the mint.

Peppermint is one of several mints within the mint family. All mints are said to strengthen the stomach and improve digestion. The pleasant aroma is soothing and invigorating. Peppermint is used against liver complaints, flatulence, nausea, seasickness, vomiting, chills, colic, fevers, dizziness, diarrhea, dysentery, cholera, influenza, and such heart problems as palpitations. It may be helpful in cases of insanity, convulsions and spasms in infants, and nervous headache. Peppermint cleanses and strengthens the entire system, including the nerves. It diffuses like alcohol and warms the whole body.

The herb tea is an excellent substitute for coffee or tea. The oil of peppermint when applied externally is useful for toothache, headache, neuralgia, burns, and rheumatism. A peppermint salve helps skin conditions. When placed in the bath, peppermint can have a calming and strengthening effect on the nerves and muscles. Peppermint enemas are excellent for cholera or for colon troubles.

[5]Richard Lucas, *Nature's Medicines* (N. Hollywood, Calif.: Wilshire Book Co., 1977), p. 189.

ROSE HIPS

Comments

Hips are the fruit of the rose, or what is left after the flower has bloomed and the petals have fallen. The ancient Greeks used the fresh hips as a food, and 1000 years before Christ, hips were referred to as the "Food of the Gods." "Gods" were believed to be men who lived so close to nature that nature whispered her secrets to them.

During World War II, the governments of England, Sweden, and Norway discovered that rose hips contained from ten to one hundred times more vitamin C than any other food. They also contain vitamins A, E, B_1, B_2, K, P, niacin, and the minerals calcium, phosphorus, and iron. Rose hip tea may be beneficial for the bladder and kidneys, and helpful in preventing colds.

SARSAPARILLA (*Smilax ornata*)

Medicinal Use

Alterative, diuretic, demulcent, stimulant, carminative, tonic.

Comments

Several years ago, researchers at Pennsylvania State College found three hormones in the sarsaparilla plant—testosterone, progesterone, and cortin. Scientists say that impotence generally results from the inability of the testicles to supply the body with a normal amount of the male hormone. Experiments have shown that testosterone tends to restore sexual power, mental alertness, and physical strength. However, the positive effects are only apparent so long as the hormone is taken. Testosterone has also been shown to improve the condition of patients with angina pectoris. Patients who used the hormone were able to tolerate more physical activity, and paroxysms were less frequent and less severe. Results have also been good when testosterone has been given for diseases of the blood vessels in the legs and feet.

The second hormone found in sarsaparilla, progesterone, is normally produced by the ovaries in the female and is essential for the development of the mammary and genital organs and for reproduction. It is also found in the corpus luteum, a yellow mass in the ovary, which aids in the preparation of the womb for pregnancy and also tends to prevent miscarriage. Progesterone has a calming effect on the womb muscles, and eases the spasmodic pains that sometimes follow childbirth.

The third hormone, cortin, is secreted by the adrenal glands. If too little cortin is secreted, the body becomes susceptible to infectious disease, nervous depression, and general weakness.

Dr. Eric Solmo, a Hungarian scientist, lived in Mexico for several years and became curious about a remedy used by the natives as a cure for physical debility, weakness, and sexual impotence. After extensive tests and studies of men and animals, he came to the same conclusion about the benefits of the hormones contained in sarsaparilla as the earlier researchers.

Philippsohn (*Derm. Wchnschr.*, vol. 93, p. 1220, 1931)[6] reported the use of a water extract of sarsaparilla in the treatment of psoriasis. One patient who previously had a very stubborn case took the treatment daily for 20 years without a single relapse. Sarsaparilla stimulates the body's defense mechanism, and is therefore a valuable treatment for syphilis. It has been used for rheumatism, gout, skin eruptions, ringworm, scrofula, internal inflammations, catarrhs, fever, colds, and dropsy. It is an excellent blood purifier. The tea may also be used as an eye wash.

SKULLCAP (*Scutellaria laterifolia*)

Medicinal Use

Tonic, nervine, antispasmodic, slight astringent, diuretic, sedative.

Comments

Skullcap is a beautiful blue-helmeted flowery plant whose name is derived from the leather helmets worn by the early Romans. By its action through the cerebrospinal centers, it is one of the best nerve tonics ever discovered. It may be used for all disorders of

[6]Ibid., p. 55.

the nervous system, including hysteria, convulsions, tremors, and palsy. It is also good for neuralgia, aches and pains, rheumatism, epilepsy, poisonous insect and snake bites, rabies, children's fever, female cramps caused by suppressed menstruation resulting from colds, fevers, functional heart troubles where cardiac action is irregular, insomnia, exhaustion, and lockjaw. It is helpful for alcoholics in delirium tremens, and relieves restlessness. It is an effective substitute for quinine. Skullcap must be taken regularly for a long period of time to be of permanent benefit.

STRAWBERRY (*Fragaria vesca*)

Medicinal Use

Mild astringent, diuretic, tonic.

Comments

Strawberry is excellent for children and for convalescents as a strengthening tonic for the entire system. It is helpful for diarrhea, dysentery, night sweats, liver complaints, gout, and jaundice. It is a good blood purifier. It may be effective against the bodily poisons that cause eczema. It should be taken internally and used as a wash externally. Strawberry is used internally for weak intestines and is also used as an enema. A gargle of the tea may be taken for sore mouth and throat. Strawberry leaves are rich in iron and also contain rutin and the minerals potassium, sodium, and magnesium.

YARROW (*Achillea millefolium*)

Medicinal Use

Diaphoretic, stimulant, tonic, astringent, alterative, vulnerary, diuretic.

Comments

Yarrow gets its botanical name *Achillea* from the legend that comrades of the Greek hero Achilles used yarrow to heal their wounds during the Trojan War. The name *millefolium* was taken because of yarrow's feathery leaves, which are so well divided that the plant appears to have a thousand leaves. Yarrow has a healing and soothing effect on the mucous membranes. It may be effective for treating bleeding from the lungs and urinary organs, diabetes, bleeding hemorrhoids, dysentery, and stomach disorders. It is helpful with typhoid and other fevers, colds, diarrhea, measles, smallpox, chicken pox, Bright's disease, colic, rheumatism, constipation, toothache, and earache. It is very good when applied externally as an ointment for cuts and wounds. Yarrow can also be used as a douche for leucorrhea and as an enema for hemorrhoids.

HERBAL PREPARATIONS

Decoction. Seeds, barks, roots, and other hard materials are prepared by decoction. Put 1 oz herb in 3 cups cold water. Cover and simmer for ½ hour. Then cover and steep for 15–30 minutes. Honey or lemon can be added. Use porcelain or glass vessels.

Fomentation. Dip cloth in the infusion or decoction, wring it out, and apply locally.

Infusion. Leaves, flowers, and some roots are prepared as teas or as infusions. Take 1 tsp per cup or 1 oz per pint. Do not boil the herb. Bring water to boil and pour the water over the herb. Cover and steep for 10–15 minutes. Honey or lemon can be added. Use porcelain or glass vessels.

Oil. Mix 2 tablespoons minced or powdered herbs with ½ cup of oil. Place in hot sun or heat daily in hot water. Shake daily. After 3 weeks, strain and use.

Ointment or salve. Take 4 parts Vaseline or like substance to 1 part herb. Stir and heat gently for 20 minutes. Cool slightly and strain. This works best if herb has been ground.

Poultice. Bruise the herb, add enough boiling water to moisten it, then apply it to the affected part of the body, covering it with a cloth wrung out in hot water.

Syrup.   Boil tea for 20 minutes, add 1 oz glycerin, and seal up in bottles as you would fruit.

Tincture.   Add 1 oz powdered herb to 8 oz alcohol and 4 oz water.   Shake daily.   Let stand for 2 weeks, then strain.

HERB GLOSSARY

ALTERATIVE   Gradually altering or changing a condition, also a blood purifier.

ANODYNE   Relieving pain.

ANTIPERIODIC   Preventing the periodic return of certain diseases.

ANTISEPTIC   Destroying infection-causing micro-organisms.

ANTISPASMODIC   Relieving or preventing involuntary muscle spasms or cramps.

APERIENT   Mild and gently acting laxative.

AROMATIC   Substance with a spicy scent and a pungent but pleasing taste.   Useful for fragrance, and often added to medicines to improve their palatability.

ASTRINGENT   Temporarily tightening or contracting the skin or tissues.   Checks the discharge of mucus and blood, etc.

CARMINATIVE   Checking formation of gas and helping to dispel whatever gas has already formed.

CHOLAGOGUE   Promoting the discharge of bile from the system.

DEMULCENT   Mucilaginous substance that soothes the intestinal tract.

DEOBSTRUENT   Clearing obstruction from the natural ducts of the body.

DEPURATIVE   Removing wastes from body, purifying blood.

DETERGENT   A cleansing action.

DIAPHORETIC   Promoting sweating.   Commonly used as an aid for relief of the common cold.

DIURETIC   Promoting flow of urine.

EMMENAGOGUE   Promoting menstruation.

EMOLLIENT   Softening and soothing skin when applied externally.

EXPECTORANT   Loosening phlegm in the mucous membrane of the bronchial and nasal passages, thus facilitating its expulsion.

HEMOSTATIC   Checking internal bleeding.

HEPATIC   Affecting the liver.

LAXATIVE   A gentle cathartic that helps to promote bowel movements.

MUCILAGINOUS   A soothing quality for inflamed parts.

NERVINE   Calming nervous irritation from excitement, strain, or fatigue.

PECTORAL   Relieving ailments of the chest and lungs.

REFRIGERANT   Generally cooling in effect, also reduces fevers.

SEDATIVE   Calming the nerves.

STIMULANT   Increasing or quickening various functions of the body, such as digestion and appetite.   It does this quickly, whereas a tonic stimulates general health over a period of time.

STOMACHIC   Strengthing and toning the stomach and stimulating the appetite.

TONIC   Invigorating or strengthening the system.

VASODILATOR   Widening blood vessels.

VERMIFUGE   Destroying and helping to expel intestinal worms.

VULNERARY   Application for external wounds.

REFERENCES

Clymer, R. Swinburne, M.D.   *Nature's Healing Agents.*   Philadelphia: Dorrance & Co., 1963.

Heinerman, John.   *Medical Doctors' Guide to Herbs.*   Provo, Utah: Bi-World Publishers, Inc., 1977.

Kloss, Jethro.   *Back to Eden.*   New York: Beneficial Books, 1971.

Lehane, Brendan.   *The Power of Plants.*   Maidenhead, England: McGraw-Hill, 1977.

Lewis, Walter.   *Medical Botany.*   New York: John Wiley & Sons, 1977.

Lucas, Richard.   *Nature's Medicines.*   N. Hollywood, Calif.: Wilshire Book Co., 1977.

Lust, Benedict, M.D.   *About Herbs.*   Wellingborough

Northants, England: Weatherby Woolnough, 1961.

Lust, John. *The Herb Book.*   New York: Bantam Books, 1974.

Meyer, Joseph. *The Herbalist.*   Glenwood, Ill.: Meyerbooks, 1976.

Null, Gary. *Herbs for the Seventies.*   New York: Robert Speller & Sons, 1972.

Rodale Herb Book.   Emmaus, Pa.: Rodale Press, 1976.

Sherborne House Book of Herbs.   Sherborne, Gloucestershire, England: Coombe Springs Press.

Thomson, William, M.D. *Herbs That Heal.*   New York: Charles Scribner's Sons, 1976.

Wren, R. W. *Potter's New Cyclopaedia.*   New York: Harper & Row, 1972.

Foods, Beverages, Supplementary Foods, and Eating Right to Feel Right

Many factors influence eating patterns and therefore affect nutrition. For example, taste preferences, states of health, and various social and cultural customs all determine what foods a person eats. Poor nutrition may be the result of consuming too little, too much, or the wrong kinds of food, because of any number of reasons.

The foods and beverages we consume should provide our bodies with the nutrients necessary for good health. Protein builds and maintains body cells, and carbohydrates, fats, and some proteins provide calories for energy. Vitamins and minerals help regulate the many chemical reactions within the body. For individual recommended dietary allowances of nutrients, see the "Nutrient Allowance Chart" on page 309.

Fresh, raw fruits and vegetables are generally more nutritious than prepared ones, although many kinds of foods are more palatable when cooked. Studies indicate that considerable losses of nutrients, especially the B complex, vitamin C, and the bioflavonoid complex, occur during storage and cooking. It is essential to select, store, and prepare foods wisely in order to obtain these nutrients. Precautions should also be taken to avoid foodborne illnesses caused by the growth of harmful bacteria. Some basic rules for storing and preparing foods in order to retain their nutrient content and to prevent food poisoning are as follows:

- Cook meats, especially pork and poultry, thoroughly in order to kill harmful bacteria.

- Guard against the growth of harmful bacteria by immediately refrigerating leftovers or foods cooked for later use. Do not allow them to cool to room temperature first.

- Keep perishable foods—especially chopped and processed meats, custards, pastries, and dairy products—in the refrigerator to avoid bacterial contamination.

- Destroy cans that bulge or canned contents that bubble out when the can is opened, in order to avoid food poisoning.

- Ensure thorough cooking of frozen foods by allowing them to thaw completely before cooking, unless otherwise stated on frozen food packages.

- Avoid soaking fruits, vegetables, or meats in water, to protect against the loss of water-soluble vitamins.

- Store fresh foods as soon as possible to minimize nutrient loss.

Supplementary foods may be useful for further increasing the nutritional value of meals. Supplementary foods must also be stored and prepared properly in order to prevent nutrient loss.

In the following section, food groups, beverages, and supplementary foods are discussed alphabetically in terms of their nutrient content and special features. This information is intended for use with the "Table of Food Composition" on page 265 and the "Nutrient Allowance Chart" on page 309.

Any reference to a body disorder or disease in connection with a food or beverage is not meant to be prescriptive, but merely represents research findings.

FOODS

EGGS

Eggs are an excellent source of complete protein; they contain all essential amino acids. (One large egg contains 7 or 8 grams of first-class protein.) Also found in eggs are vitamins A, B_2, D, and E, niacin, copper, iron, sulfur, phosphorus, and unsaturated fatty acids. The egg yolk contains the richest known source of choline, found in lecithin and necessary for keeping the cholesterol within the egg emulsified and keeping cholesterol moving in the bloodstream. The yolk also contains lecithin itself and biotin, one of the B-complex vitamins.

Eggs should be kept refrigerated at all times (at 45° to 55°F) because temperature variations will cause the whites to become thin. A soiled egg should be wiped clean with a dry cloth rather than washed, to preserve the natural protective film on the porous eggshell. This film prevents odors, flavors, molds, and bacteria from entering the egg. Eggs retain their freshness and quality better if stored large end up in their original carton.

Raw eggs should not be consumed in great quantity because the whites contain a protein called avidin, which may be harmful to the body if consumed over a long period of time, since it interferes with the use of biotin. However, avidin is inactivated by heat.

FIBER

Fiber is the part of food that is not digested by the human body, such as the skin of an apple and the husk of a wheat kernel. The normal functioning of the intestinal tract depends upon the presence of adequate fiber. A low-fiber diet has been associated with heart disease, cancer of the colon and rectum, diverticulosis, varicose veins, phlebitis, and obesity.

FISH

Fish are excellent sources of high-grade protein, polyunsaturated fatty acids, and minerals, especially iodine and potassium.

Fish are categorized as freshwater fish, saltwater fish, and shellfish. These types differ slightly in nutritive value. Freshwater fish provide magnesium, phosphorus, iron, and copper. Saltwater fish and shellfish are rich in iodine, fluorine, and cobalt. The unsaturated fat content of fish and shellfish varies with the species and season of year. Fatty fish, such as halibut, mackerel, and salmon, are good sources of vitamins A and D. Herring, oysters, and sardines contain vanadium and zinc. Shellfish are low in fatty acids but are relatively high in cholesterol.

Fish and shellfish may be purchased fresh, frozen, canned, salted, dried, or smoked. Because of the possibility of bacterial infection, fresh fish and shellfish should not remain at room temperature for more than two hours. They should be well wrapped, stored in the coldest part of the refrigerator, and used within two days.

Fish and shellfish are best cooked at low temperature (300° to 325°F) and should not be overcooked, in order to preserve flavor, juices, and nutrients.

FRUITS

Fresh fruits are good sources of vitamins and minerals, especially vitamins A and C, carbohydrates in the form of cellulose and natural sugars, and water. They are good substitutes of such high-carbohydrate foods as candy, cookies, and cakes, which contain few nutrients.

Yellow fruits, such as apricots, cantaloupe, and persimmons, are good sources of carotene, which is converted to vitamin A. Aside from acerola cherries and rose hips, the best natural sources of vitamin C are the citrus fruits, such as oranges, grapefruit, lemons, and tangerines; other sources of vitamin C are cantaloupe, strawberries, and tomatoes.

Apples and bananas contain valuable bulk fiber in the form of indigestible cellulose, which is needed for regular bowel movement. Bananas are high in magnesium and may be useful for treatment of diarrhea, colitis, ulcers, and certain cases of protein allergies. Bananas and pears are the highest in natural sugars.

Fruits may be fresh, frozen, dried, or canned, but nutrient values will decrease if fruits are not properly stored or if they are refrigerated for extended periods of time. Fresh fruits offer the richest source of vitamins and minerals as well as appetite appeal in color, flavor, and texture. Fresh fruits purchased in season will be higher in nutrient quality and more economical in price than frozen, dried, or canned fruits. It is preferable to obtain ripe rather than green fruits, since ripe fruits contain simple sugars that are very easily assimilated by the digestive system. Fruits that are not fully ripe should be allowed to ripen at room temperature and then should be stored in a cool, dark place or in the refrigerator.

Fresh fruits should always be washed prior to eating so that any possible chemical residue is removed, and should be eaten whole or peeled thinly so that nutrients found in the skin are conserved. If fruits are to be cooked, they should be cooked quickly.

Frozen fruits compare favorably in nutrient content with fresh fruits, but some loss of nutritional value may occur in the processes of drying and canning, if done improperly. Dried fruits, rich in thiamine and iron, should be softened and cooked in the same water and then stored in a cool, dry place. Home-canned fruits should be stored in a dark place to preserve their vitamin C content. Water-packed fruits are preferable to those packed in heavy syrups that contain large amounts of sugar.

FRUIT JUICES

Fresh fruit juices usually have a pleasing flavor and are easily digested. Although the nutritive value of the whole fruit is somewhat higher, juice is an excellent source of vitamins and minerals.

Juice should be extracted from chilled fruit immediately prior to serving. It should not be allowed to stand for a long period of time after extraction, because vitamin C will be lost. Juices should be refrigerated in covered containers to ensure that vitamin C will not be lost through oxidation.

GRAINS

Grains are often referred to as cereals; they are the seeds of various grasses such as wheat, rye, oats, rice, and barley. Often called the "staff of life," they provide the bulk of the world's food supply. Common foods made from these grains are flours, breads, breakfast cereals, and macaroni.

Breads, Cereals, and Pasta

The main constituent of breads is flour. Flour is the product resulting from the milling process, which involves grinding and sifting of cleaned grains. The type of flour or grain from which it originates often determines the color, texture, flavor, and nutritive value of the bread. Cereals can be made from a variety of grains, such as corn, barley, oats, wheat, rice, and rye. Nutritious pastas can be made from a variety of whole grains. Cook whole-grain pasta 12 to 15 minutes to eliminate the raw flour taste. The pasta will remain firm.

Whole-grain flour is the result of the first milling process. Whole-grain flour contains the germ of the grain, which possesses the most nutrients, and must be refrigerated to prevent rancidity. Whole-wheat flour is best for baking breads and other yeast-containing baked goods. Whole-wheat pastry flour is lighter and good for cookies, cakes, pie crusts, and other desserts. Whole-grain breads should be stored at room temperature or frozen until used. Refrigerated bread loses moisture and thus becomes stale faster than bread that is frozen or that is kept at room temperature.

All-purpose flour is a blend of different refined wheat grains. Bleached flour has been whitened to create a more uniform flour. Self-rising flour contains added salt and leavening in proper proportions. *Enriched flour* has the nutrients thiamine, riboflavin, and niacin of the vitamin B complex, and sometimes iron, returned to it. This enrichment process also applies to other "enriched" products, such as breakfast cereals and pasta.

Rice

Whole brown rice contains a generous supply of B vitamins, plus calcium, phosphorus, and iron. *Wild rice* contains twice as much protein, four times as much phosphorus, eight times as much thiamine, and twenty times as much riboflavin as white rice. *White rice,* dehulled polished rice, has no significant amount of B vitamins but may also be enriched, as are flour and cereals. *Converted rice* has undergone a process similar to milling and it has a somewhat higher vitamin content than white rice.

TOTAL NUTRIENTS IN THE KERNEL OF WHEAT*

Germ is 2½% of Kernel

Of the whole kernel the germ contains:

64% Thiamine
26% Riboflavin
21% Pyridoxine
8% Protein
7% Pantothenic acid
2% Niacin

Bran is 14% of Kernel

Of the whole kernel the bran contains:

73% Pyridoxine
50% Pantothenic acid
42% Riboflavin
33% Thiamine
19% Protein

Endosperm is 83% of Kernel

Of the whole kernel the endosperm contains:

70–75% Protein
43% Pantothenic acid
32% Riboflavin
12% Niacin
6% Pyridoxine
3% Thiamine

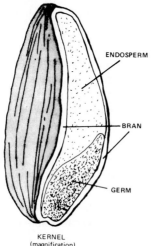

KERNEL
(magnification)

Other nutrients found in the whole wheat grain are:

Calcium	Chlorine
Iron	Sodium
Phosphorus	Silicon
Magnesium	Boron
Potassium	Barium
Manganese	Silver
Copper	Inositol
Sulphur	Folic Acid
Iodine	Choline
Fluorine	Vitamin E

And other trace materials

*Nutrition Search, Inc., *Nutrition Almanac Cookbook* (New York, McGraw-Hill, 1983), p. 8.

Whole Grains

The structure of a whole grain may be separated into three different parts (see illustration). The *germ* is the heart of the grain, which sprouts when the seed is planted. It is especially rich in the B vitamins, vitamin E, protein, unsaturated fat, minerals (especially iron), and carbohydrates. The *endosperm* constitutes the largest part of the grain. It is composed chiefly of carbohydrates in the form of starch, with some incomplete protein and traces of vitamins and minerals. The *bran* portion of the grain is the covering. It is composed chiefly of the carbohydrate cellulose, with traces of B vitamins, minerals (especially iron), and incomplete proteins.

While the entire grain is edible, the bran and germ are often removed during milling in order to reduce the chance of rancidity and to improve the storage quality of the grain. At the same time, important nutrients such as the B vitamins, vitamin E, chromium, magnesium, manganese, copper, molybdenum, selenium, zinc, silicon, iron, and numerous enzymes are lost. In order to enrich flour, bread, and cereal products, only a few select nutrients are added during processing.

LEGUMES

Legumes are plants that have edible seeds within a pod. They include peas, beans, lentils, and peanuts. Legumes are a rich source of incomplete protein, iron, thiamine, riboflavin, and niacin. When sprouted, they provide an excellent source of vitamin C.

Legumes are a hearty and versatile food. Because of their high but incomplete protein content, legumes can be used as a meat substitute when used with other complementary protein foods.

Dried legumes should be stored in tightly covered containers in a cool, dry place. They should be cooked in liquid to soften their cellulose fiber and to restore flavor and moisture that is lost in the drying process. If one adds baking soda when cooking legumes to speed up the softening of the cellulose, the thiamine content of the legumes will be destroyed.

Soybeans

Generous supplies of soybean products may serve as the major protein source in a meatless diet. However, the balance of essential amino acids in soybeans is not the same as that in meats; therefore more grams of this protein are required to supply the essential amino acids adequately. In addition, soybeans contain vitamins and minerals in a natural relationship that is similar to the human body's needs.

Soy flour, oil, and milk are used in a variety of home-cooked and commercial products. Soy flour has a creamy yellow color and a slightly nutty taste. It is a rich source of protein, the vitamin B complex, calcium, phosphorus, potassium, magnesium, and iron. Soybean oil contains large amounts of linoleic acid, an unsaturated fatty acid essential to the human body.

Soybean oil is stable against oxidation and flavor deterioration because of its lecithin and vitamin E content. Soy milk is often recommended for persons who are allergic to cow's milk. Soy milk is low in fat, carbohydrates, calcium, phosphorus, and riboflavin but rich in iron, thiamine, and niacin.

Some forms of soy protein are made into commercial imitation-meat items. Pressed soybean cakes, the product resulting from grinding the soybean residue after the soybeans have been processed for oil, can be added to a variety of cooked dishes. Sprouted soybeans contain increased amounts of vitamin C.

MEATS

"Meat" commonly refers to the flesh of animals; it is the most important source of first-class protein in the modern diet. In addition to protein, beef, lamb, and pork are good sources of the B-complex vitamins (especially thiamine and riboflavin), phosphorus, iron, sulfur, potassium, and copper. Poultry, also a good source of protein, contains the B-complex vitamins (especially niacin), iron, and phosphorus.

The quality of beef, lamb, and pork is designated by the cut—Prime, Choice, or Good—when purchased over the counter. The meat's flavor, tenderness, and ease of cooking vary with the grade and do not affect its nutritional value. In general, lean cuts with less fat are preferable. Prime and Choice cuts of meat are often not the highest in protein content because the animals were "fattened" before slaughter and the lean contains marbling, or fat granules, to increase tenderness. Good grades, therefore, may be more lean and contain more protein per pound. Luncheon meats, frankfurters, and sausages are usually high in fats and often contain nitrites which can be converted to cancer-causing nitrosamines in the stomach.

Variety, or organ, meats are usually richer in vitamins and minerals than muscle meats. Variety meats include the liver, tongue, kidneys, heart, brains, and sweetbreads (glands of calves or lambs). Liver is a very rich source of complete protein and B vitamins, especially riboflavin, niacin, and B_{12}. It is also a good source of vitamins A, C, and D; iron, phosphorus and copper. Because of the high iron and vitamin B_{12} content, liver can aid the body in combating iron-deficiency anemia and pernicious anemia.

Both raw and cooked meat should be refrigerated at a temperature of 30° to 32°F. In order to be at their best flavor and nutritive value, meats should be used within 2 or 3 days after purchase. Ground meats and variety meats should be used within 24 hours to prevent spoilage. Meat should not be soaked in water because this leads to loss of water-soluble nutrients. Nearly all meats freeze well and maintain their quality if wrapped and stored properly, although meat that is frozen for more than 6 months may show freezer burn (drying) and changes in texture. Meats should be frozen quickly and kept at temperatures of −10°F or lower to retard deterioration.

It is preferable that meats be cooked without adding fats or water; broiling and baking at moderate temperatures are recommended. Juices obtained during cooking contain valuable nutrients and should be served with the meat. Pork, or any raw product containing pork, should be cooked thoroughly to kill any trichinosis organisms that may be present. The temperature at the center of a pork roast should be at least 160° to 185°F.

Poultry that is inspected for quality is graded A, B, or C, A being the top quality. White poultry meat is especially rich in niacin and is easier to digest than dark meat, since it contains less fat and connective tissue. Dark meat, however, is superior to white meat as a source of thiamine and riboflavin.

Chilled raw poultry may be kept one or two days in the coldest part of the refrigerator. Stuffing from cooked poultry should be removed and stored separately in a covered container. The body cavity or skin of chickens and turkeys may contain a bacteria that causes food poisoning. In order to prevent a large bacterial growth due to moisture, one should store these birds with loose wrapping so that the surface of the bird will be slightly dry. It is also recommended that poultry be frozen without stuffing and stuffed immediately prior to cooking. Poultry should be thawed completely to enable thorough cooking. Poultry should be cooked thoroughly; the temperature at the center should be about 190°F.

MILK AND MILK PRODUCTS

Milk and milk products are excellent sources of calcium, complete protein, and riboflavin. Milk also contains phosphorus, thiamine, and vitamins B_6 and B_{12}, but it contains little iron or vitamin C. A glass of milk contains about 300 milligrams of calcium; three glasses of milk daily supply the needed amount of calcium for adults; children and adolescents need four or five glasses per day.

Milk is available in several forms. Most milk is pasteurized to kill bacteria and thereby to prevent the spread of milkborne diseases. The pasteurization process involves heating the milk to a high temperature and cooling it rapidly. Homogenized milk is that which has its fat content finely dispersed throughout, and because of this, it is more easily digested than nonhomogenized milk.

Whole milk usually contains about 3.5 percent fat. Skim milk is whole milk from which the fat is removed. Two percent milk contains two percent fat, which gives it more body and flavor than skim milk. Fortified milk has one or more nutrients, commonly vitamins A and D, added. Nonfat dry milk and fluid skim milk, unless fortified, contain no significant amounts of vitamin A or D because these fat-soluble vitamins are removed with the fat; but they are rich in protein, calcium, and vitamin B_2.

People who are allergic to milk may substitute buttermilk, goat's milk, yogurt, and possibly soy milk, although soy milk lacks much of the value of cow's milk because it is low in calcium and phosphorus.

Buttermilk may be obtained from the residue of the butter-making process, or it may be cultured. Most commercial buttermilk is made by the latter process, in which a harmless bacteria is added to skim milk or churned buttermilk.

Evaporated milk is whole milk with one-half of its water content removed. Condensed milk has water removed and sugar added. Dried milk results from the removal of 95 to 98 percent water from whole milk; nonfat dry milk is skim milk with the water removed.

Butter

Butter is made from milk products, contains vitamins A and D, and is high in fat content. It is a concentrated saturated fat that can cause the development of cholesterol in the arteries. Margarine made from unsaturated oils is a preferable substitute. Other saturated fats to avoid are cream, lard, the chunks of fat in meats, and the saturated vegetable oils of palm and coconut.

Cheese

Cheese is made by separating most of the curd, or milk solids, from the whey or water part of the milk. Its texture and flavor vary with ripening (aging). Most cheeses contain protein, milk, fat, calcium, phosphorus, vitamin A, and riboflavin. The best way to store cheese is by leaving it in its original wrapper in the refrigerator. If the wrapper is torn, protect the surface from drying out by covering exposed surface with waxed paper, foil, or plastic. Cheeses with a strong odor should be kept in a container with a tight cover.

Yogurt

Milk that has been fermented by a mixture of bacteria and yeasts forms a custardlike product called yogurt. The milk is defatted and soured with *Lactobacillus acidophilus* and other bacteria that are necessary for health of the intestine. Yogurt aids digestion and controls the action of the intestine in favorably stimulating the kidneys.

Yogurt contains the B-complex vitamins and has a higher percentage of vitamins A and D than does the milk it was made from; it is also high in protein.

The beneficial bacteria in yogurt make it a natural antibiotic. Yogurt has been found to be beneficial in treating high cholesterol level, arthritis, constipation, diarrhea, gallstones, halitosis, hepatitis, kidney disorders, and skin diseases.

The sugar in commercial yogurt tends to nullify its therapeutic effects. Sugar is antagonistic to the B vitamins which are made from the bacteria found in yogurt.

NUTS

Nuts are the dry fruits or seeds of some kinds of plants, usually of trees. Some readily available nuts are pecans, filberts, Brazil nuts, walnuts, almonds, and cashews. The soft inside part of the nut is the meat, or kernel, and the outer covering is the shell. Nuts are a concentrated food source of proteins, unsaturated fats, the B-complex vitamins, vitamin E, calcium, iron, potassium, magnesium, phosphorus, and copper.

Nuts may be eaten fresh, roasted, boiled, or in the form of flour or butter. Nuts may interfere with digestion unless they are chewed well or chopped into fine particles. When nuts are purchased in the shell, attention should be paid to the firmness of the seal, since partially cracked nuts soon become dry and rancid. Nuts that are shelled should be stored preferably in the refrigerator, in airtight containers, to preserve their freshness and to prevent oxidation and rancidity of their fat content.

Nut butters should contain the nut only without processing or added fats and sugar.

OILS

The term "oil" generally refers to fats in a liquid state. Vegetable oils, such as corn, cottonseed, safflower, soybean, olive, and sunflower, are widely used in cooking. These oils are important in the diet because of their content of unsaturated fatty acids, especially linoleic acid, which is necessary for growth and maintenance of the cells.

Oils may be removed from seeds, such as the safflower, or from beans, such as the soybean, by heat extraction or by pressing. Oils removed by pressing are referred to as "cold-pressed" and retain their vitamin A and E content better than those extracted by heat.

Margarine is a popular butter substitute made from solidified vegetable oils. Margarine contains some salt and flavoring compounds to make it resemble butter in taste.

Oils, margarine, and all other fats should be kept refrigerated. They should also be well covered to prevent the absorption of odors from other foods.

SEASONINGS, HERBS, SPICES, AND EXTRACTS

Seasonings, herbs, spcies, and extracts are usually derived from foods. They normally have little nutritive value because they are consumed in minute amounts.

However, they give variety to the flavor of foods, stimulate the appetite, and encourage the flow of digestive juices. Seasonings, herbs, spices, and extracts are usually derived from the bark, roots, fruits, berries, or leaves of plants, shrubs, or trees.

Salt, or sodium chloride, is the most commonly used seasoning as well as an essential body mineral. Most people, however, consume many times too much salt. The body needs only a small amount, about 2 or 3 grams per day. An excess of table salt may cause mineral imbalances in the body because the sodium in it upsets the potassium and calcium levels in the body. Salt may be plain or iodized; salt used in the home should be iodized or sea salt, from evaporated seawater, which contains many trace minerals and is an especially good source of iodine.

Pepper ranks next to salt as a common seasoning. Pepper is available in two forms, black and white. Both forms are obtained from the dried berries of the same tropical vine, but they differ in the manner of processing.

Herbs and spices lose their true bouquet and flavor after six months of shelf life. They should be stored in tightly covered containers away from heat and light so that they will not become dry and stale.

Liquid extracts, including vanilla, almond, and fruit extracts (such as lemon and orange), should be stored in a cool, dry place so as not to develop off-flavors or aromas. They must be tightly capped to prevent evaporation.

SEEDS

Seeds are the ripened ovules of plants. The most important nutritive elements of seeds are the B-complex vitamins; vitamins A, D, and E; unsaturated fats; proteins; phosphorus; calcium; and a trace of fluorine.

Edible seeds such as pumpkin seeds, sesame seeds, and sunflower seeds are rich in protein; the B complex; vitamins A, D, and E; phosphorus; calcium; iron; fluorine; iodine; potassium; magnesium; zinc; and unsaturated fatty acids. Sesame seeds are high in calcium content. Sunflower seeds contain up to 50 percent protein.

Seeds have a variety of uses and may be eaten raw, dried, roasted, or cooked. Pumpkin, sesame, and sun-

flower seeds are popular snack foods, and others, such as caraway, dill, poppy, and anise, are used as seasonings. Seeds can be especially nutritious additions to soups, salads, casseroles, and baked goods. Sunflower-seed oil may be extracted for use in cooking and baking.

Unhulled seeds have a long shelf life, provided they are kept in a cool, dry place in a tightly covered container. Hulled seeds should be refrigerated immediately and used promptly because oxidation of their fat content may make them rancid.

SWEETENERS

Sugars and other concentrated sweets furnish quick energy to the body in readily digestible form. Cane and beet sugars, jellies, jams, candy, syrup, molasses, and honey are concentrated sources of sugar. Fruits are a natural source of sugar and furnish bulk in the diet.

Sugar is a major carbohydrate source but is completely devoid of protein, vitamins, and minerals and is not considered nutritious. Refined white sugar, in granulated or powdered form, and brown sugar are made from either sugar cane or sugar beet. White sugar contains no vitamins or minerals. The B vitamins needed for its assimilation are robbed from other parts of the body. Sugar leads to an imbalance in the calcium-phosphorus relationship. Sugar may also be a contributing factor in the development of overweight, diabetes, arthritis, tooth decay, pyorrhea, asthma, mental illness, nervous disorders, and low blood sugar. Natural sources of sugar, such as fruits, usually contain adequate supplies of vitamins essential for digestion and metabolism. Brown sugar has a slightly higher nutritive value than white sugar. Honey, maple syrup, maple syrup granules, barley malt, date sugar, unrefined granulated sugar cane juice, and concentrated fruit juices are preferable sweeteners because they are not refined and contain vitamins, minerals, and enzymes to aid in their digestion. Besides sucrose (sugar), other forms of refined sugars are glucose, a light-colored syrup made from cornstarch, sorbitol, which is found in mountain ash fruits, maltose, which is formed from starches, and fructose, a sugar derived from fruits and honey. These sweeteners are extracts, just as sucrose is an extract from the sugar or beet cane. They no longer are accompanied by vitamins, minerals, and enzymes. Artificial sweeteners, including aspartame, or its trade name, NutraSweet, have been found in clinical studies to have numerous undesirable side effects.

Carob

Carob is a natural sweetener rich in B vitamins and minerals with a flavor similar to that of chocolate. It is often used as a substitute for chocolate or cocoa, especially by people who are allergic to chocolate or who wish to avoid the caffeine it contains. Carob also contains a fair amount of protein, sugar, and some calcium and phosphorus. It is available in tablet, powder, syrup, and wafer forms.

Chocolate and Cocoa

Chocolate, cocoa, and foods flavored with these substances from the cocoa bean are usually prepared with large amounts of sugar that add carbohydrates to the diet while adding no significant amounts of vitamins and minerals. Chocolate and cocoa contain two stimulants, caffeine and theobromine, which speed up the heartbeat and stimulate the central nervous system. Chocolate also contains oxalic acid, an excess of which could interfere with calcium absorption. Cocoa is lower in fat than chocolate and therefore will keep for longer periods of time. It is slightly higher in nutritive value than chocolate.

Honey

Honey is one of nature's finest energy-giving foods, consisting of carbohydrates in the most easily digestible form. Honey varies in texture, flavor, and color, depending upon place of origin and the flowers from which the nectar was gathered. Because honey is almost twice as sweet as cane or beet sugar, smaller amounts of it are needed for sweetening purposes. Honey contains large amounts of carbohydrates in the form of sugars, small amounts of minerals, and traces of the B-complex vitamins and vitamins C, D, and E.

Molasses

Molasses is a thick, sticky syrup, light to dark brown in color, with a strong, distinctive flavor. Blackstrap molasses is the residue left after the last possible extraction of sugar from the cane or beet (see "Blackstrap Molasses," p. 249). Ordinary molasses is a good mineral and vitamin source, rich in iron, calcium, copper, magnesium, phosphorus, pantothenic acid, inositol, vitamin E, and the B vitamins.

VEGETABLES

Vegetables are composed primarily of carbohydrates and water and contain very little protein. Vegetables also provide vitamins, minerals, and bulk to the diet and contribute appetite appeal through color, texture, and flavor. In general, light-green vegetables provide vitamins, minerals, and a large amount of the carbohydrate cellulose, necessary to provide bulk in the diet. Yellow and dark-green vegetables are excellent sources of vitamin A. Vegetable leaves are usually rich in calcium, iron, magnesium, vitamin C, and many of the B vitamins. The greener the leaf, the richer it will be in nutrients. Potatoes are relatively high in protein and are excellent sources of vitamin A, vitamin C, niacin, thiamine, and riboflavin as well as iron and calcium. A medium-size potato contains about 90 calories.

Vegetables are commonly available in fresh, frozen, canned, or dried forms. Fresh raw vegetables generally contain more vitamins and minerals than the processed products, although quick-freezing causes almost no nutrient loss. Properly canned vegetables usually contain as many vitamins and minerals as home-cooked fresh vegetables, but dried vegetables show a considerably greater loss of nutrients. Commercially canned vegetables are usually cooked too long, depleting nutrient value.

Before being eaten or cooked, fresh vegetables should be thoroughly washed so that chemical sprays and dirt are removed. The vegetable skins should be left on or pared as thinly as possible, so that the vitamins and minerals are preserved. Cooking time should be kept to a minimum when vegetables are boiled in water so that nutrients are conserved and flavor is retained. Baked vegetables will have a higher concentration of nutrients than boiled vegetables.

VEGETABLE JUICES

Fresh vegetable juices are an excellent source of minerals and vitamins. Juices from dark-green and yellow vegetables are especially high in vitamin A. People who want a change from raw or cooked vegetables may find juices appealing and easy to digest. Vegetable juices may also be the preferred form for persons suffering from disorders of the digestive system.

BEVERAGES

Beverages such as alcohol, coffee, cola, and tea add little nutritive value to the diet, except for water. However, milk drinks and fruit and vegetable juices contribute fair amounts of protein, fat, vitamins, and minerals to the diet.

ALCOHOLIC BEVERAGES

Alcoholic beverages may be those produced by fermentation only, such as ale, beer and most wines, and those that are distilled, such as whiskey. Alcoholic beverages supply little to the diet except calories.

CARBONATED BEVERAGES

Carbonated beverages are high in sugar content and have no nutritional value whatsoever. In order to hold the sugar in suspension and keep it from crystallizing, all soft drinks contain acid, usually orthophosphoric or citric, which eats away tooth enamel and can impair the appetite and the stomach. Certain soft drinks, especially cola, contain large amounts of caffeine, which stimulates the metabolism and leads to depletion of valuable nutrients in the body.

COFFEE

Coffee is produced from the coffee bean. It contains no nutrients but does contain caffeine. Coffee quickens the respiration process, strengthens the pulse, raises the blood pressure, stimulates the kidneys, excites the functions of the brain, and temporarily relieves fatigue or depression. If consumed in excess, coffee can cause increased nervous symptoms, aggravate heart and artery disorders, and irritate the lining of the stomach. It may also create inositol and biotin deficiencies, prevent iron from being properly utilized, and cause other vitamins to be pumped through and out of the body before they can be properly absorbed.

Coffee substitutes are powdered vegetable preparations that are used as coffee alternatives. They usually have barley or chicory-root bases and contain no caffeine.

TEA

Tea is similar to coffee in that it contains caffeine; it contains tannin, or tannic acid, and essential oils as well. The caffeine is the stimulating element; the tannin gives it its color and body; the oils give it flavor and aroma. Tannin in its concentrated form has had harmful effects on the mucous membrane of the mouth and the digestive tract, but it is generally believed that tannin does not occur in significant enough amounts in tea to be harmful. Tea actually has little nutritive value with the exception of its fluoride content. Herbal teas are preferred to commercial teas because of their therapeutic value.

SUPPLEMENTARY FOODS

Supplementary foods may be useful for individuals who wish to increase the nutritional value of their meals.

Supplements may be in the form of tablets, liquids, powders, syrups, capsules, granules, or bars; various forms may have differing nutrient characteristics. *Any information concerning ailments is not meant to be prescriptive, but merely represents research findings.*

BLACKSTRAP MOLASSES

Blackstrap molases is a truly rich source of minerals and vitamins. As the last possible extraction of the cane in refining sugar, it is the richest in nutrients of the sugar-related products. It contains more calcium than milk, more iron than many eggs, and more potassium than any food, and it is an excellent source of B vitamins. It is also rich in copper, magnesium, phosphorus, pantothenic acid, inositol, and vitamin E. One tablespoon of blackstrap molasses contains 3 milligrams of iron and over 100 milligrams of calcium. It is also a good source of natural sugar. Recommended daily dosage is 1 tablespoon dissolved in 1 cup lukewarm water or milk; one-half that amount is recommended for children. Molasses may be used as a sugar substitute in cereals and may be eaten instead of jam or jelly. Varicose veins, arthritis, ulcers, dermatitis, hair damage, eczema, psoriasis, angina pectoris, constipation, colitis, anemia, and nervous conditions may respond to supplementing the diet with this mineral-rich molasses.

BREWER'S YEAST

Brewer's yeast is a nonleavening yeast that can be added to all foods to increase their nutritional value. Brewer's yeast is one of the best sources of B vitamins and minerals. It contains sixteen amino acids, fourteen minerals, and seventeen vitamins. Brewer's yeast is high in phosphorus in relation to calcium; therefore, 8 ounces of skim milk or 4 tablespoons of dry powdered milk should be taken with every tablespoon of yeast. The recommended supplemental allowance of brewer's yeast is 1 tablespoon daily.

Wheat germ and brewer's yeast taken daily may be helpful in preventing heart trouble. Brewer's yeast may protect against toxicity of large doses of vitamin

D. It is used to prevent constipation and is a good source of enzyme-producing agents.

Brewer's yeast is one of the best sources of RNA, a nucleic acid that is important in keeping the body immune to the degenerative diseases.

Brewer's yeast is available in powder, flake, and tablet forms.

LECITHIN

Lecithin is a natural constituent of every cell of the human body and helps to emulsify cholesterol in the body. Lecithin is available both naturally in egg yolk, liver, nuts, whole wheat, unrefined vegetable oils, soybeans, and corn and as a supplement in capsule, liquid, and granule forms. Lecithin is high in phosphorus and unites with iron, iodine, and calcium to give power and vigor to the brain and aid in the digestion and absorption of fats. Lecithin also consists of ordinary fat, unsaturated fatty acids, and choline.

Lecithin may break up cholesterol and allow it to pass through arterial walls, helping to prevent atherosclerosis. It has also been found to increase immunity against virus infections and to prevent the formation of gallstones. Even distribution of body weight is also aided by lecithin. Lecithin plays an important part in maintaining a healthy nervous system and is found naturally in the myelin sheath, a fatty protective covering for the nerves. Lecithin also helps to cleanse the liver and purify the kidneys. Two tablespoons daily are recommended.

SEAWEED

Seaweed is a vegetable from the ocean which is rich in minerals. Sea plants have an advantage over land crops because they grow in seawater, in which the minerals are constantly being renewed. Seaweed is rich in all necessary minerals. There are several varieties of seaweed, including kelp, nori, and Irish moss, all of which are salty in flavor. Kelp is one of the best natural sources of iodine; it is also rich in B-complex vitamins; vitamins D, E, and K; calcium; and magnesium. It is often used as a salt substitute and is available in dried, powdered, and tablet forms.

Dulse is dark red in color and is rich in iodine. It can be used fresh in salads, but it should be soaked several times in water first. Seaweed is beneficial in maintaining the health of the mucous membranes and in treating arthritis, constipation, nervous disorders, rheumatism, colds, and skin irritations.

WHEAT GERM

Wheat germ is the heart of the kernel of wheat. It is an excellent source of protein (24 grams per one-half cup), B-complex vitamins, vitamin E, and iron. It also contains copper, magnesium, manganese, calcium, and phosphorus. It is high in phosphorus in relation to calcium, so 8 ounces of skim milk or 4 tablespoons of dry milk powder should be taken with every tablespoon of wheat germ. Wheat germ contains a vegetable oil and therefore should be tightly covered and refrigerated. Wheat-germ oil is extracted from wheat germ; it is a supplemental food high in unsaturated fatty acids and is one of the richest known sources of vitamin E.

EATING RIGHT TO FEEL RIGHT

Cooking and baking at home using wholesome ingredients need not require a drastic adjustment in preparation. Instead of sugar, honey or other unrefined sweeteners can be used; instead of butter, oil or margarine; instead of white flour, whole-grain flour. Cooking and baking from scratch or as much as possible from scratch is often preferable to preparing most prepackaged foods. Many commercially packaged and canned foods and frozen dinners contain the wrong kind of fat, sugar, and/or refined flours, although health food sections have more nutritious items. Natural foods can also be ordered by mail. Walnut Acres, Penn's Creek, Pennsylvania 17862, has a large selection. Following are some healthful hints, including sample recipes, for preparing nutritious foods. The recipes are meant to be examples of how a variety of foods can be prepared with ingredients of high-quality food value. For an expanded view, there are numerous whole-food cookbooks that can be purchased from natural food and book stores.

WHOLESOME FOODS

Food	Best Kind	Nutrients Rich in	Comments
Beverages	Herbal teas, fruit and vegetable juices, sparkling water with or without fruit juice or fruit juice concentrates, and coffee substitutes, usually made from grains.	Water, vitamins, and minerals.	Caffeine-containing beverages can cause the loss of several vitamins and minerals and overstimulate various biological systems including the nervous system and the adrenal glands.
Breads	Whole wheat, rye, corn, oat, or any combination. Whole-grain crackers, muffins, pancakes, and waffles.	Complex carbohydrates, vitamin B complex, vitamin E, potassium, magnesium, chromium, manganese, molybdenum, selenium, zinc, fiber, and unsaturated fatty acids.	Whole-grain breads usually contain a natural sweetener such as honey or raisin syrup, unsaturated oil, yeast, and salt. No dough conditioners or additives are necessary.

Food	Best Kind	Nutrients Rich in	Comments
Cereals	Whole rice, rye, wheat, oat, and corn grains.	Same as Breads.	Whole-grain cereals should be sweetened with a natural sugar such as concentrated fruit juices, honey, or barley or raisin malt.
Dairy	Unprocessed cheeses, milk, yogurt, cottage cheese, eggnog, goat milk and cheese, kefir, and ice cream.	Protein, fats, vitamin D (fortified), calcium, vitamin B_1, B_2, B_6, and B_{12}.	Ice cream and yogurt should be sweetened with an unrefined sugar such as honey or concentrated fruit juices.
Desserts	All kinds.	Same as Breads.	All cakes, pies, cookies, puddings, etc., should be made with whole-grain flour, unsaturated oil, and a natural sweetener such as honey, maple syrup, or barley malt.
Eggs	Eggs from free-running hens fed organic feed with no added drugs or hormones are preferable.	Protein, vitamin A, vitamin B_1, B_2, B_{12}, biotin, choline, pantothenic acid, vitamin E, vitamin K, iron, manganese, sulfur, and zinc.	Eggs are the highest-grade protein of any food. The yolk is extremely nutritious and contains lecithin, which keeps cholesterol moving through the bloodstream.
Fats	Unsaturated oils such as corn, peanut, safflower, sesame, soybean, sunflower, and wheat germ, margarine, and mayonnaise.	Unsaturated fatty acids.	Margarine and mayonnaise should be made from unsaturated oils. Olive oil has a higher saturated fat content than other vegetable oils. Coconut and palm oils are saturated fats.
Flours	Whole wheat, rye, corn, rice, buckwheat and soy.	Same as Breads.	Whole-wheat flour is best for baking breads and other yeast-containing baked goods. Whole-wheat pastry flour is lighter and good for cookies, cakes, pie crusts, and other desserts, although whole-wheat flour can also be used.
Fruits	Fresh, canned, frozen, and dried.	Complex carbohydrates, vitamin A, vitamin C, bioflavonoids, chromium, cobalt, iron, manganese, potassium, and fiber.	Canned fruits can be purchased packed in fruit juices.

Food	Best Kind	Nutrients Rich in	Comments
Grains	Whole barley, cornmeal, tapioca, and millet, bulgur, popcorn, brown and wild rice, and whole-grain pasta.	Same as Breads.	Cook whole-grain pastas 12–15 minutes to eliminate the raw flour taste. They will remain firm.
Meats	Lean cuts and organ meats.	Protein, vitamin A (liver), B-complex vitamins, vitamin E, cobalt, iron, molybdenum, potassium, sulfur, and zinc.	Luncheon meats and hot dogs contain nitrites which change to cancer-causing nitrosamines in the stomach.
Nuts and seeds	All kinds. All kinds of nut and seed butters.	Unsaturated fats, vitamin B_1, B_2, inositol, copper, magnesium, manganese, potassium, zinc, and fiber.	Coconut is very high in saturated fat content. Nut and seed butters should contain the nut or seed only. Many commercial peanut butters contain not only sugar but also saturated fat.
Poultry	Chicken, turkey, wild game, and organ meats.	Protein, vitamin B_1, niacin, cobalt, and iron.	The skin and dark meat contain higher amounts of saturated fats than white meat. Goose and duck are high in saturated fats.
Seafood	Fresh, canned, and frozen.	Protein, unsaturated fatty acids, vitamin A, vitamins B_1, B_{12}, biotin, choline, folic acid, pantothenic acid, vitamin D, copper, sulfur, vanadium, and zinc.	Most seafood is very rich in unsaturated fatty acids and trace minerals. Tuna is exceptionally rich in minerals and amino acids.
Sweeteners	Honey, maple syrup, molasses, barley malt, maple syrup granules, date sugar, unrefined granulated sugar cane juice, and jams sweetened with honey, fruit juice concentrates, or other natural sweeteners.	Semicomplex carbohydrates.	Natural sweeteners contain vitamins, minerals, and enzymes which aid in their assimilation. Refined sweeteners do not. Besides sucrose (sugar), glucose, sorbitol, maltose, and fructose are refined sugars.
Vegetables and legumes	Fresh and frozen.	Complex carbohydrates, vitamin A, PABA, folic acid, vitamin C, vitamin E, vitamin K, cobalt, copper, iron, magnesium, manganese, molybdenum, potassium, and fiber.	Vegetables should be steamed or sauteed lightly to preserve the nutrients. Commercially canned vegetables are usually cooked too long.

Many recipes call for some kind of fat. Unsaturated oils or margarine can be substituted for any saturated fat such as butter or lard. Margarine is less desirable because in order for the oils to become solid, they must be hydrogenated, a process that causes the loss of the essential fatty acids. However, in some margarines, usually found in natural food stores, some of the oil content is kept in liquid form.

Unsaturated oils should be unrefined; they will be called "cold-pressed," and are darker in color. Refining of unsaturated oils involves various processes that remove the lecithin and vitamins and minerals as well as the smell and flavor of the plant derivative. Safflower oil is the best all-purpose oil and the highest in essential fatty acids. Corn oil is good for popping corn and baking. Peanut oil is good for deep frying. Store all oil-containing foods in the refrigerator to prevent rancidity if kept more than a few weeks; this includes oils, nuts, seeds, nut butters, mayonnaise, and whole-grain flours.

Whenever substituting whole-wheat flour for white flour in a recipe, decrease the amount by one or two tablespoons per cup. Whole-wheat flour is best for yeast-containing breads and baked products. Whole-wheat pastry flour is made from softer wheat and has a lower gluten content, so it is good for cakes, cookies, and other desserts, although whole-wheat flour can also be used.

Plain yogurt is a good substitute for sour cream; some yogurts are not as tart as others. Creamed foods can be made with whole milk instead of cream.

WHITE SAUCE

1–3 tablespoons oil
1/4 cup whole-wheat pastry flour
2 cups whole milk
salt to taste

Heat oil; the more oil used, the richer the sauce. Whisk in flour. Slowly add the milk, stirring constantly. Bring to a boil, then lower heat and simmer 10 minutes, stirring frequently. Remove from heat and add salt to taste.

White sauce is good over grains, pasta, vegetables, crepes, and in creamed meat, poultry, and fish dishes.

Other variations to the basic white sauce:

Extrathick sauce: After removing from heat, add a few tablespoons of the sauce to 1 beaten egg, so the egg will adjust to heat and not cook. Return mixture to the sauce and cook 1 minute.

Mushroom and onion sauce: Saute mushrooms and onions in oil and add to sauce while simmering.

Yogurt sauce: For a more velvety sauce, whisk in 1/4 cup yogurt after removing from heat.

Herb or spice sauce: Nutmeg, curry spices, ginger, cinnamon, paprika, white pepper, tarragon, dill, parsley, or thyme make interesting and varied sauces. Add herbs with the milk so their flavors cook into the sauce.

Honey or maple syrup can be used instead of sugar in everything from sweet and sour sauces and barbecue sauce to cakes and dessert toppings. Unrefined granulated sugar cane juice, found in natural food stores, preserves much of the natural complex sugars, vitamins, and minerals of the sugar cane and can be substituted for refined sugar in recipes. Refined sugar is 99.9% sucrose, containing nothing but calories. In the sugar cane or sugar beet, sucrose makes up about 15% of the total ingredients. This 15% is extracted, clarified with lime, heated, filtered, spun, and treated with phosphoric acid. None of the vitamins, minerals, or enzymes are left to aid in its digestion and assimilation, and therefore it has to rob nutrient supplies from other parts of the body when ingested. Raw honey (uncooked to preserve nutrients), maple syrup, date sugar, and other natural sweeteners retain their natural supplies of vitamins, minerals, and enzymes. They are still sugars, however, and should be used in moderation.

Clover honey is the lightest of honeys and is good for baking. When substituting honey or maple syrup in a recipe, use one-half to three-fourths the amount of sugar called for and decrease the liquid by up to 1/4 cup. It can help for mixing purposes to heat honey to a runny state before adding it to a recipe. Another helpful hint is to coat the utensil used for measuring honey with oil. The honey will slide right off. Baked goods made with honey will be more moist and keep longer because of the extraordinary keeping qualities of honey. Date sugar is pulverized dates and does not dissolve but can be used in cinnamon rolls and coffee cakes, on cereal, desserts, in granolas, and in fruit salads.

Fresh home-baked breads smell magnificent and taste delightful and, especially if you have a dough hook with your mixer, are a snap to make. Quick breads or batter breads use no yeast. To keep bread fresh if not used within a few days, slice the bread so you can take out the exact amount when you need it, wrap it in a plastic bag, and place it in the freezer.

WHOLE-WHEAT BREAD

1 package yeast
1/2 cup warm water
2 1/2 cups hot water
2 tablespoons oil
3 tablespoons honey
2 teaspoons salt
5–7 cups whole-wheat flour

Dissolve yeast in warm water. Let set a few minutes. Combine hot water, oil, honey, and salt in mixing bowl. Hot water readily dissolves the salt, liquifies the honey, and creates a warm atmosphere for the yeast. Before adding the yeast mixture, make sure the water is not too warm; if it is, add a little flour to cool it down. Gradually add the rest of the flour, using just enough that the dough is not sticky. Knead (on dusted flour surface if by hand) for 10 minutes. Turn into oiled bowl, cover with wet cloth, and let rise in warm place for 90 minutes (a 150° to 200° oven turned off does fine). After raising, knead dough a few seconds, and then divide and shape into loaves or buns. Place in baking pans sprayed with a nonstick coating such as PAM and let rise 30 minutes. Bake in 350° oven for 35 to 45 minutes. Bread is done if when tapped on the bottom, it sounds hollow. For a soft crust, brush bread tops with margarine.

Any number of ingredients can be added to bread to vary the taste. Use milk instead of water. For pumpernickel, use one-half rye flour and one-half whole-wheat flour and use 1/2 cup molasses instead of honey. Add 1 cup raisins (knead in by hand at the very end of the first kneading so as not to mash them too much) and cinnamon for raisin bread. For herb bread, knead into the dough 3 to 4 tablespoons of any herb or combination, such as caraway, dill, basil, and thyme. For a scrumptious crunchy crust, after the first raising, dip shaped loaves or buns into warm water, then roll in sesame seeds. Challah can be made by dividing the dough after the first raising into three parts. Roll each part into an 18-inch long roll. Braid the pieces and pinch and tuck the ends securely. Place the challah on a large tray sprayed with PAM. Let dough rise until double. Before baking brush with beaten egg and sprinkle with sesame seeds. Bake in a 350° oven for 35 to 45 minutes.

FRENCH BREAD

1 package yeast
1/2 cup warm water
1 1/2 cups hot water
2 teaspoons salt
1 cup yogurt
5–7 cups whole-wheat flour

Follow the instructions for Whole-Wheat Bread, adding the yogurt along with the hot water, yeast, and salt. After the dough has risen the first time, shape into long loaves. Place on a French bread pan or on a rectangular cookie sheet sprayed with a nonstick coating such as PAM and sprinkled with cornmeal. Let dough rise 30 minutes. Slash tops diagonally with a sharp knife or razor. Spray with water from a spray bottle. Bake at 350° for 30 to 40 minutes. Spray the loaves with water occasionally while baking for a harder and crispier crust.

PEASANT BREAD

1 package yeast
1/2 cup warm water
2 cups hot water
3 tablespoons oil
1/4 cup blackstrap molasses
2 teaspoons salt
3 cups whole-wheat flour
1 cup cornmeal
1/2 cup rye flour
3/4 cup rolled oats or rye flakes

Follow the instructions for Whole-Wheat Bread, adding the cornmeal, rye flour, and oats or rye flakes after the whole-wheat flour. This dough is meant to be more sticky than usual, but if it's still too hard to handle, add a bit more whole-wheat flour. After raising, shape into two round loaves and place on a cookie sheet sprayed with PAM and sprinkled with cornmeal. Let dough rise 30 minutes. Bake in 350° oven for 35 to 45 minutes.

BANANA BREAD

2 cups whole-wheat pastry flour
1/2 teaspoon salt
2 teaspoons baking powder
1/4 teaspoon nutmeg
1/2 cup margarine
1/4 cup honey
2 large eggs
1 teaspoon vanilla
3 ripe bananas, mashed
1/2 cup chopped walnuts and/or sunflower seeds (optional)

Mix together honey, oil, eggs, vanilla, and mashed bananas. In another bowl, sift dry ingredients. Make a well in the center and pour in wet mixture. Stir gently until just blended. Fold in nuts. Pour into a 4- × 8-inch loaf pan or its equivalent sprayed with PAM and bake in 350° oven for 40 to 50 minutes.

BLUEBERRY MUFFINS

1 1/2 cups whole-wheat pastry flour
1 teaspoon baking powder
1/2 teaspoon baking soda
1/2 teaspoon salt
1/3 cup honey
1/4 cup oil or margarine
1/3 cup buttermilk
1 large egg
1 1/2 cup fresh blueberries

Mix together honey, oil, buttermilk, and egg. In another bowl, sift dry ingredients. Make a well in the center and pour in wet mixture. Stir gently until just blended. Fold in blueberries. Pour into a muffin tin sprayed with PAM. Fill the cups two-thirds full.

Bake in 350° oven for 20 to 30 minutes. Cool in pan 5 to 10 minutes before removing.

BRAN MUFFINS

1 cup whole-wheat pastry flour
1/4 cup cornmeal
1/2 cup bran
1/2 teaspoon salt
1 tablespoon baking powder
1/4 cup honey
2 tablespoons oil
1 cup buttermilk
1 large egg
1/2 cup raisins (optional)

Mix together honey, oil, buttermilk, and egg. In another bowl, sift dry ingredients. Make a well in the center and pour in wet mixture. Stir gently until just blended. Fold in raisins. Pour into muffin tin sprayed with PAM. Fill the cups two-thirds full. Bake in 350° oven for 20 to 30 minutes. Cool in pan 5 to 10 minutes before removing.

Homemade granola tastes much better than the packaged kind, and it's very simple to make.

GRANOLA

1/2 cup oil
1/2 cup honey
1 tablespoon vanilla
1 cup wheat germ
1 cup bran flakes
7 cups rolled oats
1 cup sesame seeds
1 cup sunflower seeds
1 cup chopped or slivered almonds
1/2 cup peanuts
2 cups raisins and/or chopped dates

In a large skillet, heat the honey, oil, and vanilla over low heat until mixture is thin. Stir in the rest of the ingredients except raisins and dates. Stir well until the dry ingredients are well-coated. Place the cereal in a large shallow pan or on a baking sheet. Bake until brown in 300° oven, about 45 minutes, stirring occasionally. Remove from oven and mix in fruit.

Fulfillment of the complete protein requirement does not necessarily involve eating meat and poultry. Complete high-quality protein can be found in dairy products, eggs, and fish. [Note: The refining of milk and milk products by removing the fat may not be as desirable as it is currently considered to be. There is nothing inherently wrong with saturated fats as long as the cells of the body are supplied with all of the nutrients necessary for fat utilization. Milk fat is essential for the absorption of several of the nutrients found in the milk, including calcium. Buildup of bad cholesterol, as opposed to good cholesterol, in the arteries is more likely to be caused by (1) a diet of refined foods from which vitamins and minerals and fiber essential for cholesterol mobilization, metabolism, and utilization are removed; (2) excess consumption of sugar, refined carbohydrates, and alcohol, which can turn into saturated body fat, causing the fat and cholesterol count of the blood to rise; (3) ingestion of extracted isolated saturated fats like cream, butter, lard, fatty meats, and the vegetable oils of palm and coconut.] Along with milk, eggs have the highest-quality protein of any foods. The yolk of egg is extremely nutritious and also contains lecithin, which emulsifies and keeps cholesterol moving in the bloodstream. Fish contains all of the essential amino acids plus generous supplies of minerals and trace elements.

Protein foods differ in nutritive value because their amino acid compositions differ. The amount of each amino acid present will vary from one protein food to another. Any one amino acid in a given protein that is not up to a certain level will cause all the rest of the amino acids to work at only a portion of their potential. This is why eating a protein food that has not only all of the essential amino acids, but each one in the proper amount, is so important. Vegetables, fruits, grains, nuts, and legumes all contain one or more of the essential amino acids below the required level. Combining grains and legumes to make up a complete protein meal, obtaining sufficient amount of the essential amino acids, must be done carefully, accurately, and consistently to ensure that the body is kept at a proper nutritional level.

PIZZA

Crust

1/2 package yeast
2 tablespoons warm water

2 tablespoons oil
1/2 teaspoon salt
1/2 cup hot water
whole-wheat flour

Dissolve yeast in warm water. Combine oil, salt, and hot water. Let cool to warm. Add the yeast and enough flour so that the dough is nonsticky and pliable. Knead 5 minutes. Cover and let rise in warm place (a 150° to 200° oven turned off does fine) for 1 hour.

Sauce

1/4 cup chopped onion
2 cloves crushed garlic
1 tablespoon oil
2 cups pureed tomatoes
1 1/2 teaspoon oregano
1/4 teaspoon basil
1/4 teaspoon thyme
1/4 teaspoon marjoram
1/4 teaspoon cayenne
1/2 teaspoon salt

Saute onion and garlic in oil. Add tomatoes and seasonings and 1/4 cup water. Simmer 30 minutes or longer, adding more water if necessary.

Toppings

sliced sauteed mushrooms
sliced sauteed green peppers
sliced sauteed onion rings
sliced olives
12 oz. shredded mozzarella or jack cheese or any cheese combination
1/4 cup grated Parmesan cheese

Roll out dough and place on pizza pan sprayed with a nonstick coating such as PAM. Brush the crust with oil and prick surface with fork. Bake in 400° oven for approximately 10 to 15 minutes. Spread sauce on dough and add vegetable toppings of choice. Return to oven and heat vegetables for approximately 5 minutes. Top with cheeses and bake until melted.

QUICHE

Crust

1/4 cup cold margarine, cut in small pieces
1 1/4 cups whole-wheat pastry flour

1/4 teaspoon salt
3–4 tablespoons cold water

Mix flour and salt. Add margarine. Use a pastry cutter, two forks, or a food processor to combine flour and margarine until the mixture resembles coarse corn-meal. Add water while stirring or while processor is running, 1 tablespoon at a time, until the dough sticks to itself. The amount of humidity in the air will determine the amount of water needed. Wrap dough and refrigerate until cold. Roll out or press into a pie plate sprayed with PAM.

Filling

1 cup grated cheese
1/2 cup chopped sauteed onions
1 large stalk chopped steamed broccoli

The outer skin of the broccoli stalk can be shaved or just the flowers can be used. Season broccoli with lemon juice and a little salt if desired. Use any cheese or mixture of cheeses. Swiss types such as Gruyère or medium to sharp cheddar are usually recommended. Spread cheese on crust. Add onions and broccoli or vegetables of choice.

Custard

3 eggs
1 cup milk
1/4 teaspoon salt

Beat together ingredients. For a large or straight-sided quiche dish, use 4 eggs and 1 1/2 cups milk. Pour custard over cheese and vegetables. Bake in 350° oven for 30 to 40 minutes.

CHILI

1 1/2 cups dry kidney or pinto beans
1 cup raw bulgur
2 cups tomato juice
1 1/2 cups chopped onion
1 cup chopped green pepper
1 cup chopped celery
3 cloves crushed garlic
1 teaspoon basil
1 teaspoon ground cumin
1 teaspoon or more chili powder
1 teaspoon salt
ground pepper to taste
2 tablespoons lemon juice or cider vinegar

Put beans into a saucepan and cover with 4 cups water. Soak for 3 to 4 hours. Add more water and 1/2 teaspoon salt. Cook until tender, about 1 hour. Add more water during cooking if necessary.

Heat tomato juice to boiling and pour over bul-gur. Let stand for 15 minutes. Bulgur is wheat kernels coarsely ground and can be found in most food stores, often in the Mideastern foods section. Bulgur will give the chili a meaty texture.

Saute garlic, vegetables, and spices in oil until vegetables are tender.

Combine all ingredients in a kettle and heat slowly. Some of the beans can be mashed for a thicker broth. Chili can also be put into a baking dish and warmed in a moderate oven. If time permits, let chili stand for an hour or so and then reheat. Serve topped with grated Colby or Jack cheese. It is good served with corn bread or over cooked brown rice.

VEGETABLE CHEESE CAKE

Vegetables

1 cup chopped onion
1 cup raw corn kernels
2 cups chopped broccoli
2 chopped green peppers
1 large diced carrot
salt and pepper to taste
1 teaspoon dill
1 teaspoon thyme
6 tablespoons melted margarine
1 heaping cup grated cheese

Saute vegetables in oil until just tender. Add season-ings. Pour melted margarine in a 9- × 13-inch pan. Spread vegetables in pan. Sprinkle grated cheese over top. Set aside.

Cake

1 2/3 cups whole-wheat pastry flour
1 teaspoon baking powder
1/2 teaspoon baking soda
1/2 teaspoon salt
2 large eggs
3 tablespoons oil
2/3 cup buttermilk
1/3 cup freshly grated Parmesan cheese

Sift dry ingredients, add cheese, and mix. Beat together wet ingredients, pour into dry mixture, and combine well. Spread carefully over vegetables as evenly as possible. Bake in a 350° oven for 25 to 30 minutes. After removing from oven, invert cake onto a tray larger than the baking pan.

TEMPURA

Tempura is vegetables or fruits coated with a batter and deep-fried. Because nutrients and juices are sealed in and the food cooked quickly, little loss occurs. Drain the tempura well to eliminate excessive oil. Tempura mixes can be found in natural food stores and are also very good.

    2 cups whole-wheat pastry flour
    1 teaspoon salt
    2 egg yolks
    1 1/2 cups water

Beat yolks into water. Add flour and salt and mix until combined. More or less water can be used, depending on desired consistency of batter. Batter is best when chilled.

   Cut pieces of any combinations of vegetables such as broccoli, cauliflower, zucchini, carrots, onions, mushrooms, and yams. Be sure vegetables are dry before dipping in batter. Drop into hot fat in a pre-heated deep fryer, being careful not to crowd vegetables. Fry until brown. Remove and drain on paper towels. Tempura can be kept warm for a few minutes in a warm oven until serving time. The following sauce can be used as a dip for the vegetables, or they may be served with thin slices of cheese.

    1/4 cup soy sauce
    1/2 cup water
    1 tablespoon oil
    1 small clove crushed garlic
    2 teaspoons grated ginger

CALZONE

Calzone is an Italian cheese-filled pastry. Besides the one listed below, fillings can be any to your liking; for example, a mixture of 1 lb ricotta cheese, 8 oz Jack cheese, 3 cups packed chopped spinach leaves, 1/2 cup minced green onion, 1/2 cup grated Parmesan, and salt and pepper to taste; or 2 cups firm cottage or pot cheese, 1 1/2 cups packed grated Jack or Muenster cheese, 1/2 cup feta cheese, 1/2 cup finely minced parsley, 1/2 cup minced onion, and salt and pepper to taste; or slices of cheese and tomato.

Dough

    1 package yeast
    1 cup warm water
    1 1/2 teaspoons salt
    whole-wheat flour

Dissolve yeast in warm water. Add salt and enough flour so dough is pliable and not sticky. Let rise in warm place for 1 hour. Punch down and divide into six portions. Roll each one out to about 1/4 inch thick.

Filling

    1 cup ricotta cheese
    1 cup pesto
    1 cup grated provolone cheese

Pesto

    6 tablespoons dried basil
    1/2 cup olive or choice of oil
    2/3 cup ground walnuts
    4 cloves crushed garlic
    2/3 cup grated Parmesan cheese

Soak basil in oil for 10 minutes. Add walnuts and garlic and saute over low heat for 5 minutes. Remove from heat. Add cheese. Combine mixture with ricotta and provolone cheeses.

   Fill one side of rolled out dough with 1/2 to 3/4 cup filling, leaving a 1-inch rim. Moisten rim with water and fold dough over. Crimp edge with a fork. Prick the top and bake on a tray sprayed with a nonstick coating such as PAM in a 375° oven until browned, approximately 15 to 20 minutes.

ORIENTAL RICE SALAD

    1 cup raw brown rice
    3/4 teaspoon salt

2 cups water
2 chopped scallions
1 cup mung bean sprouts
1 cup raw snow peas
1/2 cup sliced water chestnuts
1/4 cup lightly toasted sesame seeds
1/3 cup lightly toasted cashews

Drop rice into boiling salted water. Simmer covered for about 45 minutes, until all water is absorbed. Cool. Add rest of ingredients to rice. Mix in the following dressing:

3/4 cup unsweetened orange juice
juice of 1/2 lemon
1/2 cup oil
3 tablespoons soy sauce
1 clove crushed garlic
1/2 teaspoon grated ginger
salt to taste

POLENTA

Polenta is an Italian cornmeal mush and can be served under any combination of stir-fried, sauteed, or steamed vegetables.

1 1/2 cups whole cornmeal
1 cup water
1 teaspoon salt
4 cups boiling water
1 heaping cup grated cheese of choice

Mix cornmeal, 1 cup water, and salt. Add to boiling water. Lower heat and cook for 10 minutes, stirring constantly. Consistency will be thick. Mix in cheese. Serve hot under vegetables.

Vegetables Spanish-style

1 small eggplant, cut in cubes
2 medium green peppers, cut in cubes
1 medium zucchini, cut in cubes
1 medium onion, chopped
1 cup tomato puree
1/4 cup water
2 cloves crushed garlic
1 teaspoon cumin
1 teaspoon coriander

1/2 teaspoon chili powder
1/4 teaspoon cayenne
1 1/2 teaspoons salt

Saute garlic and onion in oil. Add eggplant, herbs, salt, tomato puree and water. Cover and simmer for 15 minutes. Add peppers and zucchini. Simmer until all vegetables are tender.

SPAGHETTI WITH GARLIC AND WALNUTS

12 oz whole-grain spaghetti
1/3 cup olive or oil of choice
1 to 1 1/2 cups walnuts
3 cloves minced garlic
1/2 teaspoon salt
1/3 cup freshly grated Parmesan cheese
pepper to taste

Put water up to boil and cook spaghetti 12 to 15 minutes. Cooking whole-grain pasta longer than refined pasta is necessary to eliminate a raw flour aftertaste. The pasta will still remain firm. Chop walnuts in large pieces and saute in oil along with garlic and salt for 5 minutes or until nuts are just lightly roasted. When pasta is done, drain and add to nut mixture. Cook over low heat for a minute or so mixing in the cheese. Sprinkle pepper on top.

Most desserts and sweets contain substantial amounts of concentrated sugar and fat, no matter what ingredients are used. For this reason, they should be consumed in moderation. Fruit is a simple and healthful dessert, eaten alone or as a fruit compote. Add dried fruits like raisins and dates and top with a dressing of yogurt and maple syrup. Yogurt can be mixed with any kind of fruit or fruits, sweetened with honey or maple syrup, flavored with vanilla extract, and sprinkled with toasted nuts or seeds such as walnuts, almonds, and sunflower seeds.

FRUIT CREPES

Crepes

1 cup whole-wheat pastry flour or buckwheat flour
1/4 teaspoon salt

2 eggs
1 cup milk

In mixing bowl, stir flour and salt together. Add beaten eggs. Slowly add milk to batter, stirring well to prevent lumping. Ingredients can also be whipped in a blender. Traditional French crepes were made with buckwheat flour, which makes a lighter pancake.

Heat crepe pan or medium-sized skillet over medium heat. Coat bottom with margarine. Ladle approximately 1/4 cup batter into pan, swirl to cover bottom. Cook both sides until just dry. Remove from heat and brush each crepe with orange liqueur if desired. Stack cooked crepes on a plate.

Filling

Fill each crepe with any fruit or combination of fruits. Roll up and top with a honey-yogurt dressing made with plain yogurt, several dashes of cinnamon, and honey to taste.

FRUIT PARFAIT

    2 cups ricotta cheese
    2 tablespoons honey or maple syrup
    1/2 teaspoon vanilla
    2 cups chopped fruit

Whip ricotta with electric beaters 5 to 7 minutes. Blend in vanilla and honey. Fold in fruit. Divide in parfait glasses and chill for 2 hours.

FRUIT COBBLER

    4 cups chopped fruit
    3/4 cup unsweetened fruit juice
    1 tablespoon cornstarch
    honey to taste

Crumb topping

    1/4 cup whole-wheat pastry flour
    1 teaspoon cinnamon
    1/3–1/2 cup date sugar or unrefined granulated cane juice
    1/4 cup margarine, in pieces

Place fruit in an 8-inch-square baking pan sprayed with PAM. Heat juice and honey to boiling, lower heat. Mix 1/4 cup liquid into cornstarch, stir until smooth, and return to juice. Cook until thickened. Pour over fruit. Blend topping ingredients until crumbly. Sprinkle over fruit mixture. Bake in a 350° oven 20 to 30 minutes, until browned.

Packages of store-bought flavored gelatin consist of nothing but sugar or artificial sweetener, gelatin, and artificial color. Gelatins made with fruit juice are not only much more healthful but more tasty and full-bodied.

REAL FRUIT GELATIN

    1 tablespoon unflavored gelatin
    1/2 cup cold water
    1 1/2 cups unsweetened fruit juice
    pinch of salt

Dissolve gelatin in cold water. Heat juice to boiling. Honey can be added for a sweeter taste. Remove from heat. Add gelatin and salt and mix well. Pour into bowl and chill. Pieces of fruit can be mixed in just before gelatin begins to congeal.

SWEDISH PUDDING

    3 cups unsweetened fruit juice
    1/2 cup honey
    1/2 cup whole-grain farina
    1/8 teaspoon cinnamon
    1 cup plain yogurt

Heat juice and honey to a boil. Any juice or combination of juices can be used. Sprinkle in farina. Farina is wheat finely ground. It is used as a hot cereal under various names, such as bear mush. Lower heat and cook slowly, stirring constantly for 10 minutes. Remove from heat. Whip mixture with electric beaters for 15 minutes; it will become very light. Fold in yogurt. Pour into custard cups and chill. Top with toasted walnuts.

FRUIT SAUCE

4 cups chopped fruit
1/4 cup water
1/2 cup honey
2 teaspoons lemon juice

Steam fruit in water until soft. Puree fruit along with remaining water in blender. Mix in honey and lemon juice. Fruit sauce can be used over desserts like ice cream, cakes, and fruit compotes.

Any cake recipe can be converted by substituting exact measure of whole-wheat pastry flour for white flour and adding 1 more teaspoon of baking powder. For a moist cake with a soft velvety texture, underbake it.

CHOCOLATE CAKE

6 tablespoons margarine
3/4 cup honey
1 oz unsweetened baking chocolate
1 egg
1 teaspoon vanilla
1 1/2 cups whole-wheat pastry flour
1 teaspoon baking soda
1 teaspoon baking powder
1/4 teaspoon salt
1/4 cup powdered cocoa
1 cup buttermilk

Melt chocolate. Cream margarine and honey. Combine all wet ingredients. Sift dry ingredients and add to wet mixture. Stir gently until just blended. Pour in a 9-inch round or square cake pan sprayed with PAM. Bake in a 350° oven 35 to 45 minutes.

Frosting

3 oz unsweetened baking chocolate
3 tablespoons margarine
1/2–3/4 cup honey
1/4 teaspoon salt
1/3 cup milk
1 teaspoon vanilla

Melt chocolate. Mix all ingredients well. Adjust honey to sweetness desired. Refrigerate until mixture is of spreading consistency.

PECAN PIE

4 large eggs
3/4 cup maple syrup or honey
1/4 cup margarine
1/2 teaspoon vanilla
1/2 teaspoon salt
2 cups pecans

(This recipe uses a 9-inch pie shell. Use crust recipe for the Quiche.) Heat margarine and honey in saucepan until runny. Mix well all ingredients except pecans. Spread pecans, chopped or whole, on unbaked pie crust. Pour on batter. Bake in 350° oven for 25 to 30 minutes or until solid.

PEANUT BUTTER COOKIES

2 cups crunchy peanut butter
2/3 cup margarine
1 1/3 cups honey
2 teaspoons vanilla
1 teaspoon baking powder
1/2 teaspoon salt
2 1/2 cups whole-wheat pastry flour

Combine wet ingredients. Sift dry ingredients. Mix wet and dry ingredients until just blended. Spoon onto cookie sheet sprayed with PAM. Press with a spatula and make a criss-cross design with a fork. Bake in a 350° oven for 10 to 15 minutes, until browned.

ICE CREAM

2 cups milk
1 1/2 cups cream
4 egg yolks
1/4 teaspoon salt
1/2 cup honey

Heat honey until runny. Combine milk, cream, beaten egg yolks and salt. Add the honey, whisking continually until mixture is well blended. Add any flavor desired such as 2 teaspoons vanilla, lemon, or almond extract, 1/3 to 1/2 cup chopped nuts, 2 oz melted unsweetened chocolate, 1 cup mashed fruit or fruit pieces, or 1 package frozen fruit. Follow directions for your ice cream machine.

CARAMEL ROLLS

Dough

1 package yeast
1/4 cup warm water
1 cup milk, scalded
3 tablespoons oil
1/4 cup honey
1 egg, beaten
1 teaspoon salt
3 1/2–4 cups whole-wheat flour

Filling

1/2 cup honey
2 teaspoons cinnamon
1/2–1 cup walnuts, coarsely chopped

Glaze

1/4 cup margarine
1/2 cup honey
1 teaspoon cinnamon

Dissolve yeast in warm water. Mix together all ingredients using just enough flour so the dough is not sticky. Knead 5 to 10 minutes. Let rise in warm place until double in size, 60 to 90 minutes. Mix filling ingredients. Roll out dough to about a 9- × 18-inch rectangle, 1/4 inch thick. Spread with filling, roll up lengthwise, and slice into 1/2-inch pieces.

Heat glaze ingredients and pour into two 9-inch round cake pans or the equivalent. Arrange dough slices flat in pans and just touching each other. Let rise in warm place for 30 minutes. Bake in 350° oven for 10 to 15 minutes or until the rolls begin to brown. Invert pan onto tray as soon as removed from the oven.

CAROB NUT FUDGE

Carob has a similar taste to chocolate and when substituted for chocolate in a recipe, often goes undetected. If substituting for cocoa, replace by an equal measure; for 1 oz unsweetened chocolate, use 3 tablespoons carob powder. Roasted carob powder has a better taste than raw powder.

2/3 cup peanut butter
2/3 cup honey
2/3 cup roasted carob powder
1/3 cup chopped lightly toasted walnuts
2/3 cup lightly toasted sunflower seeds
1/3 cup lightly toasted sesame seeds
1/3 cup raisins, soaked and drained
1/4 teaspoon peppermint oil (optional)

Heat peanut butter and honey in saucepan until runny. Remove from heat. Stir in carob powder. Mix in rest of ingredients. Press into an 8- × 8-inch pan sprayed with a nonstick coating such as PAM. Chill.

SOME RICH SOURCES OF NUTRIENTS

CARBOHYDRATES
Whole grains
Sugar, syrup, and honey
Fruits
Vegetables

FATS
Butter and margarine
Vegetable oils
Fats in meats
Whole milk and milk products
Nuts and seeds

PROTEIN
Meats, fish, and poultry
Soybean products
Eggs
Milk and milk products
Whole grains

WATER
Beverages
Fruits
Vegetables

VITAMIN A
Liver
Eggs
Yellow fruits and vegetables
Dark-green fruits and vegetables
Whole milk and milk products
Fish-liver oil*

VITAMIN B₁
Brewer's yeast
Whole grains
Blackstrap molasses
Brown rice
Organ meats
Meats, fish, and poultry
Egg yolks

Legumes
Nuts

VITAMIN B₂
Brewer's yeast
Whole grains
Blackstrap molasses
Organ meats
Egg yolks
Legumes
Nuts

VITAMIN B₆
Meats
Whole grains
Organ meats
Brewer's yeast
Blackstrap molasses
Wheat germ
Legumes
Green leafy vegetables
Desiccated liver*

VITAMIN B₁₂
Organ meats
Fish and pork
Eggs
Cheese
Milk and milk products

BIOTIN
Egg yolks
Liver
Unpolished rice
Brewer's yeast
Whole grains
Sardines
Legumes

CHOLINE
Egg yolks
Organ meats
Brewer's yeast
Wheat germ

Soybeans
Fish
Legumes
Lecithin*

FOLIC ACID
Dark-green leafy vegetables
Organ meats
Brewer's yeast
Root vegetables
Whole grains
Oysters
Salmon
Milk

INOSITOL
Whole grains
Citrus fruits
Brewer's yeast
Molasses
Meat
Milk
Nuts
Vegetables
Lecithin*

NIACIN
Lean meats
Poultry and fish
Brewer's yeast
Peanuts
Milk and milk products
Rice bran
Desiccated liver*

PARA-AMINOBENZOIC ACID (PABA)
Organ meats
Wheat germ
Yogurt
Molasses
Green leafy vegetables

PANGAMIC ACID
Brewer's yeast
Rare steaks
Brown rice
Sunflower, pumpkin, and sesame seeds

PANTOTHENIC ACID
Organ meats
Brewer's yeast
Egg yolks
Legumes
Whole grains
Wheat germ
Salmon

VITAMIN C
Citrus fruits
Rose hips
Acerola cherries
Alfalfa seeds, sprouted
Cantaloupe
Strawberries
Broccoli
Tomatoes
Green peppers

VITAMIN D
Salmon
Sardines
Herring
Vitamin D–fortified milk and milk products
Egg yolks
Organ meats
Fish-liver oils*
Bone meal*

VITAMIN E
Cold-pressed oils
Eggs
Wheat germ
Organ meats
Molasses

*Denotes supplemental form.

Sweet potatoes
Leafy vegetables
Desiccated liver*

VITAMIN K
Green leafy vegetables
Egg yolks
Safflower oil
Blackstrap molasses
Cauliflower
Soybeans

BIOFLAVONOIDS
Citrus fruits
Fruits
Black currants
Buckwheat

UNSATURATED FATTY ACIDS
Vegetable oils
Sunflower seeds

CALCIUM
Milk and milk products
Green leafy vegetables
Shellfish
Molasses
Bone meal*
Dolomite*

CHLORINE
Table salt
Seafood
Meats
Ripe olives
Rye flour
Dulse*

CHROMIUM
Honey
Grapes

Raisins
Corn oil
Clams
Whole-grain cereals
Brewer's yeast

COBALT
Organ meats
Oysters
Clams
Poultry
Milk
Green leafy vegetables
Fruits

COPPER
Organ meats
Seafood
Nuts
Legumes
Molasses
Raisins
Bone meal*

FLUORIDE
Tea
Seafood
Fluoridated water
Bone meal*

IODINE
Seafood
Kelp
Iodized salt

IRON
Organ meats and meats
Eggs
Fish and poultry
Blackstrap molasses
Cherry juice
Green leafy vegetables
Dried fruits
Desiccated liver*

MAGNESIUM
Seafood
Whole grains
Dark-green vegetables
Molasses
Nuts
Bone meal*

MANGANESE
Whole grains
Green leafy vegetables
Legumes
Nuts
Pineapples
Egg yolks

MOLYBDENUM
Legumes
Whole-grain cereals
Milk
Kidney
Liver
Dark-green vegetables

PHOSPHORUS
Fish, meats, and poultry
Eggs
Legumes
Milk and milk products
Nuts
Whole-grain cereals
Bone meal*

POTASSIUM
Lean meats
Whole grains
Vegetables
Dried fruits
Legumes
Sunflower seeds

SELENIUM
Tuna
Herring

Brewer's yeast
Wheat germ and bran
Whole grains
Sesame seeds

SODIUM
Seafood
Table salt
Baking powder and baking soda
Celery
Processed foods
Milk products
Kelp*

SULFUR
Fish
Red hot peppers
Garlic
Onions
Eggs
Meats
Cabbage
Brussel sprouts
Horseradish

VANADIUM
Fish

ZINC
Pumpkin seeds
Sunflower seeds
Seafood
Organ meats
Mushrooms
Brewer's yeast
Soybeans
Oysters
Herring
Eggs
Wheat germ
Meats

*Denotes supplemental form.

SECTION VII

Table of Food Composition

The foods in this table have been divided according to food groups and similar types of foods that do not belong to any one group. The chart runs alphabetically according to food groups, with the items in each group also being alphabetized. The first group analyzed is Bakery and Grains; the second is Beverages, and so on. If you are unable to locate a particular food in a group, this does not necessarily mean that it has not been included. Check the index in the back of the book, and look for the name indicated by an asterisk.

Food values have been calculated so as to permit easy computation. All figures are, of necessity, averages of different food samples. *The dash (—) does not indicate an absence of a particular nutrient, but rather that meaningful analysis of the food for that nutrient is lacking.* Only the zero confirms the absence of a nutrient.

There are three major factors that influence the nutrient content of foods—first, the inherent characteristics of the plant or animal; second, environmental conditions affecting the plant or animal; and third, the method of handling, processing, and cooking the plant or animal material. The content of trace minerals such as selenium, copper, and zinc depends on the soil in which they are grown and where they are grown, and will therefore vary significantly in foods from area to area.

See page 267 for the abbreviations and symbols used in the table.

One of the most important aspects of obtaining a good diet is the balancing of amino acids. There are approximately twenty-two amino acids that are the primary components of protein (see "Protein," p. 7). Eight of these amino acids, tryptophan, leucine, lysine, methionine, phenylalanine, isoleucine, valine, and threonine, are known to be "essential" because they cannot be manufactured by the body itself and must be supplied by foods in the diet.*

The amino acid content of every food differs. The amino acids in foods must be consumed in amounts and proportions that closely approximate the pattern required by the body. If *one* essential amino acid (EAA) is missing or present in a low amount, protein synthesis in the body will fall to a very low level or stop altogether. In most foods containing protein, all the EAAs are present, but in some foods one or more of the EAAs may be present in a substantially lower amount than the others, placing it out of proportion and deviating from the EAA pattern required by the body. The EAA that is absent or provides the lowest percentage of the daily Estimated Amino Acid Requirement (EAAR) (as established by

---

*Histidine and arginine are necessary for growth in children, but it is debatable whether or not they perform this function in adults.

the National Academy of Sciences) is known as the limiting amino acid (LAA) and is the factor determining the amount and quality of protein utilized by the body. For example, a food containing 100 percent of a person's lysine requirement but only 20 percent of his methionine requirement results in only 20 percent of the protein in that food being used as protein by the body. The rest is used as fuel rather than for replenishing or building of tissue.

Foods such as meat, fish, poultry, and dairy products are high in protein content and have a good proportion of EAAs. Many vegetables and fruits are low in or missing some amino acids, thus rendering the amino acids present relatively useless. Foods low in or missing a particular amino acid (the LAA) will have increased protein quality when combined in a meal with foods high in this same LAA. Macaroni and cheese, vegetable stew, and chicken chow mein are examples of how foods high in certain amino acids can be balanced with foods low or missing one or more EAA. Supplements may be used to increase the protein quality of foods.

The body's protein requirements can be easily met if the foods eaten are properly combined in order to provide *usable* protein. This means that smaller quantities of food can be consumed and the body's nutritional needs will still be taken care of. *The importance of balancing the amino acids to obtain the best possible protein from foods cannot be overstressed.*

To find exact individual amino acid requirements, simply divide body weight by 2.2 to find weight in kilograms. Then multiply this figure times the requirement for each amino acid listed under "infant," "child," or "adult." The results will appear as total milligrams of each amino acid required to carry on the daily body-building functions of protein.

Note: The amino acid content of many foods is now being determined by the U.S. Department of Agriculture. As these figures become available, they will in future printings be added to the Table of Food Composition.

REQUIREMENT (per kg of body wt), mg/day

Amino Acid	Infant (4–6 mo)	Child (10–12 yr)	Adult	Amino Acid Pattern for High Quality Proteins, mg/g of protein
Histidine	33	?	?	17
Isoleucine	83	28	12	42
Leucine	135	42	16	70
Lysine	99	44	12	51
Total S-containing amino acids (includes methionine and cystine)	49	22	10	26
Total aromatic amino acids (includes phenylalanine and tyrosine)	141	22	16	73
Threonine	68	28	8	35
Tryptophan	21	4	3	11
Valine	92	25	14	48

Source: National Academy of Sciences, *Recommended Dietary Allowances,* 9th edition, 1980, p. 43.

Contents: Table of Food Composition

WEIGHTS AND MEASURES

Weights

1 microgram	= 1/1,000,000 gram
1000 micrograms	= 1 milligram
1 milligram	= 1/1000 gram
1000 milligrams	= 1 gram
1.00 ounce	= 28.35 grams
3.57 ounces	= 100.00 grams
0.25 pound	= 113.00 grams
0.50 pound	= 227.00 grams
1.00 pound	= 16.00 ounces
1.00 pound	= 453.00 grams

Capacity Measurements

1 quart	= 4 cups
1 pint	= 2 cups
1 cup	= ½ pint
1 cup	= 8 fluid ounces
1 cup	= 16 tablespoons
2 tablespoons	= 1 fluid ounce
1 tablespoon	= ½ fluid ounce
1 tablespoon	= 3 teaspoons

Approximate Equivalents

1 average serving	= about 4 ounces
1 ounce fluid	= about 28 grams
1 cup fluid	
Cooking oil	= 200 grams
Water	= 220 grams
Milk, soups	= 240 grams
Syrup, honey	= 325 grams
1 cup dry	
Cereal flakes	= 50 grams
Flours	= 100 grams
Sugars	= 200 grams
1 tablespoon fluid	
Cooking oil	= 14 grams
Milk, water	= 15 grams
Syrup, honey	= 20 grams
1 tablespoon dry	= ⅙ ounce
Flours	= 8 grams
Sugars	= 12 grams
1 pat butter	= ½ tablespoon
1 teaspoon fluid	= about 5 grams
1 teaspoon dry	= about 4 grams
1 grain	= about 65 milligrams
1 minim	= about 1 drop water

ABBREVIATIONS AND SYMBOLS USED IN THE TABLES

avg	average
cal	calorie
C	cup
ckd	cooked
diam	diameter
enr	enriched
gm	gram
IU	International Unit
lb	pound
lge	large
mcg	microgram
mg	milligram
oz	ounce
reg	regular
sm	small
sq	square
svg	serving
t	trace
T	tablespoon
tsp	teaspoon
unsw	unsweetened
w	with
w/o	without
whl grd	whole ground
—	reliable data lacking
/	of; with; per
"	inches

BEVERAGES

	Measure	Alcoholic						Common					
		Beer	Cordials and liqueurs	Gin, rum, vodka, whiskey	Wine, dessert	Wine, red	Wine, white	Club soda	Coffee	Cola drink	Fruit-flavored drink	Diet drink	Tea
Measure		12 oz	1 oz	1 oz	3.5 oz	3.5 oz	3.5 oz	12 oz	6 oz	12 oz	12 oz	12 oz	8 oz
Weight	gm	360	34	28	103	102	102	355	180	369	372	355	240
Calories		148	97	70	153	76	80	0	3	159	179	0	0
Protein	gm	.94	—	—	.09	.21	.15	0	—	0	0	0	—
Carbohydrate	gm	13.2	11.5	—	11.4	2.52	3.4	0	.54	40	45.8	.43	.06
Fiber	gm	—	—	—	—	—	—	—	—	0	0	0	—
VITAMINS													
Vitamin A	IU	—	—	—	—	—	—	0	0	0	0	0	—
Vitamin B₁	mg	0	—	—	.02	.01	0	0	0	0	0	0	0
Vitamin B₂	mg	.07	—	—	.02	.03	.01	0	.02	0	0	0	—
Vitamin B₆	mg	.18	—	—	.05	.035	.014	0	—	0	0	0	—
Vitamin B₁₂	mcg	—	—	—	—	—	—	—	—	—	—	—	—
Biotin	mcg	—	—	—	—	—	—	—	—	—	—	—	—
Niacin	mg	1.8	—	—	.24	.08	.07	0	1.26	0	0	0	—
Pantothenic acid	mg	.169	—	—	.021	.037	.021	—	—	—	—	—	—
Folic acid	mcg	20	—	—	2	1	0	—	—	—	—	—	—
Vitamin C	mg	0	0	0	0	0	0	0	0	0	0	0	—
Vitamin E	IU	—	—	—	—	—	—	—	—	—	—	—	—
MINERALS													
Calcium	mg	14	0	0	9	8	7	18	13	11	15	14	5
Copper	mg	.292	.026	.016	.06	.026	.032	—	.007	.103	.074	.057	.026
Iron	mg	.11	.02	.01	1.61	.97	.58	—	.02	.18	.26	.46	.1
Magnesium	mg	36	0	0	4	11	8	4	13	4	4	4	5
Manganese	mg	.032	—	—	.102	.177	.205	—	.022	—	—	—	1.19
Phosphorus	mg	50	0	0	—	13	13	0	4	62	13	15	10
Potassium	mg	115	1	1	102	116	84	1	117	7	37	6	58
Selenium	mcg	.47	—	—	—	—	—	.2	—	—	—	—	.1
Sodium	mg	18	1	0	7	10	7	78	2	20	52	76	19
Zinc	mg	.18	.02	0	.06	.1	.17	—	.05	.15	.26	.78	.07
LIPIDS													
Total lipid (fat)	gm	0	0	0	0	0	0	0	.01	0	0	0	.01
Total saturated	gm	—	—	—	—	—	—	—	—	—	—	—	—
Total unsaturated	gm	—	—	—	—	—	—	—	—	—	—	—	—
Cholesterol	mg	—	—	—	—	—	—	—	—	—	—	—	—
AMINO ACIDS													
Tryptophan	gm	—	—	—	—	—	—	—	—	—	—	—	—
Threonine	gm	—	—	—	—	—	—	—	—	—	—	—	—
Isoleucine	gm	—	—	—	—	—	—	—	—	—	—	—	—
Leucine	gm	—	—	—	—	—	—	—	—	—	—	—	—
Lysine	gm	—	—	—	—	—	—	—	—	—	—	—	—
Methionine	gm	—	—	—	—	—	—	—	—	—	—	—	—
Cystine	gm	—	—	—	—	—	—	—	—	—	—	—	—
Phenylalanine	gm	—	—	—	—	—	—	—	—	—	—	—	—
Tyrosine	gm	—	—	—	—	—	—	—	—	—	—	—	—
Valine	gm	—	—	—	—	—	—	—	—	—	—	—	—
Arginine	gm	—	—	—	—	—	—	—	—	—	—	—	—
Histidine	gm	—	—	—	—	—	—	—	—	—	—	—	—
Alanine	gm	—	—	—	—	—	—	—	—	—	—	—	—
Aspartic acid	gm	—	—	—	—	—	—	—	—	—	—	—	—
Glutamic acid	gm	—	—	—	—	—	—	—	—	—	—	—	—
Glycine	gm	—	—	—	—	—	—	—	—	—	—	—	—
Proline	gm	—	—	—	—	—	—	—	—	—	—	—	—
Serine	gm	—	—	—	—	—	—	—	—	—	—	—	—

Transcribed from *Agricultural Handbook*, 1–23, U.S. Department of Agriculture.

BAKERY AND GRAINS

Breads

Bagels	Biscuit, enr	Cornbread, whl grd	Cracked wheat, enr	English muffin, enr	French or Vienna, enr	Mixed grain	Pita, whole wheat	Pumpernickel	Rolls, dinner, enr	Rolls, hamburger/ hot dog, enr	Rolls, whole wheat	Rye	Wheat	White, enr	Whole wheat	Crackers, graham
1	2″ diam	2″ sq	1 slice	1	1 slice		1	1 slice	1	1	1	1 slice		1 slice	1 slice	1
100	28	45	23	27	20	100	42	32	38	40	35	23	100	23	23	14.2
296	103	93	60	130	58	257	140	79	113	119	90	56	255	62	56	55
11	2.1	3.3	2		1.8	9.96	6	2.9	3.1	3.3	3.5	2.1	9.55	2	2.4	1.1
56	12.8	13.1	12	4	11.1	46.6	24	17	20.1	21.2	18.3	12	47	11.6	11	10.4
.22	.1	.2	.1	t	.7			.4	.1	—	.6	.1	.64	t	.4	.22
—	t	68	t	t	t	t	t	—	t	t	t	—	t	t	t	0
.38	.06	.06	.03	.23	.06	.39	.2	.07	.11	.11	.12	.04	.46	.06	.06	.01
.29	.06	.09	.02	.136	.04	.38	.068	.04	.07	.07	.05	.02	.32	.05	.02	.03
.044	—	—	.02	—	.01	.103	—	.05	—	—	—	.02	.109	.009	.04	—
—	—	—	0	—	0	0	—	0	—	—	—	0	0	t	0	—
—	—	—	—	2	—	—	—	—	—	—	—	—	—	.2	.46	—
3.53	.5	.3	.3	—	.5	4.16	2.4	.4	.8	.9	1.1	.3	4.52	.6	.6	.2
.368	—	—	.14	—	.08	.63	—	.16	—	—	—	.1	.425	.1	.174	—
24	—	—	10	2	2	65	—	—	—	—	—	6	45	9	13	—
0	t	t	t	t	t	t	t	—	t	t	t	—	t	t	t	0
—	—	—	—	—	—	—	—	—	—	—	—	—	—	.23	.3	—
42	34	54	20	20	9	104	40	27	28	30	37	17	126	20	23	6
.084	—	—	—	.1	—	.283	—	—	—	—	—	.06	.24	.05	.06	.03
2.65	.4	.5	.3	1.08	.4	3.26	1.8	.8	.7	.8	.8	.4	3.49	.6	.5	.2
20	—	—	8	4	4	49	—	23	14	14	40	10	46	5	18	5.68
—	—	—	—	—	—	—	—	—	—	—	—	.3	—	.07	—	—
67	49	95	29	—	17	212	—	73	32	34	98	34	184	22	52	21
74	33	71	31	—	18	218	—	145	36	38	102	33	138	24	63	55
—	—	—	—	—	—	—	—	—	—	—	—	—	—	6.44	15.5	—
360	175	283	122	—	116	412	—	182	192	202	197	128	539	117	121	95
.52	—	—	—	—	—	1.2	—	.365	.46	.21	—	.4	1.05	—	.5	—
2.57	4.8	3.2	.6	1	.64	3.72	2	.4	2.2	2.2	1	.3	4.1	.79	.7	1.3
—	1	.81	.1	—	.14	—	—	—	.54	.5	—	—	—	.16	.11	.3
—	3	2.25	.4	—	.45	—	—	—	1.49	1.6	—	—	—	.53	.42	.9
—	—	30	—	—	—	—	—	—	—	—	—	—	—	—	—	—
—	—	—	—	—	—	—	—	—	—	—	—	—	—	—	—	—
—	—	—	—	—	—	—	—	—	—	—	—	—	—	—	—	—
—	—	—	—	—	—	—	—	—	—	—	—	—	—	—	—	—
—	—	—	—	—	—	—	—	—	—	—	—	—	—	—	—	—
—	—	—	—	—	—	—	—	—	—	—	—	—	—	—	—	—
—	—	—	—	—	—	—	—	—	—	—	—	—	—	—	—	—
—	—	—	—	—	—	—	—	—	—	—	—	—	—	—	—	—
—	—	—	—	—	—	—	—	—	—	—	—	—	—	—	—	—
—	—	—	—	—	—	—	—	—	—	—	—	—	—	—	—	—
—	—	—	—	—	—	—	—	—	—	—	—	—	—	—	—	—
—	—	—	—	—	—	—	—	—	—	—	—	—	—	—	—	—
—	—	—	—	—	—	—	—	—	—	—	—	—	—	—	—	—
—	—	—	—	—	—	—	—	—	—	—	—	—	—	—	—	—
—	—	—	—	—	—	—	—	—	—	—	—	—	—	—	—	—

BAKERY AND GRAINS (*cont.*)
Breads (*cont.*)

	Measure	Crackers, soda	Muffins, bran, enr	Muffins, blueberry	Muffins, whole wheat	Pancakes, plain, enr	Pancakes, buckwheat	Pancakes, whole wheat	Pizza, cheese, 14"	Pretzel, twisted	Taco shell	Tortilla, corn	Waffles, enr	Zwieback
Measure		1	1		1	4" diam	4" diam	4" diam	1/8	1		6" diam	5½" diam	1
Weight	gm	2.8	40	100	40	27	27	45	65	16	100	30	75	7
Calories		12.5	104	316	103	62	54	74	153	62	453	63	209	31
Protein	gm	.26	3.1	6.09	4	1.9	1.8	3.4	7.8	1.6	8.79	1.5	7	.9
Carbohydrate	gm	2	17.2	48.8	20.9	9.2	6.4	8.8	18.4	12.1	65.7	13.5	28	5.4
Fiber	gm	.008	.72	.6	.6	.1	.2	—	.2	.05	1.9	.3	.1	.02
VITAMINS														
Vitamin A	IU	0	90	99	t	30	60	80	410	0	—	6	248	3
Vitamin B₁	mg	t	.06	.25	.14	.05	.03	.09	.04	.003	.29	.04	.13	.004
Vitamin B₂	mg	.001	.1	.18	.05	.06	.04	.07	.13	.008	.15	.015	.19	.005
Vitamin B₆	mg	—	—	—	—	—	—	—	—	.003	—	.022	—	—
Vitamin B₁₂	mcg	0	—	—	—	—	—	—	—	t	0	0	—	—
Biotin	mcg	—	—	—	—	—	—	—	—	—	—	—	—	—
Niacin	mg	.03	1.6	2.6	1.2	.4	.2	.4	.7	.1	1.72	.3	1	.1
Pantothenic acid	mg	—	—	—	—	—	—	—	—	.09	—	.016	.5	—
Folic acid	mcg	—	—	—	—	—	—	—	—	—	—	—	—	—
Vitamin C	mg	0	t	1	t	t	t	t	5	0	—	0	t	—
Vitamin E	IU	.1	—	—	—	—	—	—	—	t	—	—	—	—
MINERALS														
Calcium	mg	.6	57	34	42	27	59	50	144	4	142	60	85	.95
Copper	mg	.001	—	.08	—	.02	—	—	—	.024	.32	—	—	—
Iron	mg	.04	1.5	1.2	1	.4	.4	.54	.7	.2	2.6	.9	1.3	.04
Magnesium	mg	.81	—	11	45	6.59	13.2	—	—	—	104	32	19	—
Manganese	mg	—	—	—	—	—	—	—	—	—	—	—	—	—
Phosphorus	mg	2.5	162	200	112	38	91	—	127	21	231	42	130	5.04
Potassium	mg	3.4	172	120	117	33	66	—	85	21	—	—	109	11
Selenium	mcg	—	—	—	—	—	—	—	—	—	—	—	—	—
Sodium	mg	31	179	500	226	115	125	—	456	269	—	—	356	18.2
Zinc	mg	—	—	.5	—	.37	—	—	.79	.173	1.29	—	—	—
LIPIDS														
Total lipid (fat)	gm	.37	3.9	10.8	1.1	1.9	215	3.2	5.4	.7	19.5	.6	7.4	.6
Total saturated	gm	.075	1.2	—	—	.5	.8	—	2	—	—	—	2	.2
Total unsaturated	gm	.225	2.4	—	—	1.3	1.5	—	3	—	—	—	5	.4
Cholesterol	mg	—	—	—	—	—	—	—	—	—	—	—	—	—
AMINO ACIDS														
Tryptophan	gm	—	—	—	—	—	—	—	—	—	—	—	—	—
Threonine	gm	—	—	—	—	—	—	—	—	—	—	—	—	—
Isoleucine	gm	—	—	—	—	—	—	—	—	—	—	—	—	—
Leucine	gm	—	—	—	—	—	—	—	—	—	—	—	—	—
Lysine	gm	—	—	—	—	—	—	—	—	—	—	—	—	—
Methionine	gm	—	—	—	—	—	—	—	—	—	—	—	—	—
Cystine	gm	—	—	—	—	—	—	—	—	—	—	—	—	—
Phenylalanine	gm	—	—	—	—	—	—	—	—	—	—	—	—	—
Tyrosine	gm	—	—	—	—	—	—	—	—	—	—	—	—	—
Valine	gm	—	—	—	—	—	—	—	—	—	—	—	—	—
Arginine	gm	—	—	—	—	—	—	—	—	—	—	—	—	—
Histidine	gm	—	—	—	—	—	—	—	—	—	—	—	—	—
Alanine	gm	—	—	—	—	—	—	—	—	—	—	—	—	—
Aspartic acid	gm	—	—	—	—	—	—	—	—	—	—	—	—	—
Glutamic acid	gm	—	—	—	—	—	—	—	—	—	—	—	—	—
Glycine	gm	—	—	—	—	—	—	—	—	—	—	—	—	—
Proline	gm	—	—	—	—	—	—	—	—	—	—	—	—	—
Serine	gm	—	—	—	—	—	—	—	—	—	—	—	—	—

Cereals

	Bran flakes, 40%, Post	Corn flakes, Kellogg's	Corn grits, enr, ckd	Corn, puffed, Kix	Granola, Nature Valley	Oat flakes, fortified	Oats, puffed, Cheerios	Oatmeal, ckd	Rice, puffed	Wheat, Cream of, ckd	Wheat, flakes, Total	Wheat germ, toasted	Wheat, granules, Grapenuts	Wheat, puffed	Wheat, shredded
	1 C.	1¼ C.	1 C.	1½ C.	1 C.	1 C.	1¼ C.	1 C.	1 C.	1 C.	1 C.	1 C.	1/4 C.	1 C.	1 lg.
	47	28	242	28.4	113	48	28.4	234	14	251	33	113	28.4	12	23.6
	152	110	146	110	503	177	111	145	56	134	116	431	101	44	83
	5.3	2.3	3.5	2.5	11.5	5.3	4.3	6	.9	3.8	3.3	32.9	3.3	1.8	2.6
	37.3	24.4	31.4	23.4	75.5	20.5	19.6	25.2	12.6	27.7	26	56.1	23.2	9.5	18.8
	6.5	.3	.6	.4	4.2	1.2	1.1	2.1	.1	—	2.4	—	1.4	.4	2.2
	2072	1250	—	1250	—	2116	1250	38	—	—	5820	—	1250	—	—
	.6	.4	.24	.4	.39	.6	.4	.26	.02	.2	1.7	1.89	.4	.02	.07
	.7	.4	.15	.4	.19	.7	.4	.05	.01	.1	2	.93	.4	.03	.06
	.8	.5	.058	.5	—	.9	.5	.047	.011	—	2.3	1.1	.5	.02	.06
	2.5	—	—	1.5	—	2.5	1.5	—	—	—	7	—	1.5	—	—
	8.3	5	1.96	5	.83	8.4	5	.3	.42	1.5	23.3	6.31	5	1.3	1.08
	—	.05	—	—	.931	—	.286	.468	.045	.188	.236	1.56	.27	.062	.192
	166	100	1	—	85	169	6	9	3	9	466	398	100	4	12
	—	15	—	15	—	—	15	—	—	—	70	7	—	—	—
	21	1	1	35	71	68	48	20	1	51	56	50	11	3	10
	.321	.019	.029	.047	.367	.255	.143	.129	.024	.075	.142	.701	.094	.049	.118
	7.5	1.8	1.55	8.1	3.78	13.7	4.5	1.59	.15	10.3	21	10.2	1.23	.57	.74
	102	3	11	12	116	58	39	56	3	10	.37	362	19	17	40
	—	.023	.041	—	—	—	.765	1.37	.21	—	.495	22.5	—	—	.725
	296	18	29	39	354	176	134	178	14	42	137	1294	71	43	86
	251	26	54	44	389	343	101	132	16	43	123	1070	95	42	77
	—	—	—	—	—	—	—	—	—	—	—	—	—	—	—
	431	351	0	339	232	429	307	1	0	2	409	4	197	0	0
	2.5	.08	.17	.25	2.19	1.5	.79	1.15	.14	.33	.78	18.8	.62	.28	.59
	.8	.1	.5	.7	19.6	.4	1.8	2.4	.1	.5	.7	12.1	.1	.1	.3
	—	—	—	.18	13	—	.34	.44	—	—	.1	2.09	—	—	—
	—	—	—	.41	5.68	—	1.39	1.81	—	—	.41	9.08	—	—	—
	—	—	—	—	—	—	—	—	—	—	—	—	—	—	—
	.093	—	.019	.02	.156	.156	.058	.082	.013	.053	.063	.38	.06	.027	.049
	.171	—	.121	.088	.405	.427	.149	.211	.045	.12	.11	1.35	.106	.054	.086
	.199	—	.136	.103	.532	.5	.196	.276	.047	.168	.13	1.17	.136	.075	.101
	.354	—	.52	.325	.885	.83	.327	.461	.074	.289	.227	2.16	.235	.128	.177
	.177	—	.068	.065	.471	.583	.175	.246	.038	.098	.101	2.07	.101	.049	.079
	.083	—	.082	.055	.194	.168	.071	.101	.026	.07	.057	.624	.056	.031	.045
	.108	—	.077	.058	.287	.221	.107	.15	.015	.085	.063	.669	.066	.035	.049
	.244	—	.177	.131	.631	.47	.233	.33	.038	.206	.158	1.34	.168	.091	.124
	.159	—	.148	.102	.412	.338	.153	.215	.05	.12	.096	1.02	.102	.053	.075
	.259	—	.177	.134	.678	.538	.251	.353	.058	.183	.162	1.63	.166	.084	.127
	.314	—	.114	.112	.87	.579	.32	.452	.073	.166	.171	2.7	.169	.085	.133
	.136	—	.094	.065	.262	.219	.097	.136	.027	.088	.077	.936	.08	.046	.06
	.226	—	.295	.192	.623	.471	.23	.325	.037	.133	.128	2.11	.128	.066	.1
	.329	—	.208	.171	1.01	.962	.376	.531	.082	.178	.184	2.97	.189	.099	.144
	1.46	—	.765	.562	2.64	1.96	.98	1.38	.142	1.41	.962	5.61	1.05	.597	.75
	.264	—	.104	.093	.628	.398	.232	.328	.051	.148	.141	2.02	.144	.069	.11
	.473	—	.353	.224	.65	.554	.241	.339	.037	.464	.327	1.75	.351	.184	.255
	.273	—	.169	.122	.544	.477	.201	.283	.04	.213	.182	1.55	.18	.097	.142

BAKERY AND GRAINS (cont.)
Desserts and Sweets

	Measure	Apple or brown betty	Cake, angel food	Cake, cheese	Cake, devil's food	Cake, gingerbread	Cake, pound	Cake, sponge	Cake, white	Candied citron	Candy, caramel	Candy, chocolate bar	Candy, chocolate fudge
Measure		1 C.	1/10		2 × 3 × 2″	3 × 3 × 2″	3 × 3 × 1/2″	1/10		1 oz	1	1 oz	1″ cube
Weight	gm	215	45	100	45	117	30	50	50	28	5	28	21
Calories		325	121	302	165	371	142	149	188	89	20	147	84
Protein	gm	3.4	3.2	5.42	2.2	4.4	1.7	3.8	2.3	.1	.2	2.2	.6
Carbohydrate	gm	64	27	28.5	23.4	60.8	14.1	27	27	22.7	3.88	16	15.8
Fiber	gm	1.4	0	.45	.1	t	t	0	1	.39	.01	.112	.04
VITAMINS													
Vitamin A	IU	220	0	254	68	110	84	225	15	—	t	80	t
Vitamin B$_1$	mg	.13	.004	.03	.009	.14	.009	.03	.005	—	.002	.02	t
Vitamin B$_2$	mg	.09	.06	.13	.045	.13	.03	.07	.04	—	.009	.1	.02
Vitamin B$_6$	mg	—	—	.064	—	—	—	—	.025	—	—	—	—
Vitamin B$_{12}$	mcg	—	—	.495	—	—	—	—	—	—	—	—	—
Biotin	mcg	—	—	—	—	—	—	—	—	—	—	—	—
Niacin	mg	.9	.1	.46	.1	1.1	.1	.1	.1	—	.018	.1	t
Pantothenic acid	mg	—	—	.574	.1	—	—	—	.15	—	—	—	—
Folic acid	mcg	—	—	18	—	—	—	3	—	—	—	2	—
Vitamin C	mg	2	0	5	t	0	0	t	t	—	t	t	t
Vitamin E	IU	—	—	—	—	—	—	—	4.21	—	—	.308	—
MINERALS													
Calcium	mg	39	4	56	33	80	6	15	32	24	7.5	65	16
Copper	mg	.774	—	.06	.144	—	—	—	—	—	—	.137	—
Iron	mg	1.3	.1	.48	.4	2.7	.2	.6	.1	.2	.071	.3	.2
Magnesium	mg	14	6.76	10	—	—	—	—	—	—	—	16.2	—
Manganese	mg	—	—	—	—	—	—	—	—	—	—	—	—
Phosphorus	mg	47	10	88	62	76	24	56	46	7	6.25	65	18
Potassium	mg	215	40	98	63	531	18	44	38	34	9.64	109	31
Selenium	mcg	—	—	—	—	—	—	—	—	—	—	—	—
Sodium	mg	329	127	222	132	277	33	84	162	82	11.4	27	40
Zinc	mg	—	—	.42	—	—	—	—	1	—	—	.129	.192
LIPIDS													
Total lipid (fat)	gm	7.5	.1	19.2	7.7	12.5	8.8	2.85	8	.1	.536	9.2	.3
Total saturated	gm	2.15	—	—	—	—	—	1	2	—	.357	5	1.5
Total unsaturated	gm	2.2	—	—	—	—	—	1	5	—	.179	3	.752
Cholesterol	mg	—	—	—	—	—	—	123	—	—	—	—	—
AMINO ACIDS													
Tryptophan	gm	—	—	—	—	—	—	—	—	—	—	—	—
Threonine	gm	—	—	—	—	—	—	—	—	—	—	—	—
Isoleucine	gm	—	—	—	—	—	—	—	—	—	—	—	—
Leucine	gm	—	—	—	—	—	—	—	—	—	—	—	—
Lysine	gm	—	—	—	—	—	—	—	—	—	—	—	—
Methionine	gm	—	—	—	—	—	—	—	—	—	—	—	—
Cystine	gm	—	—	—	—	—	—	—	—	—	—	—	—
Phenylalanine	gm	—	—	—	—	—	—	—	—	—	—	—	—
Tyrosine	gm	—	—	—	—	—	—	—	—	—	—	—	—
Valine	gm	—	—	—	—	—	—	—	—	—	—	—	—
Arginine	gm	—	—	—	—	—	—	—	—	—	—	—	—
Histidine	gm	—	—	—	—	—	—	—	—	—	—	—	—
Alanine	gm	—	—	—	—	—	—	—	—	—	—	—	—
Aspartic acid	gm	—	—	—	—	—	—	—	—	—	—	—	—
Glutamic acid	gm	—	—	—	—	—	—	—	—	—	—	—	—
Glycine	gm	—	—	—	—	—	—	—	—	—	—	—	—
Proline	gm	—	—	—	—	—	—	—	—	—	—	—	—
Serine	gm	—	—	—	—	—	—	—	—	—	—	—	—

Candy, peanut brittle	Chocolate, baking	Chocolate, semisweet	Chocolate syrup	Cookies, brownies	Cookies, chocolate chip	Cookies, fig bar	Cookies, gingersnap	Cookies, macaroon	Cookies, oatmeal w/raisins	Cookies, peanut butter	Cookies, sugar	Custard, baked	Danish pastry	Doughnut, cake
1 oz	1 oz	1 oz	1 T.	2 × 2 × 3/4"	2⅓" diam	1	2" diam	1	3" diam			1 C.	1	1
25	28	28	18.7	30	10	14	7	14	14	100	100	265	42	32
119	143	144	46	146	51	50	29.4	67	63	495	494	305	179	125
1.6	3	1.2	.45	2	.55	.55	.39	.7	.9	8	4.54	14.3	3.1	1.5
23	8.2	16.2	11.7	15.3	6	10.5	5.59	9.3	10.3	58.7	65.5	29.4	19.4	16.4
.125	.7	.28	.1	.2	t	.238	t	.3	.1	.36	.12	0	t	t
0	20	10	t	60	10	15	5	0	7	152	74	930	130	26
.05	.01	t	.005	.05	.01	.005	.003	.006	.015	.19	.18	.11	.03	.05
.01	.07	.02	.015	.03	.01	.01	.004	.02	.011	.16	.12	.5	.06	.05
—	—	—	—	—	—	—	—	—	—	.082	.056	—	—	—
—	.4	.1	.1	.2	.1	.05	.03	.1	.1	3.81	2.33	.3	.3	.4
1	—	—	—	—	—	—	—	—	—	.137	.228	—	—	.12
—	—	—	—	—	1	—	—	—	—	24	9	—	—	3
0	0	t	0	t	t	t	t	0	t	0	0	1	t	t
—	3.12	—	—	—	—	—	—	—	—	—	—	—	—	.81
10	22	9	3	12	3.5	11	5.1	4	3	115	104	297	21	13
—	.748	—	.08	—	—	—	—	—	.015	.156	.043	—	—	.035
.7	1.9	.7	.3	.6	.2	.15	.16	.1	.4	1.9	1.93	1.1	.4	.4
←	81.8	—	11.8	—	—	—	—	—	—	39	8	—	8	7
—	—	—	—	—	—	—	—	—	—	—	—	—	—	—
27	109	43	17	44	10	8.5	3.3	12	14	235	189	310	46	61
43	235	92	53	57	11.8	27.8	32.3	65	52	194	68	387	48	29
9	1	1	10	75	34.8	35.3	40	5	23	566	543	209	156	160
—	—	—	.15	—	.096	—	—	—	.183	.75	.27	—	.35	2
2.6	15	10.1	.49	9.4	3	.775	.62	3.2	2.2	26.4	23.9	14.6	10	6
.5	8	5.6	t	1.5	1	.14	—	2.24	—	—	—	7	3.25	1
1.75	6	3.79	t	6	2	.42	—	.84	—	—	—	6	6.5	4
—	—	—	—	25.5	—	—	—	—	—	—	—	278	—	—
—	—	—	—	—	—	—	—	—	—	—	—	—	—	—
—	—	—	—	—	—	—	—	—	—	—	—	—	—	—
—	—	—	—	—	—	—	—	—	—	—	—	—	—	—
—	—	—	—	—	—	—	—	—	—	—	—	—	—	—
—	—	—	—	—	—	—	—	—	—	—	—	—	—	—
—	—	—	—	—	—	—	—	—	—	—	—	—	—	—
—	—	—	—	—	—	—	—	—	—	—	—	—	—	—
—	—	—	—	—	—	—	—	—	—	—	—	—	—	—
—	—	—	—	—	—	—	—	—	—	—	—	—	—	—
—	—	—	—	—	—	—	—	—	—	—	—	—	—	—
—	—	—	—	—	—	—	—	—	—	—	—	—	—	—
—	—	—	—	—	—	—	—	—	—	—	—	—	—	—
—	—	—	—	—	—	—	—	—	—	—	—	—	—	—
—	—	—	—	—	—	—	—	—	—	—	—	—	—	—

BAKERY AND GRAINS (cont.)
Desserts and Sweets (cont.)

	Measure	Doughnut, raised	Eclair, custard	Granola bars	Honey	Jams	Jellies	Molasses, blackstrap	Molasses, light	Pie, apple, 9"	Pie, chocolate cream	Pie, lemon meringue	Pie, pecan	Pie, pumpkin
Measure		1	1		1 T.	1 T.	1 T.	1 T.	1 T.	1/6		1/6	1/6	1/6
Weight	gm	30	100	100	21	20	18	20	20	160	100	140	160	150
Calories		124	239	454	64	54	49	43	50	410	264	357	668	317
Protein	gm	1.9	6.2	9.79	.1	.1	t	0	0	3.4	4.58	5.2	8.2	6
Carbohydrate	gm	11.3	23.2	66.7	17.8	14	12.7	11	13	61	29.4	52.8	82	36.7
Fiber	gm	.1	0	.86	0	.1	0	—	—	.6	.15	t	.8	.8
VITAMINS														
Vitamin A	IU	18	340	—	0	t	t	—	—	48	264	238	256	3700
Vitamin B$_1$	mg	.05	.04	.28	.002	t	t	.02	.01	.03	.1	.05	.25	.04
Vitamin B$_2$	mg	.05	.16	.11	.014	.01	.01	.04	.01	.03	.17	.11	.11	.15
Vitamin B$_6$	mg	—	—	—	.004	.005	—	.054	—	—	.047	—	—	—
Vitamin B$_{12}$	mcg	—	—	0	0	0	—	—	—	0	.366	—	—	—
Biotin	mcg	—	—	—	—	—	—	1.8	—	—	—	—	—	—
Niacin	mg	.4	.1	—	.1	t	t	.4	t	.6	.72	.3	.5	.8
Pantothenic acid	mg	—	—	.544	.04	t	—	.1	—	.176	.481	—	—	.778
Folic acid	mcg	7	—	—	1	2	—	2	—	6	9	—	—	—
Vitamin C	mg	0	t	—	t	0	1	—	—	2	t	4	t	t
Vitamin E	IU	—	—	—	—	—	—	—	—	.32	—	—	—	—
MINERALS														
Calcium	mg	11	80	60	1	4	4	137	33	1	84	20	75	76
Copper	mg	—	—	—	.008	.062	.016	.284	.2	.096	.119	—	—	—
Iron	mg	.5	.7	3.18	.1	.2	.3	3.2	.9	.5	1.08	.7	4.5	.8
Magnesium	mg	6	—	—	.6	1	.72	51.6	9.2	—	25	—	—	—
Manganese	mg	—	—	—	.006	—	—	—	—	—	—	—	—	—
Phosphorus	mg	23	112	277	1	2	1	17	9	35	109	69	165	104
Potassium	mg	24	122	326	11	18	14	585	183	128	142	70	197	240
Selenium	mcg	—	—	—	—	—	—	—	5.2	—	—	—	—	—
Sodium	mg	70	82	278	1	2	3	19	3	482	273	395	354	321
Zinc	mg	—	—	—	.016	.006	—	—	—	.143	.66	—	—	—
LIPIDS														
Total lipid (fat)	gm	8	13.6	17.6	0	t	t	—	—	17.8	15.1	14.3	36.6	16.8
Total saturated	gm	1.8	4	—	—	—	—	—	—	4.74	—	4.67	5.36	5.77
Total unsaturated	gm	5.69	8	—	—	—	—	—	—	11.8	—	8.33	28	9.23
Cholesterol	mg	—	—	—	—	—	—	—	—	156	—	130	—	91
AMINO ACIDS														
Tryptophan	gm	—	—	—	—	—	—	—	—	—	—	—	—	—
Threonine	gm	—	—	—	—	—	—	—	—	—	—	—	—	—
Isoleucine	gm	—	—	—	—	—	—	—	—	—	—	—	—	—
Leucine	gm	—	—	—	—	—	—	—	—	—	—	—	—	—
Lysine	gm	—	—	—	—	—	—	—	—	—	—	—	—	—
Methionine	gm	—	—	—	—	—	—	—	—	—	—	—	—	—
Cystine	gm	—	—	—	—	—	—	—	—	—	—	—	—	—
Phenylalanine	gm	—	—	—	—	—	—	—	—	—	—	—	—	—
Tyrosine	gm	—	—	—	—	—	—	—	—	—	—	—	—	—
Valine	gm	—	—	—	—	—	—	—	—	—	—	—	—	—
Arginine	gm	—	—	—	—	—	—	—	—	—	—	—	—	—
Histidine	gm	—	—	—	—	—	—	—	—	—	—	—	—	—
Alanine	gm	—	—	—	—	—	—	—	—	—	—	—	—	—
Aspartic acid	gm	—	—	—	—	—	—	—	—	—	—	—	—	—
Glutamic acid	gm	—	—	—	—	—	—	—	—	—	—	—	—	—
Glycine	gm	—	—	—	—	—	—	—	—	—	—	—	—	—
Proline	gm	—	—	—	—	—	—	—	—	—	—	—	—	—
Serine	gm	—	—	—	—	—	—	—	—	—	—	—	—	—

Flours

Pie crust, enr	Pudding, bread, w/raisins	Pudding, chocolate	Pudding, rice, w/raisins	Pudding, tapioca cream	Sugar, cane	Sugar, brown, packed	Sugar, confectioner's	Sugar, raw	Syrup, corn	Syrup, maple	Buckwheat	Carob	Corn	Gluten, wheat
9″	1 C.	1 C.	1 C.	1 C.	1 T.	1 C.	1 C.	1 T.			1 C.	1 T.	1 C.	1 C.
135	265	260	265	165	12	220	120	14	20	20	100	8	117	140
675	496	385	387	221	46	821	462	14	57	50	333	14	431	529
8.2	14.8	8.1	9.5	8.3	0	0	0	.06	0	0	11.7	.4	—	58
59.1	75.3	66.8	70.8	28.2	11.9	212	119	12.7	14.8	12.8	72	6.5	89.9	66.1
.3	.2	.2	.133	0	0	0	0	—	0	0	1.6	.64	—	.6
0	800	390	290	480	0	0	0	t	0	0	0	—	400	0
.27	.16	.05	.08	.07	0	.02	0	.003	0	—	.58	—	.23	—
.19	.5	.36	.37	.3	0	.07	0	.016	.002	—	.15	—	.07	—
—	—	—	—	—	—	—	—	—	—	—	.578	—	—	—
—	—	—	—	—	—	—	—	—	—	—	0	—	—	—
—	—	—	—	—	—	—	—	—	t	—	—	—	—	—
2.4	1.3	.3	.5	.2	0	.4	0	.04	t	—	2.9	—	1.6	—
—	—	—	13	3	—	—	—	—	—	—	1.5	—	—	—
—	—	—	—	—	—	—	—	—	—	—	—	—	—	—
0	3	1	t	2	0	0	0	.3	.1	0	0	—	0	0
1.17	—	1.79	—	—	—	—	—	—	—	—	—	—	—	—
19	289	250	260	173	0	187	0	7	9	33	33	28	7	56
—	.212	—	.08	.066	.002	.77	.024	.059	.072	.09	.7	—	—	—
2.3	2.9	1.3	1.1	.7	t	7.5	.1	.6	.8	.2	5	.33	2.1	—
—	—	—	—	—	—	—	—	—	—	—	—	—	—	—
—	—	—	—	—	—	—	—	—	2.8	—	2.09	—	—	—
67	302	255	249	180	0	42	0	6	3	3	347	6	92	196
67	570	445	469	223	t	757	4	—	—	26	656	—	—	84
825	533	146	188	257	t	66	1	—	—	3	1	—	1	3
.715	—	—	.82	—	.006	—	—	—	—	—	—	—	—	—
45.2	16.2	12.2	8.2	8.4	0	0	0	.07	0	0	2.5	.1	3	2.7
12	7.95	7	5.3	4	—	—	—	—	—	—	.47	—	.35	—
30	5.3	4	2.65	3	—	—	—	—	—	—	1.76	—	2.34	—
—	170	30	29	—	—	—	—	—	—	—	—	—	—	—
—	—	—	—	—	—	—	—	—	—	—	—	—	—	—
—	—	—	—	—	—	—	—	—	—	—	—	—	—	—
—	—	—	—	—	—	—	—	—	—	—	—	—	—	—
—	—	—	—	—	—	—	—	—	—	—	—	—	—	—
—	—	—	—	—	—	—	—	—	—	—	—	—	—	—
—	—	—	—	—	—	—	—	—	—	—	—	—	—	—
—	—	—	—	—	—	—	—	—	—	—	—	—	—	—
—	—	—	—	—	—	—	—	—	—	—	—	—	—	—
—	—	—	—	—	—	—	—	—	—	—	—	—	—	—
—	—	—	—	—	—	—	—	—	—	—	—	—	—	—
—	—	—	—	—	—	—	—	—	—	—	—	—	—	—
—	—	—	—	—	—	—	—	—	—	—	—	—	—	—
—	—	—	—	—	—	—	—	—	—	—	—	—	—	—
—	—	—	—	—	—	—	—	—	—	—	—	—	—	—
—	—	—	—	—	—	—	—	—	—	—	—	—	—	—
—	—	—	—	—	—	—	—	—	—	—	—	—	—	—

BAKERY AND GRAINS (*cont.*)

Flours (*cont.*)   Grains

	Measure	Pastry, wheat	Peanut, defatted	Potato	Rice	Rye, dark	Rye, light	Soy	Wheat, enr	Whole wheat	Barley, pot or scotch	Bran, wheat	Bran, rice
Measure		1 C.	1 C.	1 C.	1 C.	1 C.	1 C.	1 C.	1 C.	1 C.	1 C.	1 C.	1 C.
Weight	gm	100	60	110	125	128	80	72	110	120	200	57	105
Calories		364	223	386	479	419	286	303	400	400	696	121	278
Protein	gm	7.5	28.7	8.8	7.5	20.9	7.5	26.4	11.6	16	19.2	9	12.7
Carbohydrate	gm	79.4	18.9	87.9	107	87.2	62.3	21.9	83.7	85.2	154	35.4	60.6
Fiber	gm	.2	1.62	1.76	.2	3.07	.3	1.7	.3	2.8	2.14	5.2	2.4
VITAMINS													
Vitamin A	IU	0	—	t	0	—	—	79	0	0	0	0	0
Vitamin B₁	mg	.03	.45	.46	.52	.78	.12	.61	.48	.66	.42	.41	1.93
Vitamin B₂	mg	.03	.13	.15	.14	.28	.05	.22	.28	.14	.14	.2	.19
Vitamin B₆	mg	.045	—	.008	.2	.384	.07	.48	.066	.41	—	.468	—
Vitamin B₁₂	mcg	0	—	0	0	0	0	0	0	0	0	0	—
Biotin	mcg	—	—	—	—	—	—	49	1.1	6	—	—	—
Niacin	mg	.7	16.7	3.74	7.2	3.5	.5	1.5	3.9	5.2	7.4	12	29.6
Pantothenic acid	mg	.32	—	—	—	1.7	.58	1.22	.51	1.32	—	1.65	—
Folic acid	mcg	—	—	—	—	—	69	311	24	65	40	147	39
Vitamin C	mg	0	0	19	0	0	0	0	0	0	0	0	0
Vitamin E	IU	—	—	—	—	—	—	—	1.87	3.12	—	—	—
MINERALS													
Calcium	mg	17	62	36.3	11	69	18	143	18	49	68	67.8	72
Copper	mg	—	—	—	—	.54	.3	—	.21	.6	—	.9	—
Iron	mg	.5	2.1	18.9	6.8	5.8	.9	6	3.2	4	5.4	8.49	16.9
Magnesium	mg	26	216	—	35	147	58	178	28	136	71.4	279	—
Manganese	mg	—	—	—	—	—	—	—	—	—	—	—	—
Phosphorus	mg	73	432	196	120	686	148	402	96	446	580	727	1161
Potassium	mg	95	712	1747	—	1101	125	1195	105	444	592	639	750
Selenium	mcg	—	—	—	—	—	—	—	21.7	77.4	—	35.9	—
Sodium	mg	2	5	37.4	—	1	1	1	2	4	—	5.13	t
Zinc	mg	.3	—	—	—	—	—	—	.77	2.88	—	5.59	—
LIPIDS													
Total lipid (fat)	gm	.8	5.5	.88	.4	3.3	.8	14.2	1.1	2.4	2.2	2.6	12.8
Total saturated	gm	—	1.2	—	—	.42	—	2.5	—	t	.48	.42	2.44
Total unsaturated	gm	—	4	—	—	1	—	10.6	—	2	1.52	1.76	9.34
Cholesterol	mg	—	—	—	—	—	—	—	—	—	—	—	—
AMINO ACIDS													
Tryptophan	gm	—	—	—	—	—	—	—	—	—	—	—	—
Threonine	gm	—	—	—	—	—	—	—	—	—	—	—	—
Isoleucine	gm	—	—	—	—	—	—	—	—	—	—	—	—
Leucine	gm	—	—	—	—	—	—	—	—	—	—	—	—
Lysine	gm	—	—	—	—	—	—	—	—	—	—	—	—
Methionine	gm	—	—	—	—	—	—	—	—	—	—	—	—
Cystine	gm	—	—	—	—	—	—	—	—	—	—	—	—
Phenylalanine	gm	—	—	—	—	—	—	—	—	—	—	—	—
Tyrosine	gm	—	—	—	—	—	—	—	—	—	—	—	—
Valine	gm	—	—	—	—	—	—	—	—	—	—	—	—
Arginine	gm	—	—	—	—	—	—	—	—	—	—	—	—
Histidine	gm	—	—	—	—	—	—	—	—	—	—	—	—
Alanine	gm	—	—	—	—	—	—	—	—	—	—	—	—
Aspartic acid	gm	—	—	—	—	—	—	—	—	—	—	—	—
Glutamic acid	gm	—	—	—	—	—	—	—	—	—	—	—	—
Glycine	gm	—	—	—	—	—	—	—	—	—	—	—	—
Proline	gm	—	—	—	—	—	—	—	—	—	—	—	—
Serine	gm	—	—	—	—	—	—	—	—	—	—	—	—

	Bulgur	Cornmeal, whl grd	Cornstarch	Macaroni, enr, ckd	Millet	Noodles, egg, enr, ckd	Pasta, whole wheat	Popcorn	Rice, brown	Rice, white enr	Rice, wild	Spaghetti, enr, ckd	Tapioca
	1 C.	1 C.	1 T.	1 C.	1 C.	1 C.	4 oz	1 C.	1 C.	1 C.	1 C.	1 C.	1 C.
	170	118	8	140	228	160	113	14	196	195	160	140	152
	602	427	29	151	746	200	400	54	704	708	565	155	535
	19	10.6	t	4.8	22.6	6.6	20	1.8	14.8	13.1	22.6	4.8	.9
	129	88	7	32.2	166	37.3	78	10.7	152	157	121	32.2	131
	3	1.2	t	.1	7.3	.2	—	.3	1.6	.4	.12	.2	.15
	0	566	0	0	0	112	200	—	0	0	0	0	0
	.48	.35	0	.2	1.66	.22	.6	.055	.68	.86	.72	.2	0
	.24	.09	.006	.11	.87	.13	.85	.02	.08	.06	1.01	.11	.15
	.38	.29	t	.029	—	.04	—	.03	1	.3	—	—	—
	0	0	—	0	—	t	—	0	0	0	0	0	—
	—	t	—	—	—	—	—	—	18	5.86	—	—	—
	7.8	2.2	.002	1.5	5.24	1.9	8	.3	9.2	6.8	9.9	1.5	0
	1.12	.65	—	—	—	—	—	—	2.1	1.26	1.63	—	—
	7.7	19	—	—	—	—	—	—	32	20	—	—	12
	0	—	0	0	0	0	10.8	0	0	0	0	0	0
	—	—	—	—	4	—	—	—	3	.7	—	—	—
	49	20	0	11	45.6	16	20	2	64	47	30	11	15
	—	.156	.004	.028	—	.27	—	.04	.4	.2	—	—	.14
	6.3	2.1	.04	1.2	15.5	1.4	5.4	.4	3.2	5.7	6.7	1.3	.6
	—	125	.16	25	369	—	—	—	172	13	144	27	3
	—	—	—	—	—	—	—	—	3.2	2.1	—	—	1.04
	575	263	2.4	70	709	94	400	39	432	183	542	70	27
	389	293	.32	85	980	70	—	33.6	420	179	352	85	27
	—	—	—	—	—	—	—	—	77.2	65.1	—	—	—
	—	1	.32	1	—	3	—	t	16	10	11	1	5
	—	2.1	—	.7	—	—	—	.574	3.6	2.5	—	—	—
	2.5	4	.05	1	6.8	2.4	1	.7	3.6	1.5	1.1	.6	.3
	.34	.46	t	—	1.96	1	—	t	—	.4	—	—	—
	1.48	3	.04	—	4.1	1	—	.6	—	.9	—	—	—
	—	—	—	—	—	50	—	—	—	—	—	—	—
	—	—	—	—	—	—	—	—	—	—	—	—	—
	—	—	—	—	—	—	—	—	—	—	—	—	—
	—	—	—	—	—	—	—	—	—	—	—	—	—
	—	—	—	—	—	—	—	—	—	—	—	—	—
	—	—	—	—	—	—	—	—	—	—	—	—	—
	—	—	—	—	—	—	—	—	—	—	—	—	—
	—	—	—	—	—	—	—	—	—	—	—	—	—
	—	—	—	—	—	—	—	—	—	—	—	—	—
	—	—	—	—	—	—	—	—	—	—	—	—	—
	—	—	—	—	—	—	—	—	—	—	—	—	—
	—	—	—	—	—	—	—	—	—	—	—	—	—
	—	—	—	—	—	—	—	—	—	—	—	—	—
	—	—	—	—	—	—	—	—	—	—	—	—	—
	—	—	—	—	—	—	—	—	—	—	—	—	—

DAIRY AND EGGS
Cheese

	Measure	Bleu	Brick	Brie	Camembert	Cheddar	Cheshire	Colby	Cottage, creamed	Cottage, dry	Cottage, lowfat, 2%	Cream	Edam	Feta
Measure		1 oz	1 oz	1 oz	1 oz	1 oz	1 oz	1 oz	1 C.	1 C.	1 C.	1 oz	1 oz	1 oz
Weight	gm	28	28	28	28	28	28	28	210	145	226	28	28	28
Calories		100	105	95	85	114	110	112	217	123	203	99	101	75
Protein	gm	6.07	6.59	5.88	5.61	7.06	6.62	6.74	26.2	25	31	2.14	7.08	4
Carbohydrate	gm	.66	.79	.13	.13	.36	1.36	.73	5.63	2.68	8.2	.75	.4	1.16
Fiber	gm	0	0	0	0	0	0	0	0	0	0	0	0	0
VITAMINS														
Vitamin A	IU	204	307	189	262	300	279	293	342	44	158	405	260	—
Vitamin B_1	mg	.008	.004	.02	.008	.008	.013	.004	.044	.036	.054	.005	.01	—
Vitamin B_2	mg	.108	.1	.147	.138	.106	.083	.106	.342	.206	.418	.056	.11	—
Vitamin B_6	mg	.047	.018	.067	.064	.021	—	.022	.141	.119	.172	.013	.022	—
Vitamin B_{12}	mcg	.345	.356	.468	.367	.234	—	.234	1.3	1.19	1.6	.12	.435	—
Biotin	mcg	—	—	—	1	1	—	—	—	3	—	—	—	—
Niacin	mg	.288	.033	.108	.179	.023	—	.026	.265	.225	.325	.029	.023	—
Pantothenic acid	mg	.49	.082	.196	.387	.117	—	.06	.447	.236	.547	.077	.08	—
Folic acid	mcg	10	6	18	18	5	—	—	26	21	30	4	5	—
Vitamin C	mg	0	0	0	0	0	0	0	t	0	t	0	0	0
Vitamin E	IU	—	—	—	—	—	—	—	—	—	—	—	—	—
MINERALS														
Calcium	mg	150	191	52	110	204	182	194	126	46	155	23	207	140
Copper	mg	.011	.007	—	.022	.031	—	.012	.04	—	—	.011	.008	—
Iron	mg	.09	.12	.14	.09	.19	.06	.22	.29	.33	.36	.34	.12	.18
Magnesium	mg	7	7	—	6	8	6	7	11	6	14	2	8	5
Manganese	mg	.003	.003	—	.011	.003	—	.003	.007	—	—	.001	.003	—
Phosphorus	mg	110	128	53	98	145	131	129	277	151	340	30	152	96
Potassium	mg	73	38	43	53	28	27	36	177	47	217	34	53	18
Selenium	mcg	—	—	—	—	—	—	—	11.3	—	—	—	—	—
Sodium	mg	396	159	178	239	176	198	171	850	19[1]	918	84	274	316
Zinc	mg	.75	.74	—	.68	.88	—	.87	.78	.68	.95	.15	1.06	.82
LIPIDS														
Total lipid (fat)	gm	8.15	8.41	7.85	6.88	9.4	8.68	9.1	9.45	.61	4.36	9.89	7.88	6
Total saturated	gm	5.3	5.32	—	4.33	5.98	—	5.73	5.99	.396	2.76	6.23	4.98	4.24
Total unsaturated	gm	2.44	2.66	—	2.19	2.93	—	2.9	2.99	.182	1.37	3.15	2.49	1.48
Cholesterol	mg	21	27	28	20	30	29	27	31	10	19	31	25	25
AMINO ACIDS														
Tryptophan	gm	.089	.092	.091	.087	.091	.085	.087	.292	.279	.346	.019	—	—
Threonine	gm	.223	.25	.213	.203	.251	.236	.24	1.16	1.11	1.37	.091	.264	—
Isoleucine	gm	.319	.322	.288	.275	.438	.411	.418	1.54	1.47	1.82	.113	.371	—
Leucine	gm	.545	.636	.547	.522	.676	.635	.645	2.69	2.57	3.19	.207	.726	—
Lysine	gm	.526	.602	.525	.501	.588	.551	.561	2.12	2.02	2.51	.192	.754	—
Methionine	gm	.166	.16	.168	.16	.185	.173	.176	.789	.754	.934	.051	.204	—
Cystine	gm	.03	.037	.032	.031	.035	.033	.034	.243	.232	.287	.019	—	—
Phenylalanine	gm	.309	.349	.328	.313	.372	.349	.355	1.41	1.35	1.67	.119	.406	—
Tyrosine	gm	.368	.316	.34	.325	.341	.32	.325	1.39	1.33	1.65	.102	.413	—
Valine	gm	.442	.417	.38	.362	.471	.442	.45	1.62	1.55	1.92	.125	.513	—
Arginine	gm	.202	.248	.208	.199	.267	.25	.254	1.19	1.14	1.41	.081	.273	—
Histidine	gm	.215	.233	.203	.194	.248	.233	.236	.872	.832	1.03	.077	.293	—
Alanine	gm	.183	.19	.243	.232	.199	.187	.19	1.36	1.29	1.61	.065	.217	—
Aspartic acid	gm	.408	.45	.383	.365	.454	.426	.433	1.77	1.69	2.1	.151	.495	—
Glutamic acid	gm	1.47	1.56	1.24	1.18	1.72	1.62	1.64	5.68	5.42	6.72	.486	1.74	—
Glycine	gm	.115	.124	.112	.107	.122	.114	.116	.57	.546	.677	.042	.138	—
Proline	gm	.596	.73	.697	.665	.796	.747	.759	3.03	2.9	3.59	.195	.922	—
Serine	gm	.318	.366	.331	.316	.413	.387	.394	1.47	1.4	1.74	.113	.439	—

[1] Unsalted.

	Fontina	Gjetost	Gouda	Gruyère	Limburger	Monterey jack	Mozzarella	Mozzarella, part skim	Muenster	Neufchatel	Parmesan	Parmesan, grated	Port du salut	Provolone	Ricotta	Ricotta, part skim	Romano
	1 oz	1 oz	1 oz	1 oz	1 oz	1 oz	1 oz	1 oz	1 oz	1 oz	1 oz	1 T.	1 oz	1 oz	1 C.	1 C.	1 oz
	28	28	28	28	28	28	28	28	28	28	28	5	28	28	246	246	28
	110	132	101	117	93	106	80	72	104	74	111	23	100	100	428	340	110
	7.26	2.74	7.07	8.45	5.68	6.94	5.5	6.88	6.64	2.82	10	2	6.74	7.25	27.7	28	9
	.44	12	.63	.1	.14	.19	.63	.78	.32	.83	.91	.19	.16	.61	7.48	12.6	1
	0	0	0	0	0	0	0	0	0	0	0	0	0	0	0	0	0
	333	—	183	346	363	269	225	166	318	321	171	35	378	231	1205	1063	162
	.006	—	.009	.017	.023	—	.004	.005	.004	.004	.011	.002	—	.005	.032	.052	—
	.058	—	.095	.079	.143	.111	.069	.086	.091	.055	.094	.019	.068	.091	.48	.455	.105
	—	—	.023	.023	.024	—	.016	.02	.016	.012	.026	.005	.015	.021	.106	.049	—
	—	—	—	.454	.295	—	.185	.232	.418	.075	—	—	.425	.415	.831	.716	—
	.043	.23	.018	.03	.045	—	.024	.03	.029	.036	.077	.016	.017	.044	.256	.192	.022
	—	—	.096	.159	.334	—	.018	.022	.054	.16	.128	.026	.06	.135	—	—	—
	0	1	6	3	16	—	2	2	3	3	2	t	5	3	—	—	2
	—	0	0	0	0	0	0	0	0	0	0	0	0	0	0	0	—
	156	113	198	287	141	212	147	183	203	21	336	69	184	214	509	669	302
	—	—	—	—	—	.009	—	.008	.009	—	.101	.018	—	.007	.085	—	—
	.06	—	.07	—	.04	.2	.05	.06	.12	.08	.23	.05	—	.15	.94	1.08	—
	4	—	8	—	6	8	5	7	8	2	12	3	—	8	28	36	—
	—	—	—	—	—	.003	—	—	.003	.002	—	.006	—	.003	.024	—	—
	—	126	155	172	111	126	105	131	133	39	197	40	102	141	389	449	215
	—	—	34	23	36	23	19	24	38	32	26	5	—	39	257	308	—
	—	—	—	—	—	—	—	—	—	—	—	—	—	—	—	—	—
	—	170	232	95	227	152	106	132	178	113	454	93	151	248	207	307	340
	.99	—	1.11	—	.6	.85	.63	.78	.8	.15	.78	.16	—	.92	2.85	3.3	—
	8.83	8.37	7.78	9.17	7.72	8.58	6.12	4.51	8.52	6.64	7.32	1.5	8	7.55	31.9	19.4	7.64
	5.44	5.43	4.99	5.36	4.75	—	3.73	2.87	5.42	4.2	4.65	.95	4.73	4.84	20.4	12.1	—
	2.93	2.5	2.39	3.34	2.58	—	2.08	1.41	2.66	2.1	2.29	.47	2.86	2.32	9.87	6.33	—
	33	—	32	31	26	—	22	16	27	22	19	4	35	20	124	76	29
	—	.038	—	.119	.082	.089	—	—	.093	.025	.137	.028	.097	—	—	—	—
	—	.111	.264	.309	.209	.247	.21	.262	.252	.12	.373	.077	.248	.278	1.27	1.28	—
	—	.147	.370	.457	.346	.431	.264	.33	.325	.149	.537	.11	.41	.309	1.45	1.46	—
	—	.281	.727	.88	.593	.665	.537	.671	.641	.274	.979	.201	.704	.651	3	3.03	—
	—	.231	.752	.768	.475	.578	.559	.699	.606	.253	.937	.192	.563	.75	3.29	3.32	—
	—	.09	.204	.233	.176	.182	.154	.192	.161	.068	.272	.056	.208	.194	.69	.698	—
	—	.016	—	.086	—	.035	.033	.041	.037	.025	.067	.014	—	.033	.243	.246	—
	—	.153	.406	.494	.316	.365	.287	.359	.352	.157	.545	.112	.375	.365	1.36	1.38	—
	—	.154	.412	.503	.339	.335	.318	.398	.318	.135	.566	.116	.403	.431	1.45	1.46	—
	—	.217	.512	.636	.408	.463	.344	.430	.42	.166	.696	.143	.484	.465	1.7	1.72	—
	—	.093	.273	.276	.198	.262	.236	.295	.25	.107	.373	.077	.235	.29	1.55	1.57	—
	—	.083	.293	.317	.164	.244	.207	.259	.235	.101	.392	.08	.194	.316	1.12	1.14	—
	—	.092	.216	.272	.189	.196	.168	.21	.191	.086	.297	.061	.224	.2	1.22	1.24	—
	—	.201	.494	.466	.419	.446	.399	.498	.454	.199	.634	.13	.497	.494	2.44	2.47	—
	—	.563	1.74	1.69	1.27	1.69	1.28	1.6	1.57	.641	2.32	.477	1.51	1.76	6	6.08	—
	—	.054	.137	.151	.116	.12	.105	.132	.125	.056	.176	.036	.137	.123	.725	.733	—
	—	.334	.92	1.09	.691	.782	.567	.708	.735	.258	1.18	.243	.82	.784	2.62	2.65	—
	—	.133	.438	.487	.324	.406	.321	.401	.368	.149	.586	.12	.385	.417	1.41	1.43	—

DAIRY AND EGGS (*cont.*)

Cheese (*cont.*)   Cream

	Measure	Roquefort	Swiss	Tilsit	Processed, American	Processed, Swiss	Cheese food, American	Cheese food, Swiss	Cheese spread, American	Half and Half	Coffee	Whipping, light	Whipping, heavy	Whipped, pressurized	Sour cream
Measure		1 oz	1 oz	1 oz	1 oz	1 oz	1 oz	1 oz	1 oz	1 C.	1 T.	1 C.	1 C.	1 C.	1 C.
Weight	gm	28	28	28	28	28	28	28	28	242	15	239	238	60	230
Calories		105	107	96	106	95	94	92	82	315	29	699	821	154	493
Protein	gm	6.11	8.06	6.92	6.28	7	5.57	6.2	4.65	7.16	.4	5.19	4.88	1.92	7.27
Carbohydrate	gm	.57	.96	.53	.45	.6	2.36	1.28	2.48	10.4	.55	7.07	6.64	7.49	9.82
Fiber	gm	0	0	0	0	0	0	0	0	0	0	0	0	0	0
VITAMINS															
Vitamin A	IU	297	240	296	343	229	200	243	223	1050	108	2694	3499	548	1817
Vitamin B$_1$	mg	.011	.006	.017	.008	.004	.009	.004	.014	.085	.005	.057	.052	.022	.081
Vitamin B$_2$	mg	.166	.103	.102	.1	.078	.126	.113	.122	.361	.022	.299	.262	.039	.343
Vitamin B$_6$	mg	.035	.024	—	.02	.01	.04	—	.033	.094	.005	.067	.062	.025	.037
Vitamin B$_{12}$	mcg	.182	.475	.595	.197	.348	.363	.652	.113	.796	.033	.466	.428	.175	.69
Biotin	mcg	.8	—	—	—	—	—	—	—	—	—	.119	.071	—	—
Niacin	mg	.208	.026	.058	.02	.011	.021	.029	.037	.189	.009	.1	.093	.042	.154
Pantothenic acid	mg	.491	.122	.098	.137	.074	.277	.142	.194	.699	.041	.619	.607	.183	.828
Folic acid	mcg	14	2	—	2	—	2	—	2	6	t	9	9	—	25
Vitamin C	mg	0	0	0	0	0	0	0	0	2.08	.11	1.46	1.38	0	1.98
Vitamin E	IU	—	.098	—	.28	—	—	—	—	—	—	1.4	3	—	—
MINERALS															
Calcium	mg	188	272	198	174	219	141	205	159	254	14	166	154	61	268
Copper	mg	.01	.036	—	.017	—	—	—	—	—	.033	—	—	—	—
Iron	mg	.16	.05	.06	.11	.17	.24	.17	.09	.17	.01	.07	.07	.03	.14
Magnesium	mg	8	10	4	6	8	8	8	8	25	1	17	17	6	26
Manganese	mg	.009	.005	—	.004	—	—	—	—	—	—	—	—	—	—
Phosphorus	mg	111	171	142	211	216	113	149	202	230	12	146	149	54	195
Potassium	mg	26	31	18	46	61	103	81	69	314	18	231	179	88	331
Selenium	mcg	—	2.83	—	2.52	—	—	—	—	—	.075	—	—	—	—
Sodium	mg	513	74	213	406	388	274	440	381	98	6	82	89	78	123
Zinc	mg	.59	1.11	.99	.85	1.02	.85	1.01	.73	1.23	.04	.6	.55	.22	.62
LIPIDS															
Total lipid (fat)	gm	8.69	7.78	7.36	8.86	7.09	6.93	6.84	6.02	27.8	2.9	73.8	88	13.3	48.2
Total saturated	gm	5.46	5.04	4.76	5.58	4.55	4.35	—	3.78	17.3	1.8	46.2	54.8	8.3	30
Total unsaturated	gm	2.77	2.34	2.22	2.82	2.18	2.23	—	1.94	9.07	.95	23.8	28.7	4.35	15.7
Cholesterol	mg	26	26	29	27	24	18	23	16	89	10	265	326	46	102
AMINO ACIDS															
Tryptophan	gm	—	.114	.1	.092	.102	—	—	—	.101	.006	.073	.069	.027	—
Threonine	gm	—	.294	.255	.204	.227	—	—	.178	.323	.018	.234	.22	.087	—
Isoleucine	gm	—	.436	.421	.29	.324	—	—	.236	.433	.025	.314	.295	.116	—
Leucine	gm	—	.839	.722	.555	.62	—	—	.505	.702	.04	.508	.478	.188	—
Lysine	gm	—	.733	.578	.623	.696	—	—	.427	.568	.032	.411	.387	.152	—
Methionine	gm	—	.222	.214	.162	.181	—	—	.152	.18	.01	.130	.122	.048	—
Cystine	gm	—	.082	—	.04	.045	—	—	—	.066	.004	.048	.045	.018	—
Phenylalanine	gm	—	.471	.385	.319	.356	—	—	.264	.346	.02	.25	.236	.093	—
Tyrosine	gm	—	.48	.413	.344	.384	—	—	.252	.346	.02	.25	.236	.093	—
Valine	gm	—	.606	.497	.376	.42	—	—	.387	.479	.027	.347	.327	.129	—
Arginine	gm	—	.263	.241	.263	.293	—	—	.155	.259	.015	.188	.177	.07	—
Histidine	gm	—	.302	.2	.256	.286	—	—	.144	.194	.011	.141	.132	.052	—
Alanine	gm	—	.259	.23	.157	.176	—	—	.171	.247	.014	.179	.168	.066	—
Aspartic acid	gm	—	.445	.51	.386	.431	—	—	.313	.543	.031	.393	.37	.146	—
Glutamic acid	gm	—	1.61	1.55	1.3	1.45	—	—	.985	1.5	.085	1.08	1.02	.402	—
Glycine	gm	—	.144	.141	.103	.115	—	—	.088	.152	.009	.110	.103	.041	—
Proline	gm	—	1.04	.842	.639	.713	—	—	.658	.694	.039	.502	.473	.186	—
Serine	gm	—	.465	.395	.303	.338	—	—	.294	.39	.022	.282	.265	.104	—

Frozen Desserts   Milk

Ice cream	Ice cream, rich	Ice milk	Sherbet	Whole	Lowfat, 2%	Skim	Buttermilk	Whole, dry	Nonfat, dry	Nonfat, dry, instant	Condensed, sweetened	Evaporated	Evaporated, skim	Chocolate
1 C.	1 C.	1 C.	1 C.	1 C.	1 C.	1 C.	1 C.	1 C.	1 C.	1 C.	1 C.	1/2 C.	1/2 C.	1 C.
133	148	131	193	244	244	245	245	128	120	68	306	126	128	250
269	349	184	270	150	121	86	99	635	435	244	982	169	99	208
4.8	4.13	5.16	2.16	8.03	8.12	8.35	8.11	33.6	43.4	23.8	24.2	8.58	9.63	7.92
31.7	31.9	28.9	58.7	11.37	11.7	11.8	11.7	49	62.3	35.5	166	12.6	14.4	25.8
0	0	0	t	0	0	0	0	0	0	0	0	0	0	.15
543	897	214	185	307	500	500	81	1180	43	18.3	1004	306	500	302
.052	.044	.076	.033	.093	.095	.088	.083	.362	.498	.281	.275	.059	.057	.092
.329	.283	.347	.089	.395	.403	.343	.377	1.54	1.86	1.18	1.27	.398	.394	.405
.061	.053	.085	.025	.102	.105	.098	.083	.387	.433	.235	.156	.063	.07	.1
.625	.537	.875	.158	.871	.888	.926	.537	4.16	4.84	2.71	1.36	.205	.305	.835
—	—	—	—	5	—	5	5	17	19	—	9	3.5	—	—
.134	.115	.118	.131	.205	.21	.216	.142	.827	1.14	.606	.643	.244	.222	.313
.654	.562	.662	.062	.766	.781	.806	.674	2.9	4.28	2.2	2.29	.804	.941	.738
3	2	3	14	12	12	13	—	47	60	34	34	10	11	12
.7	.61	.76	3.86	2.29	2.32	2.4	2.4	11	8.11	3.79	7.96	2.37	1.58	2.28
.399	—	—	—	.293	—	t	.118	—	—	—	—	.37	—	—
176	151	176	103	291	297	302	285	1168	1508	837	868	329	369	280
.2	—	—	—	.5	—	.1	.047	.4	—	—	.66	.037	—	—
.12	.1	.18	.31	.12	.12	.1	.12	.6	.38	.21	.58	.24	.37	.6
18	16	19	15	33	33	28	27	108	132	80	78	30	34	33
—	—	—	—	.005	—	—	—	—	—	—	—	—	—	—
134	115	129	74	228	232	247	219	993	1162	670	775	255	248	251
257	221	265	198	370	377	406	371	1702	2153	1160	1136	382	423	417
—	—	—	—	3.17	—	—	—	—	—	—	—	1.6	—	—
116	108	105	88	120	122	126	257	475	642	373	389	133	147	149
1.41	1.21	.55	1.33	.93	.95	.98	1.03	4.28	4.9	3	2.88	.97	1.15	1.02
14.3	23.6	5.63	3.82	8.15	4.68	.44	2.16	34.2	.92	.49	26.6	9.53	.26	8.48
8.92	14.7	3.51	2.38	5.07	2.92	.287	1.34	21.4	.6	.32	16.8	5.78	.155	5.26
4.67	3.75	1.84	1.24	2.65	1.52	.132	.7	11	.28	.15	8.46	3.25	.087	2.79
59	88	18	14	33	18	4	9	124	24	12	104	37	5	30
.068	.058	.073	.03	.113	.115	.118	.088	.475	.612	.337	.341	.121	.136	.112
.217	.186	.233	.098	.362	.367	.377	.386	1.52	1.96	1.07	1.09	.387	.435	.358
.29	.25	.312	.131	.486	.492	.505	.5	2.03	2.62	1.44	1.46	.519	.582	.479
.47	.405	.506	.212	.786	.796	.818	.807	3.3	4.25	2.33	2.37	.841	.943	.776
.381	.327	.409	.171	.637	.644	.663	.679	2.67	3.44	1.89	1.92	.681	.763	.629
.12	.104	.129	.054	.201	.204	.21	.198	.845	1.08	.599	.607	.215	.241	.199
.044	.038	.048	.02	.074	.075	.077	.076	.312	.401	.221	.224	.079	.089	.073
.232	.199	.249	.104	.388	.392	.403	.427	1.62	2.1	1.15	1.16	.414	.465	.383
.232	.199	.249	.104	.388	.392	.403	.339	1.62	2.1	1.15	1.16	.414	.465	.383
.321	.276	.345	.145	.537	.544	.559	.596	2.25	2.9	1.59	1.62	.574	.644	.53
.174	.15	.187	.078	.291	.294	.302	.309	1.22	1.57	.864	.876	.311	.349	.287
.130	.112	.14	.059	.218	.22	.227	.233	.914	1.17	.647	.656	.233	.261	.215
.166	.142	.178	.075	.277	.28	.288	.292	1.16	1.49	.823	.835	.296	.332	.273
.364	.313	.392	.164	.609	.616	.634	.647	2.55	3.29	1.81	1.83	.651	.73	.601
1	.865	1.08	.453	1.68	1.7	1.74	1.57	7.05	9.08	4.99	5.07	1.79	2.01	1.66
.102	.087	.109	.046	.17	.172	.177	.178	.713	.918	.505	.512	.182	.204	.168
.465	.4	.5	.209	.778	.787	.809	.819	3.26	4.2	2.31	2.34	.831	.932	.768
.261	.225	.281	.118	.437	.442	.454	.422	1.83	2.36	1.29	1.31	.467	.524	.431

DAIRY AND EGGS (cont.)

	Measure	Milk (cont.)					Yogurt				Eggs			
		Eggnog	Malted, powder	Goat	Human	Whey, dry, sweet	Plain	Plain, lowfat	Plain, skim	Fruit, lowfat	Whole	White	Yolk	Whole, dried
Measure		1 C.	1 T.	1 C.	1 C.	1 T.	1 C.	1 C.	1 C.	1 C.	1 lge	1 lge	1 lge	1 T.
Weight	gm	254	21	244	246	7.5	227	227	227	227	50	33	17	5
Calories		342	86	168	171	26	139	144	127	225	79	16	63	30
Protein	gm	9.68	2.74	8.69	2.53	.96	7.88	11.9	13	9.04	6.07	3.35	2.79	2.29
Carbohydrate	gm	34.4	15.2	10.9	17	5.56	10.5	16	17.4	42.3	.6	.41	.04	.24
Fiber	gm	0	.13	0	0	0	0	0	0	.27	0	0	0	0
VITAMINS														
Vitamin A	IU	894	68	451	593	3	279	150	16	111	260	0	313	98
Vitamin B_1	mg	.086	.111	.117	.034	.039	.066	.1	.109	.077	.044	.002	.043	.015
Vitamin B_2	mg	.483	.142	.337	.089	.165	.322	.486	.531	.368	.15	.094	.074	.059
Vitamin B_6	mg	.127	.078	.112	.027	.044	.073	.111	.120	.084	.06	.001	.053	.02
Vitamin B_{12}	mcg	1.14	.164	.159	.111	.177	.844	1.27	1.39	.967	.773	.021	.647	.5
Biotin	mcg	—	—	5	t	—	—	—	—	—	11	2	9	—
Niacin	mg	.267	1.07	.676	.435	.094	.17	.259	.281	.195	.031	.029	.012	.012
Pantothenic acid	mg	1.06	—	.756	.549	.419	.883	1.34	1.45	1.01	.864	.08	.753	.319
Folic acid	mcg	2	10	1	13	1	17	25	28	19	32	5	26	9
Vitamin C	mg	3.81	0	3.15	12.3	.11	1.2	1.82	1.98	1.36	0	0	0	0
Vitamin E	IU	—	—	—	.55	—	—	—	—	—	.57	—	.51	—
MINERALS														
Calcium	mg	330	56	326	79	59	274	415	452	314	28	4	26	11
Copper	mg	.018	—	.095	.12	—	—	—	—	—	.1	.025	.045	.009
Iron	mg	.51	.16	.12	.07	.07	.11	.18	.2	.14	1.04	.01	.95	.39
Magnesium	mg	47	20	34	8	13	26	40	43	30	6	3	3	2
Manganese	mg	—	—	.019	t	—	—	—	—	—	.029	.013	.015	—
Phosphorus	mg	278	79	270	34	70	215	326	355	247	90	4	86	34
Potassium	mg	420	159	499	126	155	351	531	579	402	65	45	15	24
Selenium	mcg	—	—	—	—	—	—	—	—	—	3.2	1.88	2.96	—
Sodium	mg	138	96	122	42	80	105	159	174	121	69	50	8	26
Zinc	mg	1.17	.21	.73	.42	.15	1.34	2.02	2.2	1.52	.72	.01	.58	.27
LIPIDS														
Total lipid (fat)	gm	19	1.78	10	10.7	.08	7.38	3.52	.41	2.61	5.58	t	5.6	2.09
Total saturated	gm	11.3	.89	6.51	4.94	.05	4.76	2.27	.264	1.68	1.67	0	1.68	.63
Total unsaturated	gm	6.53	.8	3.07	5.3	.02	2.24	1.07	.124	.79	2.95	0	2.97	1.11
Cholesterol	mg	149	4	28	34	t	29	14	4	10	274	0	272	96
AMINO ACIDS														
Tryptophan	gm	.137	.029	.106	.041	.015	.044	.067	.073	.051	.097	.051	.041	.037
Threonine	gm	.444	.07	.398	.112	.061	.323	.489	.534	.371	.298	.149	.151	.113
Isoleucine	gm	.583	.082	.505	.137	.054	.43	.65	.709	.493	.380	.204	.16	.143
Leucine	gm	.937	.157	.765	.233	.088	.794	1.2	1.31	.911	.533	.291	.237	.201
Lysine	gm	.758	.075	.708	.168	.077	.706	1.06	1.16	.81	.41	.206	.189	.155
Methionine	gm	.222	.038	.196	.052	.018	.232	.351	.383	.266	.196	.13	.071	.074
Cystine	gm	.097	.055	.113	.047	.019	—	—	—	—	.145	.083	.05	.055
Phenylalanine	gm	.463	.092	.377	.113	.03	.43	.65	.709	.493	.343	.21	.121	.129
Tyrosine	gm	.462	.076	.437	.129	.027	.398	.601	.656	.456	.253	.134	.12	.095
Valine	gm	.643	.094	.585	.156	.052	.652	.986	1.07	.748	.437	.251	.17	.165
Arginine	gm	.378	—	.291	.105	.028	.237	.359	.391	.272	.388	.195	.193	.147
Histidine	gm	.24	.055	.218	.057	.018	.195	.295	.322	.224	.147	.076	.067	.055
Alanine	gm	.346	—	.287	.089	.045	.337	.51	.557	.387	.354	.216	.14	.134
Aspartic acid	gm	.74	—	.512	.201	.095	.625	.945	1.03	.717	.602	.296	.233	.227
Glutamic acid	gm	1.95	—	1.52	.414	.168	1.54	2.33	2.54	1.77	.773	.467	.341	.292
Glycine	gm	.213	—	.123	.064	.021	.19	.288	.314	.218	.202	.125	.084	.076
Proline	gm	.89	—	.899	.203	.059	.933	1.41	1.54	1.07	.241	.126	.116	.091
Serine	gm	.55	—	.441	.107	.046	.488	.738	.805	.559	.461	.247	.231	.174

FATS AND OILS

Fats   Oils

	Fats				Oils							
Beef tallow	Butter	Chicken	Margarine	Vegetable shortening	Corn	Olive	Peanut	Safflower	Sesame	Soybean	Sunflower	Wheat germ
1 T.	1 T.	1 T.	1 T.	1 T.	1 T.	1 T.	1 T.	1 T.	1 T.	1 T.	1 T.	1 T.
12.8	14.1	12.8	14.1	12.8	13.6	13.5	13.5	13.6	13.6	13.6	13.6	13.6
115	101	115	101	115	120	119	119	120	120	120	120	120
0	.12	0	0	0	0	0	0	0	0	0	0	0
0	.008	0	0	0	0	0	0	0	0	0	0	0
0	0	0	0	0	0	0	0	0	0	0	0	0
—	433	—	465	—	—	—	—	—	—	—	—	—
—	t	—	0	—	—	—	—	—	—	—	—	—
—	.004	—	.006	—	—	—	—	—	—	—	—	—
—	t	—	0	—	—	—	—	—	—	—	—	—
—	—	—	.012	—	—	—	—	—	—	—	—	—
—	—	—	—	—	—	—	—	—	—	—	—	—
—	.006	—	.003	—	—	—	—	—	—	—	—	—
—	—	—	.012	—	—	—	—	—	—	—	—	—
—	.375	—	.24	—	—	—	—	—	—	—	—	—
—	0	—	.024	—	—	—	—	—	—	—	—	—
.3	.223	.3	1.25	—	11.3	1.7	3.4	5.2	4	12.7	1.3	34.6
—	3.37	—	4.23	—	—	.02	.01	—	—	.01	.03	—
—	.004	—	.006	—	—	.01	.001	—	—	.056	—	—
—	.022	—	—	—	—	.05	0	—	—	0	0	—
—	.25	—	.36	—	—	0	.01	—	—	0	.03	—
—	.006	—	—	—	—	—	—	—	—	—	—	—
—	3.25	—	3.24	—	—	.16	—	—	—	.03	—	—
0	3.62	—	5.97	—	—	—	0	—	—	—	ʼ	—
—	—	—	—	—	—	—	—	—	—	—	.01	—
0	117	—	133	—	—	0	.01	—	—	0	—	—
—	.007	—	—	—	—	.01	0	—	—	0	—	.52
12.8	11.5	12.8	11.4	12.8	13.6	13.5	13.5	13.6	13.6	13.6	13.6	13.6
6.4	7.15	3.8	1.8	5.2	1.7	1.8	2.3	1.2	1.9	2	1.4	2.6
5.8	3.74	8.4	9	7.1	11.3	11	10.5	11.7	11	11	11.7	10.5
14	31	11	8.1	—	—	—	—	—	—	—	—	—
—	.002	—	.003	—	—	—	—	—	—	—	—	—
—	.005	—	.006	—	—	—	—	—	—	—	—	—
—	.007	—	.006	—	—	—	—	—	—	—	—	—
—	.011	—	.012	—	—	—	—	—	—	—	—	—
—	.009	—	.009	—	—	—	—	—	—	—	—	—
—	.003	—	.003	—	—	—	—	—	—	—	—	—
—	.001	—	0	—	—	—	—	—	—	—	—	—
—	.005	—	.006	—	—	—	—	—	—	—	—	—
—	.005	—	.006	—	—	—	—	—	—	—	—	—
—	.008	—	.009	—	—	—	—	—	—	—	—	—
—	.004	—	.003	—	—	—	—	—	—	—	—	—
—	.003	—	.003	—	—	—	—	—	—	—	—	—
—	.004	—	.003	—	—	—	—	—	—	—	—	—
—	.009	—	.009	—	—	—	—	—	—	—	—	—
—	.025	—	.024	—	—	—	—	—	—	—	—	—
—	.002	—	.003	—	—	—	—	—	—	—	—	—
—	.011	—	.012	—	—	—	—	—	—	—	—	—
—	.006	—	.006	—	—	—	—	—	—	—	—	—

FRUITS AND FRUIT JUICES

	Measure	Apple	Apple, dried	Apple juice	Applesauce, unsw	Apricot	Apricot, dried	Apricot nectar	Avocado	Banana	Blackberries	Blueberries	Boysenberries	Cherries
Measure		1	10 rings	1 C.	1 C.	3	10 halves	1 C.	1	1	1 C.	1 C.	1 C.	1 C.
Weight	gm	150[1]	64	248	244	114[1]	35	251	272[1]	175[1]	144	145	132	145
Calories		81	155	116	106	51	83	141	324	105	74	82	66	104
Protein	gm	.27	.59	.15	.4	1.48	1.28	.92	3.99	1.18	1.04	.97	1.46	1.74
Carbohydrate	gm	21	42	29	27.5	11.7	21.6	36	14.8	26.7	18.3	20.5	16	24
Fiber	gm	1.06	1.84	.52	1.3	.64	1.03	.48	4.24	.57	5.9	1.88	3.56	.58
VITAMINS														
Vitamin A	IU	74	0	2	70	2769	2534	3304	1230	92	237	145	89	310
Vitamin B_1	mg	.023	0	.052	.032	.032	.003	.023	.217	.051	.043	.07	.07	.073
Vitamin B_2	mg	.019	.102	.042	.061	.042	.053	.035	.245	.114	.058	.073	.049	.087
Vitamin B_6	mg	.066	.08	.074	.063	.057	.055	—	.563	.659	.084	.052	.074	.052
Vitamin B_{12}	mcg	0	0	0	0	0	0	0	0	0	0	0	0	0
Biotin	mcg	1.8	—	1.2	—	—	—	—	6	.6	—	—	—	.52
Niacin	mg	.106	.593	.248	.459	.636	1.05	.653	3.86	.616	.576	.521	1.01	.58
Pantothenic acid	mg	.084	—	—	.232	.254	.264	—	1.95	.296	.346	.135	.330	.184
Folic acid	mcg	3.9	—	.2	1.4	9.1	3.6	3.3	124	21.8	—	9.3	83.6	6.1
Vitamin C	mg	7.8	2.5	2.3	2.9	10.6	.8	1.4	15.9	10.3	30.2	18.9	4.1	10.2
Vitamin E	IU	1	—	—	—	—	—	—	—	.6	—	—	—	—
MINERALS														
Calcium	mg	10	9	16	7	15	16	17	22	7	46	9	36	21
Copper	mg	.057	.122	.055	.063	.094	.15	.183	.527	.119	.202	.088	.106	.138
Iron	mg	.25	.9	.92	.29	.58	1.65	.96	2.05	.35	.83	.24	1.12	.56
Magnesium	mg	6	10	8	7	8	16	13	79	33	29	7	21	16
Manganese	mg	.062	.058	.28	.183	.084	.096	—	.454	.173	1.86	.409	.722	.133
Phosphorus	mg	10	25	18	18	21	41	23	83	22	30	15	36	28
Potassium	mg	159	288	296	183	313	482	286	1204	451	282	129	183	325
Selenium	mcg	.7	—	—	.488	—	—	—	—	1.5	—	—	—	—
Sodium	mg	1	56	7	5	1	3	9	21	1	0	9	2	1
Zinc	mg	.05	.13	.07	.06	.28	.26	.23	.84	.19	.39	.16	.29	.09
LIPIDS														
Total lipid (fat)	gm	.49	.2	.28	.12	.41	.16	.22	30.8	.55	.56	.55	.35	1.39
Total saturated	gm	.08	.033	.047	.02	.029	.011	.015	4.9	.21	—	—	—	.313
Total unsaturated	gm	.166	.068	.094	.039	.262	.102	.138	23.2	.148	—	—	—	.577
Cholesterol	mg	0	0	0	0	0	0	0	0	0	0	0	0	0
AMINO ACIDS														
Tryptophan	gm	.003	.006	—	.005	.016	.023	—	.042	.014	—	.004	—	—
Threonine	gm	.01	.021	—	.015	.05	.046	—	.133	.039	—	.026	—	—
Isoleucine	gm	.011	.024	—	.015	.043	.039	—	.143	.038	—	.03	—	—
Leucine	gm	.017	.036	—	.024	.082	.075	—	.247	.081	—	.058	—	—
Lysine	gm	.017	.037	—	.024	.103	.089	—	.189	.055	—	.017	—	—
Methionine	gm	.003	.006	—	.005	.006	.006	—	.074	.013	—	.016	—	—
Cystine	gm	.004	.008	—	.005	.003	.004	—	.042	.019	—	.01	—	—
Phenylalanine	gm	.007	.017	—	.012	.055	.053	—	.137	.043	—	.035	—	—
Tyrosine	gm	.006	.011	—	.007	.031	.03	—	.098	.027	—	.012	—	—
Valine	gm	.012	.028	—	.02	.05	.047	—	.195	.054	—	.041	—	—
Arginine	gm	.008	.019	—	.012	.048	.049	—	.119	.054	—	.049	—	—
Histidine	gm	.004	.01	—	.007	.029	.021	—	.058	.092	—	.015	—	—
Alanine	gm	.01	.021	—	.015	.072	.063	—	.239	.044	—	.041	—	—
Aspartic acid	gm	.047	.104	—	.068	.333	.293	—	.569	.129	—	.075	—	—
Glutamic acid	gm	.028	.062	—	.041	.166	.129	—	.416	.127	—	.12	—	—
Glycine	gm	.011	.024	—	.015	.042	.04	—	.167	.042	—	.041	—	—
Proline	gm	.01	.02	—	.015	.107	.076	—	.155	.046	—	.036	—	—
Serine	gm	.011	.024	—	.017	.088	.074	—	.163	.054	—	.029	—	—

[1] With refuse.

	Crabapple (slices)	Cranberries	Currants, black	Dates	Elderberries	Fig	Fig, dried	Gooseberries	Grapefruit	Grapefruit juice	Grapes, slip skin	Grapes, adherent skin	Grape juice	Guava	Kiwi fruit
	1 C.	1 C.	1 C.	10	1 C.	1	10	1 C.	1/2	1 C.	1 C.	1 C.	1 C.	1	1
	110	95	112	83	145	65[1]	189[1]	150	241[1]	247	153[1]	160	253	112[1]	88[1]
	.83	46	71	228	105	47	477	67	38	96	58	114	155	45	46
	.44	.37	1.57	1.63	.95	.48	5.7	1.32	.75	1.24	.58	1.06	1.41	.74	.75
	21.9	12	17.2	61	26.6	12.2	122	15.2	9.7	22.7	15.7	28.4	37.8	10.7	11.3
	.66	1.14	2.69	1.83	10	.77	8.97	2.85	.24	—	.7	.72	—	5.04	.84
	44	44	258	42	870	91	248	435	149	—	92	117	20	713	133
	.033	.029	.056	.075	.102	.038	.133	.06	.043	.099	.085	.147	.066	.045	.015
	.022	.019	.056	.083	.087	.032	.165	.045	.024	.049	.052	.091	.094	.045	.038
	—	.062	.074	.159	.334	.072	.419	.12	.05	—	.1	.176	.164	.129	—
	0	0	0	0	0	0	0	0	0	0	0	0	0	0	0
	—	—	2.5	—	3	—	—	.7	3	1.7	3	3.2	.9	—	—
	.11	.095	.336	1.82	.725	.256	1.3	.45	.3	.494	.276	.48	.663	1.08	.38
	—	.208	.446	.647	.203	.192	.813	.429	.34	—	.022	.038	.104	.135	—
	—	1.6	1.6	10.4	—	—	14.1	—	12.2	—	3.6	6.3	6.5	—	—
	8.8	12.8	202	0	52.2	1.3	1.6	41.6	41.3	93.9	3.7	17.3	.2	165	74.5
	—	—	—	—	—	—	—	—	.26	.1	—	—	—	—	—
	20	7	61	27	55	22	269	38	14	22	13	17	22	18	20
	.074	.055	.096	.239	—	.045	.585	.105	.056	.082	.037	.144	.071	.093	—
	.39	.19	1.72	.96	2.32	.23	4.18	.47	.1	.49	.27	.41	.6	.28	.31
	7	5	27	29	—	11	111	15	10	30	5	10	24	9	23
	.127	.149	.287	.247	—	.082	.726	.216	.014	.049	.661	.093	.911	.13	—
	17	8	66	33	57	9	128	40	10	37	9	21	27	23	31
	213	67	361	541	406	148	1332	297	167	400	176	296	334	256	252
	—	—	—	—	—	—	—	—	—	—	—	—	10	—	—
	1	1	2	2	—	1	20	1	0	2	2	3	7	2	4
	—	.12	.3	.24	—	.09	.94	.18	.09	.13	.04	.09	.13	.21	—
	.33	.19	.45	.37	.73	.19	2.18	.87	.12	.25	.32	.92	.19	.54	.34
	.053	—	.038	—	—	.038	.438	.057	.017	.035	.105	.302	.063	.155	—
	.11	—	.265	—	—	.134	1.52	.553	.045	.09	.107	.307	.064	.278	—
	0	0	0	0	0	0	0	0	0	0	0	0	0	0	0
	.004	—	—	.042	.019	.004	.049	—	.002	—	.003	.005	—	.006	—
	.015	—	—	.043	.039	.015	.187	—	—	—	.016	.029	.04	.028	—
	.018	—	—	.039	.039	.015	.174	—	—	—	.005	.008	.018	.027	—
	.028	—	—	.073	.087	.021	.249	—	—	—	.012	.022	.03	.05	—
	.028	—	—	.05	.038	.019	.228	—	.019	—	.013	.024	.025	.021	—
	.004	—	—	.018	.02	.004	.047	—	.002	—	.019	.035	.003	.005	—
	.006	—	—	.037	.022	.008	.094	—	—	—	.009	.018	—	—	—
	.012	—	—	.046	.058	.012	.138	—	—	—	.012	.022	.03	.002	—
	.009	—	—	.025	.074	.02	.247	—	—	—	.01	.019	.008	.009	—
	.021	—	—	.055	.048	.018	.215	—	—	—	.016	.029	.025	.025	—
	.014	—	—	.055	.068	.011	.131	—	—	—	.042	.078	.119	.019	—
	.007	—	—	.025	.022	.007	.08	—	—	—	.021	.038	.018	.006	—
	.015	—	—	.083	.044	.029	.344	—	—	—	.024	.045	.218	.037	—
	.077	—	—	.105	.084	.113	1.34	—	—	—	.071	.13	.056	.047	—
	.046	—	—	.177	.139	.046	.552	—	—	—	.121	.221	.278	.096	—
	.018	—	—	.079	.052	.016	.193	—	—	—	.017	.032	.03	.037	—
	.015	—	—	.088	.036	.031	.376	—	—	—	.019	.035	.04	.023	—
	.018	—	—	.055	.046	.024	.282	—	—	—	.028	.051	.033	.022	—

[1] With refuse.

FRUITS AND FRUIT JUICES (*cont.*)

	Measure	Kumquat	Lemon juice	Lime juice	Loganberries	Loquat	Lychee	Mango	Melon, cantaloupe	Melon, casaba	Melon, honeydew	Mulberries	Nectarine	Orange
Measure		1	1 T.	1 T.	1 C.	1	1	1	1/2	1/10	1/10	1 C.	1	1
Weight	gm	20[1]	15.2	15.4	147	16[1]	16[1]	300[1]	477[1]	245[1]	226[1]	140	150[1]	180[1]
Calories		12	3	4	80	5	6	135	94	43	46	61	67	62
Protein	gm	.17	.06	.07	2.23	.04	.08	1.06	2.34	1.48	.59	2.02	1.28	1.23
Carbohydrate	gm	3.12	.99	1.39	19	1.2	1.59	35	22.3	10	11.8	13.7	16	15.4
Fiber	gm	.7	—	—	—	.05	.02	1.73	.97	.82	.77	1.34	.54	.56
VITAMINS														
Vitamin A	IU	57	2	2	52	151	—	8060	8608	49	52	35	1001	269
Vitamin B_1	mg	.015	.006	.003	.074	.002	.001	.12	.096	.098	.099	.041	.023	.114
Vitamin B_2	mg	.019	.001	.002	.05	.002	.006	.118	.056	.033	.023	.141	.056	.052
Vitamin B_6	mg	—	.007	.007	.096	—	—	.277	.307	—	.076	—	.034	.079
Vitamin B_{12}	mcg	0	0	0	0	0	0	0	0	0	0	0	0	0
Biotin	mcg	—	—	—	—	—	—	—	6	—	—	—	—	1.8
Niacin	mg	—	.03	.015	1.23	.018	.058	1.21	1.53	.656	.774	.868	1.34	.369
Pantothenic acid	mg	—	.014	.021	.359	—	—	.331	.342	—	.267	—	.215	.328
Folic acid	mcg	—	1.5		37.8	—	—	—	45.5	—	—	—	5.1	39.7
Vitamin C	mg	7.1	3.8	4.5	22.5	.1	6.9	57.3	112	26.2	32	51	7.3	69.7
Vitamin E	IU	—	—	—	—	—	—	3	.28	—	—	—	—	.43
MINERALS														
Calcium	mg	8	2	1	38	2	0	21	28	8	8	55	6	52
Copper	mg	.02	.006	.005	.172	.004	.014	.228	.112	—	.053	—	.099	.059
Iron	mg	.07	.02	0	.94	.03	.03	.26	.57	.66	.09	2.59	.21	.13
Magnesium	mg	2	1	1	32	1	1	18	28	13	9	25	11	13
Manganese	mg	.016	.003	.001	1.83	.015	.005	.056	.125	—	.023	—	.06	.033
Phosphorus	mg	4	1	1	38	3	3	22	45	11	13	53	22	18
Potassium	mg	37	15	17	213	26	16	322	825	344	350	271	288	237
Selenium	mcg	—	—	—	—	—	—	—	—	—	—	—	—	2.5
Sodium	mg	1	3	0	1	0	0	4	23	20	13	14	0	0
Zinc	mg	.02	.01	.01	.5	0	.01	.07	.41	—	—	—	.12	.09
LIPIDS														
Total lipid (fat)	gm	.02	.04	.02	.46	.02	.04	.57	.74	.16	.13	.55	.62	.16
Total saturated	gm	—	.006	.002	—	.004	—	.137	—	—	—	—	—	.02
Total unsaturated	gm	—	.015	.006	—	.01	—	.315	—	—	—	—	—	.063
Cholesterol	mg	0	0	0	0	0	0	0	0	0	0	0	0	0
AMINO ACIDS														
Tryptophan	gm	—	—	—	—	0	.001	.017	—	—	—	—	—	.012
Threonine	gm	—	—	—	—	.001	—	.039	—	—	—	—	—	.02
Isoleucine	gm	—	—	—	—	.001	—	.037	—	—	—	—	—	.033
Leucine	gm	—	—	—	—	.003	—	.064	—	—	—	—	—	.03
Lysine	gm	—	—	—	—	.002	.004	.085	—	—	—	—	—	.062
Methionine	gm	—	—	—	—	0	.001	.01	—	—	—	—	—	.026
Cystine	gm	—	—	—	—	.001	—	—	—	—	—	—	—	.013
Phenylalanine	gm	—	—	—	—	.001	—	.035	—	—	—	—	—	.041
Tyrosine	gm	—	—	—	—	.001	—	.021	—	—	—	—	—	.021
Valine	gm	—	—	—	—	.002	—	.054	—	—	—	—	—	.052
Arginine	gm	—	—	—	—	.001	—	.039	—	—	—	—	—	.085
Histidine	gm	—	—	—	—	.001	—	.025	—	—	—	—	—	.024
Alanine	gm	—	—	—	—	.002	—	.106	—	—	—	—	—	.066
Aspartic acid	gm	—	—	—	—	.006	—	.087	—	—	—	—	—	.149
Glutamic acid	gm	—	—	—	—	.006	—	.124	—	—	—	—	—	.123
Glycine	gm	—	—	—	—	.002	—	.043	—	—	—	—	—	.123
Proline	gm	—	—	—	—	.003	—	.037	—	—	—	—	—	.06
Serine	gm	—	—	—	—	.002	—	.046	—	—	—	—	—	.042

[1] With refuse.

Orange juice	Papaya	Passion fruit	Peach	Peach, dried	Peach nectar	Pear	Pear, dried	Pear nectar	Persimmon	Pineapple	Pineapple juice	Plantain	Plum	Pomegranate
1 C.	1	1	1	10 halves	1 C.	1	10 halves	1 C.	1	1 C.	1 C.	1 C.	1	1
248	454¹	35¹	115¹	130	249	180¹	175	250	200¹	155	250	148	70¹	275¹
111	117	18	37	311	134	98	459	149	118	77	139	181	36	104
1.74	1.86	.4	.61	4.69	.67	.65	3.28	.27	.98	.6	.8	1.92	.52	1.47
25.8	30	4.21	9.65	79.7	34.6	25	122	39.4	31.2	19.2	34.4	47.2	8.59	26.4
.25	2.35	1.97	.56	3.81	.35	2.32	9.95	.78	2.49	.84	.25	.74	.4	.31
496	6122	126	465	2812	643	33	6	1	3640	35	12	1668	213	—
.223	.082	—	.015	.003	.007	.033	.014	.005	.05	.143	.138	.077	.028	.046
.074	.097	.023	.036	.276	.035	.066	.254	.033	.034	.056	.055	.08	.063	.046
.099	.058	—	.016	.087	—	.03	—	—	—	.135	.24	.443	.053	.162
0	0	0	0	0	0	0	0	0	0	0	0	0	0	0
.8	—	—	2	—	—	.2	—	—	—	—	—	—	t	—
.992	1.02	.27	.861	5.68	.717	.166	2.4	.32	.168	.651	.643	1.01	.330	.462
.471	.663	—	.148	—	—	.116	—	—	—	.248	.25	.385	.120	.918
—	—	—	3	—	—	12.1	—	—	—	12.6	16.4	57.7	32.6	1.4
124	187	5.4	5.7	6.3	13.1	6.6	12.3	2.7	12.6	23.9	26.7	27.2	6.3	9.4
—	—	—	—	—	—	—	—	—	—	—	—	—	—	—
27	72	2	5	37	13	19	59	11	13	11	42	4	2	5
.109	.049	—	.059	.473	.172	.188	.649	.168	.19	.171	.225	.12	.028	—
.5	.3	.29	.1	5.28	.47	.41	3.68	.65	.26	.57	.65	.89	.07	.46
27	31	5	6	54	11	9	58	6	15	21	34	55	4	—
.035	.033	—	.041	.397	.047	.126	.572	.075	.596	2.55	2.47	—	.032	—
42	16	12	11	155	16	18	103	7	28	11	20	50	7	12
496	780	63	171	1295	101	208	932	33	270	175	334	739	113	399
14.9	—	—	.46	—	—	1.2	—	—	—	.93	—	—	—	—
2	8	5	0	9	17	1	10	9	3	1	2	6	0	5
.13	.22	—	.12	.75	.2	.2	.68	.16	.18	.12	.29	.21	.06	—
.5	.43	.13	.08	.99	.05	.66	1.1	.03	.31	.66	.2	.55	.41	.46
.06	.131	—	.009	.107	.005	.037	.061	.003	—	.05	.013	—	.032	—
.188	.21	—	.069	.838	.047	.295	.49	.016	—	.3	.093	—	.356	—
0	0	0	0	0	0	0	0	0	0	9	0	0	0	0
.005	.024	—	.002	.013	—	—	—	—	.017	.008	—	.022	—	—
.02	.033	—	.023	.183	—	.017	.086	—	.05	.019	—	.05	.011	—
.02	.024	—	.017	.135	—	.018	.095	—	.042	.02	—	.053	.011	—
.032	.049	—	.035	.265	—	.033	.165	—	.071	.029	—	.087	.014	—
.022	.076	—	.02	.151	—	.023	.116	—	.055	.039	—	.089	.011	—
.007	.006	—	.015	.113	—	.008	.039	—	.008	.017	—	.025	.004	—
.012	—	—	.005	.038	—	.007	.032	—	.022	.003	—	.03	.003	—
.022	.027	—	.019	.148	—	.017	.086	—	.044	.019	—	.065	.011	—
.01	.015	—	.016	.122	—	.005	.028	—	.027	.019	—	.047	.004	—
.027	.03	—	.033	.256	—	.023	.116	—	.05	.025	—	.068	.013	—
.117	.03	—	.016	.12	—	.012	.056	—	.042	.028	—	.16	.009	—
.007	.015	—	.011	.087	—	.007	.035	—	.02	.014	—	.095	.009	—
.037	.043	—	.037	.28	—	.022	.109	—	.049	.026	—	.075	.019	—
.186	.149	—	.102	.783	—	.128	.644	—	.096	.088	—	.16	.164	—
.082	.1	—	.092	.712	—	.046	.236	—	.128	.07	—	.172	.024	—
.022	.055	—	.021	.164	—	.018	.095	—	.042	.026	—	.067	.008	—
.109	.03	—	.025	.198	—	.018	.089	—	.037	.02	—	.074	.022	—
.032	.046	—	.028	.217	—	.023	.117	—	.037	.039	—	.061	.013	—

¹ With refuse.

FRUITS AND FRUIT JUICES (*cont.*)

	Measure	Prickly pear	Prune	Prune juice	Quince	Raisins, packed	Raspberries	Rhubarb	Strawberries	Tangerine	Tangerine juice	Watermelon
Measure		1	10	1 C.	1	1 C.	1 C.	1 C.	1 C.	1	1 C.	1 C.
Weight	gm	137[1]	97[1]	256	151[1]	165	123	122	149	116[1]	247	160
Calories		42	201	181	53	488	61	26	45	37	106	50
Protein	gm	.75	2.19	1.55	.37	4.16	1.11	1.09	.91	.53	1.24	.99
Carbohydrate	gm	9.86	52.7	44.6	14	12.9	14.2	5.53	10.4	9.4	25	11.5
Fiber	gm	1.87	1.72	.03	1.56	1.11	3.69	.85	.79	.28	.25	.48
VITAMINS												
Vitamin A	IU	53	1669	9	37	0	160	122	41	773	1037	585
Vitamin B_1	mg	.014	.068	.041	.018	.185	.037	.024	.03	.088	.148	.128
Vitamin B_2	mg	.062	.136	.179	.028	.3	.111	.037	.098	.018	.049	.032
Vitamin B_6	mg	—	.222	—	.037	.31	.07	.029	.088	.056	—	.23
Vitamin B_{12}	mcg	0	0	0	0	0	0	0	0	0	0	0
Biotin	mcg	—	—	—	—	7	2.28	—	1.6	—	—	4
Niacin	mg	.474	1.64	2.01	.184	1.83	1.1	.366	.343	.134	.247	.32
Pantothenic acid	mg	—	.386	—	.075	—	.295	.104	.507	.168	—	.339
Folic acid	mcg	—	3.1	1	—	5.5	—	8.7	26.4	17.1	—	3.4
Vitamin C	mg	14.4	2.8	10.6	13.8	9	30.8	9.8	84.5	26	76.6	15.4
Vitamin E	IU	—	—	—	—	—	—	—	—	—	—	—
MINERALS												
Calcium	mg	58	43	30	10	46	27	105	21	12	44	13
Copper	mg	—	.361	.174	.12	.498	.091	.026	.073	.024	.062	.051
Iron	mg	.31	2.08	3.03	.64	4.27	.7	.27	.57	.09	.49	.28
Magnesium	mg	88	38	36	7	49	22	14	16	10	20	17
Manganese	mg	—	.185	.387	—	.441	1.24	.239	.432	.027	.091	.059
Phosphorus	mg	25	66	64	16	124	15	17	28	8	35	14
Potassium	mg	226	626	706	181	1362	187	351	247	132	440	186
Selenium	mcg	—	—	—	—	—	—	—	—	—	—	—
Sodium	mg	6	3	11	4	47	0	5	2	1	2	3
Zinc	mg	—	.45	.52	—	.3	.57	.13	.19	—	.06	.11
LIPIDS												
Total lipid (fat)	gm	.53	.43	.08	.09	.9	.68	.24	.55	.16	.49	.68
Total saturated	gm	—	.034	.008	.009	.294	.023	—	.03	.018	.059	—
Total unsaturated	gm	—	.38	.072	.079	.298	.45	—	.354	.06	.188	—
Cholesterol	mg	0	0	0	0	0	0	0	0	0	0	0
AMINO ACIDS												
Tryptophan	gm	—	—	—	—	—	—	—	.01	.005	.002	.011
Threonine	gm	—	—	—	—	—	—	—	.028	.008	.015	.043
Isoleucine	gm	—	—	—	—	—	—	—	.021	.014	.012	.03
Leucine	gm	—	—	—	—	—	—	—	.046	.013	.025	.029
Lysine	gm	—	—	—	—	—	—	—	.037	.027	.017	.099
Methionine	gm	—	—	—	—	—	—	—	.001	.011	.005	.01
Cystine	gm	—	—	—	—	—	—	—	.007	.006	.01	.003
Phenylalanine	gm	—	—	—	—	—	—	—	.027	.018	.015	.024
Tyrosine	gm	—	—	—	—	—	—	—	.031	.009	.007	.019
Valine	gm	—	—	—	—	—	—	—	.027	.023	.02	.026
Arginine	gm	—	—	—	—	—	—	—	.039	.037	.084	.094
Histidine	gm	—	—	—	—	—	—	—	.018	.01	.005	.01
Alanine	gm	—	—	—	—	—	—	—	.046	.029	.027	.027
Aspartic acid	gm	—	—	—	—	—	—	—	.206	.065	.131	.062
Glutamic acid	gm	—	—	—	—	—	—	—	.134	.054	.059	.101
Glycine	gm	—	—	—	—	—	—	—	.036	.054	.017	.016
Proline	gm	—	—	—	—	—	—	—	.028	.026	.077	.038
Serine	gm	—	—	—	—	—	—	—	.034	.018	.022	.026

[1] With refuse.

MEATS
Beef[1]

	Chuck roast	Corned, brisket	Dried	Flank steak	Ground beef, lean	Ground beef, regular	Liver	Pastrami	Porterhouse steak	Rib roast	Round steak	Short ribs	Sirloin steak	Smoked, chopped	T-bone steak	Tenderloin
	1 lb	1 lb	1 oz	1 lb	4 oz	4 oz	4 oz	1 oz	1 lb	1 lb	1 lb	1 lb	1 lb	1 oz	1 lb	1 lb
	454	454	28	454	113	113	113	28	454	454	454	454	454	28	454	454
	1164	896	47	888	298	351	161	99	1289	1503	1093	1761	1179	38	1394	1095
	83	66.58	8.25	87.4	20	18.8	22.6	4.9	78.8	72.8	88	65.3	82.7	5.7	76	84.1
	0	.63	.44	0	0	0	6.58	.86	0	0	0	0	0	.53	0	0
	0	0	0	0	0	0	0	0	0	0	0	0	0	0	0	0
	130	—	—	50	22.5	40	39941	—	300	310	110	—	220	—	300	—
	.485	.195	.02	.499	.057	.043	.292	.027	.44	.349	.435	.322	.503	.024	.422	.54
	.794	.712	.09	.680	.237	.171	3.14	.048	.739	.576	.748	.535	.88	.05	.712	.97
	1.7	1.32	—	1.87	.28	.27	1.06	.05	1.62	1.39	2.02	1.34	1.71	.1	1.58	1.74
	13.7	8.07	.52	13.4	2.64	2.99	78.2	.5	11.85	12.45	12.21	11.6	12.58	.49	11.6	12
							117									
	14.6	16.6	1.06	20.6	5.1	5.06	14.4	1.44	15.3	12.4	15.97	11.6	13.9	1.3	14.8	13.9
	1.4	2.59	—	1.46	.418	.39	8.6	—	1.32	1.35	1.53	1.09	1.38	.167	1.27	1.41
	32	—	—	32	9	8	281	—	27	22	35	21	30	—	26	28
	0	0	—	0	0	0	25.3	.9	0	0	0	0	0	0	0	0
	—	—	—	—	—	—	1.59	—	—	—	—	—	—	—	—	—
	32	30	2	22	9	10	6	2	29	39	23	41	34	—	30	30
	.363	.499	.045	.327	.082	.07	3.12	—	.336	.259	.322	.24	.37	—	.322	.435
	9.44	7.66	1.28	8.9	1.99	1.96	7.71	.54	7.83	7.63	8.5	7.03	10.2	.81	7.58	10.9
	87	66	9	93	20	18	22	5	82	71	92	62	89	6	79	93
	.054	.091	—	.064	.017	.019	.298	—	.054	.054	.059	.05	.054	—	.054	.059
	779	531	49	864	154	146	360	43	770	685	846	624	798	51	703	842
	1374	1348	126	1585	295	258	365	65	1305	1180	1434	1053	1331	107	1248	1422
	—	—	—	—	—	23.5	51.5	—	—	—	165	—	—	—	—	—
	266	5519	984	321	78	77	82	348	222	241	232	224	234	357	217	223
	18.06	12.9	1.49	15.7	4.36	4.01	4.43	1.21	13.64	16.2	13.7	14.3	15.5	1.11	13.1	14.2
	90	67.6	1.11	57	23.4	30	4.34	8.27	105.6	132	79.5	164	91.5	1.25	118.5	81.6
	38.4	21.44	.45	25.6	9.39	12.18	1.69	2.95	45.15	57.4	33.73	71.5	39.15	.51	50.9	34.7
	43.5	34.99	.52	28.36	11.14	14.37	1.53	4.38	51.3	64.4	38.81	80.33	44.66	.59	57.7	39.06
	311	245	—	238	85	96	400	26	316	326	298	345	315	13	323	313
	.93	.608	.067	.98	.246	.232	.325	.045	.885	.816	.984	.73	.925	.047	.853	.943
	3.63	2.51	.346	3.82	.837	.788	1.034	.185	3.44	3.18	3.84	2.85	3.6	.24	3.33	3.67
	3.74	2.88	.338	3.9	.857	.806	1.034	.211	3.54	3.27	3.95	2.93	3.7	.234	3.42	3.78
	6.57	4.89	.616	6.9	1.6	1.5	2.13	.359	6.23	5.75	6.95	5.16	6.54	.428	6.02	6.65
	6.9	5.1	.673	7.27	1.67	1.56	1.57	.375	6.56	6.05	7.32	5.43	6.88	.467	6.33	6.99
	2.13	1.55	.199	2.24	.467	.438	.572	.113	2.02	1.86	2.25	1.67	2.12	.138	1.95	2.15
	.93	.853	.098	.98	.192	.181	.347	.063	.885	.816	.984	.73	.925	.068	.853	.943
	3.24	2.4	.309	3.4	.758	.712	1.2	.176	3.08	2.84	3.43	2.55	3.23	.214	2.97	3.28
	2.8	2.17	.249	2.9	.624	.586	.897	.16	2.65	2.44	2.95	2.19	2.78	.173	2.56	2.83
	4.04	2.93	.379	4.25	.968	.911	1.4	.215	3.83	3.58	4.27	3.18	4.02	.263	3.7	4.09
	5.25	4.1	.557	5.5	1.35	1.26	1.42	.302	4.98	4.6	5.55	4.13	5.23	.386	4.81	5.32
	2.8	2.1	.239	2.99	.636	.598	.618	.156	2.7	2.49	3.01	2.24	2.83	.166	2.6	2.88
	5.01	4.8	.545	5.27	1.3	1.23	1.4	.352	4.75	4.39	5.3	3.94	4.99	.378	4.59	5.07
	7.6	6.5	.733	7.98	1.8	1.7	2.17	.479	7.2	6.65	8.03	5.96	7.56	.508	6.95	7.68
	12.5	10.8	1.19	13.1	3.14	2.95	3.06	.796	11.8	10.9	13.2	9.8	12.4	.825	11.4	12.6
	4.5	5.56	.612	4.76	1.48	1.39	1.29	.408	4.3	3.97	4.8	3.56	4.51	.425	4.16	4.59
	3.67	4.79	.449	3.86	1.01	.953	1.19	.352	3.48	3.21	3.88	2.88	3.65	.311	3.36	3.72
	3.18	2.68	.337	3.34	.774	.727	1.09	.197	3.01	2.78	3.36	2.5	3.16	.234	2.91	3.22

[1] Beef contains approx. .63 mg vitamin E/100 gm; 13.6 mcg biotin/lb; 19 mg zinc/lb (lean, no fat)

MEATS (cont.)

	Measure	Lamb[1] Leg	Chops	Liver	Shoulder	Pork Bacon	Bacon, Canadian style	Feet	Ham, boneless	Leg	Loin, chop	Shoulder	Spareribs	Veal[2] Breast	Chuck
Measure		1 lb	1 lb	1 lb	1 lb	1 lb	1 lb	1/2	1 lb	1 lb	1 chop	1 lb	1 lb	1 lb	1 lb
Weight	gm	454	454	454	454	454	454	95	454	454	151	454	454	454	454
Calories		845	1146	617	1082	2523	714	251	827	1182	345	1249	804	828	628
Protein	gm	67.7	63.7	95.3	59	39	93.6	21	79.6	77.4	20	73	48	65.6	70.4
Carbohydrate	gm	0	0	13.2	0	.42	7.61	0	14.1	0	0	0	0	0	0
Fiber	gm	0	0	0	0	0	0	0	0	0	0	0	0	0	0
VITAMINS															
Vitamin A	IU	—	—	229070	—	0	0	0	0	.30	9	30	30	—	—
Vitamin B$_1$	mg	.59	.57	1.81	.53	1.67	3.4	.04	3.9	3.24	.948	3.08	1.74	.48	.52
Vitamin B$_2$	mg	.82	.79	14.9	.73	.472	.78	.1	1.14	.889	.294	1.19	.768	.87	.94
Vitamin B$_6$	mg	1.05	1.05	1.36	1.05	.64	1.77	—	1.52	1.81	.45	1.26	1.18	1.22	1.22
Vitamin B$_{12}$	mcg	8.2	8.2	472	8.2	4.2	3.02	—	3.75	2.79	.86	3.25	2.45	5.7	5.7
Biotin	mcg	—	—	454	—	31.8	—	—	—	—	—	—	—	22.7	22.7
Niacin	mg	19	18.5	76.5	17.1	12.6	28.2	1.05	23.8	20.5	5.33	16.8	13.6	22	23.6
Pantothenic acid	mg	2	2	32.7	2	1.6	2.36	—	2.02	3.04	.788	2.87	2.23	3.23	3.23
Folic acid	mcg	18	18	990	18	9	18	—	15	33	4	16	11	.023	.023
Vitamin C	mg	—	—	152	—	0	0	0	—	3.2	.8	3	—	—	—
Vitamin E	IU	3.6	3.5	—	3.6	1.82	—	—	—	—	—	—	—	—	—
MINERALS															
Calcium	mg	.39	35	45	35	34	36	56	.32	25	7	24	19	39	40
Copper	mg	.27	.73	25	—	.29	.204	—	.449	.295	.076	.376	.239	—	—
Iron	mg	5.1	4.7	49.4	3.9	2.7	3.07	—	4.5	3.87	.85	4.59	2.78	9.7	10.5
Magnesium	mg	61	55	64	50	39	79	7	85	91	21	77	62	—	—
Manganese	mg	—	—	1.04	—	.032	.104	—	.141	.014	.013	.05	.028	—	—
Phosphorus	mg	593	567	1583	516	646	1102	52	1122	867	224	803	671	652	722
Potassium	mg	1083	1019	916	942	631	1560	216	1508	1405	346	1325	728	1050	1126
Selenium	mcg	—	78	—	—	—	—	—	—	—	—	—	—	—	—
Sodium	mg	237	223	236	206	3107	6391	49	5974	214	63	286	212	230	246
Zinc	mg	—	—	—	—	5.23	6.31	—	9.69	8.6	2.09	11.3	7.58	—	—
LIPIDS															
Total lipid (fat)	gm	61.7	97	19.6	92	261	31.6	17.9	47.9	94.4	28.7	103	66.3	61	36
Total saturated	gm	35	54.3	6.9	52	96.4	10	6.18	15.4	34	10.3	37.3	26.3	29.3	17
Total unsaturated	gm	24	37.8	6.63	.36	150	17.2	10.3	27.9	53.7	16.3	59	36.2	28	17
Cholesterol	mg	265	270	1361	270	306	228	101	259	335	81	329	218	254	320
AMINO ACIDS															
Tryptophan	gm	—	—	—	—	.376	.93	.042	.957	.993	.256	.934	.647	—	—
Threonine	gm	—	—	—	—	1.5	3.76	.545	3.54	3.57	.923	3.38	2.26	—	—
Isoleucine	gm	—	—	—	—	1.6	3.53	.335	3.49	3.63	.939	3.43	2.32	—	—
Leucine	gm	—	—	—	—	2.73	6.6	.881	6.32	6.23	1.6	5.9	3.9	—	—
Lysine	gm	—	—	—	—	2.9	7.37	.902	6.75	7.55	1.95	7.14	4.73	—	—
Methionine	gm	—	—	—	—	.866	2.54	.21	2.1	1.86	.481	1.75	1.18	—	—
Cystine	gm	—	—	—	—	.404	1.17	—	1.2	.98	.253	.925	.624	—	—
Phenylalanine	gm	—	—	—	—	1.5	3.04	.566	3.44	3.08	.797	2.91	1.92	—	—
Tyrosine	gm	—	—	—	—	1.14	2.83	.314	2.6	2.67	.689	2.52	1.71	—	—
Valine	gm	—	—	—	—	1.89	3.73	.483	3.45	4.12	1.06	3.89	2.57	—	—
Arginine	gm	—	—	—	—	2.4	5.1	1.59	5.17	5.53	1.43	5.24	3.34	—	—
Histidine	gm	—	—	—	—	1.13	3.4	.252	2.85	3.74	.963	3.53	2.44	—	—
Alanine	gm	—	—	—	—	2.2	4.70	1.76	4.7	4.31	1.1	4.06	2.84	—	—
Aspartic acid	gm	—	—	—	—	3.24	7.8	1.46	7.54	6.75	1.73	6.36	4.46	—	—
Glutamic acid	gm	—	—	—	—	5.39	13	2.28	13	11.3	2.9	10.6	7.47	—	—
Glycine	gm	—	—	—	—	2.8	4.03	3.48	4.14	3.32	.852	3.13	2.19	—	—
Proline	gm	—	—	—	—	2.09	3.5	2.3	3.4	2.75	.708	2.6	1.82	—	—
Serine	gm	—	—	—	—	1.47	3.55	.839	3.26	2.99	.769	2.82	1.97	—	—

[1] Lamb contains approx. 13.6 mg zinc/lb (lean, no fat); 13.6 mcg biotin/lb.
[2] Veal contains approx. 12.7 mg zinc/lb (lean, no fat).

Wild Game   Luncheon and Sausage

Cutlet	Liver	Rib roast	Rump roast	Sweetbreads	Rabbit, ready-to-cook	Venison	Bologna, beef	Bologna, beef and pork	Bologna, pork	Bratwurst, ckd	Braunschweiger	Brotwurst	Frankfurter, beef	Frankfurter, beef and pork	Italian sausage, ckd
1 lb	1 lb	1 lb	1 lb	1 lb	1 lb	1 lb	1 oz	1 oz	1 oz	1 link	1 oz	1 oz	1	1	1 link
454	454	454	454	454	454	454	28	28	28	85	28	28	45	45	67
681	635	723	573	426	581	572	89	89	70	256	102	92	145	144	216
72.3	87.1	65.7	68	80.7	75	95	3.31	3.31	4.34	12	3.83	4.04	5.08	5.08	13.4
0	18.6	0	0	0	0	0	.55	.79	.21	1.76	.89	.84	1.08	1.15	1
0	0	0	0	0	0	0	0	0	0	—	0	—	0	0	0
—	102060	—	—	—	136	—	—	—	—	—	3984	—	—	—	—
.53	.9	.48	.5	.37	.29	1.03	.016	.049	.148	.429	.071	.071	.023	.09	.417
.96	12.3	.87	.9	.76	.2	2.19	.036	.039	.045	.156	.432	.064	.046	.054	.156
1.22	3.04	1.22	1.22	—	1.58	—	.05	.05	.08	.18	.09	.04	.05	.06	.22
5.7	272	5.7	5.7	63.6	—	—	.4	.38	.26	.81	5.69	.58	.74	.58	.87
22.7	—	22.7	22.7	63	—	—	—	—	—	—	2.37	.936	1.13	1.18	2.79
24.2	51.8	22	22.8	11.7	45.9	28.6	.746	.731	1.1	2.72	.96	.02	.13	.16	.3
3.23	36.3	3.23	3.23	—	2.8	—	.08	.08	.2	.27	t	t	2	2	.3
23	—	23	23	—	—	—	1	1	1	1	t	t	t	t	1
—	161	—	—	—	4.5	0	t	t	t	1	—	—	—	—	—
41	36	38	38	41	72	45	3	3	3	38	2	14	6	5	16
1.14	36	1.14	—	.27	—	—	.01	.02	.02	.08	.07	.02	.03	.04	.05
10.9	39.9	9.8	10	4.54	4.7	22.7	.4	.43	.22	1.09	2.65	.29	.6	.52	1
73	73	52	—	68	—	150	3	3	4	12	3	4	4	5	12
—	—	.136	—	—	—	—	.008	.011	.01	.039	.044	.011	.015	.014	.055
734	1510	664	699	1521	1261	1129	23	26	39	126	48	38	37	38	114
1157	1275	1051	1090	1130	1379	1525	44	51	80	180	57	80	71	75	204
—	—	—	—	—	—	—	—	—	—	—	—	—	—	—	—
253	331	230	238	281	154	318	284	289	336	473	324	315	461	504	618
—	17	—	—	—	—	—	.57	.55	.57	1.96	.8	.6	.95	.83	1.6
41	21.3	49	31	9.1	29	18	8.04	8.01	5.63	22	9.1	7.88	13.2	13.1	17.2
19.7	—	23.5	14.9	—	11	11	3.31	3.03	1.95	7.93	3.09	2.81	5.38	4.84	6.08
18.8	—	22.6	14.2	—	13	5	4.06	4.48	3.37	12.69	5.29	4.57	6.98	7.38	10.2
254	1361	254	254	1135	295	—	16	16	17	51	44	18	22	22	52
—	—	—	—	—	—	—	.03	.03	.042	.096	.041	.037	.046	.037	.108
—	—	—	—	—	—	—	.125	.145	.182	.473	.151	.17	.192	.183	.531
—	—	—	—	—	—	—	.143	.144	.188	.437	.137	.172	.219	.218	.49
—	—	—	—	—	—	—	.244	.255	.331	.802	.293	.306	.373	.369	.9
—	—	—	—	—	—	—	.254	.25	.341	.91	.258	.323	.389	.407	1.02
—	—	—	—	—	—	—	.077	.079	.117	.291	.088	.105	.118	.103	.326
—	—	—	—	—	—	—	.042	.039	.048	.121	.07	.046	.065	.058	.135
—	—	—	—	—	—	—	.119	.131	.166	.4	.157	.153	.183	.162	.449
—	—	—	—	—	—	—	.108	.102	.137	.345	.122	.126	.166	.141	.387
—	—	—	—	—	—	—	.146	.176	.209	.481	.175	.191	.223	.212	.539
—	—	—	—	—	—	—	.205	.198	.285	.706	.217	.268	.314	.382	.792
—	—	—	—	—	—	—	.105	.09	.137	.345	.091	.124	.162	.158	.387
—	—	—	—	—	—	—	.238	.207	.278	.671	.216	.262	.365	.346	.751
—	—	—	—	—	—	—	.324	.291	.398	.996	.319	.366	.497	.502	1.11
—	—	—	—	—	—	—	.54	.531	.651	1.65	.462	.598	.827	.833	1.85
—	—	—	—	—	—	—	.277	.245	.305	.726	.251	.291	.424	.371	.813
—	—	—	—	—	—	—	.238	.212	.219	.558	.217	.21	.365	.244	.624
—	—	—	—	—	—	—	.134	.144	.18	.463	.167	.167	.205	.208	.519

MEATS (cont.)
Luncheon and Sausage (cont.)

	Measure	Kielbasa	Knockwurst	Liver cheese	Liverwurst	Mortadella	Pepperoni	Polish sausage	Pork and beef sausage	Pork sausage	Salami, hard	Summer sausage	Vienna sausage
Measure		1 oz	1 link	1 oz	1 oz	1 oz	1 slice	1 oz	1 link	1 link	1 slice	1 slice	1
Weight	gm	28	68	28	28	28	5.5[1]	28	13	28	10[2]	23[1]	16
Calories		88	209	86	93	88	27	92	52	118	42	80	45
Protein	gm	3.76	8.08	4.3	4.01	4.64	1.15	4	1.79	3.31	2.29	3.69	1.65
Carbohydrate	gm	.61	1.2	.59	.63	.87	.16	.46	.35	.29	.26	.53	.33
Fiber	gm	0	0	—	—	—	0	0	0	0	0	0	0
VITAMINS													
Vitamin A	IU	—	—	4958	—	—	—	—	—	—	—	—	—
Vitamin B_1	mg	.065	.233	.06	.077	.034	.018	.142	.096	.155	.06	.039	.014
Vitamin B_2	mg	.061	.095	.631	.292	.043	.014	.042	.019	.046	.029	.069	.017
Vitamin B_6	mg	.05	.11	.13	—	.035	.01	.05	.01	.07	.05	.07	.02
Vitamin B_{12}	mcg	.46	.8	6.96	24.2	.42	.14	.28	.06	.32	.19	1.06	.16
Biotin	mcg	—	—	—	—	—	—	—	—	—	—	—	—
Niacin	mg	.816	1.86	3.33	—	.758	.273	.976	.438	.804	.487	.94	.258
Pantothenic acid	mg	.23	.22	1	.84	—	.1	.13	.06	.11	.11	.13	—
Folic acid	mcg	—	—	—	8	—	—	—	—	—	1	—	—
Vitamin C	mg	t	t	1	—	t	.018	0	—	0	t	t	0
Vitamin E	IU	—	—	—	—	—	—	—	—	—	—	—	—
MINERALS													
Calcium	mg	12	7	2	7	5	1	3	—	5	1	2	2
Copper	mg	.03	.04	.11	—	.02	0	.03	0	.02	.01	.02	0
Iron	mg	.41	.62	3.07	1.81	.4	.08	.41	.15	.26	.15	.47	.14
Magnesium	mg	5	8	3	—	3	1	4	1	3	2	3	1
Manganese	mg	.011	—	.057	—	.008	—	.014	—	—	.004	.007	.005
Phosphorus	mg	42	67	59	65	27	7	39	14	34	14	23	8
Potassium	mg	77	136	64	—	46	19	67	—	58	38	53	16
Selenium	mcg	—	—	—	—	—	—	—	—	—	—	—	—
Sodium	mg	305	687	347	—	353	112	248	105	228	186	334	152
Zinc	mg	.57	1.13	1.05	—	.6	.14	.55	.24	.45	.32	.47	.26
LIPIDS													
Total lipid (fat)	gm	7.7	18.8	7.25	8.09	7.2	2.42	8.14	4.71	11.4	3.44	6.88	4.03
Total saturated	gm	2.81	6.94	2.54	3	2.7	.89	2.93	1.68	4.1	1.22	2.77	1.48
Total unsaturated	gm	4.54	10.7	4.45	4.52	4.12	1.4	4.7	2.74	6.73	2.03	3.63	2.28
Cholesterol	mg	19	39	49	45	16	—	20	—	19	8	16	8
AMINO ACIDS													
Tryptophan	gm	.039	.073	.058	.043	.043	.011	.039	.017	.027	.021	.035	.017
Threonine	gm	.122	.326	.185	.192	.179	.047	.168	.072	.131	.096	.158	.057
Isoleucine	gm	.181	.317	.179	.187	.201	.05	.173	.069	.121	.097	.177	.089
Leucine	gm	.248	.558	.377	.326	.344	.087	.305	.127	.222	.173	.241	.128
Lysine	gm	.286	.634	.334	.331	.358	.09	.315	.141	.252	.182	.318	.127
Methionine	gm	.078	.195	.097	.081	.112	.029	.107	.043	.081	.059	.081	.042
Cystine	gm	.064	.1	.093	.043	.058	.014	.045	.018	.033	.026	.045	.028
Phenylalanine	gm	.142	.277	.203	.177	.17	.043	.153	.062	.111	.087	.133	.068
Tyrosine	gm	.139	.245	.132	.104	.15	.037	.126	.053	.096	.071	.125	.055
Valine	gm	.181	.35	.229	.246	.208	.054	.192	.077	.133	.108	.185	.092
Arginine	gm	.267	.482	.237	.232	.291	.074	.262	.111	.196	.152	.228	.113
Histidine	gm	.089	.245	.111	.128	.147	.037	.126	.054	.096	.07	.108	.044
Alanine	gm	.240	.459	.264	.237	.326	.077	.256	.106	.186	.148	.233	.104
Aspartic acid	gm	.345	.687	.383	.333	.448	.108	.367	.154	.276	.207	.331	.161
Glutamic acid	gm	.459	1.1	.52	.628	.742	.178	.6	.259	.458	.338	.507	.209
Glycine	gm	.295	.478	.265	.314	.374	.087	.281	.117	.201	.164	.254	.162
Proline	gm	.195	.367	.203	.244	.312	.067	.202	.085	.154	.119	.198	.097
Serine	gm	.15	.324	.196	.199	.188	.047	.166	.069	.128	.094	.156	.069

[1] 1/8″ thick. [2] 1/16″ thick.

NUTS AND SEEDS

Almonds	Brazil nuts	Cashews	Chestnuts, fresh	Coconut, shredded	Coconut liquid	Hazelnuts	Hickory nuts	Macadamia nuts	Peanuts	Peanut butter	Pecans	Pine nuts	Pistachios, shelled	Pumpkin seeds & squash	Sesame seeds	Sunflower seeds	Tahini	Walnuts
1 C.	1 C.	1 C.	1 C.	1 C.	1 C.	1 C.	15 sm	1 C.	1 C.	1 T.	1 C.	1 oz	1 C.	1 C.	1 C.	1 C.	1 T.	1 C.
142	140	140	160	80	240	135	15	134	144	15	108	28	128	140	150	145	15	100
849	916	785	310	277	53	856	101	940	838	86	742	180	739	774	873	812	89	651
26.4	20	24.1	4.6	2.8	.7	17	2.1	11	37.7	3.9	9.9	3.7	26	40.6	27.3	34.8	2.55	14.8
27.7	15.3	41	67.4	7.5	11.3	22.5	2	18.4	29.7	3.2	15.8	5.8	31.7	21	26.4	28.9	3.18	15.8
3.84	4.2	1.96	1.66	2.7	t	1.05	.3	7.08	3.89	.33	2.3	.31	2.4	2.66	3.6	5.5	.75	2.1
0	t	140	0	0	0	144	—	0	t	0	140	10	299	100	99	70	—	30
.34	1.34	.6	.35	.04	t	.62	.08	.469	.46	.018	.93	.36	1.05	.34	.27	2.84	.183	.33
1.31	.17	.35	.35	.02	t	.738	—	.147	.19	.02	.14	.07	.223	.442	.2	.33	.071	.13
.142	.238	.325	.527	.035	.045	.735	—	—	.576	.05	.183	—	—	—	.126	1.8	—	.73
0	0	0	0	0	0	0	—	0	0	0	0	0	0	0	0	0	0	0
25	—	—	2.1	—	—	—	—	—	49	5.8	—	—	—	—	8.1	7.8	.818	37
5	2.2	2.5	1	.4	.2	1.2	—	2.87	24.6	2.4	1	1.3	1.38	3.4		2		.9
.668	.323	1.82	.756	.16	.12	1.54	—	—	3	.147	1.7				1.02		—	.9
.136	.006	.095	—	.031	—	.097	—	—	.153	.013	.026			74	.144		0	.066
t	14	0	9.6	2	5	t	0	—	0	0	2	t			0		0	2
21.3	9.1	—	.8	.8	—	28	—	—	9.36	—	1.5							1.5
332	260	53	43	10	48	282	9	94	104	11	79	3	173	71	165	174	64	99
1.18	2.14	2.82	.67	.368		1.72	.214	.397	.62	.085	1.14	.29	1.52	1.9	2.39	2.57	.242	1.39
6.7	4.8	5.3	2.7	1.4	.7	4.6	.4	3.23	3.2	.3	2.6	1.5	8.67	15.7	3.6	10.3	1.34	3.1
386	351	374	65.6	37	67	313	24	155	252	26	142		203	738	270	57	14	131
2.7	3.9	—	5.9	1.05		5.67	—	—	2.17	.257	1.54		.419			2.9		1.8
716	970	522	141	76	31	455	49	183	586	59	312	171	644	1114	888	1214	110	380
1098	1001	650	726	205	353	950	64	493	1009	123	651	170	1399		610	1334	62	450
2.8	144	—	—	—	—	2.7	—	—	—	—	3.24		—	—	—	—	—	2
6	1	21	10	18	60	3	0	6	7	18	t	1	7	24	59	4	17	2
4.14	7.1	6.1	.95	.88	—	4	.61	2.29	4.78	.47	5.91	1.21	1.71	10.3	15.4	7.3	.69	2.26
77	93.7	64	2.7	28.2	.5	84.2	10.1	98.8	70.1	8.1	76.9	14.3	61.9	65.4	80	68.6	8.06	64
6.2	18.7	10.9	.44	24.3		4.2	.9	14.8	15.4	1.5	5.4	1.7	7.84	11.8	11.2	8.2	1.13	4.5
67	69.3	49.3	2.04	2		59	8.8	80	50.5	6.1	63.8	11.7	50	51	64	56.9	6.57	49.5
0	0	0	0	0		0	0	0	0	0	0	0	0	0	0	0	0	0
.508	.364	.325	.056	.031		.248	.2		.453	.055	.215	.086	.362	.595	.71	.5	.056	.227
1.05	.644	.813	.185	.097		.515	.06	.352	1.09	.132	.273	.216	.924	1.25	1.77	1.34	.106	.538
1.23	.841	1	.174	.105		.653	.082	.327	1.45	.177	.348	.265	1.25	1.74	1.93	1.64	.11	.679
2.2	1.66	1.76	.286	.198		1.27	.146	.619	2.8	.342	.562	.491	2.15	2.87	3.22	2.39	.195	1.19
.946	.757	1.12	.246	.118		.459	.07	.434	1.45	.176	.315	.256	1.64	2.53	1.24	1.35	.082	.466
.322	1.42	.376	.112	.05		.189	.042	.123	.384	.047	.201	.122	.488	.76	1.34	.711	.084	.336
.508	.489	.389	.118	.053		.263	.038	.129	.48	.058	.226	.124	.657	.415	.785	.649	.051	.414
1.58	1.04	1.09	.207	.135		.789	.1	.348	2.14	.26	.442	.261	1.52	1.69	2.28	1.69	.135	.754
1	.64	.673	.134	.082		.521	.064	.452	1.8	.219	.307	.249	.914	1.41	1.69	.959	.107	.527
1.46	1.28	1.43	.241	.162		.761	.1	.43	1.7	.206	.417	.352	1.8	2.72	2.22	1.9	.143	.868
3.54	3.35	2.39	.47	.437		2.48	.298	1.2	5.05	.613	1.19	1.33	2.79	5.57	4.99	3.46	.378	2.52
.792	.563	.546	.134	.062		.376	.05	.225	1.09	.133	.245	.163	.686	.94	1.02	.91	.075	.431
1.34	.798	.962	.218	.136		.814	.094	.441	1.65	.201	.365	.356	1.28	1.6	2.11	1.6	.133	.731
3.33	1.89	2.06	.93	.26		1.85	.194	1.1	5.04	.613	.765	.621	2.7	3.42	3.4	3.5	.237	1.77
8.43	4.4	4.97	.588	.609		4.07	.409	2.39	8.9	1.08	1.67	1.16	6.3	6	7.42	8.03	.569	3.37
1.75	.92	1.1	.202	.126		.81	.1	.497	2.59	.315	.407	.347	1.4	2.48	2.84	2.1	.175	.906
1.78	1.07	.946	.179	.11		.585	.081	.531	1.82	.221	.389	.366	1.2	1.4	2.04	1.7	.116	.664
1.28	1.04	1.17	.2	.138		.769	.115	.47	2.09	.255	.406	.289	1.73	1.58	1.97	1.55	.139	.938

POULTRY
Chicken[1]

	Measure	Light meat	Dark meat	Light meat, w/o skin	Dark meat, w/o skin	Back	Breast	Drumstick	Leg	Neck	Thigh	Wing	Gizzard
Measure		4 oz	5.6 oz	3 oz	3.8 oz	1/2	1/2	1	1	1	1	1	1
Weight	gm	116	160	88	109	177[2]	181[2]	110[2]	231[2]	79[2]	120[2]	90[2]	37
Calories		216	379	100	136	316	250	117	312	31	199	109	44
Protein	gm	23.5	26.7	20.4	21.9	13.9	30.2	14	30.3	3.5	16.2	8.98	6.73
Carbohydrate	gm	0	0	0	0	0	0	0	0	0	0	0	.21
Fiber	gm	0	0	0	0	0	0	0	0	0	0	0	0
VITAMINS													
Vitamin A	IU	115	273	25	78	248	121	69	206	29	136	72	80
Vitamin B_1	mg	.068	.098	.06	.084	.05	.091	.054	.112	.011	.058	.024	.013
Vitamin B_2	mg	.1	.234	.081	.201	.115	.123	.13	.274	.046	.144	.043	.07
Vitamin B_6	mg	.56	.39	.48	.36	.19	.77	.22	.48	.06	.24	.17	.05
Vitamin B_{12}	mcg	.39	.47	.34	.39	.24	.5	.25	.54	.06	.28	.15	.78
Biotin	mcg	—	—	—	—	—	—	—	—	—	—	—	—
Niacin	mg	10.3	8.33	9.33	6.8	4.78	14.3	3.97	9.07	.824	5.1	2.9	1.74
Pantothenic acid	mg	.921	1.59	.723	1.36	.811	1.16	.863	1.85	.218	.97	.375	.278
Folic acid	mcg	5	11	4	11	6	6	6	19	2	7	2	19
Vitamin C	mg	1.1	3.4	1.1	3.4	1.6	1.5	2	4.1	.5	2.1	.3	1.2
Vitamin E	IU	—	—	—	—	—	—	—	—	—	—	—	—
MINERALS													
Calcium	mg	13	18	10	13	13	16	8	17	5	9	6	3
Copper	mg	.046	.086	.035	.069	.047	.057	.043	.097	.022	.055	.02	.036
Iron	mg	.92	1.57	.64	1.12	.93	1.07	.75	1.68	.41	.93	.47	1.3
Magnesium	mg	27	30	24	25	15	36	16	34	3	19	9	6
Manganese	mg	.021	.03	.016	.023	.018	.026	.015	.033	.007	.018	.009	.024
Phosphorus	mg	189	217	164	177	112	252	113	249	23	136	65	50
Potassium	mg	237	285	210	241	142	319	151	331	35	181	76	87
Selenium	mcg	—	—	—	—	—	19.2	13.3	—	—	—	—	—
Sodium	mg	76	117	60	93	63	91	61	132	16	71	36	28
Zinc	mg	1.08	2.53	.85	2.18	1.25	1.16	1.46	2.96	.54	1.5	.65	1.11
LIPIDS													
Total lipid (fat)	gm	12.8	29.3	1.45	4.7	28.4	13.4	6.34	20.2	1.76	14.3	7.82	1.55
Total saturated	gm	3.66	8.41	.38	1.2	8.25	3.86	1.75	5.7	.45	4.08	2.19	.44
Total unsaturated	gm	7.96	18.5	.68	2.63	18.2	8.37	3.87	12.6	.99	9	4.77	.84
Cholesterol	mg	78	130	51	87	79	92	59	138	17	79	38	48
AMINO ACIDS													
Tryptophan	gm	.263	.296	.238	.256	.149	.344	.159	.341	.041	.18	.096	.06
Threonine	gm	.973	1.09	.862	.924	.564	1.26	.585	1.25	.148	.67	.363	.31
Isoleucine	gm	1.17	1.31	1.07	1.15	.66	1.54	.715	1.52	.185	.807	.421	.317
Leucine	gm	1.71	1.93	1.53	1.64	.985	2.22	1.03	2.21	.263	1.17	.632	.472
Lysine	gm	1.92	2.15	1.73	1.86	1.09	2.5	1.16	2.47	.298	1.31	.698	.465
Methionine	gm	.628	.706	.565	.606	.357	.816	.379	.81	.097	.431	.228	.176
Cystine	gm	.313	.358	.261	.28	.192	.397	.185	.402	.045	.217	.125	.088
Phenylalanine	gm	.914	1.03	.81	.869	.531	1.18	.55	1.18	.139	.630	.341	.28
Tyrosine	gm	.760	.85	.689	.739	.43	.992	.46	.982	.118	.521	.275	.205
Valine	gm	1.14	1.29	1.01	1.08	.663	1.48	.688	1.47	.174	.787	.426	.302
Arginine	gm	1.47	1.68	1.23	1.32	.9	1.87	.872	1.89	.212	1.02	.585	.484
Histidine	gm	.693	.776	.634	.679	.389	.906	.42	.895	.109	.475	.248	.136
Alanine	gm	1.36	1.57	1.11	1.19	.854	1.72	.804	1.75	.191	.951	.558	.265
Aspartic acid	gm	2.09	2.38	1.82	1.95	1.24	2.7	1.25	2.7	.313	1.44	.801	.619
Glutamic acid	gm	3.44	3.88	3.05	3.27	2	4.46	2.07	4.44	.525	2.37	1.28	1.15
Glycine	gm	1.49	1.8	1	1.07	1.08	1.78	.842	1.91	.172	1.07	.723	.353
Proline	gm	1.12	1.33	.84	.9	.759	1.38	.65	1.44	.144	.796	.502	.35
Serine	gm	.828	.946	.702	.753	.501	1.05	.493	1.06	.121	.574	.325	.302

[1] Chicken contains approx. .25 mg vitamin E/100 gm; 4.54 mcg biotin/lb.
[2] With refuse.

				Duck		Goose		Turkey				Wild Game	
Heart	Liver	Canned, boned	Liver pâté	Domesticated	Liver	Domesticated	Liver	Light meat	Dark meat	Liver	Canned, boned	Pheasant	Quail
1	1	5 oz	1 T.	10 oz	1	11.2 oz	1	6.4 oz	5.3 oz	1	5 oz	13 oz	14 oz
6.1	32	142	13	287	44	320	94	180	152	102	142	371	405
9	40	234	26	1159	60	1187	125	286	243	140	231	670	780
.95	5.75	30.9	1.75	33	8.24	50.7	15.3	39	28.7	20.4	33.6	84.2	79.4
.04	1.09	0	.85	0	1.55	0	5.94	0	0	4.21	0	0	0
0	0	0	—	0	0	0	0	0	0	0	0	0	0
2	6576	—	94	483	17559	176	29138	12	8	18403	0	655	985
.009	.044	.021	.007	.565	—	.272	.528	.101	.111	.062	.02	.267	.988
.044	.628	.183	.182	.603	—	.784	.838	.207	.307	2.21	.243	.531	1.05
.02	.24	.5	—	.55	—	1.24	.72	.86	.49	.78	—	2.46	2.43
.44	7.35	.42	—	.73	23.7	—	—	.75	.58	64.6	—	2.85	—
.8	—	—	—	—	—	—	—	—	—	—	—	—	—
.298	2.96	8.98	.977	11.3	—	11.5	6.11	9.24	4.34	10.35	9.4	23.8	30.5
.156	1.98	1.2	—	2.73	—	—	—	1.1	1.57	7.81	—	3.44	—
4	236	—	—	37	—	14	—	13	15	752	—	—	30
.2	10.8	2.8	1.3	8	—	—	—	0	0	4.6	2.8	19.6	24.6
—	—	—	—	—	—	—	—	—	—	—	—	—	—
1	3	20	1	30	5	38	40	23	26	7	17	46	52
.021	.126	—	—	.677	2.62	.864	7.07	.135	.208	.512	—	.241	2.05
.36	2.74	2.25	1.19	6.89	13.4	8	—	2.18	2.57	11	2.64	4.25	16
1	6	17	—	42	—	59	23	43	31	21	—	72	—
.005	.083	—	—	—	—	—	—	.032	.032	.294	—	.063	—
11	87	—	—	398	118	748	245	331	259	319	—	794	1112
11	73	196	—	600	—	985	216	489	396	303	—	900	874
—	—	—	—	—	—	—	—	—	—	—	—	—	—
5	25	714	—	181	—	234	132	106	108	98	663	150	215
.4	.98	—	—	3.91	—	—	—	2.82	4.49	2.53	—	3.57	—
.57	1.23	11.3	1.7	113	2.04	107	4.03	13.2	13.3	4.05	9.74	34.4	48.8
.16	.42	3.12	—	37.9	.63	31.3	1.49	3.59	3.92	1.28	2.84	10	13.7
.31	.5	6.95	—	68.1	.59	68.8	1	8.18	8.03	1.73	5.7	20.4	29
8	140	—	—	218	227	256	—	117	109	475	—	—	—
.012	.081	.345	—	.413	.116	—	.216	.43	.318	.288	.371	1.12	1.16
.043	.256	1.27	—	1.35	.367	2.26	.684	1.7	1.25	.908	1.46	4.11	3.82
.051	.305	1.54	—	1.54	.438	2.38	.818	1.95	1.44	1.08	1.68	4.55	4.1
.083	.519	2.24	—	2.58	.744	4.25	1.38	3.02	2.23	1.84	2.6	6.93	6.53
.079	.435	2.5	—	2.61	.624	4.01	1.16	3.54	2.62	1.54	3.04	7.47	6.66
.023	.136	.815	—	.835	.195	1.22	.365	1.09	.81	.483	.939	2.38	2.39
.013	.077	.422	—	.517	.111	—	.207	.428	.316	.274	.378	1.13	1.37
.042	.286	1.19	—	1.31	.41	2.12	.766	1.52	1.12	1.01	1.3	3.25	3.34
.034	.202	.993	—	1.13	.29	1.62	.541	1.47	1.09	.718	1.27	2.68	3.43
.054	.363	1.49	—	1.64	.52	2.48	.97	2.02	1.49	1.28	1.74	4.56	4.18
.061	.352	1.92	—	2.21	.505	3.15	.943	2.74	2.02	1.25	2.36	5.24	5.18
.025	.153	.903	—	.812	.219	1.41	.409	1.17	.866	.543	1	3.2	2.82
.06	.334	1.78	—	2.23	.479	3.12	.894	2.48	1.83	1.18	2.13	5.23	5.1
.092	.547	2.73	—	3.16	.784	4.56	1.46	3.75	2.77	1.94	3.22	8.11	6.69
.141	.745	4.5	—	4.9	1.06	7.54	1.99	6.2	4.59	2.64	5.34	12.2	10.2
.053	.334	1.97	—	2.66	.479	3.21	.894	2.35	1.71	1.18	2.02	4.56	6.24
.048	.285	1.47	—	1.97	.409	2.45	.763	1.81	1.33	1.01	1.55	3.48	3.5
.038	.247	1.08	—	1.4	.355	2.02	.663	1.71	1.27	.879	1.47	3.6	3.79

SALAD DRESSINGS AND SAUCES

		Salad Dressings						Sauces								
	Measure	Bleu cheese	French	Italian	Mayonnaise	Russian	Thousand Island	Barbecue	Catsup	Horseradish, prepared	Miso	Mustard	Soy	Tartar	Umeboshi	Vinegar
Measure		1 T.	1 T.	1 T.	1 T.	1 T.	1 T.	1 C.	1 T.	1 T.		1 T.	1 T.	1 T.		1 T.
Weight	gm	15.3	15.6	14.7	13.8	15.3	15.6	250	15	15	100	15	18	14	100	15
Calories		77	67	68.7	99	76	58.9	188	16	6	249	15	11	31	17	2
Protein	gm	.7	.1	.1	.2	.2	.1	4.5	.3	.2	9	.9	1.56	.1	.3	t
Carbohydrate	gm	1.1	2.7	1.5	.4	1.6	2.4	32	3.8	1.4	42.8	.9	1.5	.9	3.4	.9
Fiber	gm	0	.1	0	0	0	.3	1.5	.075	.108	2	.3	—	.042	.3	0
VITAMINS																
Vitamin A	IU	32	—	—	39	106	50	2170	210	—	0	—	0	30	0	—
Vitamin B$_1$	mg	0	—	—	0	.01	—	.075	.01	—	.1	—	.009	t	.06	—
Vitamin B$_2$	mg	0	—	—	—	.01	—	.05	.01	—	.15	—	.023	t	.09	—
Vitamin B$_6$	mg	—	—	—	—	—	—	.188	.016	.022	—	—	.031	—	—	t
Vitamin B$_{12}$	mcg	—	—	—	—	—	—	0	0	0	—	—	0	—	—	0
Biotin	mcg	—	—	—	—	—	—	—	—	—	—	—	—	—	—	—
Niacin	mg	0	—	—	—	.1	—	2.25	.2	—	1.5	—	.605	t	.6	—
Pantothenic acid	mg	—	—	—	—	—	—	—	—	—	—	—	.058	—	—	—
Folic acid	mcg	—	—	—	—	—	—	—	.001	—	—	—	1.9	—	—	—
Vitamin C	mg	.3	—	—	0	1	—	17.5	2	—	0	—	0	t	0	—
Vitamin E	IU	—	1.3	1.8	—	1.34	1.5	—	—	—	—	—	—	—	—	—
MINERALS																
Calcium	mg	12.4	1.7	1	2	3	2	48	3	9	150	18	3	3	6.1	1
Copper	mg	—	—	.105	.034	—	—	—	.089	.021	—	.06	.018	—	—	.014
Iron	mg	0	.1	0	.1	.1	.1	2.25	.1	.1	60	.3	.49	.1	2	.1
Magnesium	mg	—	—	—	—	—	—	—	—	5	—	7.2	8	—	—	.2
Manganese	mg	—	—	—	—	—	—	—	—	—	—	—	0	—	—	—
Phosphorus	mg	11.3	2.2	1	4	6	3	50	8	5	250	21	38	4	26	1
Potassium	mg	—	12.3	2	5	24	18	435	54	44	—	21	64	11	—	15
Selenium	mcg	—	—	—	—	—	—	—	—	—	—	—	—	—	—	13.3
Sodium	mg	—	213	116	78.4	133	109	2038	156	14	—	195	1029	99	9400	t
Zinc	mg	—	.01	.02	.02	.07	.02	—	.039	.16	—	.032	.036	—	—	.015
LIPIDS																
Total lipid (fat)	gm	8	6.4	7.1	11	7.8	5.6	4.5	.1	t	5.2	.9	0	3.1	.8	0
Total saturated	gm	1.5	1.5	1	1.2	1.1	.9	.67	—	—	—	—	0	—	—	0
Total unsaturated	gm	6.2	4.6	5.8	9.4	6.3	4.4	3.65	—	—	—	—	0	—	—	0
Cholesterol	mg	—	—	—	—	—	—	0	—	—	—	—	0	7	—	0
AMINO ACIDS																
Tryptophan	gm	—	—	—	.002	—	—	—	—	—	—	—	—	—	—	—
Threonine	gm	—	—	—	.008	—	—	—	—	—	—	—	—	—	—	—
Isoleucine	gm	—	—	—	.009	—	—	—	—	—	—	—	—	—	—	—
Leucine	gm	—	—	—	.013	—	—	—	—	—	—	—	—	—	—	—
Lysine	gm	—	—	—	.01	—	—	—	—	—	—	—	—	—	—	—
Methionine	gm	—	—	—	.005	—	—	—	—	—	—	—	—	—	—	—
Cystine	gm	—	—	—	.003	—	—	—	—	—	—	—	—	—	—	—
Phenylalanine	gm	—	—	—	.008	—	—	—	—	—	—	—	—	—	—	—
Tyrosine	gm	—	—	—	.006	—	—	—	—	—	—	—	—	—	—	—
Valine	gm	—	—	—	.01	—	—	—	—	—	—	—	—	—	—	—
Arginine	gm	—	—	—	.01	—	—	—	—	—	—	—	—	—	—	—
Histidine	gm	—	—	—	.004	—	—	—	—	—	—	—	—	—	—	—
Alanine	gm	—	—	—	.008	—	—	—	—	—	—	—	—	—	—	—
Aspartic acid	gm	—	—	—	.013	—	—	—	—	—	—	—	—	—	—	—
Glutamic acid	gm	—	—	—	.02	—	—	—	—	—	—	—	—	—	—	—
Glycine	gm	—	—	—	.005	—	—	—	—	—	—	—	—	—	—	—
Proline	gm	—	—	—	.006	—	—	—	—	—	—	—	—	—	—	—
Serine	gm	—	—	—	.012	—	—	—	—	—	—	—	—	—	—	—

SEAFOOD AND SEAWEED

Abalone	Agar-agar	Anchovy, in oil, drained	Bass	Bluefish	Carp	Catfish	Caviar, black and red	Clams	Cod	Crab	Dulse	Eel	Flat fish, flounder and sole species	Frog legs
3 oz		5	3 oz	3 oz	3 oz	3 oz	1 T	9 lge	3 oz	3 oz		3 oz	3 oz	4 lge
85	100	20	85	85	85	85	16	180	85	85	100	85	85	100
89	—	42	82	105	108	99	40	133	70	71	—	156	78	73
14.5	2.3	5.78	15	17	15	15.5	3.9	23	15	15.6	—	15.7	16	16.4
5	74.6	0	0	0	0	0	.64	4.62	0	0	—	0	0	0
0	0	0	0	0	0	0	0	0	0	0	.7	0	0	0
—	0	—	—	338	25	—	—	540	34	20	—	2954	28	0
.16	0	.016	.09	.049	.008	.038	—	.18	.065	.037	—	.128	.076	.14
.12	0	.073	.03	.068	.036	.09	—	.38	.055	.037	—	.034	.065	.25
—	—	.041	—	.342	.162	—	—	.14	.208	.272	—	.057	.177	.12
—	—	.176	3.25	4.58	1.3	.002	—	89	.772	9.08	—	2.55	1.29	—
—	—	—	—	—	—	—	—	2.8	.182	4.54	—	—	—	—
—	0	3.98	1.9	5.06	1.34	1.82	—	3.17	1.75	.934	—	2.98	2.46	1.2
2.55	—	—	.46	.704	.136	.424	—	.65	.13	.54	—	.204	.428	.37
4.3	—	—	—	1.4	—	—	—	4.5	1	3.6	—	—	—	—
—	0	—	—	—	1.4	—	—	—	.9	1.8	—	1.3	—	—
27	400	46	—	6	35	34	42	83	13	39	567	17	15	18
.167	—	.068	.026	.045	.048	.08	—	.619	.024	.784	—	.02	.027	—
2.7	5	.93	.71	.41	1.05	.83	1.7	25	.32	.5	6.3	.43	.3	1.5
41	—	14	—	28	25	21	—	17	27	30.8	—	16.3	27	—
.034	—	—	.013	.018	—	.013	—	.9	.013	.03	—	.03	.014	—
173	8	50	174	193	352	181	54	304	173	186	22	183	156	147
—	—	109	232	316	283	296	27	564	351	173	—	232	307	308
—	—	—	—	—	—	—	—	99	37.2	—	—	—	30.4	—
255	—	734	59	51	42	54	240	100	46	711	—	43	69	55
.69	—	.49	.34	.69	1.26	.61	—	2.46	.38	5.05	—	1.38	.39	—
.64	.1	1.94	1.98	3.6	4.76	3.62	2.86	1.75	.57	.51	3	9.9	1	.3
.127	—	.441	.431	.778	.921	.836	—	.169	.111	—	—	2	.241	—
.179	—	1.27	1.23	2.42	3.17	2.22	—	.652	.276	—	—	6.9	.478	—
72	—	—	68	50	56	49	94	60	37	35	—	107	41	40
.163	—	.065	.169	.19	.17	.173	.052	.257	.169	.217	—	.176	.179	—
.626	—	.253	.66	.746	.665	.677	.202	.99	.664	.63	—	.688	.702	—
.632	—	.266	.694	.785	.699	.712	.166	1	.698	.754	—	.723	.738	—
1.02	—	.470	1.23	1.39	1.23	1.25	.341	1.62	1.23	1.23	—	1.27	1.3	—
1.09	—	.531	1.38	1.56	1.39	1.42	.293	1.72	1.39	1.35	—	1.44	1.47	—
.328	—	.171	.446	.504	.449	.457	.103	.518	.448	.438	—	.464	.474	—
.19	—	.062	.162	.183	.162	.166	.072	.302	.162	.174	—	.168	.172	—
.521	—	.226	.588	.665	.592	.604	.171	.824	.591	.657	—	.612	.626	—
.465	—	.195	.509	.575	.512	.522	.155	.736	.511	.518	—	.53	.541	—
.635	—	.298	.777	.877	.781	.796	.202	1	.779	.732	—	.808	.825	—
1.06	—	.346	.902	1.02	.907	.925	.254	1.68	.906	1.36	—	.938	.959	—
.279	—	.17	.444	.502	.446	.455	.104	.441	.445	.316	—	.462	.472	—
.879	—	.349	.911	1.03	.916	.934	.264	1.4	.915	.881	—	.948	.969	—
1.4	—	.592	1.54	1.74	1.55	1.58	.382	2.22	1.55	1.6	—	1.6	1.64	—
1.97	—	.862	2.25	2.54	2.26	2.31	.581	3.13	2.26	2.65	—	2.34	2.39	—
.91	—	.277	.723	.818	.728	.741	.118	1.44	.727	.938	—	.752	.769	—
.593	—	.204	.533	.603	.536	.547	.192	.938	.536	.513	—	.554	.566	—
.651	—	.236	.615	.695	.619	.631	.304	1.03	.617	.612	—	.640	.654	—

SEAFOOD AND SEAWEED (*cont.*)

	Measure	Haddock	Halibut	Herring	Hijiki	Kelp	Kombu	Lobster	Mackerel	Nori	Oysters	Perch	Pike	Pollock
Measure		3 oz	3 oz	3 oz		1 T.		3 oz	3 oz		6 med	3 oz	3 oz	3 oz
Weight	gm	85	85	85	100	14.2	100	85	85	100	84	85	85	85
Calories		74	93	134	—	—	—	77	174		58	80	75	78
Protein	gm	16	17.7	15	5.6	—	7.3	16	15.8	35.6	5.9	15.8	16.4	16.5
Carbohydrate	gm	0	0	0	42.8	5.53	54.9	.43	0	44.3	3.29	0	0	0
Fiber	gm	0	0	0	13	.97	3	0	0	4.7	0	0	0	0
VITAMINS														
Vitamin A	IU	47	132	80	150	—	430	—	140	11000	282	34	60	30
Vitamin B$_1$	mg	.03	.051	.078	.01	—	.08	.368	.15	.25	.128	.08	.049	.04
Vitamin B$_2$	mg	.031	.064	.198	.2	.046	.32	.041	.265	1.24	.139	.094	.054	.157
Vitamin B$_6$	mg	.255	.292	.257	—	—	—	—	.339	—	.042	.2	.099	.244
Vitamin B$_{12}$	mcg	1.02	1	11.6	—	—	—	.786	7.4	—	16	.85	—	2.7
Biotin	mcg	.272	1.8	—	—	—	—	4.54	1.8	—	.9	41.6	—	—
Niacin	mg	3.23	11.97	2.74	4	.784	1.8	1.23	7.72	10	1.1	1.7	2.16	2.78
Pantothenic acid	mg	.108	.28	.548	—	—	—	1.39	.728	—	.155	.306	—	.3
Folic acid	mcg	1	1.8	—	—	—	—	.4	1	—	8.3	—	—	—
Vitamin C	mg	—	—	.6	0	—	11	.3	.3	10	—	2.72	3.2	—
Vitamin E	IU	.544	—	1.8	—	—	—	—	1.45	—	—	—	.18	—
MINERALS														
Calcium	mg	28	40	49	1400	156	800	26	10	260	38	91	48	51
Copper	mg	.022	.023	.078	—	t	—	1.41	.062	—	3.74	.022	.043	.043
Iron	mg	.89	.71	.94	29	.014	10	.54	1.38	12	5.63	.78	.47	.39
Magnesium	mg	33	71	27	—	104	—	15.6	64	—	46	26	27.2	57
Manganese	mg	.021	.013	.03	—	—	—	.047	.013	—	.378	.013	.018	.013
Phosphorus	mg	160	189	201	56	34.3	150	166	184	510	117	184	187	188
Potassium	mg	264	382	278	—	753	—	236	267	—	192	232	220	302
Selenium	mcg	—	—	—	—	—	—	94	—	—	44.4	—	—	—
Sodium	mg	58	46	76	—	429	2500	272	76	600	94	64	33	73
Zinc	mg	.32	.35	.84	—	—	—	2.57	.53	—	76.4	.41	.57	.4
LIPIDS														
Total lipid (fat)	gm	.61	1.95	7.68	.8	.157	1.1	.76	11.8	.7	2.08	1.39	.58	.83
Total saturated	gm	.111	.267	1.73	—	—	—	—	2.77	—	.53	.207	.1	.115
Total unsaturated	gm	.305	.165	4.98	—	—	—	—	7.48	—	.83	.894	.305	.506
Cholesterol	hg	49	27	51	—	—	—	81	60	—	46	36	33	60
AMINO ACIDS														
Tryptophan	gm	.18	.198	.171	—	—	—	.223	.177	—	.066	.178	.184	.185
Threonine	gm	.705	.775	.669	—	—	—	.647	.693	—	.255	.694	.717	.724
Isoleucine	gm	.74	.815	.704	—	—	—	.774	.728	—	.258	.729	.754	.762
Leucine	gm	1.3	1.44	1.24	—	—	—	1.29	1.28	—	.417	1.29	1.33	1.34
Lysine	gm	1.48	1.62	1.4	—	—	—	1.4	1.45	—	.444	1.45	1.5	1.52
Methionine	gm	.476	.524	.452	—	—	—	.45	.468	—	.134	.468	.485	.49
Cystine	gm	.173	.19	.164	—	—	—	.179	.169	—	.078	.17	.175	.177
Phenylalanine	gm	.627	.691	.596	—	—	—	.675	.617	—	.213	.618	.639	.645
Tyrosine	gm	.542	.598	.515	—	—	—	.532	.534	—	.19	.535	.553	.558
Valine	gm	.828	.911	.786	—	—	—	.751	.814	—	.259	.816	.843	.852
Arginine	gm	.961	1.06	.914	—	—	—	1.4	.946	—	.433	.948	.979	.989
Histidine	gm	.473	.521	.45	—	—	—	.325	.466	—	.114	.466	.482	.486
Alanine	gm	.972	1.07	.923	—	—	—	.905	.956	—	.359	.957	.99	1
Aspartic acid	gm	1.65	1.81	1.56	—	—	—	1.65	1.62	—	.572	1.62	1.67	1.69
Glutamic acid	gm	2.4	2.64	2.28	—	—	—	2.73	2.36	—	.807	2.36	2.44	2.47
Glycine	gm	.772	.849	.733	—	—	—	.964	.759	—	.371	.76	.785	.793
Proline	gm	.569	.626	.54	—	—	—	.527	.559	—	.242	.56	.579	.585
Serine	gm	.655	.722	.623	—	—	—	.629	.645	—	.265	.646	.668	.674

Salmon	Sardines, in oil, drained	Scallops	Shark	Shrimp	Smelt	Snails	Snapper	Swordfish	Trout	Tuna, in water	Wakame	Whitefish
3 oz	2	3 oz	3 oz	3 oz	3 oz	3 oz	3 oz	3 oz	3 oz	1 can		3 oz
85	24	85	85	85	85	85	85	85	85	165	100	85
121	50	75	111	90	83	117	85	103	126	216	—	114
16.9	5.9	14.3	17.8	17.3	15	20	17.4	16.8	17.7	48.8	12.7	16
0	0	2	0	.77	0	6.6	0	0	0	0	51.4	0
0	0	0	0	0	0	0	0	0	0	0	3.6	0
34	54	—	198	8.26	—	72	—	101	49	130	140	2050
.19	.019	.01	.036	.024	—	.022	.039	.031	.277	.08	.11	.128
.32	.054	.055	.053	.029	.102	.091	.003	.081	.261	.19	.14	.108
.695	.04	—	—	.088	—	.291	—	.281	1.43	.39	—	—
2.7	2.15	1.3	1.27	.987	2.92	7.7	—	1.49	6.6	1.6	—	—
1.7	5.1	.323	—	—	—	—	—	—	—	.8	—	2.72
6.68	1.26	.978	2.5	2.17	1.23	.893	.241	8.23	7.6	19	1	—
1.4	.154	.122	.59	.235	.542	.177	—	.35	1.65	.32	—	—
1.8	2.8	.4	—	2.6	—	5.4	—	—	11.3	7.8	15	—
8.2	—	—	—	—	—	—	—	.9	.4	—	—	—
10	92	21	29	44	51	48	27	4	36	20	1300	—
.18	.045	.045	.028	.224	.118	.876	.024	.107	.16	.018	—	.061
.68	.7	.25	.71	2.05	.77	4.28	.15	.69	1.27	5.28	13	.31
26.2	9	48	42	31	26	73	27	23	19	49	—	28
.009	.026	.077	.013	.043	.595	.38	.011	.016	.723	—	—	—
170	118	186	179	175	196	120	169	224	208	306	260	—
417	95	274	136	157	247	295	355	245	307	518	—	269
—	—	69.8	—	181	111	—	—	—	—	—	—	—
37	121	137	67	126	51	175	54	76	44	588	2500	43
—	.31	.81	.36	.94	1.4	1.39	.3	.97	.56	.73	—	.84
5.39	2.75	.64	3.83	1.47	2.06	.34	1.14	3.41	5.62	.83	1.5	4.98
.834	.367	.067	.786	.279	.384	.026	.242	.932	.98	.264	—	.77
3.94	2.19	.253	2.56	.784	1.3	.044	.647	2.08	4.04	.452	—	3.51
47	34	28	43	130	60	55	31	33	49	104	—	51
.189	.066	.16	.2	.241	.167	.263	.196	.189	.198	.546	—	.182
.74	.259	.614	.782	.699	.657	.908	.764	.738	.774	2.14	—	.711
.777	.272	.621	.822	.837	.69	.704	.803	.775	.813	2.25	—	.748
1.37	.48	1	1.45	1.37	1.22	1.62	1.42	1.37	1.44	3.97	—	1.32
1.55	.542	1.06	1.64	1.5	1.38	1.25	1.6	1.55	1.62	4.48	—	1.49
.499	.175	.322	.528	.486	.444	.513	.516	.498	.523	1.45	—	.48
.181	.063	.187	.191	.194	.161	.159	.187	.18	.19	.523	—	.174
.659	.231	.511	.696	.729	.585	.7	.681	.657	.689	1.91	—	.633
.57	.199	.456	.602	.575	.506	.645	.588	.568	.596	1.65	—	.547
.869	.304	.623	.919	.813	.772	.881	.898	.867	.91	2.52	—	.836
1	.354	1.04	1.07	1.51	.897	2.1	1.04	1	1.06	2.92	—	.971
.496	.174	.274	.525	.351	.441	.415	.513	.496	.519	1.44	—	.478
1.02	.357	.863	1.08	.978	.906	1.32	1.05	1.02	1.07	2.95	—	.981
1.72	.605	1.38	1.83	1.78	1.53	2.18	1.79	1.72	1.8	5	—	1.66
2.52	.882	1.94	2.66	2.95	2.24	3.12	2.6	2.51	2.63	7.29	—	2.42
.81	.283	.893	.856	1.04	.719	1.27	.836	.808	.847	2.34	—	.779
.597	.209	.582	.631	.57	.53	1	.616	.595	.624	1.73	—	.574
.689	.241	.639	.728	.68	.611	.944	.711	.687	.72	2	—	.662

SOUPS[1]

	Measure	Asparagus, cream of	Bean, black	Bean w/ frankfurters	Beef bouillon	Beef noodle	Celery, cream of	Chicken broth	Chicken, cream of	Chicken gumbo	Chicken noodle	Chicken rice	Clam chowder, New England
Measure		1 C.	1 C.	1 C.	1 C.	1 C.	1 C.	1 C.	1 C.	1 C.	1 C.	1 C.	1 C.
Weight	gm	244	247	250	240	244	244	244	244	244	241	241	244
Calories		87	116	187	16	84	90	39	116	56	75	60	95
Protein	gm	2.28	5.64	9.99	2.74	4.83	1.66	4.93	3.43	2.64	4.04	3.53	4.81
Carbohydrate	gm	10.7	19.8	22	.1	8.98	8.82	.93	9.26	8.37	9.35	7.15	12.4
Fiber	gm	.73	1.31	1.5	t	t	.38	t	.12	.24	.24	t	.27
VITAMINS													
Vitamin A	IU	445	506	869	0	629	306	0	560	136	711	660	8
Vitamin B_1	mg	.054	.077	.11	.005	.068	.029	.01	.029	.02	.053	.017	.02
Vitamin B_2	mg	.078	.054	.065	.05	.059	.049	.071	.061	.05	.06	.024	.044
Vitamin B_6	mg	.012	.094	.133	—	.037	.012	.024	.017	.063	.027	.024	.083
Vitamin B_{12}	mcg	—	.02	—	—	.2	—	.24	—	—	—	—	8.01
Biotin	mcg	—	—	—	—	—	—	—	—	—	—	—	—
Niacin	mg	.778	.534	1.02	1.87	1.06	.332	3.34	.82	.664	1.38	1.12	.961
Pantothenic acid	mg	—	.198	—	—	—	—	—	—	—	—	—	.317
Folic acid	mcg	—	24.7	—	—	4.4	2.4	—	1.6	—	2.2	1.1	3.7
Vitamin C	mg	2.8	.8	.9	0	.3	.2	0	.2	4.9	.2	.1	2
Vitamin E	IU	—	—	—	—	—	—	—	—	—	—	—	—
MINERALS													
Calcium	mg	29	45	86	15	15	40	9	34	24	17	17	43
Copper	mg	.124	.385	.395	—	.139	.142	.124	.124	.124	.195	.118	.124
Iron	mg	.8	2.16	2.34	.41	1.1	.62	.51	.61	.89	.78	.75	1.48
Magnesium	mg	4	42	49	—	6	6	2	3	4	5	1	7
Manganese	mg	.376	.642	.788	—	.273	.251	.249	.376	.251	.289	.366	.251
Phosphorus	mg	39	107	166	31	46	37	73	38	25	36	21	54
Potassium	mg	173	273	477	130	99	123	210	87	75	55	100	146
Selenium	mcg	—	—	—	—	—	—	—	—	—	—	—	—
Sodium	mg	981	1198	1092	782	952	949	776	986	955	1107	814	914
Zinc	mg	.878	1.41	1.18	—	1.54	.151	.249	.627	.376	.395	.263	.752
LIPIDS													
Total lipid (fat)	gm	4.09	1.51	6.98	.53	3.08	5.59	1.39	7.36	1.43	2.45	1.91	2.88
Total saturated	gm	1.04	.4	2.12	.26	1.15	1.4	.41	2.08	.33	.65	.46	.41
Total unsaturated	gm	2.79	1.01	4.37	.03	1.73	3.8	.92	1.9	1	1.66	1.33	2.32
Cholesterol	mg	5	0	12	t	5	15	1	10	5	7	7	5
AMINO ACIDS													
Tryptophan	gm	.029	.064	.105	—	.046	.02	—	.041	.022	.039	.041	.054
Threonine	gm	.078	.249	.413	—	.154	.059	—	.129	.083	.128	.142	.149
Isoleucine	gm	.098	.287	.488	—	.188	.078	—	.171	.1	.159	.178	.183
Leucine	gm	.163	.422	.823	—	.315	.124	—	.264	.168	.265	.27	.288
Lysine	gm	.112	.415	.68	—	.261	.073	—	.215	.161	.219	.251	.251
Methionine	gm	.041	.062	.125	—	.09	.029	—	.081	.046	.077	.092	.09
Cystine	gm	.029	.059	.11	—	.059	.02	—	.051	.017	.046	.051	.056
Phenylalanine	gm	.095	.311	.558	—	.195	.078	—	.154	.098	.164	.152	.159
Tyrosine	gm	.076	.173	.298	—	.124	.054	—	.117	.068	.106	.123	.127
Valine	gm	.115	.284	.55	—	.207	.09	—	.173	.117	.176	.188	.195
Arginine	gm	.085	.331	.525	—	.198	.059	—	.166	.122	.166	.234	.229
Histidine	gm	.049	.163	.26	—	.112	.039	—	.093	.059	.094	.101	.137
Alanine	gm	.093	.232	.498	—	.222	.061	—	.149	.151	.188	.193	.251
Aspartic acid	gm	.171	.652	1.11	—	.354	.115	—	.242	.222	.296	.318	.447
Glutamic acid	gm	.586	1.12	1.84	—	1.33	.383	—	.778	.664	1.11	.559	1.39
Glycine	gm	.068	.22	.483	—	.227	.051	—	.137	.166	.19	.171	.229
Proline	gm	.205	.217	.45	—	.312	.139	—	.256	.151	.263	.149	.183
Serine	gm	.105	.309	.495	—	.173	.076	—	.151	.09	.145	.137	.137

[1] Prepared with water.

Consomme w/gelatin	Gazpacho, ready-to-serve	Lentil w/ham ready-to-serve	Minestrone	Mushroom, cream of	Onion	Oyster stew	Pea, split, w/ham	Potato, cream of	Tomato	Turkey noodle	Vegetable w/beef	Vegetable, vegetarian
1 C.	1 C.	1 C.	1 C.	1 C.	1 C.	1 C.	1 C.	1 C.	1 C.	1 C.	1 C.	1 C.
241	244	248	241	244	241	241	253	244	244	244	244	241
29	57	140	83	129	57	59	189	73	86	69	79	72
5.35	8.69	9.26	4.26	2.32	3.75	2.11	10.3	1.74	2.06	3.9	5.58	2.1
1.76	.78	20.2	11.2	9.3	8.18	4.07	28	11.4	16.6	8.63	10.1	12
—	.78	1.4	.72	.46	.48	—	.67	—	.49	.24	.31	.49
0	200	360	2337	0	0	71	444	288	688	292	1891	3005
.022	.049	.174	.053	.046	.034	.022	.147	.034	.088	.073	.037	.053
.029	.024	.112	.043	.09	.024	.036	.076	.037	.051	.063	.049	.046
.024	.146	.223	.099	.015	.048	.012	.068	.037	.112	.037	.076	.055
0	0	.3	0	.05	0	2.19	—	—	0	—	.31	0
—	—	—	—	—	—	—	—	—	—	—	—	—
.711	.927	1.35	.942	.725	.6	.234	1.47	.539	1.41	1.4	1.03	.916
—	.171	.347	—	.293	—	—	—	—	—	—	—	—
3	—	49.6	16.1	—	15.2	—	2.5	3	14.7	—	10.6	10.6
.9	3.1	4.2	1.1	1	1.2	3.1	1.4	0	66.5	.2	2.4	1.4
—	—	—	—	—	—	—	—	—	—	—	—	—
8	24	42	34	46	26	22	22	20	13	12	17	21
.246	—	—	.123	.124	.123	1.59	.369	.251	.251	.124	.183	.123
.53	.98	2.64	.92	.51	.67	.98	2.28	.48	1.76	.94	1.11	1.08
0	—	—	7	5	2	5	48	1	8	5	6	7
.366	—	—	.366	.251	.246	.366	.67	.376	.251	.251	.315	.46
32	37	184	56	50	11	48	213	46	34	48	40	35
153	224	356	312	101	69	49	399	137	263	75	173	209
—	—	—	—	—	—	—	—	—	—	—	—	—
637	1183	1318	911	1031	1053	980	1008	1000	872	815	957	823
.366	—	—	.735	.593	.612	10.2	1.32	.627	.244	.583	1.54	.46
0	2.24	2.78	2.51	8.97	1.74	3.83	4.4	2.36	1.92	1.99	1.9	1.93
0	.29	1.12	.54	2.44	.26	2.5	1.76	1.22	.36	.56	.85	.29
0	1.86	1.61	1.8	5.93	1.4	1.06	2.43	.96	1.04	1.3	.91	1.56
0	0	7	2	2	0	14	8	5	0	5	5	0
—	—	—	.031	.034	—	—	.101	.024	.02	.037	.049	.014
—	—	—	.104	.09	—	—	.364	.061	.051	.124	.173	.075
—	—	—	.13	.112	—	—	.435	.076	.059	.151	.21	.099
—	—	—	.236	.181	—	—	.711	.117	.1	.254	.359	.147
—	—	—	.183	.127	—	—	.696	.083	.051	.212	.344	.099
—	—	—	.043	.044	—	—	.139	.029	.022	.073	.095	.024
—	—	—	.034	.027	—	—	.134	.027	.027	.046	.039	.024
—	—	—	.154	.107	—	—	.455	.083	.071	.156	.205	.099
—	—	—	.084	.088	—	—	.319	.061	.041	.102	.146	.048
—	—	—	.178	.122	—	—	.491	.093	.066	.168	.246	.099
—	—	—	.198	.095	—	—	.703	.076	.061	.159	.261	.099
—	—	—	.072	.054	—	—	.215	.039	.037	.09	.122	.048
—	—	—	.248	.093	—	—	.483	.054	.056	.181	.317	.099
—	—	—	.366	.161	—	—	1.05	.254	.161	.285	.471	.198
—	—	—	1.22	.527	—	—	1.74	.415	.773	1.07	1.4	.446
—	—	—	.393	.076	—	—	.498	.054	.054	.183	.351	.075
—	—	—	.325	.195	—	—	.468	.129	.134	.251	.32	.147
—	—	—	.145	.117	—	—	.443	.083	.078	.142	.193	.075

VEGETABLES AND VEGETABLE JUICES

	Measure	Alfalfa, sprouts	Artichoke, globe	Artichoke, Jerusalem	Asparagus	Black beans, dry	Black eye peas, ckd	Beets	Beet greens	Broccoli	Brussels sprouts	Cabbage, common	Cabbage, Chinese
Measure		1 C.	1 med.	1 C.	1 C.	1 C.	1 C.	1 C.	1 C.	1 C.	1 C.	1 C.	1 C.
Weight	gm	33	128	150	134	200	165	136	38	88	88	70	70
Calories		10	65	114	30	678	178	60	8	24	38	16	9
Protein	gm	1.32	3.4	3	4.1	44.6	13.4	2	.7	2.6	3.3	.84	1.05
Carbohydrate	gm	1.25	15.3	26	4.94	122	29.9	13.6	1.5	4.6	7.88	2.76	1.53
Fiber	gm	.54	1.36	1.2	1.1	—	—	1	.5	.9	1.3	.56	.42
VITAMINS													
Vitamin A	IU	51	237	30	1202	60	580	28	2308	1356	778	88	2100
Vitamin B_1	mg	.025	.1	.3	.15	1.1	.5	.068	.038	.058	.12	.03	.028
Vitamin B_2	mg	.042	.077	.09	.166	.4	.18	.028	.08	.1	.08	.02	.049
Vitamin B_6	mg	.011	.143	—	.2	—	.18	.06	.04	.14	.19	.066	—
Vitamin B_{12}	mcg	0	0	—	0	0	0	0	0	0	0	0	0
Biotin	mcg	—	—	—	.675	—	—	—	—	—	—	.07	—
Niacin	mg	.159	.973	1.95	1.5	4.4	2.3	.54	.152	.56	.65	.2	.35
Pantothenic acid	mg	.186	.329	—	.234	—	.66	.2	.096	.47	.27	.098	—
Folic acid	mcg	12.2	94.2	—	160	—	.168	126	.05	62	54	39	.062
Vitamin C	mg	2.7	13.8	6	44	—	28	15	—	82	74	33	31.5
Vitamin E	IU	—	—	—	2.59	—	—	—	—	—	—	.2	—
MINERALS													
Calcium	mg	10	61	21	28	270	40	22	46	42	36	32	74
Copper	mg	.052	.095	—	.2	—	—	.1	.07	.04	.06	.016	—
Iron	mg	.32	2.1	5.1	.9	15.8	3.5	1.24	1.2	.78	1.2	.4	.56
Magnesium	mg	9	60	26	24	—	90.7	28	28	22	20	10	13
Manganese	mg	.062	.426	.09	.286	—	—	.47	—	.2	.29	.11	—
Phosphorus	mg	23	99	117	70	840	241	66	16	58	60	16	26
Potassium	mg	26	434	—	404	2076	625	440	208	286	.342	172	176
Selenium	mcg	—	—	—	—	—	—	—	—	—	1.54	—	—
Sodium	mg	2	102	—	2	50	2	98	76	24	22	12	45
Zinc	mg	.3	.56	—	.94	—	3	.5	.14	.36	.36	.12	—
LIPIDS													
Total lipid (fat)	gm	.23	.26	.02	.3	3	1.3	.2	.02	.3	.26	.12	.14
Total saturated	gm	.023	.06	0	.068	—	—	.02	.004	.048	.05	.016	.018
Total unsaturated	gm	.153	.188	.008	.138	—	—	.1	.012	.17	.15	.07	.078
Cholesterol	mg	0	0	0	0	—	—	0	0	0	0	0	0
AMINO ACIDS													
Tryptophan	gm	.044	—	—	.04	—	—	.024	.012	.026	.03	.008	.011
Threonine	gm	.047	—	—	.114	—	—	.06	.02	.08	.1	.03	.034
Isoleucine	gm	.088	—	—	1.5	—	—	.06	.014	.096	.1	.04	.06
Leucine	gm	.071	—	—	.178	—	—	.08	.03	.116	.13	.044	.062
Lysine	gm	—	—	—	.194	—	—	.072	.02	.124	.13	.04	.062
Methionine	gm	—	—	—	.038	—	—	.024	.006	.03	.028	.008	.006
Cystine	gm	—	—	—	.048	—	—	.024	.006	.018	.02	.008	.012
Phenylalanine	gm	—	—	—	.096	—	—	.05	.018	.074	.086	.028	.031
Tyrosine	gm	—	—	—	.064	—	—	.05	.016	.056	—	.014	.02
Valine	gm	.048	—	—	.158	—	—	.07	.02	.112	.136	.026	.046
Arginine	gm	—	—	—	.192	—	—	.03	.02	.128	.178	.048	.059
Histidine	gm	—	—	—	.062	—	—	.028	.01	.044	.066	.018	.018
Alanine	gm	—	—	—	.192	—	—	.07	.026	.104	—	.03	.06
Aspartic acid	gm	—	—	—	.476	—	—	.14	.04	.188	—	.084	.076
Glutamic acid	gm	—	—	—	.672	—	—	.74	.084	.33	—	.19	.252
Glycine	gm	—	—	—	.132	—	—	.04	.026	.084	—	.018	.03
Proline	gm	—	—	—	.218	—	—	.05	.016	.1	—	.166	.022
Serine	gm	—	—	—	.156	—	—	.07	.022	.088	—	.05	.034

Carrots	Carrot juice	Cauliflower	Celery	Chard, Swiss	Chives	Collards	Corn	Cucumber	Eggplant	Endive	Garbanzos, dry	Garlic	Green beans
1 C.	1 C.	1 C.	1 C.	1 C.	1 T.	1 C.	1 C.	1 C.	1 C.	1 C.	1 C.	1 clove	1 C.
110	227	100	120	36	3	186	154	104	82	50	200	3	110
48	96	24	18	6	1	35	132	14	22	8	720	4	34
1	2.47	1.98	.8	.64	.08	2.9	4.96	.56	.9	.62	41	.2	2
11	22	4.9	4.36	1.34	.11	7	29	3	5	1.68	122	.9	7.85
1	2.34	.82	.82	.28	.03	1	1	.62	.82	.46	10	.05	1.2
30942	24750	16	152	1188	192	6194	432	46	58	1026	100	t	735
.1	.13	.076	.036	.014	.003	.054	.208	.032	.074	.04	.62	.01	.092
.064	.12	.058	.036	.032	.005	.119	.09	.02	.016	.038	.3	t	.116
.16	.534	.23	.036	—	.005	.125	.084	.054	.078	.1	—	—	.081
0	0	0	0	0	0	0	0	0	0	0	0	0	0
3	—	1.5	.12	—	—	—	1.95	1	—	—	—	t	—
1	1.35	.634	.36	.144	.021	.696	2.6	.321	.492	.2	4	t	.827
.216	—	.14	.2	.062	.005	.119	1.17	.26	.066	.45	—	—	.103
15	—	66	10.6	.045	—	21.4	70.6	14.4	14.4	71	.398	.1	40
10	20	71	7.6	10.8	2.4	43	10.6	4.8	.14	3.2	t	t	17.9
—	—	.15	.57	—	—	—	—	8.4	—	—	—	—	.1
30	8.3	28	44	18	2	218	4	14	30	26	300	1	41
.05	—	.032	.042	.16	.011	.484	.084	.042	.092	.05	—	.008	.076
.54	1.5	.58	.58	.64	.05	1.16	.8	.28	.44	.42	13.8	t	1.14
16	51	14	14	30	2	31	58	12	10	8	—	1	27
.156	—	.2	.164	.45	—	.686	.248	.064	.1	.21	—	—	.235
48	81	46	32	16	2	29	138	18	26	14	662	6	42
356	767	356	340	136	8	275	416	156	180	158	1594	16	230
2.2	—	.7	—	—	—	—	.495	—	—	—	—	.008	.66
38	105	14	106	76	0	52	23	2	2	12	52	1	6
.22	—	.18	.2	—	—	1.79	.7	.24	.12	.4	5.4	.038	.26
.2	—	.18	.14	.08	.02	.4	1.8	.14	.08	.1	9.6	.02	.013
.034	.066	.028	.038	—	.003	—	.28	.034	.016	.024	.9	.003	.029
.09	.192	.096	.1	—	.01	—	1.39	.058	.042	.024	8.3	.007	.071
0	0	0	0	0	0	0	0	0	0	0	0	—	0
.012	—	.026	.01	.006	.001	.037	.036	.004	.008	.002	—	.002	.021
.042	—	.072	.022	.03	.003	.102	.198	.016	.032	.026	—	.005	.087
.046	—	.076	.024	.052	.004	.119	.198	.018	.04	.036	—	.007	.073
.048	—	.116	.038	.046	.005	.18	.536	.024	.056	.05	—	.009	.123
.044	—	.108	.032	.036	.004	.14	.21	.022	.042	.032	—	.008	.097
.008	—	.028	.006	.006	.001	.039	.1	.004	.01	.008	—	.002	.024
.008	—	.024	.004	—	—	.03	.04	.004	.004	.006	—	.002	.02
.036	—	.072	.022	.04	.003	.1	.232	.016	.038	.026	—	.005	.074
.022	—	.044	.01	—	.002	.078	.19	.01	.024	.02	—	.002	.046
.048	—	.1	.032	.04	.004	.143	.28	.018	.046	.032	—	.009	.099
.048	—	.096	.024	.042	.006	.149	.2	.036	.05	.032	—	.019	.08
.018	—	.04	.014	.012	.001	.056	.138	.008	.02	.012	—	.003	.037
.064	—	.106	.026	—	.004	.125	.454	.018	.046	.032	—	.004	.092
.15	—	.234	.136	—	.008	.223	.366	.034	.146	.066	—	.015	.281
.222	—	.266	.1	—	.017	.244	.98	.16	.164	.084	—	.024	.206
.034	—	.064	.026	—	.004	.112	.196	.02	.036	.03	—	.006	.072
.032	—	.086	.02	—	.006	.125	.45	.012	.038	.03	—	.003	.075
.038	—	.104	.024	—	.004	.093	.236	.016	.036	.024	—	.006	.109

VEGETABLES AND VEGETABLE JUICES (*cont.*)

	Measure	Kale	Kidney beans, ckd	Kohlrabi	Leeks	Lentils, ckd	Lentil sprouts	Lettuce, Iceberg	Lettuce, romaine	Lima beans, ckd	Mung bean sprouts	Mushrooms	Navy beans, ckd
Measure		1 C.	1 C.	1 C.	1	1 C.	1 C.	1 C.	1 C.	1 C.	1 C.	1 C.	1 C.
Weight	gm	67	185	140	124	200	77	75	56	170	104	70	190
Calories		33	218	38	76	212	81	10	8	208	32	18	224
Protein	gm	2.21	14.4	2.38	1.86	15.6	6.9	.7	.9	11.6	3	1.46	14.8
Carbohydrate	gm	6.7	39.6	8.68	17.5	38.6	17	2.2	1.3	40	6	3	40.3
Fiber	gm	1	2.78	1.4	1.87	2.4	2.35	.35	.4	3.5	.84	.52	3
VITAMINS													
Vitamin A	IU	5963	10	50	118	40	35	250	1456	630	22	0	0
Vitamin B_1	mg	.074	.2	.07	.074	.14	.176	.05	.056	.238	.088	.072	.27
Vitamin B_2	mg	.087	.11	.028	.037	.12	.099	.05	.056	.163	.128	.3	.13
Vitamin B_6	mg	.182	—	.21	.2	—	.146	.028	—	.328	.092	.068	—
Vitamin B_{12}	mcg	0	0	0	0	0	0	0	.0	0	0	0	0
Biotin	mcg	.5	—	—	1.4	—	—	.35	—	—	—	11.2	
Niacin	mg	.67	1.3	.56	.496	1.2	.869	.148	.28	1.77	.778	2.88	1.3
Pantothenic acid	mg	.061	—	.231	.12	—	.445	.1	—	.437	.396	1.54	—
Folic acid	mcg	19.6	.068	.015	79.5	—	76.9	.02	76	—	63	14.8	—
Vitamin C	mg	80.4	—	86.8	14.9	0	12.7	5	13.4	17	13.6	2.4	0
Vitamin E	IU	8	—	—	1	—	—	—	—	—	—	.58	—
MINERALS													
Calcium	mg	90	70	34	73	50	19	15	20	54	14	4	95
Copper	mg	.194	.647	.21	.09	.54	.27	.035	—	.519	.17	.078	—
Iron	mg	1.14	4.4	.56	2.6	4.2	2.47	.4	.62	4.2	.94	.86	5.1
Magnesium	mg	23	—	27	35	—	28	5	4	126	22	8	—
Manganese	mg	.519	—	.16	.07	—	.39	.12	—	2.13	.19	0	—
Phosphorus	mg	38	259	64	43	238	133	17	26	221	56	72	281
Potassium	mg	299	629	490	223	498	248	131	162	969	154	260	790
Selenium	mcg	—	—	—	—	—	—	.675	—	—	—	8.54	—
Sodium	mg	29	6	28	25	—	8	7	4	29	6	2	13
Zinc	mg	.29	—	—	—	2	1.16	.3	—	1.34	.42	.344	1.8
LIPIDS													
Total lipid (fat)	gm	.47	.9	.14	.37	t	.43	.12	.12	.54	.2	.3	1.1
Total saturated	gm	.06	—	.018	.05	—	.044	.02	.007	.124	.048	.08	—
Total unsaturated	gm	.261	—	.077	.211	—	.249	.084	.064	.294	.052	.126	—
Cholesterol	mg	0	—	0	0	—	0	0	0	0	0	0	—
AMINO ACIDS													
Tryptophan	gm	.027	—	.014	.015	—	—	.008	.006	.151	.038	.032	—
Threonine	gm	.098	—	.069	.078	—	.253	.044	.042	.491	.08	.066	—
Isoleucine	gm	.132	—	.1	.064	—	.251	.06	.058	.745	.138	.058	—
Leucine	gm	.155	—	.094	.119	—	.484	.056	.054	.91	.182	.09	—
Lysine	gm	.132	—	.078	.097	—	.548	.06	.058	.765	.172	.048	—
Methionine	gm	.021	—	.018	.022	—	.081	.012	.012	.116	.036	.028	—
Cystine	gm	.029	—	.01	.031	—	.257	.012	.01	.141	.018	.004	—
Phenylalanine	gm	.113	—	.055	.068	—	.34	.04	.038	.571	.122	.056	—
Tyrosine	gm	.078	—	—	.051	—	.194	.024	.022	.372	.054	.032	—
Valine	gm	.121	—	.07	.069	—	.307	.048	.048	.723	.136	.068	—
Arginine	gm	.123	—	.147	.097	—	.47	.052	.05	.775	.2	.072	—
Histidine	gm	.046	—	.027	.031	—	.198	.016	.016	.393	.072	.04	—
Alanine	gm	.111	—	—	.092	—	.274	.04	.04	.493	.102	.11	—
Aspartic acid	gm	.198	—	—	.174	—	1.1	.1	.1	1.24	.498	.134	—
Glutamic acid	gm	.251	—	—	.28	—	.969	.128	.128	1.49	.168	.25	—
Glycine	gm	.107	—	—	.086	—	.246	.04	.04	.464	.066	.066	—
Proline	gm	.131	—	—	.082	—	.274	.036	.034	.172	.1	—	
Serine	gm	.093	—	—	.114	—	.381	.028	.028	.723	.034	.066	—

Okra	Onions, green	Onions, mature	Parsley	Parsnips	Peas, green	Peas, split, ckd	Peppers, sweet	Peppers, hot chili	Pickles, dill	Pimientos	Pinto beans, ckd	Potato	Potato, baking, flesh & skin
1 C.	1 C.	1 C.	1 C.	1 C.	1 C.	1 C.	1 C.	½ C.	1 lge	3 med.	1 C.	1 C.	1 lge
100	100	160	60	155	146	200	100	75	100	100	190	150	202
38	26	54	26	102	118	230	24	30	11	27	663	114	220
2	1.7	1.88	2.2	2.3	7.9	16	.86	1.5	.7	.9	43.5	3.2	4
7.6	5.5	11.7	5.1	23	21	41.6	5.3	7	2.2	5.8	121	25.7	32.8
.94	.84	.7	.9	3	3.2	.8	1.2	1.35	.5	.6	8	.66	1.2
660	5000	0	5100	50	934	80	530	578	100	2300	0	t	t
.2	.07	.096	.07	.11	.387	.3	.086	.068	t	.02	1.6	.15	.15
.06	.14	.016	.16	.12	.193	.18	.05	.068	.02	.06	.4	.06	.07
.2	—	.25	.098	.13	.247	—	.164	.21	.007	—	1	—	.7
0	0	0	0	0	0	0	0	0	0	0	0	0	0
—	—	1.5	.24	.15	—	—	—	—	—	—	4.2	2.3	2.7
1	.2	.16	.7	.2	3.05	1.8	.54	.713	t	.4	1.23	.57	1.12
.246	.144	.2	.18	.9	.152	—	.036	.046	—	.166	.41	19.2	22
88	13.8	31.8	.07	.09	95	—	16.8	17.5	—	—	—	30	31
21	45	13.4	103	16	58.4	—	128	182	6	95	t	—	—
—	—	.4	—	—	3.1	—	—	—	—	—	—	—	—
82	60	40	122	70	36	22	6	13	26	7	257	11	14
.94	.06	.064	.293	.17	.257	.5	.1	.13	—	.6	—	.388	.26
.8	1.88	.58	3.7	.9	2.14	3.4	1.2	.9	1	1.5	12.2	.9	1.1
56	20	16	24.5	40	48	—	14	19	12	—	—	51	75
.99	—	.2	.563	.75	.599	—	.14	.178	—	—	—	.394	.463
64	32	46	38	96	157	178	22	34	21	17	868	80	101
302	256	248	436	587	357	592	196	255	200	—	1870	611	782
—	—	2.5	—	—	—	.48	—	—	—	—	—	—	—
8	4	4	27	12	7	26	4	5	1428	—	19	5	6
.6	.44	.28	.44	.8	1.8	—	.18	.23	.27	—	.9	.58	.65
.1	.14	.42	.4	.8	.58	.3	.46	.15	.4	.5	2.3	.2	.2
.026	.024	.07	—	.067	.1	—	.068	.016	—	—	—	.04	.05
.036	.074	.144	—	.212	.323	—	.272	.09	—	—	—	.068	.09
0	0	0	0	0	0	—	0	0	—	—	—	0	0
.018	.02	.028	.022	—	.054	—	.012	.02	—	—	—	.048	.073
.066	.068	.044	—	—	.296	—	.03	.056	—	—	—	.1	.17
.07	.074	.068	—	—	.285	—	.028	.049	—	—	—	.12	.188
.1	.1	.066	—	—	.472	—	.044	.079	—	—	—	.186	.279
.082	.088	.09	.132	—	.463	—	.038	.067	—	—	—	.19	.283
.022	.02	.016	.01	—	.12	—	.01	.018	—	—	—	.05	.073
.02	—	.34	—	—	.047	—	.016	.029	—	—	—	.04	.059
.066	.056	.048	—	—	.292	—	.026	.047	—	—	—	.138	.206
.088	.05	.046	—	—	.165	—	.018	.032	—	—	—	.1	.172
.092	.078	.044	—	—	.343	—	.036	.063	—	—	—	.176	.263
.084	.126	.262	—	—	.625	—	.042	.072	—	—	—	.14	.214
.032	.03	.03	—	—	.156	—	..018	.031	—	—	—	.068	.1
.074	.078	.052	—	—	.35	—	.036	.062	—	—	—	.096	.143
.146	.162	.1	—	—	.723	—	.124	.215	—	—	—	.76	1.14
.272	.36	.3	—	—	1.08	—	.1	.198	—	—	—	.52	.78
.044	.086	.078	—	—	.269	—	.032	.056	—	—	—	.094	.137
.046	.1	.06	—	—	.253	—	.038	.065	—	—	—	.1	.168
.044	.078	.056	—	—	.264	—	.034	.06	—	—	—	.136	.2

VEGETABLES AND VEGETABLE JUICES (*cont.*)

	Measure	Pumpkin	Radish	Rutabaga	Sauerkraut	Soybeans, ckd	Soybean curd (tofu)	Soybean milk	Soybean sprouts	Spinach	Squash, summer	Squash, winter	Sweet potato
Measure		1 C.	10	1 C.	1 C.	1 C.	3.5 oz	1 C.	1 C.	1 C.	1 C.	1 C.	1
Weight	gm	245	45	140	235	180	100	226	70	55	130	205	130
Calories		49	7	64	42	234	72	75	90	14	25	129	136
Protein	gm	1.76	.27	1.5	2.4	19.8	7.8	7.7	9	1.8	1.4	3.7	2
Carbohydrate	gm	12	1.6	15.4	9.4	19.4	2.4	5	7.8	2.4	5.5	31.6	32
Fiber	gm	2	.24	1.4	1.6	3	.1	—	1.6	.3	.75	2.6	1
VITAMINS													
Vitamin A	IU	2651	3	810	120	50	0	90	8	4460	530	8610	26082
Vitamin B_1	mg	.076	.002	.1	.07	.38	.06	.18	.238	.06	.07	.1	.086
Vitamin B_2	mg	.19	.02	.1	.09	.16	.03	.065	.082	.11	.12	.27	.191
Vitamin B_6	mg	.139	.032	.14	.31	—	—	—	.124	.14	.186	.18	.334
Vitamin B_{12}	mcg	0	0	0	0	0	0	0	0	0	0	0	0
Biotin	mcg	—	—	—	—	—	—	—	—	3.5	—	—	—
Niacin	mg	1	.135	1.5	.5	1.1	—	.5	.804	.3	1.3	1.4	.876
Pantothenic acid	mg	1	.04	.22	.22	—	—	—	.65	.15	.468	.56	.768
Folic acid	mcg	.047	12.2	.038	—	—	—	—	120	.106	.04	—	18
Vitamin C	mg	11.5	10.3	60	33	30.6	—	—	10.6	28	29	27	30
Vitamin E	IU	—	—	—	—	—	—	—	—	1.25	—	—	—
MINERALS													
Calcium	mg	37	9	92	85	131	100	47.5	48	51	36	57	29
Copper	mg	.33	.018	.11	.235	—	—	—	.3	.32	.22	.1	.22
Iron	mg	1.4	.13	.6	1.2	4.9	5.2	1.8	1.48	1.7	.5	1.6	.76
Magnesium	mg	22	4	20	31	—	—	—	50	44	21	45	14
Manganese	mg	—	.032	.056	—	—	—	—	.492	.42	.185	—	.46
Phosphorus	mg	74	8	55	42	322	176	109	114	28	38	98	37
Potassium	mg	564	104	335	329	972	—	—	338	259	263	945	265
Selenium	mcg	—	2	—	—	—	—	—	—	—	—	—	—
Sodium	mg	3	11	7	1755	4	354	—	10	39	1	2	17
Zinc	mg	—	.13	.48	1.88	—	—	—	.82	.5	.33	.28	.36
LIPIDS													
Total lipid (fat)	gm	.17	.24	.28	.33	10.3	4.2	3.4	4.68	.2	.28	.4	.38
Total saturated	gm	.09	.014	.038	.083	1.25	—	—	.5	.03	.057	.08	.083
Total unsaturated	gm	.023	.028	.158	.17	7.68	—	—	3.1	.088	.137	.21	.216
Cholesterol	mg	0	0	0	0	0	—	—	0	0	0	—	0
AMINO ACIDS													
Tryptophan	gm	.022	.002	.018	—	.27	—	—	.126	.022	.014	.041	.026
Threonine	gm	.051	.013	.064	—	.886	—	—	.32	.068	.036	.082	.107
Isoleucine	gm	.056	.014	.07	—	.977	—	—	.276	.082	.055	.112	.107
Leucine	gm	.083	.017	.053	—	1.59	—	—	.464	.124	.09	.125	.157
Lysine	gm	.096	.016	.055	—	1.33	—	—	.386	.098	.085	.09	.105
Methionine	gm	.02	.003	.014	—	.27	—	—	.062	.03	.022	.031	.053
Cystine	gm	.005	.002	.015	—	.203	—	—	.03	.02	.016	.02	.017
Phenylalanine	gm	.056	.01	.043	—	1	—	—	.222	.072	.053	.112	.129
Tyrosine	gm	.074	.006	.032	—	.797	—	—	.182	.06	.04	.089	.088
Valine	gm	.061	.014	.067	—	.988	—	—	.3	.09	.069	.122	.14
Arginine	gm	.096	.018	.207	—	1.79	—	—	.266	.09	.065	.158	.1
Histidine	gm	.027	.006	.042	—	.6	—	—	.148	.036	.033	.041	.04
Alanine	gm	.049	.01	.046	—	1	—	—	.26	.08	.081	.121	.117
Aspartic acid	gm	.181	.022	.122	—	2.6	—	—	.8	.134	.187	.302	.367
Glutamic acid	gm	.326	.059	.199	—	4.18	—	—	.784	.192	.164	.522	.209
Glycine	gm	.047	.01	.038	—	.925	—	—	.214	.076	.057	.1	.096
Proline	gm	.047	.008	—	—	1.04	—	—	—	.062	.048	.1	.094
Serine	gm	.078	.009	.049	—	1.24	—	—	.414	.058	.062	.103	.111

	Tomato	Tomato juice	Tomato paste	Turnips	Turnip greens	Vegetable juice cocktail	Water chestnuts	Watercress	Yams	Yellow wax beans
	1	1 C.	1 C.	1 C.	1 C.	1 C.	4 avg	1 C.	1 C.	1 C.
	123	243	262	130	55	242	25	35	200	125
	24	46	215	39	15	41	20	7	210	28
	1.1	2.2	8.9	1.3	.83	2.2	.4	.8	4.8	1.8
	5.3	10.4	48.7	8.6	3	8.7	4.8	1.1	48.2	5.8
	.57	.4	2	1.15	.44	.8	.2	.35	1.8	1
	1394	1940	8650	t	4180	1690	0	1720	t	290
	.074	.12	.52	.05	.039	.12	.04	.03	.18	.09
	.062	.07	.31	.09	.055	.07	.05	.06	.8	.11
	.059	.366	.996	.117	.145	.338	—	.045	.51	.098
	0	0	0	0	0	0	0	0	0	0
	2	—	—	.13	—	—	—	.14	—	—
	.738	1.9	8.1	.8	.33	1.9	.2	.3	1.2	.6
	.304	.607	1.97	.26	.21	—	—	.108	.5	.172
	11.5	.017	—	.026	107	—	—	.017	42	.042
	21.6	39	128	47	33	22	1	28	18	16
	.55	—	—	.026	1	—	—	—	—	—
	8	17	71	51	105	29	1	53	8	63
	.095	.246	—	.09	.193	.484	—	.032	.44	—
	.59	2.2	9.2	.7	.61	1.2	.2	.6	1.2	.8
	14	20	50	25	17	26	2.4	6.5	62	—
	.15	.188	—	.052	.256	.242	—	.189	—	—
	29	44	183	39	23	53	16	19	100	46
	254	552	2237	348	163	535	125	99	1508	189
	.8	—	—	.78	—	—	—	—	—	—
	10	486	100	64	22	484	5	18	17	4
	.13	.1	2	—	.1	.48	—	—	.43	—
	.26	.2	2	.13	.17	.2	.1	.04	.4	.3
	.037	.02	.332	.014	.039	.03	—	.01	.063	—
	.146	.08	1.3	.077	.077	.12	—	.014	.13	—
	0	0	0	0	0	0	0	0	0	—
	.009	.012	.068	.012	.014	—	—	.01	.018	—
	.027	.042	.226	.033	.045	—	—	.046	.081	—
	.026	.036	.192	.047	.043	—	—	.032	.078	—
	.041	.052	.276	.043	.075	—	—	.056	.144	—
	.041	.054	.282	.047	.054	—	—	.046	.089	—
	.01	.01	.05	.014	.019	—	—	.006	.032	—
	.015	.01	.058	.007	.009	—	—	.002	.029	—
	.028	.04	.2	.022	.051	—	—	.038	.107	—
	.018	.024	.134	.017	.032	—	—	.022	.06	—
	.028	.036	.2	.039	.056	—	—	.046	.093	—
	.027	.036	.2	.031	.052	—	—	.052	.191	—
	.016	.03	.158	.018	.02	—	—	.014	.051	—
	.031	.058	.3	.046	.057	—	—	.046	.095	—
	.151	.232	1.24	.082	.087	—	—	.064	.233	—
	.402	.74	3.95	.169	.112	—	—	.064	.272	—
	.027	.03	.16	.033	.05	—	—	.038	.08	—
	.021	.042	.218	.034	.039	—	—	.032	.081	—
	.03	.044	.236	.038	.034	—	—	.02	.122	—

SECTION VIII

Nutrient Allowance Chart

The following chart is designed to give you a better understanding of the calories and nutrients your body requires daily. The figures are based on the Recommended Dietary Allowances (RDA) of the National Research Council.[1] RDA should not be confused with United States Recommended Daily Allowances (USRDA), a set of values derived from RDA by the Food and Drug Administration as standards for nutritional labeling.

The chart is divided into three categories: children, girls and women, and boys and men. The sections are further divided into different ages and weights.

Level of Activity

Resting Metabolic Rate. Represents the minimum energy needs for day and night with no exercise or exposure to cold.

Sedentary. Includes occupations that involve sitting most of the day, such as secretarial work and studying.

Light. Includes activities that involve standing most of the day, such as teaching or laboratory work.

Moderate. May include walking, gardening, and housework.

Active. May include dancing, skating, and manual labor such as farm or construction work.

The Nutrient Allowance Chart includes the require-

[1]National Academy of Sciences, *Recommended Dietary Allowances.* 1980, 9th edition.

ments for resting metabolic rate and for light activity. The chart below is included to allow calculation of calories for requirements for sedentary, moderate, and active levels. Although calorie requirements vary with the level of activity, nutrient requirements, as stated under an individual's desirable weight in the Nutrient Allowance Chart, remain the same.

DAILY CALORIE REQUIREMENTS FOR LEVELS OF ACTIVITY

Metabolic Rate	Men	Women
Resting	See "Nutrient Allowance Chart"	See "Nutrient Allowance Chart"
Sedentary	16 cal/lb body weight	14 cal/lb body weight
Light	See "Nutrient Allowance Chart"	See "Nutrient Allowance Chart"
Moderate	21 cal/lb body weight	18 cal/lb body weight
Active	26 cal/lb body weight	22 cal/lb body weight

It can be seen from the above chart that a moderately active man of 180 pounds requires approximately 3780 calories per day. This figure is obtained by multiplying 180 pounds by 21 calories. These estimates do not take into account body build and height, which also affect calorie requirements.

The "Desirable Height and Weight Chart" is included so that dieters may estimate their ideal weight, based on sex, height, and body frame. This information should be used in connection with the "Nutrient

Allowance Chart" so that one may determine what nutrients and calories are required and cut calories accordingly.

The carbohydrate, fat, and protein allowances given in the "Nutrient Allowance Chart" apply to only those persons with light activity patterns. The amount of protein should not fall below the figure given, since this is considered the amount needed by the average healthy person in order to repair and build the body.

Charts 1 and 2 were the generally accepted height and weight charts for many years. Charts 3 and 4 are new tables based on a mortality study of 4 million healthy adults over a 22-year period. These tables set forth the weights at which men and women of various heights and bone structures can expect to live a long life. The new tables allow for higher weight than the old ones, but many people feel that these may not be ideal. Therefore both sets are included.

DESIRABLE HEIGHT AND WEIGHT CHART

Chart 1
Desirable Weights for Men Aged 25 and Over*

Height with Shoes (1-in. heels) Feet	Inches	Small Frame	Medium Frame	Large Frame
5	2	112–120	118–129	126–141
5	3	115–123	121–133	129–144
5	4	118–126	124–136	132–148
5	5	121–129	127–139	135–152
5	6	124–133	130–143	138–156
5	7	128–137	134–147	142–161
5	8	132–141	138–152	147–166
5	9	136–145	142–156	151–170
5	10	140–150	146–160	155–174
5	11	144–154	150–165	159–179
6	0	148–158	154–170	164–184
6	1	152–162	158–175	168–189
6	2	156–167	162–180	173–194
6	3	160–171	167–185	178–199
6	4	164–175	172–190	182–204

*Weight in pounds according to frame (in indoor clothing). For nude weight, deduct 5 to 7 lb. This chart prepared by Metropolitan Life Insurance Company.

Chart 2
Desirable Weights for Women Aged 25 and Over*

Height with Shoes (2-in. heels) Feet	Inches	Small Frame	Medium Frame	Large Frame
4	10	92–98	96–107	104–119
4	11	94–101	98–110	106–122
5	0	96–104	101–113	109–125
5	1	99–107	104–116	112–128
5	2	102–110	107–119	115–131
5	3	105–113	110–122	118–134
5	4	108–116	113–126	121–138
5	5	111–119	116–130	125–142
5	6	114–123	120–135	129–146
5	7	118–127	124–139	133–150
5	8	122–131	128–143	137–154
5	9	126–135	132–147	141–158
5	10	130–140	136–151	145–163
5	11	134–144	140–155	149–168
6	0	138–148	144–159	153–173

*Weight in pounds according to frame (in indoor clothing). For nude weight, deduct 2 to 4 lb. This chart prepared by Metropolitan Life Insurance Company.

Chart 3

Height Feet	Inches	Small Frame	Medium Frame	Large Frame
5	2	128–134	131–141	138–150
5	3	130–136	133–143	140–153
5	4	132–138	135–145	142–156
5	5	134–140	137–148	144–160
5	6	136–142	139–151	146–164
5	7	138–145	142–154	149–168
5	8	140–148	145–157	152–172
5	9	142–151	148–160	155–176
5	10	144–154	151–163	158–180
5	11	146–157	154–166	161–184
6	0	149–160	157–170	164–188
6	1	152–164	160–174	168–192
6	2	155–168	164–178	172–197
6	3	158–172	167–182	176–202
6	4	162–176	171–187	181–207

*Weights at ages 25–59 based on lowest mortality. Weight in pounds according to frame (in indoor clothing weighing 5 lb, shoes with 1-inch heels).

Chart 4

Height Feet	Inches	Small Frame	Medium Frame	Large Frame
4	10	102–111	109–121	118–131
4	11	103–113	111–123	120–134
5	0	104–115	113–126	122–137
5	1	106–118	115–129	125–140
5	2	108–121	118–132	128–143
5	3	111–124	121–135	131–147
5	4	114–127	124–138	134–151
5	5	117–130	127–141	137–155
5	6	120–133	130–144	140–159
5	7	123–136	133–147	143–163
5	8	126–139	136–150	146–167
5	9	129–142	139–153	149–170
5	10	132–145	142–156	152–173
5	11	135–148	145–159	155–176
6	0	138–151	148–162	158–179

*Weights at ages 25–59 based on lowest mortality. Weight in pounds according to frame (in indoor clothing weighing 3 lb, shoes with 1-inch heels).

Source: 1979 Build Study, Society of Actuaries and Association of Life Insurance Medical Directors of America, 1980.

NUTRIENT ALLOWANCE CHART

	Children (Boys and Girls)					Girls			Women
	0–6	6–1	1–3	4–6	7–10	11–14	15–18	19–22	23–50
Age	mo	mo yr	yr	yr	yr	yr	yr	yr	yr
Weight, lb	14	20	28	44	66	97	119	128	128
Weight, kg	6	9	13	20	30	44	54	58	58
Calories required for									
Resting metabolic rate									1620
Light activity	770		1100	1600	2200	2300	2300	2000	2000
Carbohydrates, g	115		165	240	330	345	345	346	300
Fats, g	28		38	58	80	80	78	79	66
Protein, g	14	14	23	30	34	46	46	44	44
MINERALS									
Calcium, mg	360	540	800	800	800	1200	1200	800	800
Iodine, mcg	40	50	70	90	120	150	150	150	150
Iron, mg	10	15	15	10	10	18	18	18	18
Magnesium, mg	50	70	150	200	250	300	300	300	300
Phosphorus, mg	240	360	800	800	800	1200	1200	800	800
Potassium, mg	350–925	425–1275	550–1650	775–2325	1000–3000	1525–4575	Adequate daily intake 1875–5625 mg.		
Sodium, mg	115–350	250–750	325–975	450–1350	600–1800	900–2700	Adequate daily intake 1100–3300 mg.		
VITAMINS									
Vitamin A, IU	1400	2000	2000	2500	3300	4000	4000	4000	4000
Vitamin B complex									
Thiamine (B_1), mg	0.3	0.5	0.7	0.9	1.2	1.1	1.1	1.1	1.0
Riboflavin (B_2), mg	0.4	0.6	0.8	1.0	1.4	1.3	1.3	1.3	1.2
Pyridoxine (B_6), mg	0.3	0.6	0.9	1.3	1.6	1.8	2.0	2.0	2.0
Cyanocobalamin (B_{12}), mcg	0.5	1.5	2.0	2.5	3.0	3.0	3.0	3.0	3.0
Biotin, mcg	35	50	65	85	120	100–200	Adequate daily intake 150–300 mcg.		
Choline, mg*		Average daily intake 500–900 mg					Average daily intake 500–900 mg.		
Folic acid, mg	.03	.045	0.1	0.2	0.3	0.4	0.4	0.4	0.4
Inositol, mg*							Average daily intake 1,000 mg		
Niacin, mg	6.0	8.0	9.0	11	16	15	14	14	13
Para-aminobenzoic acid (PABA), mg		No Recommended Dietary Allowance					No RDA		
Pantothenic acid, mg	2.0	3.0	3.0	3–4	4–5	4–7	Adequate daily intake 5–10 mg		
Vitamin C (ascorbic acid), mg	35	35	45	45	45	50	60	60	60
Vitamin D, IU	400	400	400	400	400	400	400	300	200
Vitamin E, IU	4.0	6.0	7.0	9.0	10	12	12	12	12
Vitamin K, mcg	12	10–20	15–30	20–40	30–60	50–100	Adequate daily intake 70–140 mcg		
TRACE MINERALS									
Chromium, mg	.01–.04	.02–.06	.02–.08	.03–.1	.05–.2	.05–.2	Adequate daily Intake .05–.2 mg		
Copper, mg	.5–.7	.7–1.0	1.–1.5	1.5–2.0	2.0–2.5	2.0–3.0	Adequate daily intake 2–3 mg		
Fluoride, mg	.1–.5	.2–1.0	.5–1.5	1.0–2.5	1.5–2.5	1.5–2.5	Adequate daily intake 1.5–4 mg		
Manganese, mg	.5–.7	.7–1.0	1.0–1.5	1.5–2.0	2.0–3.0	2.5–5.0	Adequate daily intake 2.5–5 mg		
Molybdenum, mg	.03–.06	.04–.08	.05–.1	.06–.15	.1–.3	.15–.5	Adequate daily intake .15–.5 mg		
Selenium, mg	.01–.04	.02–.06	.02–.08	.03–.12	.05–.2	.05–.2	Adequate daily intake .05–.2 mg		
Zinc, mg	3	5	10	10	10	15	15	15	15

*Robert S. Goodhart and Maurice E. Shils, *Modern Nutrition in Health and Disease,* 5th ed. (Philadelphia: Lea and Febiger, 1973), p. 263.

Age	Women			Boys			Men	
	Preg-nant	Lactat-ing	51 and over	11–14 yr	15–18 yr	19–22 yr	23–50 yr	51 and over
Weight, lb			128	97	134	147	154	154
Weight, kg			58	44	61	67	70	70
Calories required for Resting metabolic rate								
Light activity	+300	+500	1850	2800	3000	3000	2600	2600
Carbohydrates, g			277	—	—	—	390	390
Fats, g			59				87	87
Protein, g	+30 g	+20 g	44	45	56	56	56	56
MINERALS								
Calcium, mg	1200	1200	800	1200	1200	800	800	800
Iodine, mcg	175	200	150	150	150	150	150	150
Iron, mg	30–60	18+	10	18	18	10	10	10
Magnesium, mg	450	450	300	350	400	350	350	350
Phosphorus, mg	1200	1200	800	1200	1200	800	800	800
Potassium, mg	Average daily intake 1875–5625 mg			1525–4575	Average daily intake 1875–5625 mg			
Sodium, mg	Average daily intake 1100–3300 mg			900–2700	Average daily intake 1100–3300 mg			
VITAMINS								
Vitamin A, IU	5000	6000	4000	5000	5000	5000	5000	5000
Vitamin B complex								
Thiamine (B$_1$), mg	+.4	+.5	1.0	1.4	1.4	1.5	1.4	1.2
Riboflavin (B$_2$), mg	+.3	+.5	1.2	1.6	1.7	1.7	1.6	1.4
Pyridoxine (B$_6$), mg	+.6	+.5	2.0	1.8	2.0	2.2	2.2	2.2
Cyanocobalamin (B$_{12}$), mcg	4.0	4.0	3.0	3.0	3.0	3.0	3.0	3.0
Biotin, mcg	Adequate daily intake 150–300 mcg			100–200	Adequate daily intake 150–300 mcg			
Choline, mg*	Average daily intake 500–900 mg				Average daily intake 500–900 mg			
Folic acid, mg	0.8	0.5	0.4	0.4	0.4	0.4	0.4	0.4
Inositol, mg*	Average daily intake 1,000 mg				Average daily intake 1,000 mg			
Niacin, mg	+2	+5	13	18	18	19	18	16
Para-aminobenzoic acid (PABA), mg	No RDA				No RDA			
Pantothenic acid, mg	Adequate daily intake 5–10 mg				Adequate daily intake 5–10 mg			
Vitamin C (ascorbic acid), mg	80	100	60	50	60	60	60	60
Vitamin D, IU	400	400	200	400	400	300	200	200
Vitamin E, IU	15	15	12	12	15	15	15	15
Vitamin K, mcg	Adequate daily intake 70–140 mcg			50–100	Adequate daily intake 70–140 mcg			
TRACE MINERALS								
Chromium, mg	Adequate daily intake .05–.2 mg			.05–.2	Adequate daily intake .05–.2 mg			
Copper, mg	Adequate daily intake 2–3 mg			2.0–3.0	Adequate daily intake 2–3 mg.			
Fluoride, mg	Adequate daily intake 1.5–4 mg			1.5–2.5	Adequate daily intake 1.5–4 mg			
Manganese, mg	Adequate daily intake 2.5–5 mg			2.5–5.0	Adequate daily intake 2.5–5 mg			
Molybdenum, mg	Adequate daily intake .15–.5 mg			.15–.5	Adequate daily intake .15–.5 mg			
Selenium, mg	Adequate daily intake .05–.2 mg			.05–.2	Adequate daily intake .05–.2 mg			
Zinc, mg	20	25	15	15	15	15	15	15

*Goodhart and Shils, *Modern Nutrition in Health and Disease*, 5th ed., p. 263.

UNITED STATES RECOMMENDED DAILY ALLOWANCES (USRDA)

Vitamins and Minerals	Unit of Measurement	Infants	Children under 4 Years of Age	Adults and Children 4 or More Years of Age	Pregnant or Lactating Women
Vitamin A	International units	1500	2500	5000	8000
Vitamin D	International units	400	400	400	400
Vitamin E	International units	5	10	30	30
Vitamin C	Milligrams	35	40	60	60
Folic acid	Milligrams	0.1	0.2	0.4	0.8
Thiamine	Milligrams	0.5	0.7	1.5	1.7
Riboflavin	Milligrams	0.6	0.8	1.7	2.0
Niacin	Milligrams	8	9	20	20
Vitamin B_6	Milligrams	0.4	0.7	2.0	2.5
Vitamin B_{12}	Micrograms	2	3	6	8
Biotin	Milligrams	0.05	0.15	0.30	0.30
Pantothenic acid	Milligrams	3	5	10	10
Calcium	Grams	0.6	0.8	1.0	1.3
Phosphorus	Grams	0.5	0.8	1.0	1.3
Iodine	Micrograms	45	70	150	150
Iron	Milligrams	15	10	18	18
Magnesium	Milligrams	70	200	400	450
Copper	Milligrams	0.6	1.0	2.0	2.0
Zinc	Milligrams	5	8	15	15

Bibliography

Adams, Ruth and Frank Murray. *Body, Mind, and the B Vitamins.* New York: Larchmont Books, 1972.

——— and ———. *Vitamin E, Wonder Worker of the 70's.* New York: Larchmont Books, 1972.

Airola, Paavo. *Cancer Causes, Prevention, and Treatment.* Phoenix, Ariz.: Health Plus, 1972.

———. *Are You Confused?* Phoenix, Ariz.: Health Plus, 1974.

———. *How to Get Well.* Phoenix, Ariz.: Health Plus, 1974.

Altschul, A. M. *Proteins, Their Chemistry and Politics.* New York: Basic Books, 1965.

American Journal of Obstetrics and Gynecology, Vol. 61, June 1951.

Ancowitz, Arthur. *Strokes and Their Prevention.* New York: Jove Publications, 1982.

Anderson, Linnea, Marjorie Dibble, Helen S. Mitchell, and Hendrika Rynbergen. *Nutrition in Nursing.* Philadelphia: J. B. Lippincott Co., 1972.

Atkins, Robert C. *Dr. Atkins' Nutrition Breakthrough.* New York: Bantam Books, 1981.

Bailey, Herbert. *Vitamin E: Your Key to a Healthy Heart.* New York: Arc Books, 1970.

Basu, T. K. *About Mothers, Children and Their Nutrition.* London: Thorsons Publ., 1971.

Bender, A. E. *Dietetic Foods.* New York: Chemical Publ. Co., 1967.

Benjamin, Harry. *Your Diet in Health and Disease.* Croyden, Great Britain: Health for All Publ. Co., 1931.

Bennett, Hal Zina. *Cold Comfort.* New York: Clarkson N. Potter, 1979.

Berkeley, George E. *Cancer, How to Prevent It and How to Help Your Doctor Fight It.* Englewood Cliffs, N.J.: Prentice-Hall, 1978.

Bieler, Henry G. *Food Is Your Best Medicine.* New York: Random House, 1965.

Bogert, L. J., George M. Briggs, and Doris H. Calloway. *Nutrition and Physical Fitness,* 9th ed. Philadelphia: W. B. Saunders Co., 1973.

Borsaak, Henry. *Vitamins.* New York: Pyramid Books, 1940.

Bowerman, William J. and W. E. Harris. *Jogging.* New York: Grosset & Dunlap, 1967.

Brennan, R. O. *Nutrigenetics.* New York: New American Library, 1977.

Brewster, Dorothy Patricia. *You Can Breastfeed Your Baby.* Emmaus, Pa.: Rodale Press, 1979.

Brunner, L. W., C. P. Emerson, Jr., L. K. Ferguson, and D. S. Suddarth. *Textbook of Medical-Surgical Nursing,* 2d ed. Philadelphia: J. B. Lippincott Co., 1970.

"Cancer News Journal." *Prevention,* December 1971.

Carey, Ruth L., Irma B. Vyhmeister, and Jennie S. Hudson. *Commonsense Nutrition.* Omaha: Pacific Press, 1971.

Carroll-Clark, E. H. *How to Save Your Teeth.* London: Thorsons Publ., 1968.

Chaney, Margaret S. and Margaret L. Ross. *Nutrition,* 8th ed. Boston: Houghton Mifflin Co., 1971.

Cheraskin, E., W. M. Ringsdorf, and J. W. Clark. *Diet and Disease.* Emmaus, Pa.: Rodale Books, 1968.

Clark, Linda. *Get Well Naturally.* New York: Devin-Adair Co., 1965.

———. *Know Your Nutrition.* New Canaan, Conn.: Keats Publ. Co., 1973.

Clark, Michael. "Vitamin E—The Better Treatment for Angina." *Prevention.* December 1972.

Clarke, J. H. *The Prescriber,* 8th ed. Rustington, England: Health Science Press, 1968.

Clymer, R. Swinburne. *Nature's Healing Agents.* Philadelphia: Dorrance Co., 1963.

Collins, Daniel A. *Your Teeth, a Handbook of Dental Care for the Whole Family.* Garden City, N.Y.: Doubleday & Co., 1967.

Corrigan, A. B. *Living with Arthritis.* New York: Grosset & Dunlap, 1971.

Crain, Lloyd. *Magic Vitamins and Organic Foods.* Los Angeles: Crandrich Studios, 1971.

Crook, William G. *Are You Allergic?* Jackson, Tenn.: Professional Books, 1978.

Darling, Mary. *Natural, Organic, and Health Foods.* USDA Extention Folder No. 280. St. Paul: University of Minnesota, 1973.

Davidson, Stanley, R. Passmore, and J. F. Brack. *Human Nutrition and Dietetics,* 5th ed. Baltimore: Williams and Wilkins Co., 1972.

Davis, Adelle. *Let's Eat Right to Keep Fit.* New York: Harcourt, Brace & World, 1954.

———. *Let's Have Healthy Children,* 2d ed. New York: Harcourt, Brace & World, 1959.

Davis, Adelle. *Let's Get Well.* New York: Harcourt Brace and World, 1965; New York: New American Library, 1972.

———, and Marshall Mandell. *Let's Have Healthy Children.* New York: New American Library, 1979.

Deutsch, Ronald M. *The Family Guide to Better Food and Better Health.* Des Moines, Iowa.: Meredith Corp., 1971.

Dubos, Rene and Maya Pines. *Health and Disease.* New York: Time-Life Books, 1965.

Ebon, Martin. *The Truth about Vitamin E.* New York: Bantam Books, 1972.

Ellis, John M. and James Presley. *Vitamin B$_6$: The Doctor's Report.* New York: Harper & Row, 1973.

Ehrlich, David, and George Wolf. *The Bowel Book.* New York: Schocken Books, 1981.

Feingold, Ben F. *Why Your Child Is Hyperactive.* New York: Random House, 1975.

Fleck, Henrietta. *Introduction to Nutrition,* 2d ed. New York: Macmillan Co., 1971.

Fredericks, Carlton. *Nutrition—Your Key to Good Health.* North Hollywood, Calif.: London Press, 1964.

———. *Eating Right for You.* New York: Grosset & Dunlap, 1972.

——— and Herbert Bailey. *Food Facts and Fallacies.* New York: Arco Publ. Co., 1965.

Furgurson, Jill E., and Halvor L. Harley. *Herpes Sufferers Get H.E.L.P.* Denver: Royal Publications, 1982.

Galton, Lawrence. *The Silent Disease: Hypertension.* New York: New American Library, 1974.

Garrison, Omar V. *The Dictocrats' Attack on Health Foods and Vitamins.* New York: Arc Books, 1971.

Goldberg, Philip, and Daniel Kaufman. *Natural Sleep.* Emmaus, Pa.: Rodale Press, 1978.

Gomez, Joan. *A Dictionary of Symptoms.* New York: Bantam Books, 1967.

Goodhart, Robert S. and Maurice E. Shils. *Modern Nutrition in Health and Disease,* 5th ed. Philadelphia: Lea & Febiger, 1973.

——— and Michael G. Wohl. *Manual of Clinical Nutrition.* Philadelphia: Lea & Febiger, 1964.

Graham, Judy. *Multiple Sclerosis.* Wellingborough, England: Thorsons Publishers, 1982.

Gray, Madeline. *The Changing Years.* New York: Doubleday, 1981.

Guthrie, Helen A. *Introductory Nutrition,* 2d ed. St. Louis: C. V. Mosby Co., 1971.

Heinz Nutritional Data, 6th ed. Pittsburgh: Heinz International Research Center, 1972.

Heritage, Ford. *Composition and Facts about Food.* Mokelumne Hill, Calif.: Health Research Center, 1968.

Herting, David C. "Perspective on Vitamin E."

American Journal of Clinical Nutrition, Vol. 19, pp. 210–216, September 1966.

Hill, Howard E. *Introduction to Lecithin.* Los Angeles: Nash Publ., 1972.

Hoffer, Abram, and Morton Walker. *Nutrients to Age Without Senility.* New Canaan, Conn.: Keats Publishing, 1980.

——. *Orthomolecular Nutrition.* New Canaan, Conn.: Keats Publishing, 1978.

Holvey, David (ed.). *The Merck Manual,* 12th ed. Rahway, N.J.: Merck & Co., 1972.

Hoover, John E. (ed.). *Remington's Pharmaceutical Sciences,* 14th ed. Easton, Pa.: Mack Publ. Co., 1970.

Howe, Phyllis S. *Basic Nutrition in Health and Disease,* 5th ed. Philadelphia: W. B. Saunders Co., 1971.

Hunter, Beatrice T. *The Natural Foods Primer.* New York: Simon and Schuster, 1972.

Illustrated Medical and Health Encyclopedia. New York: H. S. Stuttman Co., 1959.

Industrial Medicine and Surgery, Vol. 21, June 1952.

Jensen, Bernard. *Seeds and Sprouts for Life.* Escondido, Calif.: Jensen's Nutrition & Health Products, undated.

Johnson, Harry J. *Creative Walking for Physical Fitness.* New York: Grosset & Dunlap, 1970.

Jolliffe, Norman (ed.). *Clinical Nutrition,* 2d ed. New York: Harper & Brothers, 1962.

Journal of the American Dental Association, August 1955.

Kloss, Jethro. *Back to Eden.* New York: Beneficial Books, 1972.

Kotschevar, Lendal H. and Margaret McWilliams. *Understanding Food.* New York: John Wiley and Sons, 1969.

Krause, Marie V. and Martha A. Hunscher. *Food, Nutrition and Diet Therapy,* 5th ed. Philadelphia: W. B. Saunders Co., 1972.

Kuhne, Paul. *Home Medical Encyclopedia.* Greenwich, Conn.: Fawcett, 1960.

Kuntzleman, Charles T. (ed.). *The Physical Fitness Encyclopedia.* Emmaus, Pa.: Rodale Books, 1970.

Lappé, Francis L. *Diet for a Small Planet.* New York: Ballantine Books, 1971.

Lesser, Michael. *Nutrition and Vitamin Therapy.* New York: Grove Press, 1980.

Locke, David M. *Enzymes—The Agents of Life.* New York: Crown Press, 1971.

Macia, Rafael. *The Natural Foods and Nutrition Handbook.* New York: Harper & Row, 1972.

Marsh, Dorothy B. (ed.). *The Good Housekeeping Cookbook.* New York: Good Housekeeping Book Division, 1963.

Martin, Ethel A. *Nutrition in Action,* 2d ed. New York: Holt, Rinehart & Winston, 1967.

McDermott, Irene E., Mabel B. Trilling, and Florence W. Nicolas. *Food for Better Living,* 3d ed. Chicago: J. B. Lippincott Co., 1960.

Miller, Fred D. *Healthy Teeth Through Proper Nutrition.* New York: Arco Publishing, 1978.

Mitchell, Helen S., Hendrika J. Rynbergen, Linnea Anderson, and Marjorie V. Dibble. *Cooper's Nutrition in Health and Disease.* Philadelphia: J. B. Lippincott Co., 1972.

Morales, Betty Lee. *Cancer Control Journal,* March 1973.

Moyer, William C. *Buying Guide for Fresh Fruits, Vegetables and Nuts,* 4th ed. Fullerton, Calif.: Blue Goose, 1971.

Moyle, Alan. *Nature Cure for Asthma and Hay Fever.* Croyden, Great Britain: Health for All Publ. Co., 1951.

Murray, Frank. *Program Your Heart for Health.* New York: Larchmont Books, 1978.

"New in Print/Sound/Film," *Journal of the American Dietetic Association,* September 1972, p. 340.

Newbold, H. L. *Dr. Newbold's Revolutionary New Discoveries About Weight Loss.* New York: New American Library, 1979.

——. *Mega-Nutrients for Your Nerves.* New York: Berkley Publishing, 1981.

Norris, P. E. *About Vitamins.* London: Thorson's Publ., 1967.

Nuernberger, Phil. *Freedom from Stress.* Honesdale, Pa.: Himalayan International Institute, 1981.

Null, Gary and Steve Null. *The Complete Handbook of Nutrition.* New York: Robert Speller & Sons, 1972.

Nutrition Almanac, 2d ed. Minneapolis, Minn.: Nutrition Search, 1973.

Nutrition Almanac Cookbook. Bismark, N.D.: Nutrition Search, 1983.

"Nutritive Value of Foods," *USDA Home and Garden Bull.* 72, 1971.

O'Brien, Edward J. *Cigarettes: Slow Suicide!* New York: Exposition Press, 1968.

Page, M. E. and H. L. Abrams. *Your Body Is Your Best Doctor.* New Canaan, Conn.: Keats Publ. Co., 1972.

Passwater, Richard A. *Selenium as Food and Medicine.* New Canaan, Conn.: Keats Publishing, 1980.

Pauling, Linus. *Vitamin C and the Common Cold.* New York: Bantam Books, 1971.

_____. *Vitamin C, the Common Cold and the Flu.* New York: W. H. Freeman, 1976.

Pearson, Durk, and Sandy Shaw. *Life Extension—A Practical Scientific Approach.* New York: Warner Books, 1982.

Pfeiffer, Carl C. *Mental and Elemental Nutrients.* New Canaan, Conn.: Keats Publishing, 1975.

Philpott, William H., and Dwight K. Kalita. *Brain Allergies.* New Canaan, Conn.: Keats Publishing, 1980.

Pike, Ruth L. and Myrtle L. Brown. *Nutrition: An Integrated Approach.* New York: John Wiley & Sons, 1967.

"Potassium: The Neglected Mineral," *Let's Live,* October 1973.

Prevention Magazine Staff. *The Complete Book of Minerals for Health.* Emmaus, Pa.: Rodale Press, 1981.

_____. *The Complete Book of Vitamins.* Emmaus, Pa.: Rodale Press, 1977.

_____. *The Encyclopedia of Common Diseases.* Emmaus, Pa.: Rodale Press, 1982.

_____. *No More Headaches.* Emmaus, Pa.: Rodale Press, 1982.

Price, Joseph M. *Coronaries Cholesterol Chlorine.* New York: Pyramid Books, 1969.

"Problem: Lead and What To Do About It," *Prevention,* October 1973.

Rainey, Jean. *How to Shop for Food.* New York: Barnes & Noble, 1972.

Recommended Dietary Allowances, 9th ed. Washington, D.C.: National Academy of Sciences, 1980.

Reuben, David, M.D. *The Save Your Life Diet.* New York: Ballantine, 1975.

Robinson, Corinne H. *Basic Nutrition and Diet Therapy,* 2d ed. New York: Macmillan Co., 1970.

_____ *Normal and Therapeutic Nutrition,* 14th ed. New York: Macmillan Co., 1972.

Robley, Spencer H. *Emphysema and Common Sense.* West Nyack, N.Y.: Parker Publ. Co., 1968.

Rodale, J. I. *The Health Builder.* Emmaus, Pa.: Rodale Books, 1957.

_____. *The Complete Book of Food and Nutrition.* Emmaus, Pa.: Rodale Books, 1961.

_____. *The Health Seeker.* Emmaus, Pa.: Rodale Books, 1962.

_____. *Best Articles from* Prevention. Emmaus, Pa.: Rodale Books, 1967.

_____. *The Complete Book of Vitamins.* Emmaus, Pa.: Rodale Books, 1968.

_____. *The* Prevention *Method for Better Health.* Emmaus, Pa.: Rodale Books, 1968.

_____. *Cancer Facts and Fallacies.* Emmaus, Pa.: Rodale Books, 1969.

_____. *The Encyclopedia of Common Diseases.* Emmaus, Pa.: Rodale Books, 1969.

_____. *My Own Technique of Eating for Health.* Emmaus, Pa.: Rodale Press, 1969.

_____. *The Encyclopedia for Healthful Living.* Emmaus, Pa.: Rodale Books, 1970.

_____. *Magnesium: That Nutrient that Could Change Your Life.* New York: Pyramid Books, 1971.

_____. *Complete Book of Minerals for Health.* Emmaus, Pa.: Rodale Books, 1972.

_____. *Vitamin A: Everyone's Basic Bodyguard.* Emmaus, Pa.: Rodale Press, 1972.

_____. *Be a Healthy Mother, Have a Healthy Baby.* Emmaus, Pa.: Rodale Press, 1973.

Rosenberg, Harold, and A. N. Feldzamen. *The Doctor's Book of Vitamin Therapy.* New York: G. P. Putnam's Sons, 1974.

Rothenberg, Robert E. *The New American Medical Dictionary and Health Manual.* New York: New American Library, 1968.

_____. *Health in the Later Years,* rev. New York: Signet Books, 1972.

Samuels, Mike and Hal Bennett. *The Well Body Book.* New York: Random House, 1973.

Schauss, Alexander. *Diet, Crime and Delinquency.* Berkeley, Calif.: Parker House Publishing, 1981.

Seaman, Barbara, and Gideon Seaman. *Women and the Crisis in Sex Hormones.* New York: Rawson Associates, 1977.

Shackelton, Alberta D. *Practical Nurse Nutrition Education,* 3d ed. Philadelphia: W. B. Saunders Co., 1972.

Sheinkin, David, Michael Schachter, and Richard Hutton. *Food, Mind and Mood.* New York: Warner Books, 1980.

Shute, Evan. *The Heart and Vitamin E.* London, Canada: Evan Shute Foundation, 1963.

Shute, Wilfrid E. and Harold J. Taub. *Vitamin E for Ailing and Healthy Hearts.* New York: Pyramid House, 1969.

————. *Health Preserver.* Emmaus, Pa.: Rodale Press, 1977.

Sidhwa, Kekir. *Fit for Anything.* Lewes, Sussex, England: Health for All Publ. Co., 1964.

Smith, Dorothy W., Carol P. Hanley Germain, and Claudia D. Gips. *Care of the Adult Patient.* Philadelphia: J. B. Lippincott Co., 1971.

Smith, Lendon. *Feed Your Kids Right.* New York: McGraw-Hill, 1979.

"Smoking Depletes Vitamin C," *Prevention,* February 1971.

Sokoloff, Boris. *Cancer: New Approaches, New Hope.* New York: Devin-Adair

Stein, Mendel. *Vitamins.* Edinburgh: Churchill, Livingstone, 1971.

Stone, Irwin. *The Healing Factor: "Vitamin C" Against Disease.* New York: Grosset & Dunlap, 1970.

"Summer Cold; Vitamin C . . . ," *Prevention,* July 1970.

Swan, Dr. Roy. *The Multiple Sclerosis Diet Book.* New York: Doubleday, 1977.

Synder, Arthur W. *Vitamins and Minerals.* Los Angeles: Hansens, 1969.

Thomas, Clayton L. (ed.). *Taber's Cyclopedia Medical Dictionary,* 12th ed. Philadelphia: F. A. Davis Co., 1973.

Toxicants Occurring Naturally in Foods. Washington, D.C.: National Academy of Sciences, 1973.

Vitamins Explained Simply, The, 5th ed. Melbourne: Science of Life Books, 1972.

Wade, Carlson. *Magic Minerals.* West Nyack, N.Y.: Parker Publ. Co., 1967.

————. *Health Food Recipes for Gourmet Cooking.* New York: Arco Publ. Co., 1969.

————. *Helping Your Health with Enzymes.* New York: Universal—Award House, 1971.

Watt, B. K. and A. L. Merill. "Composition of Foods—Raw, Processed, Prepared," *USDA Handbook* 8, 1963.

Wayler, Thelma J. and Rose S. Klein. *Applied Nutrition.* New York: Macmillan Co., 1965.

Webster, James. *Vitamin C, The Protective Vitamin.* New York: Universal—Award House, 1971.

Wheatley, Michael. *About Nutrition.* London: Thorsons, 1971.

White, Philip (ed.). *Let's Talk about Food,* 2d ed. Chicago: American Medical Association, 1970.

Williams, Phyllis S. *Nourishing Your Unborn Child.* New York: Avon Books, 1982.

Williams, Roger J. *Nutrition against Disease.* New York: Pitman Publ., 1971.

Williams, Roger J. *Alcoholism—The Nutritional Approach.* Austin: University of Texas Press, 1980.

————, and Dwight K. Kalita, eds. *A Physician's Handbook on Orthomolecular Medicine.* New Canaan, Conn.: Keats Publishing, 1977.

Williams, Sue R. *Review of Nutrition and Diet Therapy.* St. Louis: C. V. Mosby Co., 1973.

Wilson, Eva D., Katherine H. Fischer, and Mary E. Fugue. *Principles of Nutrition,* 2d ed. New York: John Wiley & Sons, 1965.

Winter, Ruth. *Beware of the Food You Eat,* rev. ed. New York: Signet Books, 1971.

————. *Vitamin E: the Miracle Worker.* New York: Arco Publ. Co., 1972.

Wintrobe, M. M. et al. *Harrison's Principles of Internal Medicine,* 6th ed. New York: McGraw-Hill Book Co., 1970.

Yudkin, John. *Sweet and Dangerous.* New York: Peter H. Wyden, 1972.

Index

[An asterisk (*) following an entry refers to the Table of Food Composition]